New Concept and New Way of Treatment of Cancer

New Concept and New Way of Treatment of Cancer

Xu Ze Xu Jie Bin Wu

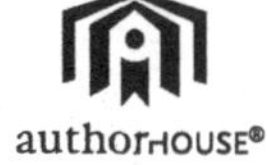

AuthorHouse™
1663 Liberty Drive
Bloomington, IN 47403
www.authorhouse.com
Phone: 1-800-839-8640

Published by AuthorHouse 03/26/2013

ISBN: 978-1-4817-3270-3 (sc)
ISBN: 978-1-4817-3271-0 (e)

Library of Congress Control Number: 2013905617

Contents

Part IV: Experimental Research

Part V: Clinical Demonstration

Part VI: Scientific Research

Introduction to the book

Bin Wu and Sitthipol Tovanich

Cancer therapy is complicate because cancer cells can change themselves to adapt to the environment easily and to grow very fast. Currently cancer therapy includes multiple methods such as surgery, bioimmunotherapy, chemotherapy and radiologic therapy, etc. The immune system, especially such as central immune organs such as bone marrow and thymus in the hosts play extremely important roles in getting rid of all of the pathogens such as the cancer cells, bacteria and virus etc. Dr. Xu, etc in China develops his own therapy concepts and ways of the treatment of Cancer after his 20 years of animal research and 50 years of the clinical experiences. In this book, he wrote down his basic and clinical research results and point out the new ways to treat the cancer, which is his third book of the cancer therapy. He has strong confidence that we can prevent and treat cancer happen as we can control and treat the chickpox through our immune system function, etc. According to his animal and clinical researches, he concluded that Thymus shrink and the immune function decrease are one of the important reasons which can cause the caners because the naïve T cells are from thymus and naïve T cells can produce specific CD8 killer cells when they meet the new antigens in the peripheral immune organs such as the lymph nodes etc to get rid of the particular tumor cells and other foreign antigens so that if we increase our thymus and bone marrow immune function, the cancer growth can be completely controlled. The most important thing is that he developed a series of anticancer traditional medicines which can protect and improve thymus and bone marrow functions and have amazing clinical effects on his cancer patients and developed his new unique and independent and new concepts and new ways of treatment of cancer such as: 1. For the long term therapy, the bioimmunological therapy of improving the immune regulation is the best supplemental treatment after the surgery because the tumor cells can exist in our body as **three forms**: primary site tumor cells, metastastic site tumor cells and the tumor cells or tumor thrombus on the ways to the metastasis site. 2. For the short term therapy: Radiotherapy and chemotherapy is using from the short term therapy because of their strong side effects. These new ways already produce significant benefits on advanced patients in China.

The immune system in the hosts is extremely important to protect the hosts from all kinds of different diseases such as HIV, other virus and cancers, etc. To improve our immune functions such as thymus and bone marrow and spleens and livers is the keys to conquer the cancers and other diseases. Dr. Xu developed a series of clinical surgerical technical skills and a series of traditional Chinese medicines which can protect our immune systems to inhibit the cancer cell growth. The following parts are the summary of these concepts and ways from Dr. Xu Ze, etc:

1. **The theory of the XZ-C anticancer therapy is based on the following animal and clinical research: on XZ animal experimental research, the results showed that removing thymus can make the animal tumor models. When the tumors grew big, thymus will gradually shrink which proved that thymus shrinking and the immune system decreases are the causes of the cancer occurrence so that Dr. XU Ze, etc posted that the cancer therapy experimental basis are to improve and to protect the thymus function such as XZ-C's immune regulation and control therapy medicines**

which he produced the unique medication products: XZ-C immune regulation and control medications from 1 to 10. After using these medications on 12,000 patients and following up with them more than 18 years, the curative effects are satisfied such as some advanced cancer patients survive more than 18 years which showed us that these new medicines and new ways are great.

2. Dr. Xu Ze, etc developed the following new ways to conquer the cancer cells and so far many cancer patients in the advanced stages, after using his surgery skills and taking his anticancer medications, are still alive or can survive more than 18 years and live with the cancers.
   a. Surgery and bioimmunotherapy will be the main treatment for the patients and the radiology and chemotherapy are the assistant treatment for the patients. The anticancer therapy should be focused on enhancing the host immune regular system against the cancer instead of only focusing on killing the cancer cells.
   b. Chemotherapy can be used in the individual organs instead of the whole body organs.
   c. Drug sensitivities in the cancer cells should be tested for Chemotherapy medicine
   d. XZ-C tradition medicines from 1 to 10 have the selections for different patients such as Z-C1 can significantly inhibit the cancer cells growth, however will not affect the normal cells;Z-C4 can improve thymus functions and increase the immune function; Z-C8 can protect the bone marrow. Also XZ's TG medicine can inhibit the cancer new microvascular growth.
   e. The tumor samples should be cultured which should be done by individuals and selections
   f. The operation of the tumors should pay attention to the cancer-free techniques such as preventing the blood to spread the tumor cells in the body instead of the traditional lymph system transferring ways.
   g. It is better to do chemotherapy by the surgeons and the surgery nurses because they are familiar with the chemotherapy pumps. The following are the comparation of the XZ new anticancer therapy concepts and the traditional concepts:

Table 1. The comparation between XZ anticancer theropy concepts and the traditional concepts

The principles	Improve the immune function to get rid of the cancer cells	Kill the cancer cells
Cancer Pathogenesis	Thymus shrink Immune function decreases	no
The experimental results and evidences	Improve the immune functions And increases the immune functions	no
The therapy rules	Build up enter pictures	Partially and only kill the cancer cells.

The therapy models	The enter therapy: surgery and bioimmunology The short therapy: radiotherapy and chemotherapy because of the side effects so that it is not good to be used too long and too strong	Chemotherapy+ radiotherapy
The therapy medications	XZ-C improve the immune functions, which combined the western and Chinese tradition medicine together on the molecular level.	Has the cell toxicities(kill the cancer cells and the normal cells)
The side effects	No	More side effects, some have the more toxicities, even the immune function failure. The radiotherapy damage is perminant.
The therapy effects	To improve the life qualities and to extend the survival times	Several months of recovery, then recurrence and development again.
The medical costs	Cheaper than radioactive and chemotherapy	Cost more money.
The prospects	It is very safe and a new way against the cancers.	The therapy effects is only 5% and have limit future.

Note: Xu Ze, etc on his reform and innovation of research on treatment of cancer.

3. Dr. Xu's new concepts are the following, which can conquer the cancers:
   1). The cancer's main etiology and pathogenesis are the decreases of thymus and immune functions.
   2). XZ-C immune regular therapy medications are to increase the thymus functions, which is the anticancer basic therapy and the evidence of his experiment.
   3). The goals of the anticancer therapy are to pay attention to the relationship of the cancer and the host to build up the whole pictures.
   4). The scientific models of the long-term anticancer therapy are the operations +the biological therapy + the immune therapy. The short-term therapy should be the radiology +chemotherapy.
   5). Local organs chemeotheray should be more effective than the whole body vein chemotherapy.

4. The medications which were made by XZ-C etc groups based on metastasis procedures and treatment:

Table 2 Metastasis procedures and treatment measures

Metastasis procedures	Z-C immunity control treatment
Proliferation of primary cancer	Z-C1 inhibits cancer cells
	Z-C4 protect thymus and improve immunity
	Z-C8 protects bone marrow to generate blood vessel
Growth of newly generated tumor Blood vessels	Z-C2-TG resists formation of blood vessels
Attack basement membrane	Z-C2-CA resists adhesion
	Z-C2-MD resists movement
Penetrate into blood vessels or Lymphatic vessels	Z-C2-MD resists penetration into blood vessels
In the blood of circulationg system	Z-C1+4 immunity regulating
	Z-C2-LM
Form blood thrombus	Z-C2-SAP dissolves cancer clot
	Z-C1+4 immunity regulation
Pass out blood vessels	Z-C2-MD resist passing out of blood vessels
Form metastatic focus	Z-C1+4 immunity regulating
	Z-C2-TG inhibits growth of blood vessels
Metastatic lymph node YaDan emusion	

In brief, this book is the scientific summary of the author's treatment experience on oncology surgery during his 50 years of oncology surgical practice and of the auther's research achievement during his 20 years of animal cancer experiment and clinical research. The author demonstrated the innovative concepts of cancer therapy including the new cognition of cancer etiology and pathogenesis and the new concepts and the new methods of cancer therapy and anticancer metastasis and the experimental information and analysis of clinical testified results and the new ways of conquering the cancers. In this book the contents are creative and the ideas are new and the theories are related to the practices. There are extremely high scientific value and clinical application. It includes the whole(entire) new concepts and creative concepts and has both the experimental research basis and clinical testified "anticancer therapy new concepts".

In order to introduce the author's contents and concepts to all over the world, thank authorhouse help press great help to publish this book internationally. Thanks again.

This book was completely translated during such shortly several months, which all depends on the cooperation of the translators. It isn't easy to translate this book which is full of many new knowledge and the innovative concepts into English so that maybe there are mistakes which we please can be forgiven for this.

Brief Introduction to Author

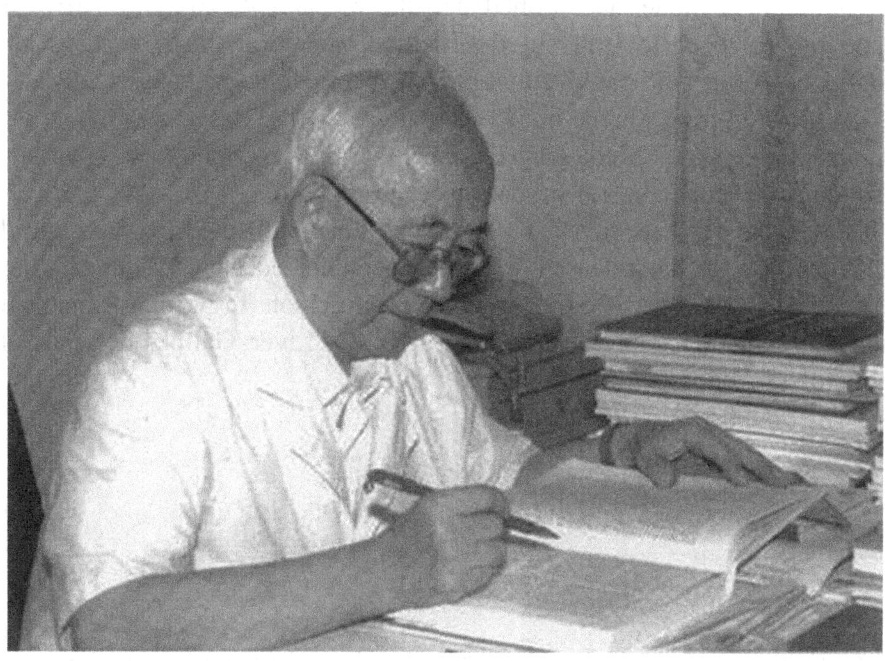

Xu Ze, male, born in Leping County of Jiangxi Province in Oct. 1933, gradated from Tongji Medical University in 1956, successively held the post of director of department of surgery of Affiliated Hospital of Hubei College of Traditional Chinese Medicine, professor, chief physician, tutor of postgraduate and doctoral student, President of Experimental Surgery Restitute Institute of Hubei College of Traditional Chinese Medicine, Director of Abdominal Tumor Surgery Research Room and Director of Anti Carcinomatous Metastasis and Reoccurrence Research Room. in addition, he held concurrent posts of Standing Director of China Medical Association Wuhan Branch, Vice President of Wuhan Micro-circulation Academy, Academic Member of International Liver Disease Research, Cooperation and Exchange Center, Member of International Surgeon Union, Standing Member of 1st, 2nd, 3rd and 4th Editorial Board of China Experimental Surgery Journal, Standing Member of 1st, 2dn and 3rd Editorial Board of Abdominal Surgery Journal. Enjoying Special Allowance of State Council.

He has been engaged in surgery work for 49 years and accumulated rich experience in radical operation of lung cancer, esophageal carcinoma, liver cancer, carcinoma of gallbladder, adenocarcinoma of pancreas, gastric carcinoma and intestinal cancer as well as in clinical therapy with Chinese Traditional Medicine combined with Western Medicine of prevention of reoccurrence and metastasis after operation.

He has been engaged in scientific research of surgery for 15 years and obtained many fruits, among which the task of Experimental Study and Clinical Application of Self-made Type Z-C1 Abdominal Cavity—Vein Flow Turning Unit in Therapy of Chronic Ascites of Hepatic Cirrhosis issued by Science Commission of Hubei Province was awarded Second Prize of Scientific Fruit by People's Government of Hubei Province and was popularized and applied in 38 hospitals in 12 provinces all over the country in 1982. The task "Experimental Study on Physiological Mechanism and Pathogenesis of Schistosome with Method of Experimental Surgery", issued by

National Natural Fund Commission was awarded Second Prize of Scientific Fruit by People's Government of Hubei Province in 1986.

He began to study the tumor experience, established the tumor animal model and metastasis and reoccurrence animal model and probed into the mechanism and rules of carcinomatous metastasis and reoccurrence to find out the method to inhibit the metastasis. 48 kinds of Chinese traditional herbs that could counteract the intrusion, metastasis and reoccurrence were found and selected from a large number of natural herbs. Based on this, he invented and developed China Xu Ze (Z-C) Medicine Treating Malignancy, which had remarkable curative effects through over 10 years' clinical validation of many cases.

He has been engaged in teaching for 40 years and has cultivated many young doctors, 10 masters and 2 doctors. He has released 126 papers, published New Understanding and New Mode of Therapy of Cancer as the editor in charge; participate in writing 8 medical exclusive books including Therapeutics of Liver Disease, Surgery of Liver, Gallbladder and Pancreas and Surgical Operation of Abdomen.

A Brief Introduction to the Second Author

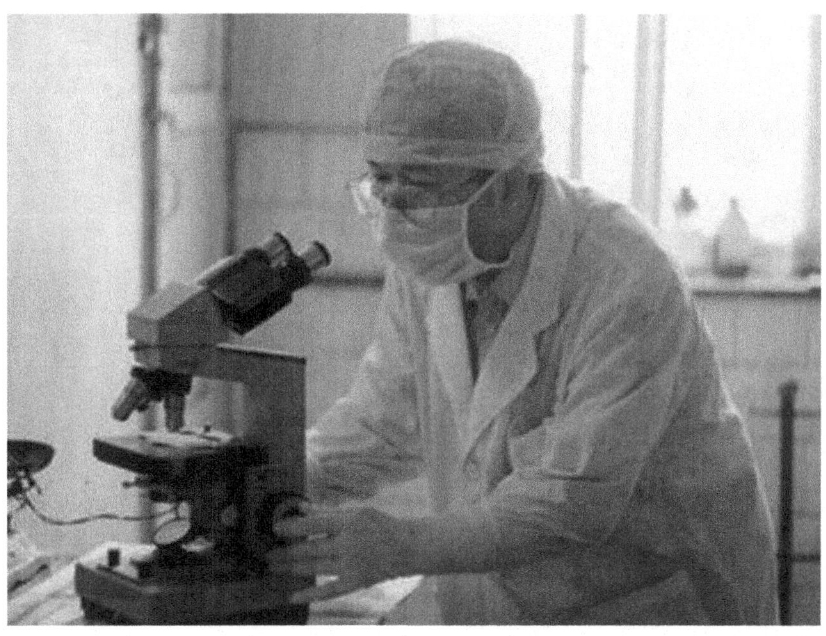

Xu Jie, male, graduated from Department of Traditional Chinese Medicine of Hubei University of Chinese Medicine in 1992 and from Department of Clinical Medicine of Hubei Medical University (now the Medicine School of Wuhan University) in 1996, serving as the associate chief physician of the surgery in Affiliated Hospital of Hubei University of Chinese Medicine, namely Hubei Hospital of Traditional Chinese Medicine and engaged in study on experimental tumor of experimental surgery and the clinical work of general surgery and urinary surgery.

Since 1992, he has participated in study on the experimental tumor in Research Institute of Experimental Surgery of Hubei University of Chinese Medicine, made the transplantation of cancer cells, established the tumor animal model, carried out a series of study on experimental tumor; probed in the mechanism and rules of cancerous reoccurrence and metastasis, screened and studied through the in vivo tumor-inhibiting experiment on the tumor-bearing animal model over 200 kinds of traditional Chinese herbs that may play a role in anticancer and cancer inhibition held by the literature and found and screened 48 kinds of traditional Chinese herbs with the role in preventing cancerous invasion, metastasis and reoccurrence from a large number of natural herbs.

He has participated in the clinical verification of XZ-C Medicine and the follow-up survey, completed the experimental study and clinical verification, data processing, collection and summary of this book.

A Brief Introduction to the Main Translator and Main Editor

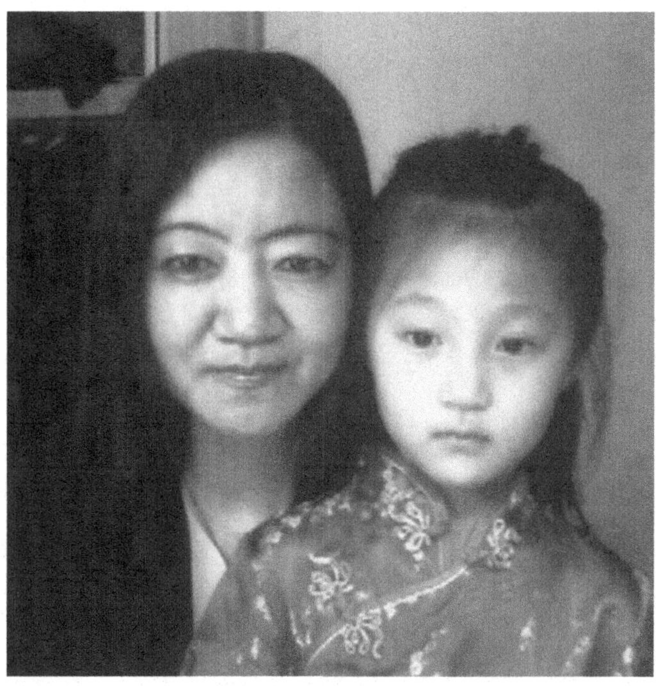

Bin Wu, MD, Ph.D., graduated from College of Yunyang of Tongji University of Medical Sciences for her MD degree; Studied her Master degree and her Ph. D degree in Sun Yat-Sen University of Medical Sciences. After she received her Ph.D., she worked as a Post-doctoral Follews in the Johns Hopkins Medical School and University of Maryland Medical School. She pasted her USMLE tests and is going to do her residency training in America. She dedicate herself to oncology clinical and research. Her goal is to conquer cancer, which she believe this great contribuation to our health. She has a daughter.

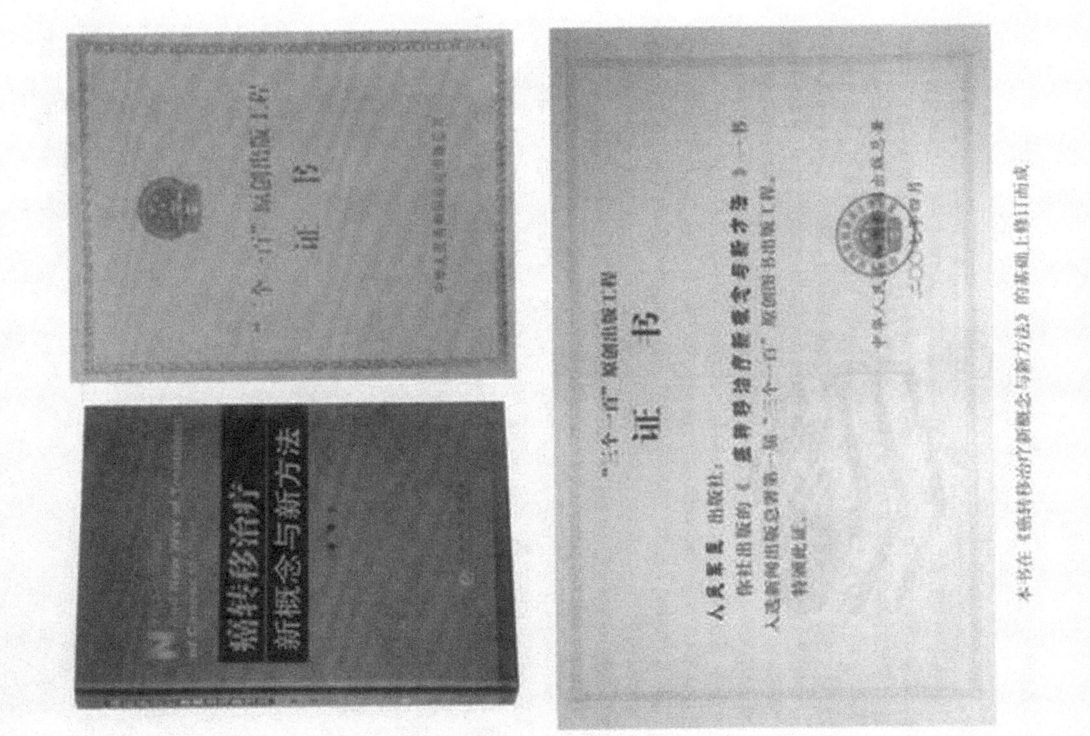

Content Abstract

This book is the scientific summary of the author's treatment experience on oncology surgery during his 50 years of oncology surgical practice and of the author's research achievement during his 20 years of animal cancer experimentation and clinical research. The book is divided into 38 chapters in which the author demonstrates innovative concepts of cancer therapy including a new cognition of cancer etiology and pathogenesis, new concepts and methods of cancer therapy and anti-cancer metastasis and recurrence. The author also demonstrates experimental information and analysis of clinically testified results and new ways of conquering the cancers from many aspects. The cancer existing in the human body has three forms: the two points and a line, and "eight steps" and "three stages" of carcinoma metastasis, the third field of anti-carcinoma-metastasis and recurrence treatment, three Steps of therapy of carcinoma metastasis, etc. It includes both the review and recall of traditional surgical and chemotherapy and radioactive therapy and the summary and analysis of the experimental information and clinical testifying results for XZ-C immunologic regulation and control anti-carcinoma traditional Chinese's medicine which the author purified from the Chinese herbs. In addition, in this book the author added the scientific methods of the cancer therapy and the strategies and suggests for the overcoming the cancer development. Some part contents of this book have generated great attention in the international field of oncology. In this book the contents are creative and the ideas are new and the theories are related to the practices. There are extremely high scientific value and clinical application, which is a value reference for clinical oncologist, oncology specialists and oncology scientific researcher and the family and caregivers of the cancer patients.

Preface

In 1985, I, by letters and calls, visited over 3000 patients after radical treatment of the carcinomas in thoracic surgery department an general surgery department by me. Finally, I found that most of the patients experienced recurrence and metastasis within 2 to 3 years after the operation or even within several months for some patients, from which I deeply realized that the operation was successful and standard, but the long-term effect was unsatisfactory or even unsuccessful. It also suggested that to prevent from recurrence and metastasis is the key to prolong the survival period after the operation. Therefore, we must make clinical fundamental research in depth and it will be difficult to improve the clinical curative effect without the breakthrough in fundamental clinical research. As a result, we build the Institute of Experimental Surgery of anticancer recurrence and metastasis, and spent 24 years on doing a series of experimental research and clinical testifying work from the following aspects:

1. The experimental research on Pathogenic factor, pathogenesis and pathological Physiology of carcinoma to seek for effective medications and control measures.

   My colleagues and I had spent four years making the experimental research on tumor in the research lab. The selected topics of the research items were wholly from the clinic, in this way, we wanted to interpret or settle some clinical problems through experimental research. All of these were the clinical experimental research.

2. New Drugs experimental research on seeking for the drugs of ant-cancer, ant-metastasis and ant-recurrence.

   The existing anticancer drugs, kill the cancer cells and the normal cells as well, with great toxic action and adverse reaction. This lab searched for the new drugs only inhibiting the cancer cells but not affecting the normal cells from the Chinese herbal medicines of the natural medicines thrugh the cancer-inhibiting experiment on the cancer-bearing mouse. This lab had spent three years making the cancer-inhibitig and screeing experiment on the cancer-bearing animals from the common traditional anti-cancer prescriptions and 200 kinds of Chinese herbal medicines in the anti-cancer prescriptions reported in each province one by one. Finally, we screened 48 kinds of Chinese herbal medicines with relatively good tumor-inhibition rate and relatively good immunity-upgrading action and found the Chinses herbal medicine TG inhibiting the regenerate micrangium.

3. Clinical Verification

Through the above-mentioned fundamental experimental research on the recurrence and metastasis for four years and the experimental research on the screened herbs from the Chinese herbal medicines of the natural medicines for 3 years, we found a batch of $Z\text{-}C_{1\text{-}10}$ medicines; and then, through clinical verification of over 12,000 patients in metaphase and advanced stage of the carcinomas or suffering from the metastasis after operation for 16 years of the application of Z-C medicine, the relatively good effect had been obtained, the quality of life had been improved, the symptom had been improved and survival time had been obviously prolonged.

Recently, I have sorted out, summarized and collected the review, analysis, reflection and understanding of the clinical practical cases in the past 50 years as well as outcomes and findings of the experimental research on the cancer-bearing animals over 10 years and the experimental research and clinical verification data and finally pubished two exclusive books: 1. <<New Understanding and Mode of Carcinomatosis Treatment>>, published by Hubei Science and Technology Press, written by Xu Ze, Jan. 2001. 2. <<New Concept and Way of Treatment of Cancer Metastasis>>, published by Beijing People's Military Medical Press, written by Xu Ze, Jan. 2006, which was granted Certificate for Three-one-Hundred Original Books by General Administration of press and Publication of People's Republic of China in Apr. 2007.

This book is the author's third book, which is the true record of scientific research from experiment to clinic, then from clinic to experiment. Also it is the summary of the experimental research and clinical testifying information, then up to the theory levels, which points out the new discovery, new recognition such as practical clinical oncology theory, cancer therapy and cancer research development and reformation and all of these clinic practical innovative theory can guide the clinical therapy.

Because all of the clinical treatment, medication application, diagnosis must have the theory basis, it is necessary to create the clinic practical theory. During my 50 years of

Clinic oncology surgery practice, I realized that because the cancer etiology, pathogenesis are not clear, the oncology become the last scientific specialty so that it need to be developed on the basic scientific research, clinic testifying research and the research of the combination of the basic and the clinics.

During seven years we conducted a series of basic clinical experimental research and basic problem investigation on 6000 animal models and selected anticancer drugs from 200 tranditional herbs on the animal models one by one, which were finished by my graduate students together. "Experimental Study of the effects on the growth of tumor from spleen and the medication of improvement of the spleen function", finished by Dr. Zhushiping; "Experiment on Adoptive Immunologic Reconstitution of Fetal Liver, Spleen and Thymus Cells through Combined Transplantation", finished by Dr. Qingshaoming; "the experiment research of the inhibition of herb medicine to the tumor cells in S_{180} mouse", finished by Dr. Lizhengguong; "'TG'S INHIBITION ON ANGIOGENESIS OF TRANSPLANTATION TUMOR OF MICE", finished by Dr. Luliling. All of the above researches are my research projects which are the basic problems closely related to the clinical practice. All of my students worked hard and completed these difficult and careful experimental research projects and contribute the development of cancer prevention and anticancer and experimental oncology medicine.

This book includes the experimental research and clinical testifying patient cases, up to the theory of the new concepts and new theories and new models of cancer therapy, which are the first and creative opinions. Because the oncology develops very fast and is involved in many science specialties such as molecular biology and molecular immunology and has the wide knowledge, it is difficult to avoid mistakes so that we ask the readers to forgive these.

Xu Ze
January 8, 2011 in Wuhan
Email: xuze88cn@yahoo.com.cn
Tel:027-88049526

Acknowledgements

This book is for all of people who concern human being health. Thanks and appreciation to Dr. Sitthipol Tovanich, who graduated from University of Washington Medical School in Seattle in USA and is an anesthesiologist, for his advice and encouragement to get this book published soon. Also thanks to all of authorhouse staffs.

Bin Wu, M.D., Ph.D.

CHAPTER 1

The Concept of Traditional Cancer Therapeutics Should Renew Thought and Change Conception

I. Cancer therapeutics should be established based on the understanding of the concept of cancer

After the Second World War, oncology has developed greatly at home and abroad for half a century. The traditional three therapies and operative tumor therapy have a history of over one hundred years, while radiotherapy and chemotherapy have a history of 80 years and nearly 60 years respectively. In 1980s, biotherapy and immunotherapy arose. Quite great progress has been made in the curative effect of tumor and relatively better curative effect has been achieved for many tumors, however, the curative effect of an abundance of tumors are still in extremely poor state.

In 1985, the author made follow-up survey to over 3000 patients who had experienced general surgical and chest cancer operations performed by the author, and found that most the patients experienced recurrence and metastasis within 2 to 3 years after the operation or even within several months for some patients, from which I deeply realized that the operation was successful and standard, but the long-term effective was unsatisfactory or even unsuccessful.

Since 1970s, in view of the extremely high recurrence and metastasis rate after operation, to prevent the recurrence and metastasis after operation, a series of assistant chemotherapy has been adopted after operation or even before operation (such as mastocarcinoma), but the results have been not satisfactory. Recurrence and metastasis still appear in or after the course of assistant chemotherapy after operation or appear along with chemotherapy; I have observed from a great many of patients in our tumor special clinic that assistant chemotherapy after operation fails to prevent recurrence and metastasis and intensive recurrence and metastasis causes the failure of immunologic function to some cases. The clinicians should seriously, calmly, objectively and practically consider, review, analyze and turn over to think the above facts. Many basic concepts and theories are still not clear and the curative effect is not high, therefore, we must make clinical fundamental research in depth and it will be difficult to improve the clinical curative effect in case of no breakthrough in fundamental clinical research.

(I) Review of the history of traditional therapeutic method

The establishment of scientific basis of modern medicine for cancer only has a history of over one hundred year. The traditional cancer therapeutics, i.e. three therapies, have taken shape gradually in the past one hundred years and is established on the basis of traditional mode concept of cancer. We will briefly review the formation of traditional mode concept of cancer and cancer therapeutics of modern medicine and their contributions to anti-cancer achievements of human beings.

The classical tumor mode concept was established based on the understanding of integrated level of cytology, pathology, cell biology, microbiology and anatomy and cellular level in the end of 19th century and the first half 20th century. In those days, the subjects concerning cellular level really accelerated the great development in medical science. They held that the tumor cells were converted from normal cells which would have abnormal formation, metabolism and functions after converted to tumor cells. Tumor cells grew vigorously and continuously, lacked coordination with the whole organism of host, and disabled it from maturation to different extent. They held that tumor originated from individual cell, that is to say, tumor was originated from clone, cancer cells were able to regenerate autonomously and were divided and reproduced continuously, one to two and two to four, therefore, cancer cells were the arch criminal and the root of canceration, and they must be killed. All of the cancer cells must be killed for therapy. The scientists at the beginning of 20th Century sought the method to kill cancer cells.

1. In 18th Century, distinguished doctors held that cancer was local disease and could be cured by surgical operation. In 1881, Billroth firstly performed the surgical radical operation on tumor, i.e. partial gastrectomy. In 1888, Langen Buch successfully resected pedicel bearing tumor on the left lobe of liver. In 180, Halsted performed radical mastectomy, illuminated the principle of en bloc resection for the first time, i.e. primary tumor was resected together with local lymphatic vessel and lymph nodes, laying the foundation for the most modern tumor surgical operations. The technology of surgical tumor resection operation was developed along with the development of surgical medicines; after the middle period of 20th Century, the range of tumor surgical opcration became larger due to the progress in the technology of surgical operation, a series of super radical operations, such as expanded radical mastectomy. It was proved by the practice over years that the expanded surgical removal range could not improve the tumor-free survival time and total survival time for most cancerous protuberances, such as lung cancer, liver cancer and cancer of pancreas.
2. In December, 1898, Curie found radium, a new trace element that she had been seeking for a long time, and obtained Nobel Prize in 1911, and radium had been extensively researched and applied in medical science since then. However, radium had a certain lethal action. In 1930s, the doctors observed that when the workers in clock and watch factories painted the radium pigment on the figures on dial plate, they had the habit of licking the stylus, and many of them caught bone cancer. Furthermore, Curie died of leukemia in July, 1934; unquestionably, this was the direct result of radiation of radium. It was proved by facts that radium was quite effective to massive tumor, any tumor would shrink rapidly after injection with syringe needle painted with radium on the tip, and the "radium therapy" was the main method for cancer treatment for decades of years. 800-1000kV X-ray machine was developed in 1932 and cyclotron and induction accelerator were developed subsequently. Radicisotope was applied to tumor treatment step by step. At present, although the radiotherapy has certain effect on the treatment of various tumors, the effect is still not ideal in general, and the main reasons of unsuccessful treatment include recurrence and metastasis.
3. After the Second World War (1946), it is found that the cell toxicant (Nitrogen mustard) and its derivation in the chemical warfare have obvious inhibitory action on tumor, however, due to its poor selectivity, it is called cytotoxic drug, it can kill cancer cells and kill the normal cells of host at the same time, so the toxic side effect is relatively large. The existing therapy design is still established on the basis of logarithm value—cells—killing, which is derived

from growing mode of L_{1210} leukemia cell strain. It is embarrassing that the killing mode of one logarithm only indicates the resistance of host rather than therapy. As to the vital cancer cells, after each therapy, there are still some left and they can't be thoroughly killed.

The above-mentioned three therapies of traditional therapeutic method have made great accepted contributions to anti-cancer achievements of human beings. However, up to the beginning of 21st Century, cancer is still very rampant, the incidence rate of cancer grows continuously, the death rate is still quite high, and the recurrence and metastasis still cannot be prevented, even though many patients receive normal and systematic radiotherapy and chemotherapy after operation. Why the traditional therapy cannot obviously reduce the death rate? Whether it is presented that the traditional therapy does not conform to the actual conditions of the biological characteristics of the carcinomatosis? What is the matter with the traditional concept and the traditional therapy? What is the defect? How to correct the defect in concept or understanding so as to make it more perfect and more coincidental with the actual conditions of molecular biological characteristics of the carcinomatosis?

In view that the concept of cancer therapeutics is established based on the understanding of the cancer concept, it is necessary to research the new progress in cancer concept so as to research the concept of cancer therapeutics.

As to the understanding of the concept of carcinomatosis, Harvey Schipper had incisively elaborated it.

(II) Traditional mode of cancer

Fundamental principles of traditional mode: the contents of the traditional mode of cancer can be divided into five fundamental principles.

1. Cancer is of asexual reproduction (clone): the formation of carcinoma stems from the canceration in the single cell, so no matter how the canceration is induced, the tumor is endowed with all characteristics of tumor by this cell.
2. Autonomy of malignant tumor: the cancer cells are continually divided and proliferated and they do not obey the regulation and control, they are autonomous in behavior, the tumor cells grow as per the index, so it is thought that the growth rate is stable.
3. Irreversibility of canceration process: the canceration process has shown its irreversibility in a certain stage before clinic. The cellular aberration not only advances continually but also accumulates, resulting in failure of treatment, as is the natural development of canceration process.
4. Relation between tumor and host: the reaction of the host to the tumor is objective, however, its impacts on the natural disease process of the tumor is not inevitable.
5. It is required by the heal to kill the last cancer cell: if the canceration process is irreversible, autonomous and lethal, the only way to healing is to kill off all cancer cells. In case of remained cancer cells, they will be proliferated again; in case of remained tumor or unapparent tumor, it is regarded that the treatment fails and the patient will meet with death.

(III) Concept of traditional cancer therapeutics

It is held by the traditional concept that cancinoma is the continual division and proliferation of cancer cells, so the treatment must target killing the cancer cells, so these three goals of traditional cancer therapeutics are determined based on the concept of traditional mode of killing off the cancer cells.

The principle of current cancer therapeutics is based on the following precondition: in order to achieve the goal of heal, it is necessary to kill or eliminate the last cancer cells. As a result, people adopt the expanded operation and strengthen chemotherapy and radical radiotherapy. However, the curative effects are not so satisfying. At the beginning of 1960s, the extent of surgical operation on tumor tended toward expansion and a series of super-radical operations had been developed. Subsequently, it has been proven by the practice for years that the expansion of extent of surgical removal of the cancer cells, such as breast cancer, lung cancer, liver cancer and pancreatic cancer, has not improved the cancer-free survival time and total survival time. In 1980s, the one receiving intensive chemotherapy and radical radiotherapy could not achieve the improvement of survival quality or elongation of survival time. Since the hematopiesis function and immunologic function of the bone marrow are seriously restricted, some complications endangering the life are coming out. Therefore, it is necessary to establish a new mode to probe into the cancer, strive for opening a new way and renew the concept from the clinical and experimental data.

The classic concept of tumor mode is derived from microbiology. Penicillin was discovered by Fleming in 1929 and streptomycin was discovered in 1944. The clinical application of antibiotics has played an important role in controlling or eliminating a few of contagious diseases and infectious diseases. Microbiology veritably protests at thorough elimination of the exotic disease disseminators. When the patient suffers from the seriously infectious disease, such as lobar pneumonia, acute tonsillitis and so on, it is necessary to kill the bacillus for treatment with antibiotics, if the curative effect is not so good, the antibiotics sensitive to pathogenesis will be selected, the dosage will be increased or the combined administration will be adopted to thoroughly eliminate the pathogenesis. However, infection is quite another thing from tumor, the latter stems from the host body. When treatment of cancer with radiotherapy and chemotherapy is not ideal, it is possible to increase the dosage as the anti-cancer cytotoxic drug differs from the antibiotics: ① The anti-cancer cytotoxic drug kills the cancer cells as well as the normal cells, inhibits hematopiesis function and immunologic function of the bone marrow and has the side effects on the liver and the kidney, if the dosage is increased, the host cannot withstand it; ② Generally, anti-cancer cytotoxic drug cannot be used for drugsensitive test or drug resistant test and it is only blindly administered by experience while the antibiotics can be used for drugsensitive test so as to select the sensitive antibiotics.

To sum up, the concept of traditional cancer therapeutics holds the tumor is based on the maniac division and proliferation of the cells, so the cancer cells are the arch criminal, as a result, the target of the treatment goal of the traditional cancer therapeutics is the cancer cell, namely killing-off of the cancer cells.

II. Heal shall be realized through regulation and control instead of killing

(I) Assumptive new mode of cancer therapeutics

The assumptive new mode of cancer therapeutics includes some new examples and its predominant idea holds that cancer is a kind of disease, the regulation and signal transmission among the cells are disrupted instead of loss and the carcinogenesis is a continuous entity with possibility of reversion.

The understanding of the cancer by the new mode is based on information transfer and regulation and control. It is convinced that the canceration is a process of evolvement step by step, however, it holds that they may be potentially reversed. The last step of healing the cancer is to mobile the reappearance of the regulation and control role of the host instead of eliminating the last cancer cells. This mode refers to the experience and phenomena of clinical lab and epidemiorlogy as well as the modern molecular biology and traditional concepts. Based on the viewpoint of new mode, the mechanism that the cancer is healed through regulation and control may be presented and other pending issues may be explained.

The cancer cells do not always differ from the normal cells greatly. It has been clearly convinced from the present and previous observation that autonomy of tumor is very limited. Through the clinical observation over one century and the analysis in the past 20 years, the biological findings have definitely convinced that the cancerization course can be reversed. We had treated the cancer through killing off the cancer cells to the utmost extent, but we had not made great achievements. When it looks as if the condition is controlled, new cancerization may take place again. It has been proven by the past experience and the progress of modern science that the cancer cells can coexist with the host and they do not always damage the host.

All of these facts tell us that it is time to reconsider the mode of cancer treatment, which needs adjusting out understanding of cancer. Maybe our understanding is established on the concept that it is necessary to kill off the canceration cells as they can not be reversed, restricting our ability of understanding and treating cancer in an all-round way. Based on the above-mentioned, a new mode of cancer treatment is gradually formed.

(II) Fundamental principle of new mode

1. Clone: cancer is an evolvement process instead of a morphological solid, formation of tumor individual stem from the single cell in the organism, however, the tumor cells have been making the accommodation to the local environment.
2. Most of the structure of the cancer cells is normal: its malignancy characteristics result from the change in few genes and (or) environment. Except the lost genes, all signals of the other cell genes will be remained and the abnormality of the genes is mainly caused by the abnormality of regulation and control of expression. At present, it is shown by the increased facts that each functional part of the canceration is related to the characteristic gene product, which is consistent with the clinical observation. It can be reasonably inferred that the tumor grows, infiltrates and transfers under the proper conditions and the evolvement at each step depends on the exiguous reaction of the gene product with characteristic code. Now a kind of metastasis inhibiting gene (nm23) and its product have been discovered, which further indicate that the canceration has the intrinsic reversibility.

3. Unbalance of regulation and control: **the reaction of host determines the final results.** It is shown by the above-mentioned that the canceration results from the unbalance of regulation and control instead of the adequate autonomy. It is indicated by the clinical and experimental experience that the tumor keeps a certain response relation with the host. When the tumor results from the unbalance of regulation and control instead of the autonomy of the tumor, some clinical phenomena can be easily understood. Clinically, it is known by us that the cancer cells can make adaptative response to the environment of the host at high level. The long-term application of immunosuppressant may induce the tumor, when the immunosuppressant is suspended, the tumor can be entirely released. Although the factors inducing the tumor have not been proven, the reaction of host determines the final results. The kidney transplantation tumor with metastasis to the lung will be entirely released after suspension of the antirejection therapy. It looks as if the pregnancy improves the relation between the tumor and the host. Now people have focused on killing the tumor, developed so many therapeutic methods and developed many anti-cancer cytotoxic drugs in the past half a century, however, they cannot prevent the attack and metastasis of tumor. Viewed from the data, the cytotoxic drugs as the assistant of radiotherapy after operation also cannot prevent the reoccurrence and metastasis of the cancer because most of them severely inhibit the immunity even the non-immunological part of the host reaction. When people increase the concentration and dosage of the chemotherapeutic drugs to make them more aggressive to the cancer cells (such as intensified radiotherapy), we right lead the mechanism of long-term survival or healing to the more dangerous way, even bring about the artificial or iatrogenic immunologic function breakdown.

4. Reversibility of cancer cells: reversibility and anti-metastasis of tumor

   As above-mentioned, since the tumor arises from the normal tissues, then, whether are the cancer cells reversed to the normal cells? It was regarded as a mirage scores of years ago, however, the history of scientific advance has proven for times that the mirage can be realized. Just because of this, at present, the scientists are seriously studying this task so as to control the cancer cells artificially by all means to make it free of malignant growth, recover and change the cancer cells into normal cells.

   If the canceration is gradually induced and is not lethal immediately, the canceration cells possibly have the reversibility. The cancer cells can be reversed to the normal cells by means of a series of approaches including the change of a batch of processes before reversion induces the canceration; blockade of the incomplete or false signal transmission role; control over ineffective enzyme and accepter or the way of inducing metabolism dromotropic action. However, the metabolism of most of the cells has the capacity of keeping balance, in addition, in order to heal the patient suffering from the tumor, it is not required that the canceration meet with the reversion in all directions, it is only necessary to regulate the key steps such as proliferation, infiltration and metastasis of cancer cells again or make the key steps reversed.

   Viewed from molecular biology, the cancer results from the change in DNA structure. It is the unbalanced differentiation of the cells caused by the genetic information that introduces the normal nucleic acid to the cancer cells via the genetic engineering, inducing the tumor cells to differentiate to the normal cells. Shanghai Tumor Research Institute had extracted RNA from the normal hepatic cells, then incubated and cultivated it together with the liver cancer cells to correct the abnormal genetic activities of the liver cancer cells through the regulation and control reaction of normal liver RNA so as to make it reversed to the normal cells. The scientists now are looking for the bioactive substances related to the genetic information, for example, the normal mRNA can induce the cancer cells to reverse to the normal cells.

Some drug has the probability of inducing the cancer cells to differentiate to the normal cells.

In recent years, a kind of cell fusion technology has been developed, which can make two kinds of different somatic cells fuse with each other. If the fibrocytes of the mouse fuse with the cancer cells of the mouse, the hybrid cell obtained become a kind of intermediate cell, with the intermediate texture and biological characteristics.

The work to induce the cells to differentiate to the normal cells to reverse the tumor cells is just remaining in the early stage, no matter the rule of regulating and controlling the cell differentiation with nucleic acid or the rule of regulating and controlling the cell differentiation with drugs, is not made clear and it needs further study. Therefore, the burden is heavy and the road is long!

Some scientists hold that it is possible to realize the reversion of the tumor in the early stage of the canceration while the tumor becomes an irreversible canceration in the late stage of the cancer, therefore, they put forward a suggestion: it is not necessary to induce the tumor to return to the normal state, but it is necessary to induce the tumor to differentiate to mature or make for apoptosis and death. It looks as if this is a more realistic assumption, in this way, it is likely to make the patients suffering from the advanced cancer enjoy the achievements of studying on tumor induction and reversion.

5. Killing tumor cells: the precondition of adopting the cytotoxic drugs to treat the tumor is the understanding that the it is not only possible but also necessary to kill the last cancer cell until it is proven by the clinic application and the lab that the tumor has been entirely eliminated, as is the prerequisite of healing the patient suffering from the tumor. However, according to our experience over 20 years, this argumentation is contradictory. Some clinical cases show that killing can shrink or subside the tumor, however, it cannot directly heal the tumor. Although the dosage of cytotoxic drug is increased and most of the cancer cells are subsided, the survival rate of the patient is not improved. Soon after, it will reoccur and the tumor will be enlarged.

All the obviously healed patients do not seem to adopt the mode of killing the cancer cells. For example, the treatment of tumor with platinum-based drug seems to be related to the induced cell differentiation. The action of interferon and interleukin to the sensitive cells is realized by the regulation and control mechanism. As to the levamisole as the adjuvant for carcinoma of large intestine, it is deemed that its effects are from the change in host reaction.

We had tried out best to kill the cancer cells to treat the cancer before, however, no great achievements had been made. Later, enlarged radical operation, intensified chemotherapy and radical radiotherapy were adopted. However, the results were not ideal and they could not improve the survival quality of the patient suffering from cancer and the survival time of the patient suffering from cancer after operation.

In the recent 50 years, the treatment of cancer by traditional Chinese medicine has made great achievements. A large number of data indicate that the cancer cells can coexist with the host and they may not always damage the host. In the recent 16 years, among 12000 patients suffering from metaphase and advanced cancer treated by Shuguang Tumor Research Institute and Wuchang Shuguang Tumor Special Clinic, some reoccurrence and metastasis patients, such as the patients with anastomotic stoma reoccurrence cancer and gastric carcinoma that cannot be ablated or treated through radiotherapy and chemotherapy, after taking Z-C medicine for a long time over 3-5 years, the conditions are controlled and stabilized, they can survive with tumor (coexist with the tumor) and take care of themselves, the survival quality is good and the survival quality is obviously prolonged.

Conclusions: this mode is not completely new, it is mainly the response to the new knowledge challenging the traditional concept and tries to conceptualize the canceration of the cell based on this. Now the most effective killing therapy we know at present is the most potential factor inducing the tumor and resulting in cell resistance. In the past scores of years, we have been catching a sight of epigamic circumstance that the treatment without cell toxicant can heal the tumor once in a while. Despite all this, the therapeutic direction that the people strive for is to kill the last cancer cell. If the therapeutic direction meets with new conversion, maybe our visual field will be broader. We should open a new road to reform and innovate the therapeutic concept.

It is deemed by us that undoubtedly we should kill the foreigners invading the body, however, as to the cancer cells, we shall make a differential treatment just because they are only the variant tissues in the normal body of the host, here we reaffirm that the cancer shall be treated through regulating the control over them by the mechanism instead of the necessary and impossible killing-off of all cancer cells.

Since we have a new cognition of the cancer concept, then, the concept of cancer therapeutics shall renew the thought, the understanding and the concepts and innovate the therapeutic theory and technology.

In view of the experience and lessons of the author over half a century, now we should research the urgent problems in the current cancer study, seek for the breakthrough for clinical research from the weak link of the modern medicine and find the breakthrough of prevention and control from the invasion, reoccurrence and metastasis, look for the anti-reoccurrence and anti-metastasis drugs from the chemical drugs and the natural herbs and deepen the new understanding of the cancer concept at the molecular level, genetic level, integrated treatment level and targeted treatment.

III. New progress of research on cancer and new trend of therapy

(I) New progress of fundamental research on cancer

Most research on tumor is conducted combining with clinic work. To overcome cancer, it is necessary to get a deep understanding of the nature of cancer, recognize cancer from the perspective of pathogenic factor, pathologic physiology, pathogenesis, pathology, heredity and immunity, and reveal the nature of carcinoma. The solider the fundamental theoretical research on carcinoma is, the richer are the specific measures of anti-cancer.

1. What is the origin of carcinoma? Scientists in ancient and modern times, in China and elsewhere, have explored the question for hundreds of years, but it remains an unrevealed mystery. How does a normal cell changes into a cancer cell? How can cancer cell itself

evolves into tumor? Why cancer cell can pass down its character of excessive growth to the coming generations, and lead to human death?

To reveal the secret of excessive growth of tumor and passing it down to the coming generations, many scientists in the past have done much work, but most of it is rather rough restricted by historical conditions and what has been observed is often superficial. Until sixty years ago, i.e. 1950s, an unexpected experiment result was found that when a toxic diplococcus pneumoniae, killed at high temperature, was mixed with a nontoxic diplococcus pneumoniae and injected into the body of a mouse, the mouse would die of disease, and toxic diplococcus pneumoniae could be separated out of the dead mouse. This was a revealing experiment. How dead diplococcus pneumoniae recovered? How nontoxic diplococcus pneumoniae became toxic? It could not be explained at that time. Ten years later, someone cultivated the extract of toxic diplococcus pneumoniae together with nontoxic diplococcus pneumoniae, it turned out that nontoxic diplococcus pneumoniae became toxic. The extract was DNA. It was demonstrated by experiment for the first time that the basic substance of heredity was DNA. How DNA controlled heredity? It proved that the genetic code existing in DNA molecule controlled all hereditary characters.

How genetic code transfers genetic information? There are two approaches, one is DNA self-duplication, the other is NDA controls protein synthesis through RNA, i.e. DNA transfers genetic information to RNA and controls protein synthesis through delicate matching of three RNAs. DNA duplication and DNA's controlling protein synthesis through RNA is a very close and rigorous process. Normal cells follow this rule strictly and maintain normal functions. However, some link of the complex process may mutate or go wrong disturbed by internal and external factors of the organism, triggering changes in DNA structure and function, some of which become "malignant information" and incur canceration. Previous theories of carinogenic factors are divergent and controversial. Currently, the studies on carinogenic factors begin to converge, whether chemical carinogenic factors such as benzene and nitrosamine, physical carinogenic factor such as radioactive rays, or biological carinogenic factor such as virus. They all acknowledge only by affecting DNA genetic information can cancer be incurred. DNA is damaged by these factors at first and incompletely rehabilitated, disturbing the sequence of nucleotide on helix chain, i.e. incur error of genetic code. As the wrong code is passed down, normal cells cannot retain their original genetic characters, changing the cells of the next generation into cancer cells and triggering crazily growing carcinoma.

Since mid-1970s, with the new progress of life science, establishment and development of DNA recombination, gene transfer and hydridoma technology, genetic engineering, protein engineering technology, it is possible to study the nature and characteristics of cancer cells by a combination of molecular level and cellular level, and find out anti-cancer approaches and reverse and differentiation or cancer gene treatments. Development of these special technologies accelerates revelation and recognition of malignant behavior of tumor cells, lays a foundation for controlling tumor occurrence, reduce the rate of suffering from cancer and death rate.

The basic biological character of tumor cell is manifested as disorderly regulation of cell proliferation and differentiation. In recent years, owing to the discovery of growth factor and growth inhibitory factor, people have got an understanding of regulation of cell proliferation and differentiation.

As is known to all, cell growth, death and differentiation are the most fundamental physical activities of the cell and basic issue of life science. Whether for growth factor, hormone or oncogene products, apoptosis, their effects of promoting cell proliferation and inducing cell death come down to affecting operation of the cell cycle, which is under the control of cell cyclin dependent kinase and its inhibitors. Cell continuous proliferation, apoptosis and reduction caused by abnormal regulation mechanism of cell cycle are the core of uncontrolled growth of the tumor cell. Hence, tumor can also be deemed as a cell cycle disease.

In mid-1980s, the research on tumor occurrence mechanism has made great advances. Most tumors are monoclonal, need to go through several steps to change from normal cells into malignant cells, which manifested as obviously different development stages. More importantly, the application of molecular biological technologies reveals that there is a close relationship between tumor occurrence and abnormal gene: ①about 5% human tumors are inherited from the family; ②the occurrence of all tumors is accompanied by somatic cell mutation, tumor development involves abnormal expression of multiple genes; ③multiple carcinogenic factors such as virus, radioactive ray, chemical carcinogen, can all cause gene mutation; ④ the gene involved in tumor occurrence and evolution are often related with such basic life activities as cell proliferation, differentiation and apoptosis. Hence, it is recognized that tumor is a gene disease.

After 1976, the scientists discovered and recognized the nature of oncogene such as V-src, ras myc. Ten years later, they noticed the functions of tumor suppressor gene such as Rb, P_{53} and P_{16}, opening up a new era of recognition of tumor in all aspects. Given the boom of research on gene therapy and apoptosis emerging at the end of 1980s and beginning of 1990s, the relationship between apoptosis or programmed cell death (PCD) and tumor drew more attention. It was believed multicellular organism maintains self-stability through cell proliferation and apoptosis, and the imbalance of them can cause tumor occurrence. It has been proved that inhibited apoptosis may be one of the tumor pathogenesis. However, it should be pointed out that proliferation, differentiation and apoptosis of normal cells are under strict control of gene. Therefore, uncontrolled cell proliferation, differentiation obstacle and apoptosis hindrance are just representation of tumor occurrence. To reveal tumor occurrence mechanism in essence, it is necessary to explore the change in gene structure or abnormal gene expression behind these representations on gene level.

2. The contact of human body with carcinogenic factors, even occurrence of cancer cells in human body, will not necessarily cause carcinoma.

As a matter of fact, not a few abnormal cells occur in healthy human body everyday, but they are not likely to grow and proliferate on a large scale and eliminated by immune system of the body. To ensure relative stability of its own genetic information, eliminate harmful mutation of DNA molecule, kill cancer cells in the body, human body has a whole set of immune defense system, which will give out alarm signals in case of occurrence of abnormal cells. In 1980s, the scientists separated out an alarm signal of malignant tumor, referred to as recognition factor, which was a kind of protein, gave out alarm, announced the occurrence of cancer cells in the body and summoned leukocyte responsible for cleaning to attack cancer cells. They also found that fewer recognition factors in the body of the cancer patient meant more serious tumor.

Carcinoma tends to occur to a few people whose immunologic function is damaged. Some people with congenital immunodeficiency tend to suffer from cancer. Behind the breast bone there is a glandular organ called thymus, which is an important immune organ of the body. Seniors' immunologic function degenerates due to thymus atrophy, increasing the rate of carcinoma occurrence. In 1985 while the author was conducting the experimental study of modeling of animal inoculated with tumor cells, he made over 400 modeling experiments, which all failed, and later ablated the mice's thymus first, leading to complete success in modeling. The conclusion of the experimental study confirmed there was a relationship between immunologic function organs and tumor occurrence.

Therefore, carcinogenic factor is an aspect of tumor occurrence, i.e. the external factor, while immune defense capacity of the organism is another aspect of tumor occurrence, i.e. the internal factor. The external factor effects through the internal factor, and the organism's internal factor finally controls tumor occurrence. A seed cannot take root, geminate and grow without suitable soil. As what is soil to the seed, cancer cell cannot evolve into tumor before escaping from the monitoring of the body's alarm system and breaking through the immune defense line of the organism. Far-sighted medical scientists and clinic scientists all have expectations of the field. We predict that future cancer treatment will derive from the immune defense system and adopt the approach of immunologic regulation, rather than just killing cancer cells by mere surgical operation and radioactive or chemical therapy.

According to our current recognition, the formation of most tumors in the body can be generalized as three procedures: first, carcinogenic factor (physical, chemical and biological) acts on the organism, disturbs cellular metabolism; second, disturb DNA genetic information within the nucleus, hereditary variation of the cell triggers canceration; third, cancer cells escape from immune alarm monitoring and defense system of the body, begin to split and proliferate, forming carcinoma.

The theoretical basis of therapeutics stems from the above theoretical basis. In view of the above new recognition, cancer should be treated through regulation rather than injury.

There have been two views of cancer occurrence and evolution:

> One view is that cancer occurrence and evolution is an "independent process" basically unrestricted by any defense mechanism, treatment should focus on tumor itself while paying little attention to regulating effects of immune system of the organism. The other view is that cancer occurrence and evolution is a "dependent process" or "controlled process" regulated by multiple factors within the body, especially immune factors, which entails that treatment should pay equal attention to "eliminating the pathogenic factors" and "reinforcing the vital qi". We hold that the process cannot be controlled effectively unless combine and apply the principles of "reinforcing the vital qi and eliminating the pathogenic factors" in a medical sense.

(II) New trend of therapy

The research on tumor biology and therapeutics must be consistent with the latter based on the theoretical basis of the former. Until now, tumor biology has developed to the level of molecular biology, cytokine and gene, while the theoretical basis of tumor therapeutics remains at the cytology level half a century ago, which is constant proliferation of cancer cells aimed at killing cancer cells. The traditional method is killing cancer cells, so using cell toxicant is not very effective, which is solved by increasing the dosage and adding several drugs for combination. Since 1980s, with the rapid development of molecular medicine, molecular immunology and cytokine study, new biological therapeutics emerges and tumor therapeutics advances.

It can be deemed that the research on anti-cancer medicine has entered a new stage, facing updated theories, technologies and ideas. The traditional idea and work method based on cell toxicant is under attack, research scope of anti-tumor drugs has not been limited to traditional cell toxicant drug, differentiation inducer and biological reaction moderator, immunologic regulatory Chinese medicines combining Chinese and western medicine are emerging.

1. Immunological therapy: as the clinic evidence related with immunity and immune index such as spontaneous extinction of individual tumor indicate that immunologic function of the organism is declining with the evolution of tumor, enlightening us to expect much of immunologic therapy of tumor. Many scholars and clinic doctors were once committed to pioneering this field with great interest, to make break-through progress in cancer treatment. However, after several booms and peaks, until the end of 1970s, although the research on cancer immunologic therapy achieved some results in animal experiment and in vitro experiment, the treatment effects in clinic experiment are not satisfactory enough.

   Since the beginning of 1980s, the rapid development of cell biology, molecular biology and biological engineering technology has brought about new opportunities for cancer immunological therapy. The theory of biological response modifier (BRM) renews the recognition of traditional tumor immunological therapy and establishes the fourth tumor treatment formula beyond operation, radioactive therapy and chemical therapy, i.e. biological treatment of tumor. The establishment of BRM theory provides theoretical basis for biological treatment of cancer, and the development and utilization of biological engineering technology makes possible the clinic application of biological treatment of tumor. The use of cell engineering technology can produce large quantities of cell toxicant active cells such as macrophages, cell toxicant T lymphocyte, killer cell capable of naturally killing cells and lymphokine activation, as well as hybridoma cell excreting monoclone antibody. Genetic engineering technology can produce tens of cytokines for BRM such as interleukin, interferon, tumor necrosis factor, immunoglobulin factor and colony stimulating factor in large quantity.

   The progress of the above biological technologies and deep understanding of cellular immunity provides opportunities for humans to develop immunological treatment of malignant tumor. For one thing, adoptive immunity therapy transfers cell toxicant active lymphocyte with anti-tumor activity to tumor host. For another, combination of TIL, LAK/IL-2 and IFN/IL-2 may lead to the development of new therapies effective to human malignant tumor.

2. Inducement and differentiation therapy: Inducement and differentiation therapy for tumor is a new area of tumor therapeutics. The therapy is different from traditional chemical therapy and radiotherapy. The difference does not lie in that it does not kill tumor cells, but that it induces the tumor cells to differentiate towards mature phase under the effect of differentiated inducement agent, recover the normal or approximately normal representation and functions of the cell. Since the active mechanism of differentiated inducement is different from radiotherapy and chemical therapy, the experimental research

of differentiated inducement focuses on research on proliferation and differentiated inducement. Clinic application is divided into inducement and differentiation therapy of tumor and inducement and extinction therapy of tumor. Inducement and differentiation therapy adopts the following inducement and differentiation agents: vitamin D3, phorbol, cytokine, ATRA, inducement and extinction is $A_{s2}O_{3.}$ In 1986, Ruijin Hospital of Shanghai Second Medical University first applied ATRA inducement and differentiation therapy to APL, obtaining a high remission rate. In 1992, Harbin Medical University used $A_{s2}O_3$ "173" traditional Chinese medicine solution to treat APL, obtaining a very high remission rate. Later on, through further research, it was found that using ATRA and $A_{s2}O_3$ to treat APL offered successful examples for tumor treatment by inducement and differentiation and extinction.

3. Biological therapy: One of the major achievements in life science and medical science in 1980s is the rapid emergence of a new study—"biological therapy" or "bioregulator therapy" based on the development of medical molecular biology, molecular immunity, oncology and cytokine. Modern biological therapeutics is deep and broad in research content and scope. The basic characteristics of scientifically grounded modern biological therapeutics are: the preparations used in biological therapy are "self substances" in the organism, its radical differences from radiotherapy and chemical therapy lie in: it has no progressive damage on normal tissues and cells of the organism, especially immune structure and function, but has regulatory and enhancing effect. As is known, radiotherapy and chemical therapy are different in this aspect. As a non-selective "damage therapy", it injures normal histiocyte of the organism while damaging cancer tissue, and tend to cause serous consequences due to serious damage on marrow hematopiesis system and immune structure and function.

   The research on anti-cancer biological therapy focuses on basic theories and clinic application technologies of biological therapies such as "anticancer cell therapy", i.e. anticancer cell system (NK cell group, K cell group, TK cell group, LAK cell group, macrophage, etc); "anticancer cytokine therapy", i.e. anticancer cytokine system (IFN, IL-2, TNF, etc); "anticancer gene therapy", i.e. anticancer gene system (R_b gene, P_{53} gene, other genes, etc), and anticancer antibody.

4. New tumor vaccine research and development and gene therapy in recent years offers more promising prospect

More efforts will be undoubtedly made to develop more reasonable and effective comprehensive therapies for tumor treatment in the future. Biological therapy will plays a more vital role in treatment with development of the times. With the change of traditional ideas, tumor therapy will leap forward in quality.

(1) Biological response modifier will be applied more widely, so will immunological control therapy.
(2) Cell differentiation and inducement agent open a new path for tumor treatment.
(3) Gene therapy will have broad prospect.
(4) Blood vessel growth inhibitor will be applied.
(5) Comprehensive therapy will become the direction of tumor treatment.

With the rapid development of biological technology in medical field, coupled with further understanding of tumor pathogenesis on cellular element level, tumor treatment has entered a new era, shifting from the ear of cell toxicant treatment to the era of targeting treatment. The so called "targeting treatment" means that drugs are aimed at the intended target, without injuring other normal cells, tissues or organs. Targeting treatment is classified into three types: first, aiming at a particular organ, for example, some drug is only effective to the tumor in a particular organ, which is called organ targeting; second, cell targeting, which refers to exclusively aiming at the tumor cells of a particular type; third, molecule targeting, which means aiming at some part of a particular protein family in tumor cells, or segments of a nucleotide or a gene product for treatment.

In light of the overall strategy, tumor treatment is designed to eliminate the tumor cells below a particular order of magnitude by various methods (it is reported that this order of magnitude is 10^6 for mice, $3.5x10^9$ for human cells, approximately equivalent to globular node with the diameter of 1.5cm), re-motivate, reactivate and recover immunological functions of human body itself under the condition, fulfilling the purpose of long-term peaceful coexistence with tumor, which is the tumor treatment in the 21st century.

CHAPTER 2

Thymic Aplasia and Inferior Immunologic Function: One of the Possible Pathogenic Factors of Cancer

[**Abstract**]
Objectives: Probe into the pathogenic factors and pathophysiology of cancer.
Method: Firstly we probe into the relation between thymus removal and inferior immunologic function and the establishment of cancer-bearing animal models so as to make the experimental study on cancer-bearing animal models.
Results: The cancer-bearing animal model can be established after removal of the thymus of the mouse and it is helpful to establish the cancer-bearing animal model through injection of immunosuppressant.
Conclusions: The occurrence and development of cancer has obviously affirmative relation with the thymus of the immune organ of the host and its functions.
Keywords: thymic aplasia, immunologic function, cancer-bearing animal model

This lab has made a series of experimental study on animal to probe into the pathogenic factors and pathophysiology of cancer. Through analyzing and reflecting the results of experimental study, we obtain new findings, new thinking and new enlightenments: one of the pathogenic factors may be thymus atrophy, damaged thymus function and inferior immunologic function. Therefore, Professor Xu Ze initiated that one of the pathogenic factors may be thymus atrophy, damaged function of central immune organ, inferior immunologic function, inferior immunological surveillance and immunologic escape. However, what causes the thymus atrophy of the host? Through repeated consideration and inference, the author holds that maybe the solid tumor produces one factor to inhibit the thymus, which shall be further studied by experiment and is called cancer-based thymus-inhibiting factor temporarily by us.

I. Experimental study to probe into pathogenic factors and physiopathology of cancer

This lab has made a series of experimental study on animal to probe into the pathogenic factors and pathophysiology of cancer. Firstly, we made intravital specimen of aseptic tumor into homogenate unicell suspending liquid and tried to transplant it on the experimental animal, but we failed time and again. Subsequently, we ablated the thymus of the mouse and then we succeeded in the transplantation. Some mouse was injected with cortisone to reduce the immunity of the mouse, in this way, the transplantation was successful. The method of thymus removal: take one Kunming white rat aged 8-10 weeks, 21±2g, no matter it is female or male, incise the skin at the breast, cut off 2nd, 3rd and 4th rib, separate them slightly to expose the thymus to quickly remove it and then close the chest cavity rapidly. Then we raised the rat and made the formal experiment after 2 weeks and established the cancer-bearing animal model. Establishment of cancer-bearing animal model: take the fresh tumor from the tumor-bearing rat to make the unicell suspending liquid, after dyeing the cancer cells with lichenin and counting (1x10^6/ml), make the hypodermic inoculation at the left side of each rat with 0.2ml physiological saline for cancer cells.

Observation index: weigh the rat every 3 days and measure the diameter of the tumor with vernier caliper, measure the immunologic function and determine the blood picture. Finally, after removal of the thymus of 30 rats, the inoculation was successful.

Through transplantation in 5th days after thymus removal, the node as large as a soybean came out after 5-6 days and the tumor as large as a finger came out after 10-21 days, the transplanted cancer could survive for 3-4 weeks, however, the passage failed.

Experimental study to probe into the pathogenic factors and physiopathology—new findings

This lab has the following findings from the experimental tumor study:

Experiment 1: this lab excises the thymus (TH) of 30 mice and establishes the cancer-bearing animal model. It is helpful to establish the cancer-bearing animal model through injecting the depressant. It is proven by the study conclusions: the occurrence and development of the cancer has remarkably affirmative relation with the thymus of the immune organ of the host and its functions.

Experiment 2: Does the inferior immune lead to the cancer or the cancer lead to the inferior immune at all? Our experimental results: the inferior immune leads to the occurrence and development of the cancer, without the descent of immunologic function, it is not easy to realize the successful inoculation. It is suggested by the experimental results: improving and maintaining the good immunologic function and protecting the good thymus of the central immune organ are the important measures for preventing the occurrence of cancer.

Experiment 3: in studying the relation between the metastasis of cancer and the immune, this lab establishes 60 animal models for liver metastatic carcinoma, which are divided into two groups including Group A applied with immune depressant and Group B not applied with immune depressant. Results: the metastatic lesions in the liver in Group A are obviously more than the ones in Group B. It is suggested by the experimental results: metastasis is related to the immune and inferior immunologic function or application of immune depressant may promote the tumor metastasis.

Experiment 4: When making experiments to probe into the effects of tumor on immune organ, this lab finds that the thymus meets with progressive atrophy with the advance of the cancer (600 cancer-bearing animal model mice). The thymus of the host meets with the acute progressive atrophy after the cancer cells are inoculated, the cell proliferation is prevented and the volume is obviously shrunk. It is suggested by the experimental results: the tumor may inhibit the thymus, resulting in the atrophy of the immune organ.

Experiment 5: we also find through experiment that if some experimental mice are not successfully inoculated or the tumor is very small, the thymus is not obviously shrunk. In order to understand the relation between the tumor and the atrophy of the thymus, we excise the transplanted solid tumor of one group of mice when it grows up to the size of a thumb. After one month, through anatomy, we find the thymus does not meet with progressive atrophy again. Therefore, it is inferred by us that maybe the solid tumor produces one kind of unknown factor to inhibit the thymus, which shall be further studied through experiment.

Experiment 6: it is proven by the above-mentioned experimental results: the advance of the tumor makes the thymus meet with progressive atrophy, then, can we take some measures to prevent the atrophy of the thymus of the host? Therefore, we further perfect the design to seek for the method or drug to prevent the atrophy of the thymus of the cancer-bearing mice through the experimental study on animal. So we make the experimental study to recover the function of the immune organ through cell transplantation of the immune organ. We discuss the atrophy of the thymus of the immune organ in preventing the advance of tumor, seek for the method to recover the functions of the thymus and reconstruct the immune, carry out the cell transplantation of foetal liver, spleen and thymus with the mice and establish the immunologic function through adoptive immunity. It is shown by the results: through the joint transplantation of three groups of cells, namely S, T and L (200 experimental mice), the entire extinction rate of the tumor in the long term is 46.67% and the one with the entire extinction of the tumor get a long survival life.

Experiment 7: in the experiment to probe into the effects of tumor on the immune organ such as spleen, we find: the spleen can inhibit the growth of the tumor in the early stage of the tumor, however, in the late stage, the spleen meets with the progressive atrophy. It is suggested by the study results: the effects of spleen on the growth of the tumor are embodied into bi-direction, in the early stage, it can inhibit the tumor to a certain extent, however, in the late stage, it fails to inhibit the tumor. The cell transplantation of the spleen can enhance the role of inhibiting the tumor.

Experiment 8: it is suggested by the results of the follow-up survey: control over the metastasis is the key to cancer treatment. Now it is well known that the cancer cell metastasis has multiple steps and links. In order to try to interrupt one link so as to prevent the metastasis, we consider the formation of the regenerative blood vessel of tumor is one of the links in which the metastatic cancer cells can nidate, root and grow into the cancer node or not. In 1986, this lab was making the microcirculation study and we observed the formation of the blood capillary of transplanted tumor node of cancer-bearing mice and its flow rate and flow with the micro-circle microscope; then we tried to seek for the drugs for prevention of the formation of the tumor blood vessel from the natural herbs, observed the formation process of the regenerative blood vessel with Olympus micro-circle microscope photograph system and counted the flow rate and flow of the arteriole and venule, found Common Threewingnut Root acetic ether extract (TG) from the traditional Chinese herbs and carried out the blood vessel inhibition test. It was found from the results: in the first day of inoculation there was no regenerative blood vessel and in the second day it was found that the fine micro regenerative blood vessel grew up. TG can reduce the density of the regenerative blood capillary of the tumor.

Experiment 9: we also found from a large batch of tumor-bearing animal models in the lab that the more the hypodermically inoculated solid tumor of some cancer-bearing experimental mice, the more different the cancer cells of the central tissue of the transplanted solid tumor from the peripheral cancer cells. The center of the node is mostly aseptically necrosed or liquefied its periphery is still surrounded with active cancer cells. Therefore, in the clinical treatment, we adopted the measures to treat the aseptic necroses.

II. Probing into the method of progressive atrophy of thymus of central immune organ and reconstructing the immune in preventing the advance of tumor

From the above-mentioned experimental study, it is analyzed and held by us that one of the pathogenic factors and the physiopathology may be the thymus atrophy, blocked proliferation of thymus cells, damaged thymus functions and inferior immunologic function, resulting in immunologic escape of the canceration cells.

The experimental results were very exciting. In those days, I considered to use it for clinical probation and attempted to extract the thymus from the dead fetus receiving the induction of labor with water bag to prepare the homogenate so as to try out the cell transplantation of homogeneous xenogenous thymus, however, which has not been allowed up to today, so it cannot be carried out. Then, what could we do to prevent the atrophy?

In 1986, I got enlightened from the discussion in the satellite meeting of one international micro-circulation academic conference to seek for the micro-circulation drug from the natural herbs and then transplanted the adoptive immune from the biological cells to reconstruct the immune and then sought for a kind of drug from the natural herbs of traditional Chinese herbs that can activate the cytokine, enhance the immunological surveillance, inhibit the tumor and prevent the atrophy of the thymus. All drugs must be subject to the animal experiment and clinical verification, as a result, we made the cancer-bearing animal model and made the in vivo tumor-inhibiting screening experiment on the cancer-bearing animal with over 200 kinds of natural traditional Chinese herbs one by one. Results: the anti-cancer immune-regulating TCM with relatively good tumor-inhibiting rate had been screened. From experimental screening to clinical observation and verification and then to further screening and concentration from the angle of immunopharmacology of TCM, we prepared XZ-C1-10 medicine, which can promote the thymus hyperplasia, prevent the thymus atrophy, improve the immune, protect the bone marrow and promote the function of lymphocyte T and cytokine, with relatively high tumor-inhibiting rate. XZ-C1-10 medicine only inhibits and kills the cancer cells, does not affect the normal cells and can be used for oral administration for a long time. Since cancer is a kind of chronic disease, the division, proliferation and clone of the cancer cells is a long, sustainable and progressive process, so it's better to select the orally administered traditional Chinese herbs with long-term curative effects, without toxin and with slow release. The treatment of cancer with traditional Chinese herbs is carried out after the pathogenic factors are judged on the human body. It shall kill the cancer cells as well as improve the immunologic functions of the organism as well so as to strengthen the anti-cancer capability of the organism, as a result, some refractory cancer with wide metastasis can be controlled, the life of the patient is prolonged, the pain of the patient is reduced, which opens up a new way to further probe into the treatment of the cancer.

In view that it was found by this lab from the experimental tumor that the thymus met with the progressive atrophy with the advance of tumor, then, what could we do to intervene and prevent its atrophy? Therefore, we improved the design further and tried to seek for the method or drug to prevent the thymus atrophy of the tumor-bearing mice through the animal experiment. Then we adopted the experimental study to recover the function of the immune organ through cell transplantation of the immune organ. We were probing into the method for preventing the thymus atrophy of the immune organ in advance of the tumor, recovering the function of the thymus and reconstructing the immune and making the experimental study on reconstruction of the immunologic function through homogeneous xenogenous cell transplantation of fetal liver, spleen and thymus and adoptive immune. Great achievements had been made: through joint transplantation of three groups of cells namely S, T and L, the extinction rate of the tumor in the near term was 40%, the entire extinction rate of tumor in the long term was 46.67% and the one with the entire extinction of the tumor got a long survival life.

In the past one century, there has been little fundamental study and experimental study on cancer, all of which targeted the cancer cell test to seek for the drugs to kill the cancer cells and were affected by the mode of killing the bacillus by the antibiotics and strived for killing the cancer cells. Despite great efforts, the death rate of cancer is still taking the first place. The classic tumor treatment mode concept is derived from the microbiology and the microbiology holds thoroughly kills off the bacillus of foreign infectious diseases in deed. The current principle of cancer therapy is to kill the cancer cells, in order to cure the cancer, it is necessary to kill off or eliminate the last cancer cells. Therefore, the expanded operation, intensified chemotherapy and radical radiotherapy have been adopted. However, the results are not ideal and they cannot improve the survival quality or prolong the survival time.

Since the hematopiesis function and the immunologic function of the bone marrow are severely inhibited, some complications endangering the life come out. Therefore, it is suggested that it is necessary to establish a new treatment mode, try to probe into and update the concept from other concepts and open up a new way.

On Dec. 12, 2009, upon invitation of Stehlin Tumor Research Institute in Houston in U.S.A, we paid a visit to it for academic exchange, which was established in 1969 and the president was an old professor aged 86 years. One of the main scientific research achievements of that institute was the invention of the Swiss depilous immune mouse firstly in the world, which was used for the cancer study and became the standard animal model for tumor study in U.S.A. At the beginning of 1970s, the scientists firstly implanted the tumor on the human body into the thymus-free mouse, Dr. Giovanella from that institute was among those scientists, resulting in great breakthrough by the research institute firstly. Thymus-free mouse is a relatively ideal experimental animal because its immune system is relatively weak and cannot resist the tumor.

The thymus-free nude mouse found by Stehlin Tumor Research Institute was the animal model of transplanted cancer and now has become the golden standard of the animal model in the world through the practice in animal experiments all over the world over scores of years.

The animal experiment room in this research institute, began to seek for the animal and method of cancer-bearing model in 1985. At that moment, I was the director of clinical surgery and the director of the animal lab of experimental surgery concurrently, so it was very convenient for work coordination. At that time, we thought so simply and we prepared the cancer specimen excised in the clinical operation room into the cancer block tissue homogenate (cell suspension) and then transplanted it into the rats swiftly within 30s, totally we transplanted it into 60 rats, but we failed entirely. Later, we firstly excised the thymus of Kunming white rat cultivated in pure line and then we carried out the transplantation and inoculation, we got a success.

Viewed from the results of Stehlin Lab in Houston in U.S.A and this lab in Wuhan, China, the key to successful transplantation experiment is no thymus, the animal without thymus or the one with thymus excised can be successfully transplanted, therefore, it is suggested that the thymus is key and it is the key regarding growth of the transplanted cancer cells or not.

The above-mentioned two points are the common understanding of both Stehlin and us, so we consider releasing the above-mentioned analysis conclusions. One of the pathogenic factors of cancer may be the thymus atrophy and inferior immunologic function, which become the theoretical basis or experimental basis of XZ-C immune regulation and control therapy (similar BRM).

Therefore, based on the enlightenment from the study results of a series of animal study regarding pathogenic factors and pathophysiology of the cancer by this lab, we put forward: thymus resection—immunologic deficiency—descent of immunological surveillance—immunologic escape may be one of the pathogenic factors of the cancer and one key of the pathogenesis. It is the new progress of tumor theory in 21st century, offering direction and basis to the cancer therapeutics in 21st century and offering theoretical basis and experimental basis of the immune regulation and control targeted therapy of the cancer. The new finding, enlightenment and thinking is the original innovation and it has not been mentioned in the textbooks and literatures at home and abroad.

One of the pathogenic factors mentioned above by us may be the thymus atrophy and the inferior immunologic function. In case that this new theory and hypothesis is argued and recognized, it will lead to a series of reform and innovation of cancer therapeutics, for example, the reform and innovation of the cognition of cancer therapeutic concept, the reform and innovation of cognition of cancer treatment objective or target; the one of cancer diagnostic procedure and curative effect judgment standard, the one of cancer treatment way and treatment mode and the one of research and development of anti-metastasis drug.

An Introduction to Author:

1. Xu Jie, Hospital Affiliated to Hubei University of Chinese Medicine, Department of Surgery of Hubei Hospital of Traditional Chinese Medicine
2. Xu Ze, Research Institute of Experimental Surgery of Hubei University of Chinese Medicine, xuze88cn@yahoo.com.cn

CHAPTER 3

XZ-C Therapeutics of Immunity Regulation and Control—Theoretical and Experimental Basis of Thymus Protection for Immunity Improvement and Bone Marrow Protection for Hematogenesis

I. Enlightenment from animal experiments by this lab

It is found by this lab that the cancer-bearing rats are confronted with the progressive atrophia and damage to the central immune organ, which shall be protected to protect the thymus so as to improve the immunity.

Based on the above-mentioned enlightenment from the results of experimental study on the pathogenic factor and pathogenesis of carcinomatosis by this lab, the new theory and new ways of XZ-C targeted therapeutics of immunity regulation and control initiated by Professor Xu Ze have the theoretical and experimental basis because the findings from the experimental study by this lab indicate that the cancer-bearing rats are confronted with progressive atrophia, damage to the central immune organ, descent of immunologic function and inferior immunological surveillance, so its curative principles shall be based on prevention of progressive athophia, promotion of thymus hyperplasia, improvement of immunity, protection of hematopiesis function of bone marrow, improvement of immunological surveillance and control over the immunologic escape of the canceration cells.

As is now well known, the immune organs include the central immune organs and peripheral immune organ, the former includes the thymus and the bone marrow and the latter includes the spleen and the lymph node. It is validated by the literature and the work in this lab that when the cancer comes, the tumor will produce a factor inhibiting the immune organ, which is temporarily called thymus-inhibiting factor by us and inhibits the thumus, causing the thymus to be progressively atrophic and inhibiting the functions of the central immune organ, in this way, the immunologic function descends and the immunological surveillance of the tumor is lost or weakened, resulting in the further progress of the tumor.

Therefore, the therapeutic theory of the curative principles of thymus protection for immunity improvement and bone marrow protection for hematogenesis initiated by us is reasonable and scientific and has the theoretical and experimental basis. The clinical verification and observation of over 12000 patients suffering from metaphase and advanced cancer in Shuguang Tumor Special Clinic over 16 years, has indicated that the curative principle of thymus protection for immunity improvement and bone marrow protection for hematogenesis initiated, clinically verified, observed by us over 16 years through clinical application is correct and reasonable and the curative effects are satisfying and worth of the patients' confidence.

XZ-C therapeutics of immunity regulation and control was initiated by Professor Xu Ze in 2006 in his monograph New Concept and New Way of Treatment of Cancer Metastasis. He holds that the cancer and the defense of the organism are in the dynamic balance in the normal conditions and the occurrence and development of the carcinomatosis is caused by the disturbance of the dynamic balance. If the disturbed state can be artificially regulated to the normal state, it can control the growth of cancer and subside the cancer.

As is now well known, occurrence, progress and development and treatment prognosis of the cancer are determined by the contrast of two factors: biological characteristics of the cancer cells and the inhibition and defensive capability of the host organism to the cancer cells, if both of them are in balance, the cancer can be controlled; otherwise, the cancer will advance.

Under the normal conditions, the host organism has a certain capability in inhibiting the cancer cells, however, the inhibition and defensive capabilities are suppressed and damaged to different extent, resulting in the loss of the immunological surveillance and the immunologic escape of the cancer cells, leading to development and metastasis of the cancer cells.

II. The human body has a complete set of anti-cancer immune system and it shall be protected, regulated and activated.

In probing into the curative principle of cancer, we should research which anti-cancer immunological cell line, which anti-cancer cell sub-line, which anti-cancer gene system and which humoral immunity system exists in the human body so as to strengthen the anti-cancerometastasis.

1. Which anti-cancer immunological cells in the human body may be activated and strengthened so as to realize the anti-cancerometastasis? The immunological cells engaged in anti-cancer in the human body include:

   (1) Cytotoxic lymphocyte (CTL): it plays a primary role in anti-tumor immunity, CTL in the human body includes CD_3 and CD_8, and CTL has a high content in peripheral blood and spleen and a certain content in thoracic duct, thymus and bone marrow. Under a certain condition, it can produce IL-2, IL-4 and IFN to activate other anti-cancer immunological cells and lethal macrophages, NK cells and lethal B cells to jointly exert the anti-tumor role.

   (2) Natural killer cell (NK cell) with the anti-tumor role: NK cells are a group of broad spectrum anti-cancer cells. They do not rely on the antibody or the thymus to kill the activity and their main role is to surveil and remove the canceration cells in the human body. It is found by the clinical observance that the ones with activity insufficiency of NK have obviously increased incidence rate of malignant tumor. NK cells are an important part in the organism with anti-cancer immunological surveillance function in the early stage.

   (3) LAK cells: LAK cells are the most important cancer cells in the modern biological therapeutics and peripheral mononuclear cells in the human body can remarkably kill so many kinds of tumor cells in the human body with the induction of IL-2. LAK cells have a wider anti-cancer spectrum than NK cells while LAK cells can kill the tumor cells that cannot be killed by NK cells.

   (4) Macrophage (MO): it plays an important role in anti-tumor immunity in the human body.

2. Which anti-cancer cytokine in the human body may be activated and strengthened so as to realize the anti-cancerometastasis? The anti-cancerometastasis cytokines engaged in anti-cancer in the human body include:
   (1) Interferon (IFN): it has the function of anti-cell differentiation and immunoloregulation. It plays a role in anti-proliferation of some tumor cells and its anti-cancer role may be related to the immunoloregulation. It can strengthen the activity of NK cells and MO.
   (2) Interleukin-2 (IL-2): this kind of lymphocyte is a kind of T-cell growth factor, with strong function of regulating intrinsic immunity. It can promote the activation of T-cells, NK cells and monocytes as well as the release of INF-a and TNF.
   (3) Tumor necrosis factor: its role in cell is the cell toxicant role and it can affect the micrangium of the tumor, resulting in the necrosis of the central portion of the tumor.

In recent years, with the rapid development of molecular biology, molecular immunology, molecular immunological pharmacology and gene engineering, the foundation of molecular level of "anti-cancer organ" and the clinical study are continuously expanded and deepened, its outlook of anti-cancerometastasis is very attracting.

At present, the study on immunotherapy of anti-cancer molecular biology is mainly centralized on "four sub-systems" of "anti-cancer organ", namely "anti-cancer cellular therapy", "anti-cancer cytokine therapy", "anti-cancer gene therapy" and "anti-cancer anti-body therapy".

The basic characteristics of these molecular biological and immunological therapies are as follows: all pharmaceutics of molecular biological and immunological therapies are the inherent substances in the organism and fundamental differences from radiotherapy and chemotherapy are: it has no progressive damage to the normal histiocytes of the organism, especially the cells and the functions of the immune system and the structure and the function of the hemopoietic system of the bone marrow and plays a role in regulation and reinforcement of immunological reaction. As is now well known, radiotherapy and chemotherapy are entirely different from it, the chemotherapy is a kind of non-selective traumatic therapy, killing the cancer cells as well as the normal cells at the same time, which damage the normal histiocytes of the organism, resulting in severe damage to the hemopoietic system and the immunological structure and function, with the severe consequence.

The biotherapy is a kind of therapy stabilizing and balancing the vital mechanism by means of the regulation on biologic reaction. The American scholar Oldham (1984) initiated biological regulation and mediation (BRM) theropy and then initiated the concept of tumor biotherapy based on the therapy.

III. Overview of Study on Similar BRM Anti-cancer Regulation and Control Medicine

Through study on animal experiments by us for 4 years and the clinical verification by the tumor special clinic over 16 years, it is indicated that XZ-C medicine has the roles and curative effects similar to BRM and it is screened from the traditional Chinese herb resources with role similar to BRM.

XZ-C medicine is screened from 200 kinds of traditional Chinese herbs through experiments by Professor Xu Ze (ZU ZE-China, Z-C) in the lab. Firstly, we adopt the culture in vitro of cancer cells and screen 200 kinds of traditional Chinese herbs in vitro one by one, observe the experimental study on the direct damage to the cancer cells in the culture tube by each drug and make the check experiment on tumor-inhibiting rate between the chemotherapy drug CTX and the control group of normal cells in the culture tube. Finally, we select a batch of herbs with a certain tumor-inhibiting rate of proliferation of cancer cells. Then we further establish the tumor-bearing animal model and carry out the experimental study on the 200 kinds of traditional Chinese herbs for the in vivo tumor-inhibiting rate of the tumor-bearing animal model and screen, analyze and evaluate the herbs scientifically, objectively and strictly one by one. It is proven by the results that only 48 kinds of herbs have relatively good tumor-inhibiting rate and another 152 kinds of traditional Chinese herbs are the traditional Chinese herbs commonly used by the herbalist doctors, through experimental screening of tumor-inhibiting rate in vivo by the tumor-bearing experiment, it is proven that they have no anti-cancer role or the tumor-inhibiting rate is very slight.

The screening by this lab is mainly the in vivo tumor-inhibiting experiment of the tumor-bearing animal model. The in vivo chronic experiment on every traditional Chinese herb is observed by one experimental group for 3 months, after screening, 48 kinds of traditional Chinese herbs are selected and then 2 and 3 kinds of dried medicinal herbs are arranged in groups to carry out the tumor-bearing experiments in vivo on the tumor-bearing animal and then it is found by us that the tumor-inhibiting effect of a single dried medicinal herb is not better than the one of the dried medicinal drug compound through tumor-inhibiting experiments. It seems that the single dried medicinal herb only play a role in inhibiting the proliferation of the tumor while the dried medicinal herb compound can inhibit the proliferation of the tumor-bearing rats and play a role in regulating and controlling the organism, enhancing the physical power, improving the immunity, promoting the generation of tumor-inhibiting cytokines, protecting the normal cells and promoting the anti-cancer cytokines as well.

Based on the screening of the single traditional herbs through the in vitro experiments and the tumor-inhibiting experiment screening on the tumor-bearing animal model over 4 years, through experimental optimization and combination and then experiment, this lab finally recombines Z-$C_{1\text{-}10}$ compound of anti-cancer, anti-metastasis and anti-reoccurrence through immunity regulation and control and finally it is subject to the clinical verification. Since 1992, we have established the cooperation group to carry out the clinical verification. Up to today from then on, through the clinical verification and observation of over 12000 patients suffering from the cancer in Shuguang Tumor Special Clinic over 16 years, the condition has been stable and improved, the symptom has been improved, the survival quality has been improved and the survival time has been obviously prolonged. So the lesions of many patients suffering from metastasis have been stabilized and have not further spread, as to some patients after operation cannot receive the chemotherapy due to the descent of leucocytes, the metastasis has been controlled after taking the medicine and no metastasis occurs again. Good curative effects have been obtained.

IV. Similar BRM Functions and Effects of XZ-C Medicine

Biological response modifier (BRM) is first put forward by Oldham in 1982 to describe BRM. It refers to the ability of regulating the organism's response or reply to surface "attack" by biological response modifier.

The cells and humoral factors of the organism's immunity system are under subtle control, the organism's ability of response or reply will be affected significantly in case of imbalance.

Biological response modifier is used to restore the unbalanced organism to normal balance, fulfilling the purpose of preventing diseases.

BRM opened the new field for biological treatment of tumor. At present, BRM is widely recognized in the medical circle as the fourth model of tumor treatment.

BRM is designed to regulate the immunologic function of the organism and restore the function of immune system of the contained organism. Such drug has manifold function mechanisms, but all of them exert regulating functions by activating the organism's immune system.

Biological response modifiers, most of which drive from microorganisms and plants, were previously referred to as immunopotentiator, immunostimulant, immunologic cordial or immunomodulator, now collectively named as biological response modulator or modifier(BRM).

The author screened out XZ-C medicine with good inhibition rate through in vivo experiment on mice inoculated with tumor. It has the functions of improving immunity, protecting centrum immune organ thymus, improve cellular immunity, protecting thymus tissue, protecting hematogenesis of bone marrow, increasing the number of akaryocyte and leukocyte, activate immunologic cytokine, the main pharmacological action of XZ-C improving the immunological surveillance in blood is protecting thymus and improving immunity. 48 types of immunologic drugs with high inhibition rate are screened out by four-year animal experiment, among which 26 types are identified through immune and cytokine level detection as capable of enhancing phagocytic function, or enhancing cellular immunity, or enhancing humoral immunity, or enhancing thymus weight, or promoting proliferation of bone marrow cells, or enhancing T cell function, or enhancing LAK cytoactive; or inhibiting blood platelet coagulation and resisting embolus; or resisting tumor poison and metastasis; or removing free radical. The anticancer mechanism of the above XZ-C medicine is:

1. Activating the organism's immunocyte system, promoting the enhancement of the host's defense mechanism and effect, achieving the capacity of immune response to cancer.
2. Activating immune cytokine system of anticancer mechanism of the organism, enhancing the host's immune defense mechanism and improving immunological surveillance of immunocyte of the organism's blood circulation system.
3. Protecting thymus and improving immunity, protecting bone marrow for hematogenesis, stimulating hematogenesis of bone marrow, promoting recovery of marrow inhibition, increasing leukocyte and akaryocyte.
4. Mitigating toxicant and side effects of chemotherapy and radiotherapy, enhancing the endurance of the host.
5. Cancer progress is caused by imbalance between biological characteristics of cancer cells and the organism's pharmaceutical capacity for cancer, XZ-C medicine is used to improve immunity and make them regain balance.
6. Regulating directly the growth and differentiation of tumor cells.
7. Increase the volume and weight of thymus, keeping thymus from progressive atrophy, for thymus will go through progressive atrophy when cancer evolves.
8. Stimulating the host's immune response to anticancer, enhancing the organism's anticancer ability, strengthening the sensitivity of cancer cells to the organism's anticancer mechanism, favorable for killing cancer cells on the way of metastasis.

XZ-C medicine can enable the host to make powerful immune response to cancer cells, achieving the purpose of treating cancer. XZ-C medicine can trigger the following immune responses of the host: enhancing regulation or restoring the host's immune response to tumors; stimulating inherent immunologic functions of the host, activating the host's immune defense system; restoring immunologic functions.

As described above, XZ-C medicine has similar function mechanism to BRM, can have the same treatment effects with BRM in clinic application.

V. Clinic Application and Applicable Scope of XZ-C Medicine

1. Application principles of XZ-C medicine

   XZ-C medicine with BRM and similar BRM function can enhance immune response of the organism and strengthen the tumor immunologic surveillance of the organism, producing good effects in the case of cell mutation or small tumor, the best effects when tumor is shrunk to the minimum through surgical operation or radiotherapy, or medication.

   Immunotherapy is effective to a certain degree for those losing the opportunity of operation, having too poor condition to endure chemotherapy and radiotherapy through mitigating symptoms and prolonging survival time.

   After radical resection of tumors, XZ-C medicine treatment is feasible to reduce recurrence and metastasis. After resection of large tumors by operation, XZ-C medicine treatment is also feasible to eliminate potential remaining cancer cells and cancer cells far away likely to spread.

   If tumor cannot be resected, radiotherapy or chemotherapy can be used to injure tumor cells in large quantity, and then XZ-C medicine is used for treatment after in vivo tumor load is reduced.

2. Clinic observation and applicable scope of XZ-C medicine

(1) Metastasis after anticancer operation: restore and improve immunity after operation, improve the life quality after operation, kill remaining cancer cells after operation, prevent metastasis, inhibit cancer cell proliferation, prevent recurrence, consolidate and enhance long-term effect. Applicable scope: ①after radical operations of cancer of metaphase and late stage;②after palliative excisions of cancer;③after operation of late cancer cannot be excided by exploratory operation; ④at the stage where only gastroenterostomy or colostomy can be done; ⑤late cancer cannot be excided and losing operation indication; ⑥after tumor excision + cannula drug pump operation.

(2) Improve the life quality of patients of late cancer in an all-around way, prolong the survival time, inhibit mitochysis of cancer cells, control proliferation of cancer cells, and enhance overall immunity, for the sake of resisting diffusion metastasis. Applicable scope: ①those subject to near-term or long-term metastasis, or recurrence after cancer operations; ②liver metastasis, lung metastasis, brain metastasis, or complicated by cancer pleural effusion or ascites.

(3) Relieve cancer pain: Z-C medicine to be taken orally or for external application is used to treat intractable pains of late cancer and soften and shrink metastasis tumor on body surface.

(4) Combine interventional therapy or cannula drug pump therapy, protect of liver, kidney, marrow hemopoietic system and thymus and other immune organs, enhance immunity, improve overall immune condition after medicine injection treatment, maintain, consolidate and enhance the effects of interval of medicine injection and long term, prevent metastasis, diffusion and recurrence, improve and enhance the survival quality of liver cancer patients after interventional or cannula treatment, prolong survival time.

(5) Combine radiotherapy and chemotherapy to mitigate toxicant and side effects, enhance treatment effects, protect liver, kidney, marrow hemopoietic system and immune system, enhance immunologic function and increase leukocyte.

(6) Combine XZ-C medicine and decoction of herbal medicine: for example, combine anticancer decoction for clearing liver and eliminate liver edema to treat liver cancer complicated by ascites or metastasis cancer ascites in abdominal cavity; combine with jaundice curing decoction to treat liver cancer complicated by jaundice; combine with decoction for reducing enzyme and transferring negative to treat liver cancer complicated by high aminopherase and positive HBsAg.

3. The occasion of applying XZ-C medicine

Most cancer patients have poor immunologic function and should be treated immediately after being diagnosed. Three major therapies, i.e. operation, chemotherapy and radiotherapy may further reduce the patients' immunologic function, reducing the patients' endurance to operation or chemotherapy and radiotherapy, and reducing immunological surveillance in immune cell system in the patients' body. Hence, immunotherapy should be started in the period of operation or radiotherapy and chemotherapy. XZ-C medicines are all taken orally, and the patients can take XZ-C medicine only if they can eat. They are generally taken 1-2 weeks after operation. Taking XZ-C medicine before radiotherapy and chemotherapy, at the interval of period of radiotherapy and chemotherapy and upon completion of radiotherapy and chemotherapy may help reduce or control recurrence and metastasis. It helps mitigate toxicant and side effects of chemotherapy and radiotherapy, prevent chemotherapy from causing poor immunologic function and enhance immunity, promote marrow hematogenesis function and protect marrow for hematogenesis, activate the organism's immunocyte system and immune cytokine system, improve immunological surveillance, help prevent recurrence and metastasis.

CHAPTER 4

Principles and Characteristics of Xu Ze's New Concept of Cancer Treatment

It has been seen from the clinical medical practice in about 100 years that the three traditional therapeutics including operation, radiotherapy and chemotherapy have made relatively good curative effects in treating the malignant tumor and so many patients have obtained CR/PR curative effects throaty radiotherapy and chemotherapy and the tumor has been obviously shrunk. However, it is a pity that the tumor meets with reoccurrence, enlargement and metastasis later. Although radiotherapy or chemotherapy is made again, the curative effects on most patients are extremely bad and they die of metastasis and reoccurrence.

In 1985, the author carried out the follow-up survey over more than 3000 patients after operation on cancer in general surgery and chest surgery, finding that most of the patients met with reoccurrence and metastasis in 2-3 years, some patients event met with reoccurrence in several months after operation. That's to say, the operation was successful, however, the long-term curative effects were failing. As a result, the author deeply understands that the anti-cancerometastasis is the key to overcome the cancer at present.

The author summarizes the experience and lessons positive and negative from the clinical practice cases over 54 years, forms the following new understanding, puts forward the new theoretical concept and launches the new therapeutic strategies through combining the long-term experimental study with the clinical practice.

I. Anti-cancerometastasis, the key to overcome the cancer

Anti-cancerometastasis, is the key to overcome the cancer because the metastasis is the first cause of the death caused by cancer.

If the cancer does not meet with metastasis, the patient will not die to a great extent, the metastasis is the cause of the death and anti-metastasis is the core to overcome the cancer.

In the past one century from 20th century, the goal of tackling the key problem is to kill the cancer cells aiming at the primary carcinoma lesion and metastatic carcinoma lesion. Although the efforts have been made for a century, the cancer mortality has been always taking the first place. The main reason why the mortality is so high is the metastasis. Obviously, the previous traditional therapeutics cannot reduce the stubbornly high mortality. The first cause of its failure is that the goal cannot target the metastasis and control the metastasis.

At the beginning of 21st century, the uppermost problem of cancer treatment is still how to prevent the metastasis. In case that the metastasis after radical operation of cancer cannot be successfully prevented, the cancer treatment cannot get a great-leap-forward development.

Now we deeply realize that the key problem to be tackled is to prevent the metastasis at present. The core of cancer treatment is to prevent the metastasis.

Therefore, one of the goals of cancer treatment in 21st century is anti-metastasis.

The above-mentioned problems impel us to update the thoughts and change the ideas to open a new road to find the new therapeutics for preventing metastasis and overcome the cancer while improving the curative effects of the traditional therapeutics as per the traditional ideas. Therefore, we raise: analyzing and understanding the immune state of the host and the multiple steps and links of cancerometastasis based on the biological characteristics of the cancer and the biological behaviors of the cancerometastasis to find a new treatment mode for anti-cancerometastasis.

Viewed from the above-mentioned, the necessity of establishing Anti-cancerometastasis and Reoccurrence Institute by us can be illuminated.

The academician of Liver Cancer Research Institute of Fudan University, Tang Zhaoxian, raised in *On Clinical Research on Carcerometastasis* on Nov. 9, 2007: "if the cancerometastasis is not studied, the improvement of curative effects is a soap bubble".

Great attention has been paid to the tumor metastasis since 1990s in the world. Metastasis Research Society was established, Clinical and Experimental Metastasis was issued. Cancerometastasis Research Society was established in Tokyo, Japan.

The study on metastasis in China starts relatively late, Professor Gao Jin published *Cancer Invasion and Metastasis—Fundamental Research and Clinic* based on a large quantity of rich experimental data in 1996, which was the first monograph on cancerometastasis and was excellent in both the pictures and their accompanying essay. In 2003, the academician Tang Zhaoxian published his monograph Foundation and Clinic of Metastasis and Reoccurrence of Liver Cancer and he raised in the monograph: "the next important goal of study on primary liver cancer is to prevent and control reoccurrence and metastasis", in addition, he said: "metastasis and reoccurrence have become one bottle-neck of further improving the survival rate of liver cancer and one of the most important difficulties in overcoming the cancer". These monoprahies accelerate the attention to and study on the metastasis by the scholars in China. In 2006, Professor Xu Ze published New Concept and New Way of Treatment of Cancer Metastasis and put forward some theoretical innovations, which was granted with "Three-One-Hundred Original Book" by General Administration of Press and Publication of the People's Republic of China.

(I) Reflection on traditional therapeutics: why it cannot prevent reoccurrence and metastasis of cancer cells?

In virtue of the experimental observation on the tumor-bearing animal in the lab for 7 years, the clinical case history of over 12000 cases in the tumor special clinic and the follow-up survey over 16 years, we have analyzed and evaluated these valuable experimental clinical data, summed up the experience and lessons from the success and the failure and thought why the traditional therapeutics cannot reduce the death rate remarkably and control reoccurrence and metastasis? And thought what's matter with the traditional therapeutics concerning the recognition and concept?

It is held by the author that the traditional therapeutics of cancer has the following weak links:

(1) The traditional therapeutics inhibits the immunologic function and inhibits the hematopiesis function of the bone marrow.

(2) Traditional intravenous chemotherapy is the interrupted therapy, in this way, the therapy cannot be carried out in the intermission while the cancer cells are continuously proliferated and divided in the intermission;

(3) The traditional therapeutics damages the host because the chemotherapy cells have no selectivity, so it is actually a two-edged sword, killing not only the cancer cells but also the normal cells, especially the immunological cells of the bone marrow.

(4) The traditional therapeutics damages the central immune organ. When cancer comes, the thymus is inhibited, meanwhile, the chemotherapy inhibits the bone marrow, in this way, one disaster after another, the whole central immune organ is damaged and cannot be effectively protected.

(5) The goal of the traditional therapeutics only pays attention to killing the cancer cells by the chemotherapy while ignores the resistance and restriction of the host itself to the cancer. In facts, the occurrence and development of the tumor depends on the immunologic function of the host and the biological characteristics of the tumor itself, namely the balance between the biological characteristics of the tumor cells and the effects of the host on the restriction factors, if both of them are balanced, it can be controlled; otherwise, it will make progress. The traditional chemotherapy makes the immunologic function drop down and makes the cancer cell free from the immunological surveillance and control, resulting in metastasis while chemotherapy and more metastasis while more chemotherapy.

(6) The traditional therapeutics ignores the anti-cancer capability of the human body itself and the roles of anti-cancer cell cluster of the anti-cancer system in the host body (NK cell cluster, LAK cell cluster, macrophage cluster and TK cell cluster) and anti-cancer cytokine system IFN, IL-2 and TNF; ignores the roles of cancer-inhibiting gene and cancerometastasis-inhibiting gene in the host body (the cancer gene and the cancer-inhibiting gene exist in the human body, the same to the cancerometastasis gene and cancerometastasis-inhibiting gene) and ignores the roles of nervous body fluid system in the host body and the incretion; all of these organs and their affectois play an important role in regulation, balance and stabilization, so we shall try to protect and activate these intrinsic anti-cancer factors in the human body.

(7) The goal of the traditional therapeutics is relatively unsophisticated, just to kill the cancer cells, which does not conform to the biological characteristics known at present, such as adhesion, invasion and movement of the cancer cells and the activity of hydrolytic enzyme as well as the actual conditions of the biological behaviors such as metastasis links and multi-step, molecular immune mechanism and angiogenesis factors and so on.

The above-mentioned existing problems impel us to make the further study and update thoughts and ideas and make progress in reform and be brave in innovation while in continuously improving the traditional therapeutics according to the traditional ideas. Innovation must challenge the traditional idea, it is not to replace the traditional idea but to overcome its disadvantages and correct its shortages to make it more perfect. Innovation shall open a new road to find the new way to overcome the cancer. Therefore, it is suggested by the author: analyzing and understanding the immune state of the host and the multiple steps and multiple links of cancerometastasis as well as the molecular metastasis mechanism based to the biological characteristics of the cancer and the biological behaviors of the cancerometastasis to put forward the new mode of anti-cancerometastasis treatment.

(II) Formation and characteristics of Xu Ze's new concept of cancer treatment

Based on the reflection on the traditional therapy, we have cognizance that the cancer is based on data transmission and mediation and control, although canceration is a gradually progressive process, it is potential to realize reversion. The last step of cancer treatment is to mobilize the host to recover the mediation and control role instead of killing off the final cancer cells. In this way, Xu Ze's new concept of cancer treatment was formed. This concept mode refers to the experience and phenomena of the clinical lab and the epidemiology as well as the modern molecular biology and traditional concept. Viewed from the new therapeutic concept, the mechanism that the cancer is cured through mediation and control may be illuminated.

The differences between the cancer cells and the normal cells are not always so great.

Through the clinical observation over one century and the analysis over 10 years, to our surprise, it is clearly found that the tumor is limited in autonomy and the cancerization course can be reversed. Previously, we tried out best to treat the cancer by killing off the cancer cells, however, we did not make great achievements. When it looks as if the condition is under control, the new canceration may meet with reoccurrence and metastasis.

Since 1970s, in view of the high reoccurrence and metastasis rate of the cancer after operation, in order to control the reoccurrence after operation, the assistant chemotherapy after operation has been adopted, even the chemotherapy before operation (for example, on breast cancer) has been made, however, the results have not been so satisfactory and the assistant chemotherapy after operation on the patients cannot prevent the reoccurrence and metastasis. As to some cases, the chemotherapy is intensified, resulting in adynamia of immunologic function. All these issued shall be seriously and calmly thought, reviewed, analyzed and reflected by the clinicians so as to find how to prevent the reoccurrence and metastasis to treat the cancer.

In the recent 20 years, the understanding of the molecular metastasis mechanism of cancer has made great progress, however, there have been no actually effective measures for preventing the metastasis of the cancer cells at home and abroad. Although some new anti-cancer drugs have come out in recent years, the curative effects cannot be improved to our satisfaction. The reason why some cancer cells cannot be radically cured by the exploration in the middle and late stage is that the lymph node meets with the remote metastasis. It is important and key to inhibit the cancerometastasis so as to reduce the death rate of cancer and improve the curative effects.

The goal of tackling the key problem is relatively simple, just to kill the cancer cells, which does not entirely conform to the actual condition of the biological characteristics of the cancer at present, for example, the invasion behaviors of the cancer cells, metastasis link and multi-step, molecular biological mechanism of metastasis, immunoreactivity of the organism and inducement of reoccurrence and reoccurrence after incubation for several months even several years. Now it is known by the people at present that the anti-cancer drug does not always prevent the metastasis or kill the cancer cells.

Therefore, it is held by the author that now it is key to prevent the metastasis so as to overcome the cancer and it is core to study how to prevent the metastasis so as to cure the cancer.

Main characteristics of Xu Ze's cancer therapeutics: control over metastasis, protection of immunity of the patient instead of simply killing the cancer cells.

II. Principle of Treatment of Cancer

At present, the principle of treatment of cancer is based on the following precondition: it is necessary to kill or eliminate the last cancer cells so as to cure the cancer. As a result, the expanded operation, intensified chemotherapy and radical radiotherapy are adopted by the people. However, the results are not so ideal. At the beginning of 1960s, the scope of operation of tumor surgery tended expansion and a series of super-radical operations were developed. Later, it had been proven by the practice for years that the expansion of the scope of surgical removal (such as breast cancer, lung cancer, liver cancer and cancer of pancreas) had not improved the survival quality or prolonged the survival time. In 1980s, the patients receiving intensified chemotherapy or radical radiotherapy did not get an improved survival quality or prolonged survival time. The hematopiesis function and the immunologic function of the bone marrow are seriously inhibited, resulting in some complications endangering the lives. Therefore, many therapists deem necessary to establish a new mode and principle to probe the prevention of metastasis and update the idea and open up a new way from other ideas.

(I) Principle of traditional treatment of cancer

The principle of treatment of the traditional chemotherapy drug killing off the cancer cells is derived from the microbiology. Its principle holds: when the human body is infected with bacteria, the antibiotics shall be used to kill the source bacteria; accordingly, if the human body suffers from the cancer, the chemotherapy drug shall be used to kill off the cancer cells. Penicillin was found in 1929 by Fleming and streptomycin was found in 1944. The clinical application of antibiotics plays an important role in controlling or eliminating a lot of infectious diseases. Indeed, microbiology claims to thoroughly eliminate the foreign disease disseminators. When the human body suffers from the seriously infectious disease, such as lobar pneumonia and acute tonsillitis, it is necessary to kill off the bacteria with antibiotic for treatment, in case of insufficient curative effects, the antibiotic sensitive to the pathogenic bacteria will be selected and the dosage will be increased or the drug combination shall be adopted to eliminate the pathogenesis bacteria thoroughly. However, the infection is quite another thing to the tumor and the latter comes from the host body. When curative effects of radiotherapy and chemotherapy are not so good, it is impossible to increase the dosage just because the anti-cancer cytotoxic drug differs from the antibiotics:

(1) The antibiotics only selectively kills the bacteria instead of the cells while the cytotoxic drug for chemotherapy has no selectivity and it kills the cancer cells as well as the normal cells, especially, it easily kills the immunological cell, inhibits the hematopiesis function and immunologic function of the bone marrow and has the side effects on liver and kidney. In case that the dosage is increased, the serious side effects will come, as a result, the host cannot stand it.

(2) Before application of antibiotics, the drug sensitivity test can be made to select the sensitive antibiotics, meanwhile, as to the anti-cancer drug for chemotherapy, generally the drug sensitivity test or the drug resistance cannot be made and it is used by experience, in this way, it has a certain blindness.

In a word, the principle and goal of traditional treatment is to kill the cancer cells and the method adopted by them is to kill the cancer cells with radioactive rays and their common disadvantage is that they have no selectivity, killing the cancer cells as well as the normal cells of the host, especially the hematopoietic cells and the immunological cell of the bone marrow. However, the radiotherapy is of local treatment, so the scope of the normal cells of the host damaged by it is relatively small while the chemotherapy is of systemic treatment and it damages the normal cells of the host in the whole body, in this way, the side effects are serious and the patient suffers from the serious damage. If the chemotherapy drug applied is not sensitive to the cancer cells of the patient or has drug resistance, it kills off the normal cells, especially the immunological cells of the cancer patient rather than the cancer cells. As a result, it will aggravate the patient's condition instead of playing a role in treatment.

In addition, in chemotherapy, especially in the assistant chemotherapy after radical operation on cancer, no one knows whether the cancer cells exist in the body of the patient, how many cancer cells exist in the body of the patient and where they are in the body at all. After one or more treatment courses of chemotherapy, no one knows whether the cancer cells and how many cancer cells are killed off, so the curative effects cannot be judged.

(II) Basic principle of Xu Ze's new concept of cancer treatment

1. Design the therapeutic scheme and research on the medical specialty aiming at the biological characteristics of the cancer cells That is to say, to inhibit their division and proliferation. It is not always necessary to kill off the cancer cells to inhibit the division and proliferation of the cells. As to the cancer cells in the early stage, its division and proliferation can be inhibited and the differentiation and reversion can be induced; as to the ones in the advanced stage, we should try to accelerate their apoptosis. It is certainly good to selectively kill off the cancer cells; in case of no selectivity, the drug shall be administered carefully so as to protect the patient from damage in treatment. **We should research the intelligent anti-cancer drugs with selectivity**, which only have effects on the special molecule in the cancer cells and do not damage the normal cells of the host. **The medication of cancer shall be people-oriented and it is necessary to study how to change the chemical anti-cancer drug with very great side effects to the intelligent anti-cancer drugs with very small side effects. The intelligent anti-cancer cells shall have very definite target, only killing the cancer cells instead of the normal cells. XZ-C Medicine independently researched and developed by us only kills the cancer cells instead of the normal cells.**
2. The unique behaviors of invasion and metastasis aiming at the biological behaviors of the cancer cells Metastasis is a malignant behavior. It is well known that the fundamental difference between the benign tumor and the malignant tumor is that the former meets with metastasis while the latter does not meet with the metastasis. If we can take measures to prevent the metastasis of the cancer cells, is the malignant tumor becoming the benign tumor? 85%~95% of the patients die of the metastasis of the cancer. In case of no metastasis, most of the patients will not die. In case that the metastasis does not happen or it is controlled, the cancer is not so terrible. Therefore, the principle of treatment of cancer is to prevent the metastasis, design the therapeutic scheme and intervention scheme of anti-metastasis, research and develop the anti-metastasis drug, try to obstruct and intercept

the cancer cells in metastasis and cut off or block one or more links of metastasis so as to control the metastasis.

(III) Three goals of treatment of cancer

Based on the review, reflection, analysis and evaluation of the clinical cases about cancer treatment, according to the experience and lessons of success and failure of cancer treatment, it is held by the author that the goal of cancer treatment is to **eliminate the tumor, protect the organism and regain health**. Therefore, the specific therapeutic goals include the following three aspects.

1. Effectively inhibit the division and proliferation of the cancer and selectively kill off the cancer cells. **We should research and develop the intelligent anti-cancer drug**. At present, the cytotoxicity of the chemotherapy drug is large and it has no selectivity, killing the cancer cells as well as the normal cells of the host, especially the hematopoietic cells and the immunological cells of the bone marrow, damaging the organism and doing harm to the patients. The scientists and the pharmacologists shall make efforts to research the drugs and try to find the intelligent anti-cancer drugs. At American Tumor Annual Meeting held in New Orleans in U.S.A on Mar. 26, 2004, the experts advocated to research and develop the intelligent anti-cancer drugs. **What is the intelligent anti-cancer drug? The intelligent anti-cancer drug only affects the special molecules in the cancer cells and it is the new drug only killing the cancer cells but not damaging the normal cells, with very small side effects and very strong target to the cancer cells.**
2. How to prevent metastasis. The biological characteristics and behaviors of the cancer cells are invasion and metastasis. The reason why the cancer is malignant is mainly the wide harm of invasion and metastasis to the human body. Over a century, the goals of the three traditional therapies have been always aiming at the primary lesion cancer and metastatic carcinoma lesion and ablating the primary carcinoma lesion by operation or treat the metastatic carcinoma lesion with radiotherapy and other local treatment. It is commonly held that the primary carcinoma lesion and the metastatic carcinoma lesion can be seen or touched and they are local, so they can be treated with operation or radiotherapy. Reviewing and reflecting the clinical practice for 54 years, I had made so many radical operation on chest and abdomen based on the above-mentioned understanding, however, after the follow-up survey of 3000 patients after operation made by me in 1985, I was discerning and apprehending quickly and completely that how to prevent the reoccurrence and metastasis after operation is the core to determine the long-term curative effects of the cancer. The primary carcinoma lesion or the metastatic carcinoma lesion may be represented locally while the remote metastasis is systemic.
3. How to improve the immunologic function of the host, protect, activate and improve the anti-cancer capability of the anti-cancer organ in the human body. **The course of treatment of cancer shall be always focusing on strengthening the body resistance and eliminating pathogenic factors. Strengthening the body resistance refers to protect the immunological recognition capability of the organism, mobilize the positive anti-cancer factors in the human body and improve the anti-cancer capability of the organism; Eliminating pathogenic factors refers to inhibiting and killing off the cancer cells and eliminating the tumor.** Strengthening the body resistance and eliminating

pathogenic factors as well as protecting the immunologic function and killing off the cancer cells are dialectical and united. However, at present, the chemotherapy only pays attention to killing the cancer cells, ignoring the protection of the host and damaging the immune system of the host and the hemopoietic system of the bone marrow, resulting in eliminating pathogenic factors while damaging the body resistance. In case that the chemotherapy drug has drug resistance, it may do harm to the body resistance while not eliminating the pathogenic factors. One scientific scheme shall be designed for the treatment of tumor. Unbalance between the immunity of the organism of the patient and the tumor as well as the inferior immunological surveillance capability make the tumor develop further. Therefore, it is necessary to pay attention to its function of the immune system in treatment and try to recover its balance. The principle of treatment is to improve the immunologic function of the host and activate the functions of anti-cancer cell system, anti-cancer cytokine system and anti-cancer gene system of the human body.

III. Force for Cancer Treatment

As to the force used to kill or control cancer cells in human body, two different thoughts lead to two different kinds of understanding.

(I) Traditional therapy

The three traditional therapies for cancer treatment including operative therapy, radiation therapy and chemotherapy kill cancer cells in human body by foreign force.

The three therapies have made great contributions to the history of human's fighting against cancer and have saved innumerable cancer patients, furthermore, they will do so in the future, so they are effective for cancer treatment. However, nearly all anticancer drugs kill normal histiocyte at the time of killing cancer cells, especially bone marrow hematopoietic cells and gastrointestinal cells with exuberant proliferation, which usually result in reduction in patient's immunologic function. This practically attacks or damages the immunity of inner treatment of human being to different extents.

(II) Xu Ze's new concept of cancer treatment

Killing cancer cells in human body should resort to two kinds of force: one is foreign force from operation, radiation therapy and chemotherapy, the other is intrinsic force from patient's autoimmunity. Although medicament, operation and therapeutic techniques are important to patient's therapy, intrinsic immunity of human body is more important. Many problems must depend on patient's self force, such as nutrition problem, it is hard to attain the object if the patient organism can't absorb and utilize despite given sufficient nutriment. Take healing of incision as another example, it must rely on patient's intrinsic healing function and exogenous factor can only influence or accelerate its healing.

Intrinsic immunity of human body can kill cancer cells. Literature material shows that a tiny tumor (1-8g) can release several millions or hundreds of thousands of cancer cells to blood within 24h, but most (99.99%) of them will be killed by human body immune system can kill cancer, only less than 0.1% can survive and grow to metastatic carcinoma. The data from our own laboratory show that Kunming mouse can kill 99% of cancer cells by its autoimmunity within 24h when injected 10^5 S_{180} malignant cells to caudal vein. More cancer cells will be killed if the mouse takes XZ-C-$_1$ and XZ-C_4 immunization regulation and control traditional Chinese medicine. Anti-cancer Metastasis Lab of Wuhan Shuguang Tumor Special Clinic has implied XZ-C_1 and XZ-C_4 to patients regularly in recent 10 years, it is shown by clinical data statistics that certain amount of cancer cells in metastasis can indeed be killed.

Human body has certain anti-cancer ability and there is a complete anti-cancer mechanism and system in host body with the anticancer effect of anticancer cell cluster (NL cell cluster, K cell cluster, LAK cell cluster, macrophage cluster and TK cell cluster), the anticancer effect of anticancer cytokine system, FN, IL-2, TNF and LT, and the effect of anti-oncogene and inhibiting cancer metastasis gene, therefore, it must be protected, activated and brought into play.

The generation and development of cancer is close related to immunologic hypofunction of the body. The carcinoma can directly infringe immune organ to worsen or inhibit immunologic function and can release immunosuppressive factor to bring down the immunity of host or to induce the intracorporeal suppressor cell to increase. The Thymus of host has been inhibited in case of cancer and chemotherapy inhibits bone marrow, just like one disaster after another. Traditional therapy neglects the intrinsic anticancer ability of human body and the anticancer force of anticancer cell, anticancer cytokine, antioncogene and anti-metastasis gene in anticancer system, in this way, the whole central immune organ shall be damaged and can not be effectively protected, which is why the curative effect of traditional therapy can't be improved.

Consequently, the author suggests attaching great importance to exerting and relying on the intrinsic force of anticancer system of the host.

CHAPTER 5

Xu Ze Proposes: Cancer Treatment Should Update the Idea, Change the Concept and Establish Treatment Outlook in An All-round Way

Theory guides clinic: carry out the treatment in an all-round way aiming at the cancer cells and the host synchronously.

Professor Xu Ze holds: the treatment of cancer shall get rid of the one-sided treatment outlook of simply killing the cancer cells and we should update the idea, change the concept and establish the treatment outlook in an all-round way. Since the cancer is opposite to the cancer cells and the host, the impaired anti-cancer force of host leads to the occurrence and development of the tumor while the intensive anti-cancer force of the host can control the development of the cancer, just like the "teeter-totter", as one falls, another rise. Therefore, the treatment of cancer is not only to kill the cancer cells, but also to protect the host and does not harm the host so as to enhance the anti-cancer force of the host and establish the cancer treatment outlook in an all-round way.

I. The objective of traditional therapy is relatively simple, just to kill the cancer cells, which is only one aspect of cancer treatment.

It does not conform to the actual conditions of biological characteristics and behaviors of cancer cells understood nowadays.

The traditional cancer therapy holds that the cancer is the continual division and proliferation of the cells, so the cancer cells are the arch criminal. Its treatment objective must be to kill the cancer cells.

Objective of chemotherapy: to kill the cancer cells, only to kill the cancer cells.

Objective of radiotherapy: to kill the cancer cells, only to kill the cancer cells.

Since 1930s, the radiotherapy, namely "radium therapy" has been used to kill the cancer cells and since the middle of 1940s the cytotoxic drug for chemotherapy has been used to kill the cancer cells. At that time, the principles of cancer treatment was to kill or eliminate the last cancer cell so as to heal the cancer.

Therefore, people adopted the expanded operation and strengthened the chemotherapy and the radical chemotherapy. At the beginning of 1960s, the operation range of tumor surgery tended to expansion and developed a series of super-radical operations. Subsequently, after the practice over years, it was proven that it could not improve the total survival time. In 1980s, the patients receiving intensive chemotherapy and /or radical radiotherapy, did not improve their survival quality or prolong the survival time. The hematopoietic function of the bone marrow and the immunologic function were severely restrained, resulting in increased complications endangering the life. In view that the cancer often meets with recurrence and metastasis after surgical radical operation, the assistant chemotherapy after operation was prevailing at the beginning of 1990s. However, whether the assistant chemotherapy after operation prevents recurrence and metastasis? 10 years ago before 21st century, although so many cancer patients received the correct and systemic chemotherapy and radiotherapy after operation, recurrence and metastasis could not be prevented.

Why the traditional therapy with the objective of simply killing the cancer cells cannot reduce the death rate? Why it cannot prevent recurrence and metastasis? Why it only can play a role in a short-term remission? Why it only can remit the cancer but cannot heat the cancer patients? Is it real that the cancer cannot be cured? Or only simple radiotherapy and chemotherapy cannot cure the cancer? What is the problem in chemotherapy and radiotherapy? What are the defects and the disadvantages? Or is the therapeutic strategy with the objective of simply killing the cancer cells wrong? Are the cancer cells killed in chemotherapy? How many cancer cells are killed? How many cancer cells are remained in the body of the patient? Whether is the chemotherapy drug sensitive or not? Whether does it have drug tolerance? All of these things are remained unknown. Whether it is presented that the traditional therapy does not conform to the actual conditions of the biological characteristics of the cancer cells? It only kills the cancer cells while ignores the host.

II. Why the traditional therapy with the objective of simply killing the cancer cells cannot prevent recurrence and metastasis?

1. Because the cytotoxic drugs for chemotherapy and the radiation have no selectivity. Each coil has two sides. It kills not only the cancer cells but also the normal tissue, especially the hematopoietic cells and immunological cells of the bone marrow, harming the host.

   The traditional therapy harms the nervous organs, the thymus is restrained by the cancer while chemotherapy and radiotherapy restrain the bone marrow, resulting in one disaster after another, in this way, the whole nervous immune organ is damaged and it cannot be effectively protected. The decrease of immunologic function reduces the immune surveillance to a certainty, resulting in immunologic escape of canceration cells, finally resulting in metastasis after chemotherapy and metastasis in chemotherapy.

2. The anti-cancer drug killing the cancer cells is only of the first order kinetics. That is to say, it only kills the cancer cells no matter how many cancer cells exist, the drug with a certain dose only can kill the cells at a certain rate and the drug with an increased dose cannot kill all of the cancer cells.
3. The chemotherapy drug cannot cure the cancer once and for all. The lethality of the cytotoxic drug only is valid in these days when the chemotherapy drug is delivered and after that the drug will entirely lose the drug effect. The remained cancer cells will be continually divided, proliferated and cloned, resulting in recurrence and metastasis.
4. The cytotoxic drug killing cancer cells is related to the cyclic sensitivity of the cancer cells. If a certain drug reacts on the sensitivity of Stage S or M_1, in the period of intravenous injection to the patient, some cancer cells are beyond Stage S or M_1, so it is invalid.
5. Production of drug tolerance. As above mentioned, the chemotherapy drug kills the cancer cells as per the first order kinetics, so it is unlikely to kill the cancer cells with chemotherapy drug, it will take some periods of treatment repeatedly to reduce the cancer cells to below 10^6, in this way, the drug resistance produces easily. At this moment, if the dose is increased, the bone marrow and the epithelial tissue of the patient mostly cannot withstand its toxic reaction.

III. The objective of traditional therapy only pays attention to radiotherapy and chemotherapy killing cancer cells and ignores the resistance and inhibition of the host itself to the cancer

Actually, the occurrence and development of the tumor, is dependent on the immunologic function of the host and the biological characteristics of the tumor, namely the balance between the biological characteristics of the tumor cancers and the influences of the host on the confinement factors, if both of them are balanced, it is controlled; otherwise, it will be developed.

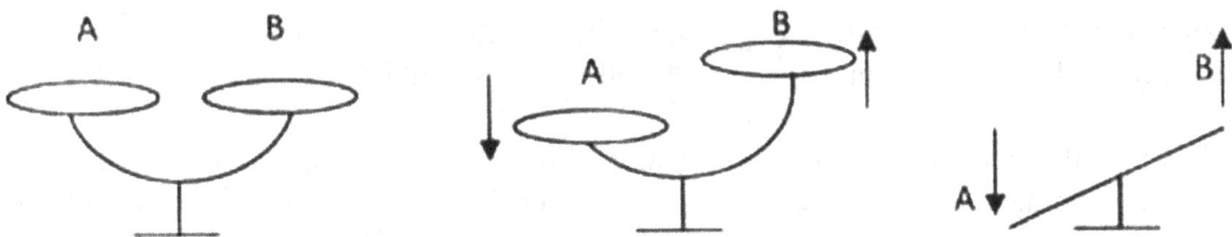

Fig. 1 balance and stability:
A: host—immunologic function
B: tumor—biological characteristics

Fig. 2 unbalance decrease of immune
tumor development

It was found from the animal experiments made by us in the lab that the occurrence and development of the cancer is definitely and affirmatively related to the anti-cancer capability of the immunologic function of the host and the immunologic function of the host is an important confinement factor of tumor control, if both of them are balanced, it is controlled; otherwise, it will be developed.

In the past half a century, the researchers at home and abroad had been focusing on the test on cancer cells to seek the drugs to kill the cancer cells, their ideas were affected by the mode of antibiotics killing the bacteria so as to kill the cancer cells. However, they did not know that they were two entirely different things: the antibiotics only kill the bacteria install of the normal cells and they can be used to make experiments on drug susceptibility while the chemotherapy drug can kill the cancer cells as well as the normal cells, however, it cannot be used to make the experiments on drug susceptibility.

IV. The objective of the traditional therapy only pays attention to radiotherapy and chemotherapy killing cancer cells and ignores the anti-cancer system of the host

The human body itself has a complete set of anti-cancer cell system while radiotherapy and chemotherapy ignore the anti-cancer cells in the host (NK cell group, K cell group, LAK cell group, macrophage group and TK cell group), the reaction of anti-cancer cell sub-systems IFN, IL-1 and TNF; ignores the reaction of cancer-inhibition gene and cancer-inhibition transfer gene in the host (cancer gene and cancer-inhibition gene as well as cancer transfer gene and cancer-inhibition transfer gene exist in the human body) and ignores the reaction of nervous body fluid system and the incretion system in the host. These organs and their affectois play an important role in adjustment, balance and stabilization of the host organism. These intrinsic anti-cancer factors in the human body shall be protected and activated by all means.

V. Professor Xu Ze proposes the objective or target of cancer treatment should establish the treatment outlook in an all-round way aiming at the cancer cells and the host synchronously.

Since the traditional therapeutic mode with the objective of simply killing the cancer cells has not settle the problem in the past half a century, it is necessary to establish a new treatment mode, update the idea and open a new way.

Through deep consideration and analysis, Professor Xu Ze proposes the concept of "balance theory" affecting recurrence and development of cancer:

Biological characteristics of cancer } ⇄ if both of them are balanced, it is controlled;
Restriction capability of host on it } ⇄ otherwise, it will be developed

Therefore, the objective or target of the cancer treatment must aim at the cancer and the host,

Namely treatment of ① host—immunity—biological factor, cytokine and traditional Chinese medicine for immune regulation and control target of cancer ②carcinoma—cancer cells—operation, radiotherapy and chemotherapy

Professor Xu Ze holds: if the treatment objective or target only kills the cancer cells, it only focuses on one side, which is unilateral. If the treatment objective or target only focuses on the immune regulation and control, it only stresses on one side, which is unilateral. The above-mentioned treatment outlook is unilateral and is not comprehensive and it is impossible to conquer the cancer. If the treatment objective or target focuses on both the host and the cancer, which can kill the cancer cells, protect the host, strengthen the immunity, protect the chest and the bone marrow, produce the blood and enhance the anti-cancer capability of the host, which is an all-round treatment outlook and it is possible to conquer the cancer.

As to the concept of current traditional therapy, the treatment objective or target only killing the cancer cells is the unilateral treatment outlook, which does not protect the anti-cancer force of the host, but damages the immunity of the host, therefore, it cannot conquer the cancer. It is necessary to establish cancer treatment outlook in an all-round way, that is to say, the objective or target is to focus on both the host and the carcinoma, which not only kills the cancer cells but also strengthen the immunity of the host, conforming to the actual conditions of the biological characteristics of cancer cells, so it is possible to conquer the cancer.

Through reviewing and reflecting the experience and lessons from clinical tumor surgery over 54 years, Professor Xu Ze holds: in order to conquer the cancer, it is necessary to simply kill the cancer cells as well as strengthen the immunity of the host to inhibit the tumor, bring the anti-cancer organ functions of the human body into play and exert their anti-cancer capability to make the anti-cancer resistance of the host stronger, in this way, it can inhibit the tumor for a long time and prevent its development to realize the cancer-bearing survival. Its treatment objective:

1. To control occurrence and development of the tumor, firstly the host shall be taken into consideration, stressing on how to strengthen the anti-cancer capability of the host to inhibit occurrence and development of the tumor.
2. Strengthen the anti-cancer force of the host to inhibit the development of the tumor so as to realize the cancer-bearing survival and prolong the survival period.

3. Try to make the anti-cancer force of the host stronger to inhibit the development of the tumor for a long time to make it stable and dormant, in this way, it will not be developed, resulting in the long-term cancer-bearing survival and becoming a chronic disease.

VI. Why Professor Xu Ze proposes the treatment outlook in an all-round way? Stressing on inhibiting occurrence and development of tumor through strengthening the anti-cancer capability of the host

This lab has been carrying out a series of experimental study for 16 years to probe into the possible etiologic factor and nosogenesis of the cancer, research the pathophysiology through animal experiment and probe in invasion, recurrence and metastasis mechanism of the cancer so as to find the effective measures for regulation and control. The following new experimental findings offer the theoretical basis and experimental basis for proposing the treatment outlook in an all-round way.

Experiment 1: this lab excises the thymus of the rat and establishes the cancer-bearing animal model, the injection of the immunosuppressive agent is helpful to establish the cancer-bearing animal model. It is proven by the research conclusions that the recurrence and development of cancer has obviously affirmative relation with the thymus of the immune organ of the host and its functions.

Experiment 2: whether the low immunity leads to the cancer or the cancer leads to the low immunity at all? Our experimental results: the low immunity leads to the occurrence and development of the cancer, without the decrease of the immunologic functions, it is not easy for successful inoculation. It is presented by the experimental results that improvement and maintenance of the good immunologic functions and protection of the good central immune organ is one of the important measures to prevent the occurrence of the cancer.

Experiment 3: in researching the relation between the metastasis of cancer and the immunity, this lab establishes the animal model of liver metastatic carcinoma and it is found by us that if the patient is administered with immunosuppressive agent, the metastasis lesion in the liver. It is shown by the experimental results that: metastasis is related to the immunity, the low immunologic functions or administration of immunosuppressive agent may promote the metastasis of the tumor.

Experiment 4: when making the experiment to probe into the effects of the tumor on immune organs of the organ, it is found by us that the thymus meets with progressive atrophy with the development of cancer. It is shown by the experimental results that the tumor may suppress the thymus, resulting in the atrophy of the immune organ.

Through analyzing and thinking the experimental research results, we obtain the new findings, new concept and new enlightenment. Therefore, Professor Xu Ze firstly proposes in the world that one of the etiologic factors and nosogenesis of cancer may be the atrophy of thymus, decrease of immunologic function and immunologic escape. So the treatment outlook in an all-round way must stress on strengthening the anti-cancer force of the host to enhance the immunologic functions so as to suppress the occurrence and development of the tumor.

VII. How to establish the cancer treatment outlook in an all-round way? Stressing on killing the cancer cells as well as strengthening the anti-cancer immunity of the host

The objective or target of cancer treatment outlook in an all-round way aims at both the tumor and the host and research the clinical treatment scheme of cancer from the biological characteristics of the cancer cells and the reaction of the host organism. And then, how to realize the objective?

1. It must be made clear that the human body has a complete set of anti-cancer organ, so it is necessary to bring the reaction of the immune system into play, enhance the immune surveillance and prevent the escape of canceration cells. In fact, the radiotherapy and the chemotherapy cannot kill off all of the cancer cells, the remained cancer cells will be continually divided, proliferated and cloned in geometrical progression, such as one into two, two into four, in this way, it leads to recurrence and metastasis.
2. Radiotherapy and chemotherapy must pay attention to improvement of the immunologic functions of the host synchronously. In order to kill the cancer cells, it cannot simply rely on the chemotherapy drug, it is necessary to rely on the anti-cancer capability of the organism to eliminate the remained cancer cells, why? Because the cytotoxic drug for chemotherapy has limited capability to kill the cancer cells, in addition, the drug effect only lasts a short period.
   (1) The chemotherapy reaction timc is limited and momentary and the chemotherapy drug cannot kill off the cancer cells once and for ever, it only has the drug effect on killing the cancer cells in the days of intravenous injection for chemotherapy, after chemotherapy, the drug effect disappears and it has no reaction again and it only has the drug effect within 2-3 months even though the chemotherapy is made 4 times even 6 times, after that, it must rely on the anti-cancer capability of the immunologic functions of the host.
   (2) The capability of chemotherapy to killing the cancer cells is limited, it cannot kill off all of the cancer cells as per the first order kinetics, it only can kill a part and another part remains again. For example, the patient suffering from acute lymphoblastic leukemia has over 10^{12} cancer cells before administration of chemotherapy drug, after treatment, there are about 10^{7} cancer cells surviving, even though the dose is increased, the lethality will not be increased, subsequently, it must rely on the anti-cancer capability of the immunologic functions of the host to eliminate the remained cancer cells.
   (3) The chemotherapy is a two-sided sword, which kills the cancer cells as well as the hematopoietic cells and immunological cells of the bone marrow, promoting the decrease of the immunologic function, therefore, it is necessary for the chemotherapy to recover or strength the immunologic functions of the host.
   (4) After radiotherapy and chemotherapy, the remained stem cells of tumor are still continually divided, proliferated and cloned, so it is still necessary to improve the anti-cancer capability of the host to suppress the development of tumor for a long term.

Therefore, Professor Xu Ze proposes the current radiotherapy or chemotherapy should be combined with immunological therapy, biological therapy and XZ-C anti-cancer medicine for immune regulation synchronously. It is necessary to reform it to immune + chemotherapy and immune + radiotherapy.

3. How to improve the immunologic functions of the host to suppress the development of tumor for a long time. Viewed from a short term, the radiotherapy kills the cancer cells with chemotherapy drugs, viewed from a long term, it shall rely on the immunologic functions and the immune surveillance of the host to eliminate the remained cancer cells. So the treatment outlook in an all-round way must stress on protecting the chest and improving the immunity to improve the immunologic functions of the host so as to suppress the development of the tumor.

The cancer is a kind of general disease, so it is necessary to research the cancer and consider the clinical treatment scheme from the biological characteristics and behaviors of the cancer. The immune system is specially suitable for eliminated the remained cancer cells, especially the cells in resting stage of the stem cells of the tumor which are difficult to be eliminated by radiotherapy or chemotherapy, which is helpful to prolong the cancer-free survival time. Radiotherapy and chemotherapy only can kill a part of the cancer cells instead of all cancer cells, the rest 10^7 cancer cells are slowly eliminated by the immunological cells of the host organism, so it is difficult to conquer the cancer by radiotherapy and chemotherapy.

Immunological therapy of tumor is an important part of biological treatment of the tumor and it is the key of the treatment outlook in an all-round way. Biological treatment of tumor is based on biological response modifier (BRM), namely BRM theory created by Oldham in 1982. Based on this, Oldham put forward four modality of cancer treatment of tumor treatment in 1984, namely the biological treatment. According to BRM theory, in normal conditions, the tumor and the defense of the organism are in dynamic balance, the occurrence, invasion and metastasis of the tumor are entirely caused by the maladjustment of the dynamic balance. If the maladjusted state can be artificially adjusted to the normal level, it can control the growth of the tumor and make the tumor extinct.

The biological treatment is to adjust the biological response through supplementing, inducing or activating the intrinsic biological active cells (or) factors with cell toxic cytoactive in BRM system in the body in vitro. The biological treatment is different from the three largest traditional therapies, including operation, radiotherapy and chemotherapy, the radiotherapy and the chemoyherapy targets directly attacking the tumor.

The biological treatment of the tumor mainly includes: (1) adoptive infusion of immunologic living cells; (2) application of lymphokine/cytokine; (3) specific active immunity, including tumor vaccine and monovalent vaccine.

The cells and the humoral factors of the organism reaction system are in delicate regulation and control, when they are unbalanced, the reaction or response capability of the organism will be remarkably affected, the adoption of biological reaction moderator is to recover the unbalanced organism state to the normal state so as to realize the objective of preventing the tumor.

The biological reaction moderator is to moderate the immunologic function of the organism, recover the suppressed functions of the immune system of the organism. The reaction mechanism of the drugs is to activate the immune system of the organism to bring its regulation function into play, most of them are from microorganism and the plants.

VIII. Immune regulation and control therapy is the key of the all-round cancer treatment

It has been proven by 4-year's experimental study and 16-year's clinical verification that XZ-C medicine has the similar reaction and curative effect to BRM and it is the one with the similar reaction to BRM screened from the resources of Chinese traditional herb.

XZ-C medicine is screened through experiment by Professor Xu Ze in China (XU ZE-China, XZ-C) in the lab from 200 kinds of Chinese herbal medicines. Firstly we adopt the culture in vitro of cancer cells, screen 200 kinds of Chinese herbal medicines one by one in vitro, observe the direct damage to cancer cells by the medicines in the culture tube through experimental study and make the check experiment of tumor-suppression rate with the normal cells cultured with chemotherapy drug CTX and in the test tube as the control group. Finally, we select a batch of drugs with the rate of tumor-suppression of the proliferation of cancer cells. Then we further create the tumor-bearing animal model and make the experimental study on 200 kinds of Chinese herbal medicines for in vivo tumor-suppression rate and then screen, analyze and evaluate them one by one scientifically and objectively. It is proven by the experimental results that only 48 kinds of medicines have relatively good tumor-suppression rate while another 152 kinds of Chinese herbal medicines are the common anti-cancer Chinese traditional medicines used by the herbalist doctors, through experimental screening for tumor-suppression rate in the tumor-bearing experimental tumor, which are proven no anti-cancer reaction or little tumor-suppression rate.

XZ-C medicine with relatively better tumor-suppression rate screened through the tumor-bearing rats in the lab by us can improve the immunity, protect the thymus of the central immune organ, improve the cellular immunity, protect the function of the thymus, improve the immunity, protect the hematopiesis function of the bone marrow, increase the erythrocytes and white blood cells, activate the immunocyte factors and improve the immune surveillance in the blood. The main pharmacological action of XZ-C medicine is anti-cancer and improvement of immunity. This group screens 48 kinds of medicines with relatively high tumor-suppression rate through 4-year's animal experiment and then it detects 26 kinds of medicines through immune and cytokine level detection, that can enhance the phagocytic function, or cellular immunity; or humoral immunity; or increase the weight of the thymus; or promote the proliferation of bone marrow cells; or enhance T cellular functions; or increase LAK cytoactive; or increase the active level of the interferon IFN; or increase the active level of TNF; or increase the stimulating factors of CSF colony or inhibit the thromboxane of the blood platelets.

1. Application principles of XZ-C medicine. BRM and XZ-C medicine with similar reaction to BRM can strengthen immunological reaction of the organism, strengthen the immune surveillance reaction of the organism and they have relatively good effects when the cells meet with catastrophe or the tumor is very small. Through surgical operation or radiotherapy or medication, it will realize the best curative effect when the tumor is minimized.

As to the patient losing the opportunity of operation, with bad body condition, not withstanding radiotherapy and chemotherapy, the immunological therapy has a certain curative effect and reduces the symptom and prolongs the survival time.

After radical excision of the tumor, in order to reduce the recurrence and metastasis, XZ-C medicine can be administered for treatment; when large tumor is excised with operation, in order to eliminate the remained cancer cells and the ones that may be spread remotely, XZ-C medicine can also be administered.

If the tumor cannot be excised, the chemotherapy or the radiotherapy can be made firstly to kill a large number of tumor cells, after the tumor load in the body is reduced, XZ-C medicine can be administered for treatment.

In a word, the host is opposite to the host and the contradiction exists all along the whole process of occurrence and development of the tumor. When the functions of the immune system of the organism are complete, the organism can restrain and eliminate the tumor through cellular immunity and humoral immunity reaction. On the other hand, the growing tumor has so many effects on the immune system of the organism, inhibiting the immunologic functions of the organism and promoting the development of the tumor.

So the cancer treatment scheme must aim at the host and the tumor synchronously. The theory shall be used to guide the clinic; at the same time, the all-round anti-cancer treatment shall be made aiming at the cancer cells and the anti-force forces of the host and the treatment outlook in an all-round way shall be established. The regulation and control shall be used to cure the patients instead of simple killing.

CHAPTER 6

XU ZE Proposes New Combinational Mode of Multi-disciplinary Comprehensive Treatment

Professor Xu Ze holds the combination of multi-disciplinary comprehensive treatment must have reasonable theoretical basis, and the new recognition that the host affects tumor progress and metastasis is of important theoretical value and clinic guiding significance. Two factors including tumor and host shall be considered in formulating anti-carcinoma and anti-metastasis strategies and making comprehensive treatment. Organic integration of discipline, method, technology and medicine with reasonable theoretical basis must be the treatment outlook in an all-round way.

At the beginning of 21st century, carcinoma treatment has entered into the era of multi-disciplinary comprehensive treatment.

Current situation of comprehensive treatment: it takes three traditional therapies as the main body. In most cases, the way of comprehensive application depends on the clinical department for initial diagnosis. Most patients are initially diagnosed in chemotherapy department, in which case they will be subject to chemotherapy firstly and then radiotherapy. If the patients are initially diagnosed in radiotherapy department, then they will be subject to radiotherapy followed by chemotherapy. If the patients are initially diagnosed in surgery department, they will be subject to operation with the presence of operation indications, followed by chemotherapy or radiotherapy, and will be subject to radiotherapy or chemotherapy with the absence of operation indications. The result of such comprehensive treatment is that many patients still fail to prevent recurrence and metastasis, and some even promote the failure of immunologic function.

Biotherapy, immunotherapy, differentiation-inducing therapy, cytokine therapy and immunologic regulation and control therapy of Chinese medicine combined with western medicine have not been incorporated into the treatment scheme of most tumor therapist.

I. The Reason why we put forward the new treatment mode of scientific organic integration

The study on carcinoma therapeutics must be based on tumor biology, both of which must be consistent with each other. Unit now, in the early years of 21st century, the tumor biology has developed into the level of molecular biology, cytokine and gene while the theoretical basis of the traditional cancer therapeutics has been still remaining the cellular level over 50 years which is based on the unceasing proliferation aiming at killing off carcinoma cells. Traditional radiotherapy and chemotherapy aims at killing cancer cells, so cytotoxic drug is used, but the effect is poor which requires increasing the dosage and adding several medicines for combination. In the recent decade, the trend of research on antitumor drugs and status of clinical application indicate the clinical application of traditional anticancer drugs was subject to more limitations due to great side effects, low targeting, the patients' tolerance to drugs, etc.

It can be deemed that the research on anticancer drugs has entered a new stage, facing updating of theories, technologies and ideas. The traditional idea and working method merely aiming at simply eliminating cancer cells by cytotoxic drug as the theoretical basis is under attack.

Since 1980s, with the rapid development of medical molecular, molecular immunology, immunopharmacology, TCM immunopharmacology and cytokine, new bio-therapeutics has emerged, driving the advancement of cancer therapeutics. Biotherapy, immunologic therapy, differentiation inducer, biological reaction regulator, immunological regulation and control TCM at molecular level combined with western medicine are coming out in succession. New tumor vaccine development and gene therapy in recent years presents a more fascinating prospect.

The author holds that cancer therapy needs a scientifically designed treatment plan. In case of cancer, further development of tumor is contributed to imbalance between anticancer immunocompetence and tumor development of the organism and the absence of immune surveillance. Hence, both of them must be recovered to balance and stability through therapy.

II. How to carry out organic, integrated and multi-disciplinary treatment scheme

1. **Professor Xu Ze proposes that carcinoma treatment needs a scientifically designed "organic, integrated and multi-disciplinary treatment scheme". And the scientifically designed organic integration must be consistent with the actual conditions of the patient:**
   (1) Biological characteristics and behaviors of cancer cells, which means that the malignant cells in the organism will be continually progressively divided, proliferated and cloned once becoming cancer cells, from one to two, two to four . . . . throughout the whole course of cancer occurrence, evolvement, metastasis and recurrence. Hence, treatment measures must stress on control and treatment in the whole course, rather than a certain stage of the course of disease.
   (2) Immunologic state of the host. Cancer is in continual evolvement. Cancer cells are featured in uncontrolled infinite proliferation; their canceration results from imbalance in control. A response relationship must be kept between tumor and host, and the response of the host determines the final results.
   (3) According to the biological behaviors of cancer cells, multiple-step and multi-link of cancer cell metastasis and its "eight steps", "three stages" and "two points and one line", intervene and intercept cancer cells on the way to metastasis and adopt a new, scientific, organically integrated treatment mode in an all-round way.

2. **The combination of comprehensive multi-disciplinary treatment must have reasonable theoretical basis, that is to say, an all-round treatment outlook and the new recognition of host affecting tumor progress and metastasis must be of great theoretical value and clinical guiding significance.** In working out the strategies of anticancer attack and metastasis and selecting comprehensive treatment, we should consider adopting which discipline, method, technology and medicine to realize the organic integration with reasonable theoretical basis in light of tumor and host.

What is the primary determining factor during occurrence, development and metastasis of cancer? Is it tumor or host? Is it immunological anticancer competence of the host organism or attack and metastasis competence of cancer cells? In the past half century, the research has focused on cancer cell itself, all countries aim at the way of killing the cancer cells. Therefore, traditional treatment is killing cancer cells, which is the single objective. Despite some remarkable progresses, they all fail to solve the problem radically, just addressing secondary symptoms rather than primary ones.

In recent years, more attention is shifted to host factor. Our lab has spent four years in experimental study on tumor origin, pathogenesis pathologic physiology and cancer attack and metastasis mechanism to explore anticancer immunocompetence and tumor interaction and to seek the control effects on cancer cell attack and metastasis. Through four-year clinic experiment and basic research in our lab, it is found that thymus removal can produce tumor-bearing animal model; with the progress of transplanted tumor, thymus will go through progressive atrophy, which can be prevented by tumor removal; injecting immunologic inhibitor facilitates production of mice tumor-bearing animal model; injecting immunologic inhibitor into tumor-bearing animal mode will increase lung metastasis and liver metastasis lesion; through careful analysis and further consideration, it is found that the relationship between host and tumor and vice versa is the regulation function of the mutual influence between host microenvironment and tumor cells to tumor-bearing animal model. The interaction between cancer cells and host microenvironment finally determines whether and when metastasis lesion can be formed. These indicate the interaction between host microenvironment and tumor cells. **Hence, Professor Xu Ze proposes the "balance" theory which holds that cancer will evolve if the relation between the biological characteristics of cancer cells and the immunological anticancer competence of the host organism is unbalanced; it will be under control and stabilized if the balance is recovered. Thus the treatment must be targeted at two aspects, namely host and tumor, so as to recover them to a balanced and stable state.**

Through experimental exploration of the interaction, interrelationship between host and tumor coupled with clinic practice experience and lessons, we analyze whether cancer cells or host determines the occurrence, development and metastasis and recurrence of cancer. What is behind the death of cancer? Why cancer tumor causes death? **Our current understanding is that the death of tumor patients is mainly contributed to metastasis and recurrence, but how recurrence and metastasis leads to death? According to our preliminary analysis, consideration and understanding, it is contributed to complication and immunologic failure.** So the final result shall be considered as both tumor itself and host.

According to analysis and understanding in our lab, poor immunological function of host organism —(plus some factor causing cell mutation)→ malignant mutation of cells most → of them are phagocytized by immunologic cells of the organism → the rest malignant cells will be continually divided, proliferated and cloned →

tumor formation —(Inhibit immunity / Th atrophy, further drop in immunity)→ metastasis —(Immunologic escape / Immunologic failure)→ widespread metastasis.

Professor Xu Ze holds: based on the findings of experimental study in our lab and the data of clinic verification and clinic observation, it is the interaction between cancer

cells and host microenvironment and anticancer immunological competence that finally determines cancer progress and that whether and when the metastasis lesion can be formed. The revelation of this regulatory mechanism of interaction is of great theoretical value and clinical significance. As regards formulation of anticancer metastasis strategies and development of new medicines, we should consider tumor and host factors, which provide theoretical basis for seeking effective intervention methods and developing new medicines. XZ-C medicine developed by us for immunological enhancement through thymus protection and hematopoiesis through spinal marrow protection takes strengthening host factor as the theoretical and experimental basis.

Based on the above analysis, the strategies of diagnosis, treatment, medicine development, anticancer control, antimetastasis should be considered from the perspectives of tumor and host. This may be deemed as the principle of radically changing the current partial treatment scheme with the single aim of killing cancer cells and establishing the treatment outlook in an all-round way previously described.

III. Professor Xu Ze proposes the specific scheme for new combination mode of comprehensive multi-disciplinary treatment Advocated

How to combine multi-disciplinary for comprehensive treatment?

At first, we should transform the idea and update the approach, establish treatment outlook in an all-round way, arrange intervention, regulation, control and treatment measures in the whole course of disease, i.e. the whole process of cancer occurrence, development, recurrence and metastasis. Now we comprehensively divide the responsibilities of the main treatment methods of all disciplines commonly used at present and coordinate them organically as per overall therapy or short-term therapy.

1. Overall therapy: mainly based on radical operation treatment, tumor removal and lymph node elimination are followed by biotherapy, immunotherapy, cytokine therapy, differentiation inducement, gene, immunotherapy with Chinese medicines combined with western medicine, XZ-C medicine in a long term or the whole course, to strengthen anticancer immunocompetence of the host, regulate or control recurrence and metastasis. They can be used in the whole course of cancer disease.
2. Short-term therapy: mainly based on radiotherapy and chemotherapy as the primary form, which is in phases or intermittent, or killing cancer cells suddenly in a short course, but not and cannot cover the overall course or a long course. In this case, the duration of cancer cell elimination can be only four cycles or six cycles, longer duration will produce drug resistance.

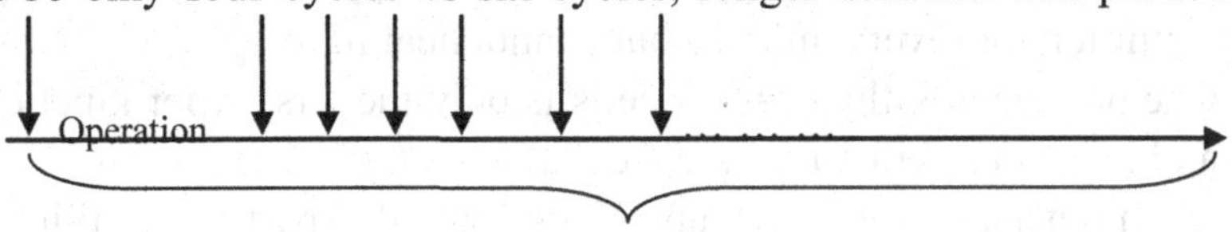

Operation

Overall therapy

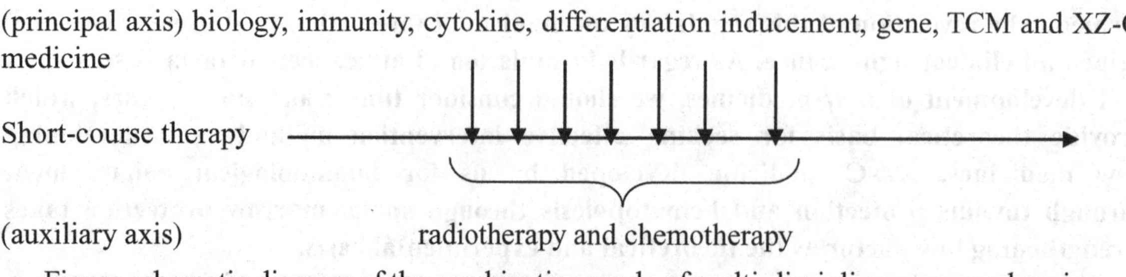

Figure schematic diagram of the combination mode of multi-disciplinary comprehensive treatment

(1) When working out the strategies of the above overall therapy and short-course therapy, we should take tumor and host into account, which may thoroughly change the partial treatment merely killing cancer cells at present. Currently, radiotherapy and chemotherapy only aim at cancer cells, which are partial and incomplete, and fail to consider treatment approaches in light of tumor and host as described above. Apart from this, radiotherapy and chemotherapy will also injure and kill hematopoietic cells and immunological cells of the bone marrow of the host, undermining the immunological function of the host and damaging the host.

(2) Short-course therapy just covers a short stage in the whole course of disease for cancer patients, so it should be deemed as an adjuvant therapy (or referred to as auxiliary axis), for it merely aims at a single aspect of cancer cells.

① Biological characteristics of cancer cells. Cancer stems from malignant mutation of a single cell, the cancer cells are progressively divided and proliferated, from one to two, from two to four . . . . Cancer is a development process rather than a form or entity. Therefore, the therapy to kill off cancer cells cannot eliminate all cancer cells. As long as several cancer cells remain, they can be continually divided, proliferated and recurred. Moreover, chemotherapy cannot injure tumor stem cells, which are bound to constant division, proliferation, resulting in cancer cells. Hence, the treatment method solely relying on killing cancer cells fails to comply with biological characteristics and biological behavior of cancer cells.

② The effective time of cytotoxic drug is limited. It is only effective during the period of application, and ineffective beyond the period, so it cannot be done once and for all. Its effective time is limited, so the remaining $10^{6\text{-}7}$ cancer cells still need to be eliminated by immunological competence of the host. Moreover, tumor stem cells will continue to form cancer cells. Therefore, radiotherapy and chemotherapy can only relieve the condition for several months but cannot heal it.

③ Chemotherapy killing cancer cells is only the first order kinetics, its lethality is limited and it can only kill $10^{6\text{-}7}$ cancer cells.

④ Chemotherapy drug is a double-edged sword. Apart from killing cancer cells, it can also kill normal cells, hematopoietic cells and immunological cells of the bone marrow of the host, causing drop in immunological function of the host.

Traditional chemotherapy and radiotherapy are only targeted at the factor of cancer cell tumor, which is limited, partial and incomplete, thus it is difficult to conquer the cancer. Because canceration process is the result of regulation imbalance, it must be targeted at host and tumor, and the reaction of the host decides the final result. It should be cured by regulation instead of injury alone.

(3) Overall therapy. It covers the whole course of cancer disease from cancer occurrence, development, recurrence, metastasis, progress, targeted at these two factors, i.e. tumor and host. It applies radical operation to remove cancer lesion entity, and applies biotherapy, immunotherapy, gene treating cytokine, immunological regulation TCM and so on to the host, so as to improve anticancer competence of the organism. Such scientific and organic integration is targeted at two aspects, i.e. cancer cells and host. It is an all-round treatment outlook, which is comprehensive, reasonable and scientific, complies with pathogenesis, pathological physiology, biological characteristics and biological behaviors of cancer cells, and is likely to conquer cancer. Therefore, overall therapy should be the principal axis of cancer treatment, with operation treatment as the main form, biotherapy, immunotherapy, gene therapy, and differentiation inducement therapy, TCM immunological regulation therapy, improving immunity by chest protection and hematogenesis by bone marrow protection distributed and applied in the whole course of cancer treatment.
It is a scientific, reasonable and all-round treatment outlook and a radical method.

Short-course therapy should be auxiliary axis of cancer treatment, with chemotherapy and radiotherapy as the main form. It is only designed to kill off cancer cells and should be combined with overall therapy.

The new treatment mode of scientific and organic integration must have a reasonable theoretical basis, with the theory guiding clinic practice.

Xu Ze holds: the new mode of multi-disciplinary comprehensive treatment described above has a reasonable theoretical basis, comply with the realities of the patient's condition and is rational and scientific.

1. The experience and lessons of clinic treatment practice demonstrate killing cancer cells cannot control cancer or overcome cancer. It is partial and incomplete to merely target at one aspect of cancer cell.
2. The objective or target of cancer treatment should be both host and tumor. As regards which is the main side and who decides the final destiny of the cancer patient, both tumor itself and host should be considered.
3. We must update the approach and transform the idea, fist establish a treatment outlook in an all-round way, scientifically arrange intervention, regulation and treatment measures with the whole course of cancer occurrence, development, recurrence and metastasis.
4. We should work out design and arrangement of "principal axis" and "auxiliary axis" new treatment mode, which is appropriate and scientific, with theoretical basis and in line with the realities of the patient.
5. We must orient human firstly, manage to eliminate toxicant and side effects of radiotherapy and chemotherapy as possible, increase patient safety, study the toxicity and safety of each medicine and technology, which must have appropriate theoretical basis guiding clinic practice.

In short: cancer treatment, whether in early, middle or late stage, requires multi-disciplinary comprehensive treatment and appropriate theoretical basis guiding clinic practice.

Operation is a method of local treatment. Tumor surgeons hold that cancer first occurs in local part, and then attacks the surrounding tissues, shifts to other places through lymphatic vessels and blood vessels. Therefore, they often focus on local part in treatment, i.e. control local growth and diffusion, and especially carry out operation to eliminate lymph nodes shifting through lymph. Although operative treatment has seen constant improvement over the years, its long-term effects fail to be increased significantly. Recurrence and metastasis after operation pose a grave threat to prognosis of the patient, which has attracted great concern of the medical circle, but effective good practice remains absent.

Radiotherapy is also local treatment. Its effect local tumor is to kill off cells with the index of unit dosage. The effects of chemotherapy are greatly affected by cell oxygenation, type of the tumor, cell repair and other factors, and it cannot resist metastasis and recurrence.

Biological characteristics of cancer are attack, recurrence and metastasis, which are vital reasons for failure of operative and chemotherapy treatment.

In recent years, some argues cancer deals with the whole body, so whole body treatment should take chemotherapy as the primary form. Unfortunately, although new medicines come out continually over the past decade, treatment schemes and methods update constantly, the effects of chemotherapy are unsatisfactory. As cell toxicant drug is unselective, it can kill off both cancer cells and normal cells of the host, especially tend to injure immunocytes, with serious toxicant and side effects, inhibiting hematopiesis function of spinal marrow and reduce immunity. Therefore, the writer holds that traditional chemotherapy does not completely comply with the real situation of biological behavior of cancer as we recognized today, for example, attack behavior, metastasis of cancer cells deals with multiple links and steps. Currently, people have realized that antitumor medicine does not necessarily resist metastasis and recurrence.

The biotherapy of tumor newly emerging in 1980s, such as immunotherapy, cytokine therapy, differentiation inducement therapy and gene tumor vaccine therapy, has proved some therapies can regulate the immunity of the patients, but has not proved which immunological preparation or method can induce tumor extinction.

In the last two decades, there are many reports on cancer treatment by tradition Chinese medicine. Its prospect is of concern. Especially with further research on medicine and immunology, it has been recognized that confusion of immunological system is closely related with occurrence and development of tumor. Traditional Chinese medicine has its own characteristics and advantages in treating tumor by regulating immunological function of the organism. Immunological regulation of traditional Chinese medicines and the development of Chinese medicine immunomodulator will be concerned and favored across the world. If combined with operation, radiotherapy and chemotherapy, SZ-C medicine can give full play to its immunological regulation function during treatment, obviously prolong survival time and improve survival quality, displaying characteristics and advantages of traditional Chinese medicine. Its disadvantage lies in that it cannot cause evident change on tumor itself.

Since the methods above are different in action mechanism and effects of cancer treatment, and have their own disadvantages, thus it is necessary to evaluate the advantages and disadvantages of the therapies, "gains" and "losses" of the patients, for example, what are the advantages and disadvantages of adopting this therapy, what will the patients gain or lose? We can draw from the advantages of each therapy to offset their disadvantages, combine the therapies in an organic and appropriate way, forming a comprehensive plan of cancer treatment. Only in this way can we significantly reduce toxic and side effects of the medicine, improve survival quality of the patients and prolong overall survival time. Over the past 16 years,

Shuguang Tumor Clinic has applied the comprehensive treatment mainly involving operation +XZ-C medicine to more than 12000 cancer patients at middle and late stage. Most of them have achieved the effects of improving survival quality, stabilizing disease lesion, controlling metastasis, existence with tumor and significantly prolonging life.

CHAPTER 7

The Main Forms of Existence of Carcinoma in a Body

[Abstract]

Objective: Probe into the main forms of cancer existing in human body.

Methods: This paper, sums up the positive and negative experience and lessens in clinical practice cases for 49 years, combines with the long-term practice and study as well as the understanding of clinical practice, holds the following new understanding and puts forward the new theoretical concept, proposes to implement the new treatment strategy.

Results: it finds and puts forward that the existence of cancer in human body has three forms and the third manifestation is the cancer cell in metastasis.

Conclusion: The traditional therapeutic concept holds that there are only two forms (primary lesion and metastases). It is firstly found and put forward by us in the world that there are three forms: 1. primary lesion; 2. metastases; 3. cancer cell in the route of metastasis. The goal of cancer treatment should be oriented to these three forms. New concept, oriented to these three forms, is a complete concept of therapeutics and it is possible to overcome the cancer. The traditional concept, oriented to the former two forms and it is difficult to overcome the cancer.

Introduction

It can be seen from the clinical medical practice about one hundred years that the traditional three therapies of treatment, namely operation, radiotherapy and chemotherapy for treatment of carcinomas have obtained relatively good curative effects and many patients have obtained CR and PR curative effects with obvious shrinkage of tumour. However, it is a pity that the tumour recurs, enlarges and transfers before long. Although the secondary radiotherapy or chemotherapy is carried out, most of the effects are bad, finally resulting in death due to metastasis and reoccurrence.

In 1985, the author carried out the follow-up survey on over 3000 patients after general surgical operation and thoracic cancer operation made by myself with the findings that most of the patients met with reoccurrence and metastasis on average in 2~3 years, some of them even met with reoccurrence in several months after operation, which indicated that the operation was successful, but the long-term curative effect was unsuccessful. Therefore, the author deeply realizes that anticancer metastasis is the key to overcome the cancer at present.

The author, summing up the experiences and lessons of the clinical practice cases in the past 49 years from positive and negative aspect and combining the long-term experimental research and clinical practice, gets the following understanding, puts forward the new theoretical concept and initiates new treatment strategy.

1. Traditional Cancer Therapeutics Holding Two Forms Exist

There are two forms of cancer existing in human body: one is the primary lesion of primary tumor and another is the metastatic node or metastases. No matter the primary or metastatic tumor, some can be visible or touched (such as breast carcinoma, thyroid carcinoma and metastases of supraclavicular lymph nodes), some can be seen through the endoscope and some can be seen that the occupying lesion exists through X-ray, ultrasonic, CT, MRI and other imaging examination.

Carry out clinical diagnosis on primary tumor or metastatic tumor according to the above-mentioned signs or physical examination, and then further carry out the pathological section or paracentesis cytology examination on cancerous protuberance to form a correct diagnosis.

The goal or target of treatment of traditional cancer therapeutics aims at these two existing forms, namely the primary tumor or metastatic tumor just because no matter the primary tumor or metastatic tumor is composed of cancer cell while the goal of treatment is to kill the cancer cell. How to kill the cancer cell? The traditional therapy of treatment mainly depends on the surgical operation, radiotherapy and chemotherapy.

The standard for judging the curative effect of traditional cancer therapeutics is remittance, shrinkage of tumor, CR and PR.

The reason why the traditional therapy of treatment fails is mainly the recurrence and metastasis.

2. XU ZE New Concept of Cancer Treatment Holding Three Forms Exist

Why the recurrence or metastatic tumor happens after the primary tumor or metastatic tumor is ablated? Through long-term experimental research and clinical practice, the author holds that the cancer existing in the human body has three forms: the first one is the primary lesion of primary tumor; the second one is metastatic node or metastatic tumid lymph node; the third one is the cancer cell and cancer cell group and micro-metastasis in metastasis routing. The first two forms may be visible or touched or seen through endoscope or has the occupying lesion that can be seen through imaging. The third manifestation is the thousands of cancer cells or cancer mill groups or slight cancer embolus in metastasis routing, which cannot be seen or touched. These potential, hidden and roving metastatic cancer cells, which cannot be examined through endoscope, ultrasonic, CT and MRI and so on, is the largest threat to the life of the patient suffering from cancer. The manifestation of this kind of cancer existing in the human body is not manifested in the body surface or viscera organs. In the past, it had not been found or considered and at present, various examination approaches cannot examine it. In operation, it cannot be seen by eyes, for example, in radical operation for carcinoma of stomach, the phyma of stomach cancer and metastatic tumid lymph nodes can be seen by us, however, whether the cancer cell exists in the vein of stomach wall or portal vein blood stream cannot be seen? And how many cancer cells exist? And where the cancer cells in the vein blood stream go? Whether the cancer cell groups touched and extruded into the vein flood stream arrive at the stomach vein or the portal vein even the portal vein branch in the anus? It is impossible to not touch the cancer phyma in operations research and abscission of phyma of stomach cancer and cleaning down of lymph node, since the operation by hand necessarily makes a large number of cancer cells extruded and exfoliated, flowing into the blood circulation through out-neoplasm vein and rushing into the blood stream of portal vein, however, which cannot be seen by the operation doctor. These cancer cells rushing into the blood stream of portal vein will flow into the portal vein system in the anus. Generally, the various immunological cells in the portal vein will carry out the immune surveillance over the cancer cells in the blood circulation of the portal vein and will phagocytize them. However, in a short time, the immunological cells in the portal vein system cannot phagocytize these cancer cells rushing abruptly. After a period of time, some cancer cells escape the immune surveillance, the cancer cells surviving after impact of blood stream may implant in the sinus hepaticus, the blood vessel produces and forms the intrahepatic metastasis, which is a phenomenon as well as a fact, however, it has not been thought and discovered that it is a dynamic manifestation of the cancer cell existing in the human body. The anti-cancer metastasis and recurrence lab of this experimental surgical research institution, through analysis and research of the metastasis rule of over 10000 clinic patients suffering from cancer, has been aware of this phenomenon and find it, that is to say that the essence of the metastasis is the cancer cells in the metastasis routing and the goal of anti metastasis and the target of treatment should aim at the cancer cells in metastasis routing, namely the third manifestation of cancer existing in human body; in the past, since the people had not been aware of this point, they only cured the primary lesion and metastasis and tried to shorten or eliminate it, but not knew that the shrinkage of the phyma did not mean that it did not transfer. The traditional therapy of treatment fails in reoccurrence and metastasis in a long term.

3. Research and Cognitive Process of the Third Manifestation of Cancer in Human Body

Since it is cognized by us that the key to cure the cancer is to anti-metastasis, how to realize the anti-metastasis? And how to cognize the detailed process, step and mechanism of the metastasis of cancer cells? How these cancer cells move? What is their movement rule? Where is the weak link of the cancer cell in metastasis routing? Which link(s) should be stricken or blockaded? The goal of striking the cancer metastasis must be objectified.

In order to settle the above-mentioned problems, the experimental surgical anti-metastasis and recurrence lab was established by us to carry out the fundamental research of experimental tumor, implant the cancer cells, establish the animal model of tumor and develop a series of experimental tumor research: probing into the mechanism and rule of cancer invasion and metastasis; probing into the relationship between the tumor and immunity and the immune organ as well as the one between the immune organ and the tumor; finding the effective measures to regulate and control the invasion and metastasis of cancer. This lab has spent 3 years in the experimental research on the animal model of cancer metastasis and the experimental observation for observing and tracing the fortune and rule of the cancer cells in the metastasis routing.

It is easy to find some new approaches through the animal experiment and some experimental achievements are obtained. However, it is difficult to verify many experimental results just because that the clinical verification must last 3~5 years before the long-term curative effect can be evaluated. Usually, good effect is obtained in the experimental research, however, it is difficult to observe the remarkable clinical effect just because that the subject investigated in the lab is the mouse while the clinical object is the patient, the experimental results are not always be applied to clinic and it must be subject to the clinical verification and observation for 3~5 years even 8~10 years before the long-term reoccurrence and metastasis of cancer can be understood. Why the patients meet with the occurrence even wide metastasis and spreading where-after or before long even after the primary lesion or metastasis of these patients are appropriately even satisfactorily cured? Where these metastasis and reoccurrence cancer cells exist in which form? What causes the difference in metastasis time from several months to several years? We remain perplexed despite much thought. Where are these cancer cells hidden in the human body? Why are they so pertinacious? The popular explanation of the patients' families is that "the cancer is alive and it can move". With the enlightenment of this popular explanation, combining with the clinical practice for 49 years and the experience in diagnosis and treatment of the patients subject to metastasis and reoccurrence in the tumor outpatient service, the author realized and found that the forms of the cancer cell in human body were not only the primary lesion and metastasis; the third manifestation, namely the cancer cell and cancer cell group exist in the metastasis routing. The third manifestation has been not mentioned in the literatures and teaching books up to today. Just because that the people have not cognized it, resulting in ignore of the special manifestation of the cancer cell in the metastasis routing.

Many patients are subject to the comprehensive treatment such as radiotherapy and chemotherapy over the primary lesion or metastasis tumor by means of various traditional therapeutic methods, the cancer cell meets with metastasis chronically and duratively, thus where these cancer cells exist or hide? Through research, it is deemed by us that these cancer cells has slow or quick metastasis speed in the metastasis routing; under a certain conditions, they may meet with dormancy and rest in GO stage; sometimes, the cancer cells are active, entering the cell cycle. The so-called "condition" may be relevant to the factors such as the cancerous protuberance and local micro-environment of the host; it also be related to the cyto-dynamics of the cancer cells. In facts, these thousands of cancer cells in metastasis routing are most dangerous. They are the hidden enemy; the cancer cells with metastasis potential surviving in the metastasis routing will slowly and gradually form the new metastasis. They are in the active and slow attack. However, the presently traditional therapeutic method is to wait for the new metastasis and then cure it.

The reason why the cancer cells survive in the metastasis routing is because that it can escape the immune surveillance of the immunological cell in the blood circulation. If the cell toxicant chemotherapy is used to cure the metastasis, it is possible to kill many immunological cells, resulting in further weakening the immune surveillance of the immunological cells in the blood circulation of the patient and surviving of more cancer cells in the metastasis routing due to escaping the immune surveillance, forming more new metastasis.

So then, who kills the cancer cells transfused? Through analysis and presumption, it is possible that some cells transfused into the circulation system are killed because they do not adapt the environment or they are damaged due to the impact of the rapid blood stream or are obstructed by the impediment micro-circulation, however, most of the cancer cells entering the blood circulation, are mainly the immunizing ability of the mouse, which are killed by a large number of immunological cells in the blood circulation of the mouse. Therefore, in the treatment of anti-metastasis, the treatment of cancer cells and cancer cell groups in the metastasis routing must protect the immunizing ability of the host body and it is necessary to try to mobilize, recover and activate its immunologic function of the immune system, instead of striking, damaging and reducing or avoiding striking, damaging and reducing the immunizing ability and functions of immune system of the host body as much as possible. How to try to protect, mobilize and activate the immune functions of the host to deal with the cancer cells in metastasis routing is an important anti-metastasis strategy.

4. The Goal of Cancer Treatment Aiming at These Three Forms of Cancer

In the above, it is put forward by us there are three forms of cancer in human body, the first one is the primary lesion, the second one is the metastasis. These two forms have been cognized by us for one century, however, the third manifestation found by us is the cancer cell, cancer cell groups and micro-cancer embolus in the metastasis routing. If the new theory put forward by the author is discussed and widely accepted, it would give rise to a series of reform and renovation; for example, the reform and renovation in concept of cancer treatment; the one in goal or target of cancer treatment; the one of diagnosis method of cancer; the one of treatment methods and treatment mode of cancer and the one of research and development of the medicine for anti cancer and anti-metastasis.

Therefore, XU ZE New Concept of Cancer Treatment holds that the goal or garget of cancer treatment should synchronously aim at these three forms of cancer in human body, namely primary lesion, metastasis and the cancer cell in metastasis routing.

Why do we ablate the primary lesion? When an early tumor is just about several centimeters even below 1 cm, no symptom or sign appears and no severe damage to the parenchymatous viscera happens, why do we ablate the primary lesion?

One of the goals of surgical removal is to prevent the metastasis. This understanding is very important for the surgeons. With this understanding, they can attach great importance to the non-tumor idea in operation, can do well in the non-tumor technology and do well preventing the reoccurrence and metastasis after operation and start from the operation.

To sum up, The treatment of cancer should include not only the surgical removal of the primary lesion and treatment of metastasis by means of operation, radiotherapy or immunity chemotherapy aiming at the first two forms, but also the goal or target of the treatment aiming at the third manifestation, namely obstructing and intercepting the cancer cell groups in metastasis routing to strengthen the immune surveillance of the host body and disturb the metastasis of the cancer cells. According to the metastasis routing, the molecule metastasis mechanism of multi-step, multi-factor and multi-link of metastasis routing, design the new anti-metastasis treatment mode to disturb and intercept the cancer cell.

Why the third manifestation of cancer cell, namely the cancer cell groups in metastasis in human body is not cognized by the doctors or patients? Because that the cancer cell groups in human body in metastasis routing cannot be seen and touched or pried by the endoscope; furthermore, it cannot be examined by ultrasonic, CT, MRI and circumferential routine blood test, as a result, it cannot bring about the great attention.

In the past 100 years, generally, people attach great attention to the first manifestation, namely the primary lesion and the second manifestation, namely the metastasis existing in the human body; at present, the teaching texts at home and abroad only discuss these two forms, namely clinical manifestation, symptom and sign. However, the third manifestation found and put forward by us at home and abroad is the cancer cell groups and micro-metastasis in metastasis routing, although no clinical manifestation exists, it exist exactly. Only when it reaches up to molecule organism level, gene level and molecule immune level, can it be found and cognized, such as the various excessive expressions of the tumor signs developed at present, the change of molecule immune gene and the existence of micro-metastasis. The existence of individual cancer cell in the blood and bone marrow can be detected at molecule level; the indexes, molecule immune indexes, cytokine and sign of tumor can be detected by the new examination method at molecule level so as to improve the diagnosis and treatment level of the cancer metastasis. We believe in the coming future, the early diagnosis of precancer and micro-metastasis and the early treatment at gene level will be realized surely.

The author holds that the traditional fundamental theory of cancer, diagnosis and treatment of cancer metastasis are at the cell level. In the 21 century, the fundamental theory, examination and diagnosis as well as treatment of the cancer and cancer metastasis will reach up to the level of molecular biology, gene and molecule immune and other molecule oncology.

References

1. Xu Ze, New Understanding and New Modes of Carcinomatous treatment. Wuhan: Hubei Science and Technology Press, 2001, 3-6
2. Xu Zhe, New Concepts and New Methods of Treatment of Carcinomatous Metastasis. Beijing: People's Military Medical Press, 2006, 1-3

CHAPTER 8

Two Points and One Line of Carcinoma Development

[Abstract]

Objectives: To probe into the whole process of carcinoma development and metastasis.

Methods: To deeply analyze the mutual relations, subordinate relationship and dynamic relations among the primary lesion, the metastasis and the cancer cell in metastasis routing in the process of carcinoma metastasis.

Results: Finding and putting forward one new idea or concept, namely two points and one line of carcinoma metastasis and putting forward that it is necessary to attach great importance to the two points and cut off one line in treatment.

Conclusions: the new concept put forward by us attaches importance to the surgical removal or radiotherapy and chemotherapy of primary lesion and metastasis as well as the interception and killing of the cancer cells in the metastasis routing. This new idea, called "Two Points and One Line" is very significant just because it opens up one new field for fundamental experiment and clinical practice research of carcinoma.

[Keywords] Primary Carcinoma; Metastatic Carcinoma; Metastasis; Cancer Cell

Introduction

It is put forward by us that the carcinoma existing in human body has three manifestations, including primary carcinoma, metastatic carcinoma and the cancer cell groups in metastasis routing, then, what is the mutual relations among these three manifestations and how do they interact each other? What are the dynamic relations among them in the whole process of carcinoma development? It is advantageous to further illuminate the specific concept and work of anti-metastasis through deeply probing into the dynamic relations among them in the whole process of the carcinoma development.

The carcinoma development is a gradual, orderly, dynamic, continuous, multi-step, multi-link, multi-link and complicated process of cellular molecular biology. Through study and analysis, one new idea is put forward by the author, namely Two Points and One Line of Carcinomas Development.

1. One of the objectives of carcinoma treatment is to prevent metastasis

Why the malignant tumor should be treated? Just because of its hazardness. In case that it is not treated, it will meet with evolution, invasion, metastasis and transmission from head to foot. Why the primary carcinoma should be subject to surgical removal? Just because that if it is not removed, it will meet with evolution, invasion, metastasis and then transmission with the blood from the head to foot. Therefore, it is necessary to remove the original place of the cancer cell metastasis. Why the metastatic carcinoma should be treated or removed? (The single metastatic carcinoma can be removed; however, however, the metastatic carcinomas are mainly composed of many single metastatic carcinoma, most of which cannot be removed and then treated with radiotherapy or chemotherapy or intervention, radio frequency and ultrasound focusing and so on). Because that the metastatic carcinoma is not treated, it will continue to transfer, in this way, every metastatic carcinoma is another original place of new metastasis.

Therefore, one of the essential objectives of treatment of primary carcinoma or metastatic carcinoma through surgical removal or radiotherapy and chemotherapy is to prevent the metastasis so as to try to remove the original place of cancer cell metastasis.

In the past dozens of years, what has been done by us has been in this manner, however, the textbooks have not clearly pointed out that one of the essential objectives is to prevent the metastasis as early as possible. Based on this know understanding, attention must be paid to that all administer drugs or technical measures shall be advantageous to prevent the metastasis of cancer cell but not promote or increase the opportunity of cancer cell metastasis in operation or radiotherapy or chemotherapy so as to result in the iatrogenic metastasis and dissemination. For example, the removal of tumor through surgical operation, no matter the operation is large or small, it is necessary to attach great importance to and abide by the ideal and technology of no tumor and the surgeons should pay equal attention to the idea of no tumor and the idea of no bacteria. Even the technology of non-tumor is more strict that the abacterial technology. It is possible for the surgical knife, the surgical scissor, the needle and the thread in operation as well as every operation technology to promote the metastasis of cancer cell, as may increase with the bad operations by the operator on the tumor body or tumor organization such as excessive extrusion, eversion, needle threading and cutting and so on. These probabilities of implantation, diffusion and metastasis of iatrogenic cancer cells caused by operation have been proved by the molecular biology or immunohistochemical method up to today: when not a few of cases are in operation, the cancer cells can be found in the blood circulation or the transformation of cancer cell from Yin to Yang before operation shows that the operation has the possibility to bring about the diffusion of cancer cells. Meanwhile, it shows that some recurrence and metastasis cases may be caused by the improper operation, such as the implantation of incision and so on. Therefore, it is necessary to do some work in the operation so as to prevent the recurrence and metastasis after operation.

When the primary carcinoma or metastatic carcinoma is only 1cm large, no symptom appears, no discomfort happens, no damage to the function of the organ happens, then why it should be removed? Just because of removal of it as early as possible so as to prevent the metastasis. Why should the tumor completely be removed as early as possible? Just for thoroughly preventing the metastasis as early as possible.

Why should the metastasis of the tumor be prevented? The metastasis is the characteristic of malignant tumor; the reason why the malignant tumor is malignant is that the cancer cells of the malignant tumor are transferred and diffused. It is well-known that the main discrimination between the venign tumor and the malignant tumor is that the former is transferred while the latter is not transferred. If both of them are surgically removed, the former will not recur and meet with the metastasis while the latter will recur and meet with metastasis frequently.

2. Two Points and One Line of Carcinoma Development

Through the experiments on animals for anticancer and anti-metastasis made by us for 15 years and the analysis, reflection and experience in the personal clinical practice cases of the author for 50 years, an understanding or idea of the carcinoma development has been gradually formed, which is the so-called "Two Points and One Line". What is "Two Points and One Line"? "Two Points" means the starting point of metastasis, namely the primary carcinoma and the end point of metastasis, namely the metastatic carcinoma. "One Line" means one route of the cancer cells transferring to the remote organs through trudge between these two points, namely the primary carcinoma and the metastasic carcinoma. See Fig. 3-1.

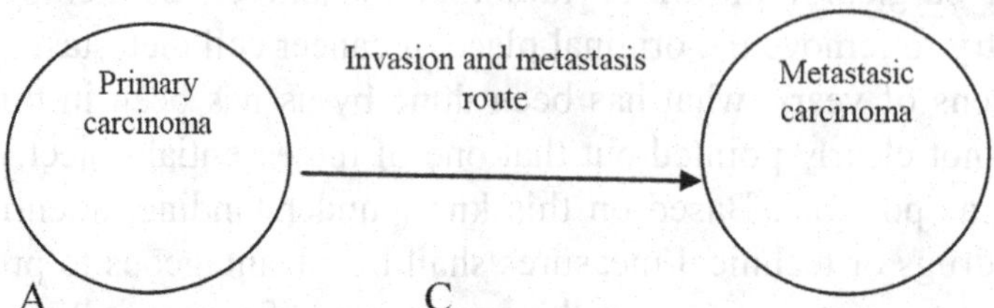

Fig. 3-1 Sketch Map of Two Points and One Line of Carcinoma Development

Note: A. Primary carcinoma, the starting point of metastasis; B. Invasion and metastasis route; C. Metastasic carcinoma, the end point of metastasis

The metastasis rule of the biologic behavior of one cancer cell shall be:

Dropping out of the primary carcinoma, transferring through lymph path and (or) the route of blood circulation, trudging to the amphi position target organ of the metastasic nidation and settling down and growing into the metastasic tumor node.

In the two points in Fig. 3-1, Point A is the starting point of metastasis and Point C is the end point of metastasis, however, these two points have different means and their treatment methods shall be different from each other. The starting point is the primary carcinoma and it is the metastasis place of protogenesis, generally speaking, there is only one starting point; while Point C is the end point and it is also the subsequent metastasic carcinoma; sometimes there are many metastasic carcinomas; of course, it is possible that one metastasic carcinoma appears firstly and then another metastasic carcinomas appear. As to the primary carcinoma within the operative indication, it can be treated with surgical removal; however, as to the metastasic carcinoma, if only one local metastasic carcinoma that can be removed, it can surely be removed. However, in the clinical work, there are sometimes many metastasic carcinomas which occur in different periods successively, in this way, it is impossible to remove them through surgical operation, let alone the radical treatment.

No matter the primary carcinoma as the starting point or the metastasic carcinoma as the end point, when the carcinoma grows into a certain size, it will also become the new source of the metastasis of the deciduous cancer cells. These metastasic carcinoma can meet with metastasis again and become the starting point of the metastasis in the second round, in this way, the former Pont C becomes Pint A' which arrives at C', the end point of the metastasis in the second round via one line. If this metastasis lasts gradually, it will finally endanger the patient's life. See Fig. 3-2:

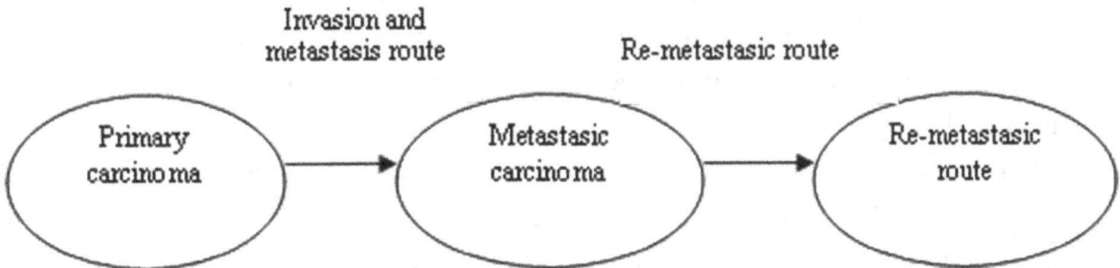

Fig. 3-2 Sketch map of re-metastasis of metastasic carcinoma

Note: A' is the new starting point; B' is the re-metastasic route; C' is the new end point

3. Traditional carcinoma therapeutics only paying attention to "Two Point" but neglecting "One Line"

In the past one century, the three traditional therapies, including surgical operation, radiotherapy and chemotherapy, only pay attention to Two Points. When one primary tumor of the patient is found, it shall firstly take the surgical removal of the primary carcinoma into account; if it can be removed, remove it. In case of failure to surgical removal, the radiotherapy and chemotherapy shall be carried out. In case of the metastasic carcinoma, it shall take the surgical removal of the metastasic carcinoma into account (in fact, most of them cannot be surgically removed). In case of failure to surgical removal, radiotherapy, chemotherapy and other local treatment shall be taken into account. The above-mentioned therapies are correct, however, their goal or target mainly focuses on Two Points but neglects One Line, namely not considering how to take prevention and treatment measures for the cancer cells in the route of metastasis. Actually, it is key to cut off One Line so as to overcome the carcinoma. Anti-metastasis is the core of carcinoma treatment.

4. XU ZE New Concept of Carcinoma Treatment holding attention shall be paid not only to Two Points but also to cutting off One Line

It is well-known that although carcinoma is not infectious, one of the joint biological characteristics of cancer cell is metastasis. Generally, the cancer cell has one biological behavior or habit: it can be separated and dropped out of the carcinoma tumor, enter lymph path or blood circulation, transfer and migrate to another amphi position organ via a certain metastasic path and route and nidate and grow into the metastasic carcinoma.

Through analysis of the experimental data in the lab for probing the metastasis rule and the clinical information of many metastasis cases in the specialized tumor outpatient combining traditional Chinese medicine and Western medicine, it can be summarized by us that the metastasis flow of cancer cell is quite similar with the one of the infectious diseases.

1. The three largest factors of infectious diseases include: ① source of infection; ②channel of infection; ③ the crowd liable to infection. The metastasis of cancer cell also has three largest factors: ① source of metastasis; ②channel of metastasis; ③ the organ liable to infection.

2. Countermeasure to cure the infectious diseases: ① isolate to cure the patient suffering from infectious diseases; ② cutting off channel of infection; ③ enhance the immunity of the crowd liable to infection. It is held by the author that the countermeasures for curing the metastasis of carcinoma can also adopt the similar principle: ① Curing primary carcinoma,

(surgical removal or radiotherapy); ② cutting off channel of metastasis, interfering, intercepting and killing the cancer cells in route of metastasis; ③ enhancing the immune surveillance ability of the organism and improving the anticancer ability of the human body. However, the control over the infectious disease (for example, control over SARS) is the epidemiologic control in the macro-environment in the society while the control over the metastasis of cancer cell is to interfere the metastasis of cancer cell in the micro-environment of organism of the host. The above-mentioned therapeutic methods can be summarized as Fig. 3-3:

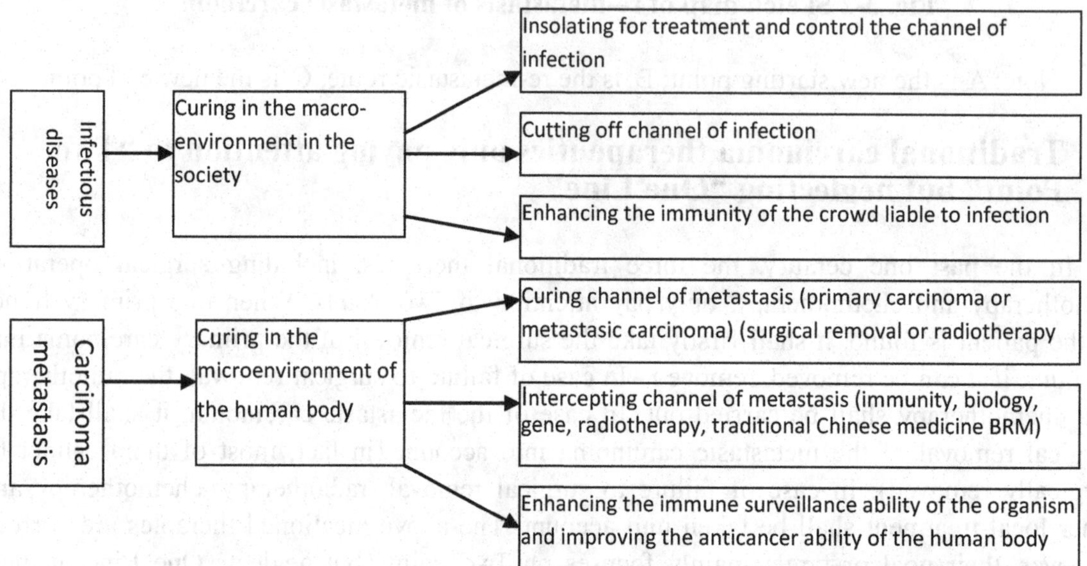

Fig. 3-3 Therapeutic method of infectious diseases and carcinoma metastasis

To sum up, it can be seen that XU ZE New Concept of Carcinoma Treatment pays attention not only to the surgical removal, radiotherapy and chemotherapy of primary carcinoma and metastasic carcinoma but also to intercepting and killing the cancer cells in the route of metastasis. This new theory called "Two Points and One Line" has the following important significance:

(1) Making the goal or target of anti-metastasis more clear and specific;
(2) Further supplementing an perfecting the countermeasures or strategy of traditional carcinoma therapeutics;
(3) Emphasizing that the anti-metastasis shall pay attention not only to "Two Points" but also "One Line". Only the cancer cells in the route of metastasis are cut off, can the curative effect of carcinoma treatment can be improved.
(4) Making the people relatively clearly understand the metastasis of carcinoma, putting forward a new theoretic basis, which is advantageous for the clinicians to reasonably design and make use of the existing various therapeutic methods and probe into the new therapeutic methods.
(5) Opening up a new field for fundamental experimental research and clinical practice research of carcinoma.

References

1. Xu Ze, New Understanding and New Modes of Carcinomatous treatment. Wuhan: Hubei Science and Technology Press, 2001, 3-6
2. Xu Zhe, New Concepts and New Methods of Treatment of Carcinomatous Metastasis. Beijing: People's Military Medical Press, 2006, 15-18

CHAPTER 9

Three Steps of Therapy of Carcinoma Metastasis

Xu Ze[1] Xu Jie[2]

[Abstract]

Objectives: Probing into the detailed strategies of therapy of carcinoma metastasis.

Methods: Deeply analyzing "Eight Steps" and "Three Stages" of carcinoma metastasis and trying to destroy the metastasis steps respectively.

Results: Putting forward the three countermeasures for therapy of carcinoma metastasis, namely "Three-Steps" through analysis.

Conclusions: The space allocation of XU ZE Three Steps of Therapy of Carcinoma Metastasis is in blood circulation and its time allocation is in three different stages. XU ZE Three Steps of Therapy of Carcinoma Metastasis attach importance to the immunity of the host and improvement of immune surveillance of the immunological cells in blood circulation on the cancer cells in the routing of metastasis.

[Keywords]: Anti carcinoma metastasis; three steps; immune surveillance

1. Try to Do Well in Each Step

As to how to make clearer the extremely complicated dynamic and continuous biological process of carcinoma metastasis with multi-step and multi-element, through repeated thinking and carefully analysis, we summed up and put forward Eight Steps of Metastasis of Cancer Cells in the aforesaid. Based on Eight Steps, we tried to make clearer and more particular of the concept of extremely complicated dynamic and continuous biological process of carcinoma metastasis with multi-step and multi-element with respect to understanding. In order to take scientific measures to obstruct and intercept each metastasis step and destroy it one by one, it is necessary to make clear the concept of each step in the metastasis process. Only when the target of each step is made clear, can the prevention and cure countermeasures be carried out, researched and probed into.

In the above, we have mentioned "Three Stages" of carcinoma metastasis and illuminated it in details. The reason why "Three Stage" is put forward is that one of the keys to therapy of cancer is to anti metastasis, however, at present, the understanding of the concept of metastasis

1 Xu Ze, male, Dr. tutor, Professor of surgery,; Chief of the Dept. of Surgery Affiliated Hospital Hubei College of Traditional Chinese Medicine; Director of Institute of Experimental Surgery of Hubei College of Traditional Chinese Medicine; Member of the International Liver Research Center; Chief of Hubei Branch of China Anti Cancer Research Society of Traditional Chinese Medicine and West Medicine.

2 Xu Jie, Department of Surgery Affiliated Hospital College of Traditional Chinese Medicine Correspondence to: xuze88cn@yahoo.com.cn

is still ambiguous and it is not clear and particular. People only understand the severity of the harm of the metastasis to the patients, however, it lacks of effective prevention and therapeutic countermeasures with clear concept and detailed profile. In order to take scientific measures to obstruct and intercept each metastasis step, based on the Eight Steps, Three Stages and the molecular mechanism of carcinoma metastasis, we try to establish the preventive and therapeutic countermeasures for each stage and called it Xu Ze Three Steps of Therapy of Carcinoma Metastasis.

2. Trying to Get a Good Idea about the Object

The basic process of carcinoma metastasis is: the cancer cell falling from the primary tumor—degrading the basement membrance—migrating into blood capillary and small vein—survived cancer cell adhering to endothelial cell of blood capillary or basement membrance under the exposed endothelium—passing through wall—growing up in the remote target organ and forming the metastatic carcinoma, which is an extremely complicated, dynamic and continuous biological process, composed of several relatively independent but interlocked steps. In each step, a series of molecular biological events will happen between cancer cells, and between the cancer cells and the host cells, finishing the whole metastatic process and finally forming the metastatic carcinoma.

That is to say, it is necessary for the cancer cells to be subject to and finish the whole metastatic process before forming the metastatic carcinoma. any failure of each step will result in the stop of the whole metastatic process, which presents that if we take measures to destroy the metastatic steps one by one and carry out the strategy and tactics of obstruction and interception of the cancer cells in the routing of the metastasis, it is certainly possible to break or intercept the metastatic routing and intercept and kill the cancer cells in the routing of metastasis.

Xu Ze New Concept and Mode of Therapy of Carcinoma and Carcinoma Metastasis are to try to intercept one or several steps or links of the above-mentioned metastatic process so as to control the metastasis.

In order to realize the above-mentioned objectives, what measures shall be taken by us for anti metastasis? With which theory? Which technology and which drug? In which step or in which stage and link to intercept the cancer cells in the routing of the metastasis?

3. Three Steps of Therapy of Carcinoma Metastasis

1. First step of anti carcinomatous metastasis: in this stage, the metastatic process of cancer cells is as follows: cancer cells falling from the primary carcinoma—adhering to the stroma outside the cells—degrading ECM to open up a road for cancer cells—carrying out cell movement via the adherence of degraded stroma or the degraded stroma for adherence—then arriving at the external wall—degrading basement membrane of blood vessel—doing Amoeba movement, firstly stretching out the pseudopodium—then passing through the wall.

   Prevention and cure countermeasures: this stage is the intervention and repression countermeasure before the cancer cell falls from the primary carcinoma and enters the blood vessel. In this stage, the therapeutic "targets" are mainly anti-adherence, anti-degradation, anti-movement and anti cancer cell attack. The therapeutic goal is to prevent the cancer cells from entering the blood vessel so as to realize the goal of "turning the enemy back at the border".

2. Second step of anti carcinomatous metastasis: in this stage, the metastasis process of cancer cell: it will pass through the wall and enter the blood circulation. The cancer cell will be interweaved in various blood cell components including blood plasma and blood or will be adhered to cancer cell group together with homo-cancer cell, or will be adhered to slight cancer embolus together with the alloplasm such as blood platelet and white blood cell and float in venous system→turn back to the right ventricle→circulate→enter pulmonary vein→turn back to left ventricle together with the venous blood, some cancer cells can stay in the pulmonary microcirculation blood vessel (forming the pulmonary metastasis lesion), some will enter the pulmonary vein→turn back to the left ventricle via the pulmonary microcirculation. The cancer cell, interweaved in the blood, enters the aorta and then jets into the small artery of the parenchymatous viscera and then enters the microcirculation of each organ (especially the parenchymatous organ, such as liver, kidney, brain and porotic substance of bone through the impact force and vertex flow and pump flow of the heart valve blood. Most of the cancer cells in the circulation will be damaged and killed by the immunological cells in the circulation or the strong blood impact force and shearing force, the tiny minority of the survived cancer cells form the micro-cancer embolus, adhering to the endothelial cell of the micrangium, degrading the basement membrance and passing through the blood vessel.

   In this stage, the cancer cell will contact various immunological cells in floating in the blood circulation and cannot survive possibly due to being captured and phagocytized by various immunological cells in the blood. Few survived cancer cells will be adhered to the endothelial cell of the blood vessel due to escaping from the monitoring of the immunity in the blood circulation.

   Prevention and cure countermeasures: in this stage, the "target" of therapy of carcinoma metastasis is to protect and enhance the immunologic function of various immunological cells in the blood circulation, activate the immunological cytokine and resist adherence (homogenous adherence of cancer cells and cancer cells, alloplasmatic adherence of cancer cells with blood platelet and so on), resist movement, resist aggregation of blood platelet, resist high coagulation and resist cancer embolus.

   Therapeutic goal: activating the immunological cell, protecting function of thymus organization, improving immunity, protecting the bone marrow and producing the blood and promoting the cancer cells floating in the blood circulation to be captured, phagocytized, surrounded and annihilated and intercepted by the immunological cell group.

   The second step is the main battlefield to kill off the cancer cells floating in the blood circulation as well as the main countermeasures to interfere and repress the carcinoma metastasis.

3. Third Step of anti carcinomatous metastasis: the metastasis process of the cancer cell in this stage: the cancer cell escapes the monitoring of the immunological cell in blood circulation and the annihilation of the immunological cell, passes through the wall and anchors itself in the organs with agreeable local microenvironment for settlement, in this way, the new blood capillary of tumor forms and then it gradually forms the metastatic carcinoma.

Prevention and cure countermeasures: the interference and repression countermeasures, mainly aiming at improving the histogenic immunity of the local microenvironment and regulating the local microenvironment to make it adverse to the survival and nidation and repress the angiogenesis factor and the new angiogenesis.

To sum up, space allocation of Xu Ze Three Steps of Therapy of Carcinoma Metastasis is in the blood circulation and the time allocation is in three different stages. It attaches importance to improvement of the host immunity. It can be summed up and concluded as Table 10-1

Table 10. 1 Xu Ze Three Steps of Therapy of Carcinoma Metastasis

Metastasis stage of cancer cell	Metastasis process	Prevention and cure countermeasures
The stage before the cancer cell intrudes the circulation First step of anti metastasis	Separating the cancer cell from the primary cancer→degrading ECM→adherence and de-adherence→movement→before entering the blood vessel.	• anti-adherence anti-degradation anti-movement anti stroma metal protease
Transportation stage of cancer cell in blood circulation Second step of anti-metastasis	The cancer cell group and micro cancer embolus float in the blood circulation and are damaged due to being phagocytized and captured by the immunological cell and be subject to the shearing force of the blood.	• enhancing and activating various immunological cells in circulation, improving the immunologic function as the main battlefield of killing off the cancer cells in the routing of the metastasis
The stage in which Cancer cell escapes the blood circulation and anchors "target" organ Third step of anti metastasis	After cancer cell escapes from the blood vessel, it anchors the organ for nidation, forms the new blood vessel and forms the metastatic lesion.	• anti-adherence anti-aggregation of blood platelet anti cancer embolus • TG • Inhibiting angiogenesis factor • Inhibiting angiogenesis • Improving immunological regulation • Improving the immunity of local microenvironment.

The metastatic lesion is not the terminal. When the metastatic lesion grows up to a certain size, it has the cancer cells separated, intruded and transferred, in this way, it will become a new original place of the cancer cell metastasis. At this moment, the primary lesion and metaststic lesion will become the original place of the ablation and metastasis of the cancer cells via blood metastasis. Therefore, the more and larger the metastatic carcinoma is, the more the cancer cells in the blood circulation are. The number of the immunological cells in the blood circulation of the body of the patient is far insufficient for controlling a large number of cancer cells falling from the carcinoma lesion and entering the blood circulation. The immunologic function of the organism will be severely unbalanced, even the immunologic function will break down, resulting in the hematogenous dissemination. At this time, the organism of the patient will meet with the functional crisis of the immunologic cells. As to how to perfect and deal with this situation, there are only two methods, one is foreign aid and another is endogeny. The foreign aid is the transplantation of stem cell and the endogeny is bioremediation, immunological therapy, genetherapy, molecular biological therapy, treatment by Chinese herbs, Z-C immunologic regulation therapy by Chinese herbs and BRM therapy.

References

1. Xu Ze, New Understanding and New Modes of Carcinomatous treatment. Wuhan: Hubei Science and Technology Press, 2001, 3-6
2. Xu Zhe, New Concepts and New Methods of Treatment of Carcinomatous Metastasis. Beijing: People's Military Medical Press, 2006, 53-55

CHAPTER 10

Pioneer the Third Field of Anti-carcinoma-metastasis

[Abstract]

Objectives: probe into and pioneer the third field of therapy of carcinoma metastasis

Methods: through reviewing, analyzing, evaluating and thinking a large number of cases in the clinical medical practice for half a century, put forward the new findings, new understanding and new theoretical concept in clinical basic theory.

Results: it is found that the new specific measures for therapy of carcinoma metastasis are to obstruct and intercept the cancer cells in routing of metastasis. Furthermore, it puts forward the necessity and feasibility of pioneering the third field of therapy of carcinoma metastasis.

Conclusions: finding and putting forward the third field of therapy of carcinoma metastasis. The main battlefield for killing off the cancer cells in routing of metastasis is in the blood circulation and the most important is to improve the immune regulation and immune surveillance.

[Keywords]: Carcinoma metastasis; Cancer cells in routing of carcinoma metastasis; Immune regulation

Introduction

We have discussed the three forms of existence of carcinoma in a body in another paper, including primary tumor, namely primary lesion, the secondary tumor, namely metastatic lesion, which have attracted attention from the people for a century up to today and are the target of various therapeutic measures, operations, radiotherapy and chemotherapy. While the third form, namely the cancer cells in routing of metastasis, has not been recognized and reported in the literatures by the people up to today and is firstly put forward by us through the experimental study for years and after analysis and thinking of clinical practice. The first two forms of existence are the existence of big or small tumors, most of which are the cancer cells that can be seen or palpated or can be seen with endoscope or have space occupying lesions through X-ray photograph or B-ultrasonic, CT and MRI or can be seen through pathological examination such as slice of operation specimen, aspiration biopsy or examination of exfoliated cells and so on. The therapeutic measures adopt surgical removal of tumor in early stage and radiotherapy and chemotherapy of tumor in middle and late stage to shrink and remit the tumor. The third form of existence of the cancerous protuberance in a body, namely the cancer cells in routing of metastasis cannot be seen or palpated or examined by B-ultrasonic, CT and MRI, which are potential and hidden. Then, how to prove the scientificalness of the existence?

I. Odd carcinoma cells can be found in blood, medulla and lymph node

1. The adhesive force between the carcinoma cells is relatively smaller than the one between the normal cells, in this way, the carcinoma cells will easily drop out from the corpus carcinosus and invade the lymphatic vessel and blood vessel. The phenomenon that the cancer cell easily drops out was found in 1930s and the cancer cell could be found in the blood, later it was found that when the corpus carcinosus was pressurized, the venous blood of the drainage tumor had a large number of cancer cells.
2. As to the patient suffering from carcinomatosis not accompanied with distant metastasis, the individual tumor cells (ITC) can be detected in the bone marrow of 20%~50% cases. Since the tumors are in different places, the above-mentioned circumstances differ from each other greatly. The positive detectable rate of the individual tumor cancer in the bone marrow and the regional lymph node has a certain relation with the location of the primary tumor.
3. In the recent 10 years, since molecular biology and molecular immunology have made great progress, many marks of tumor have been found, the detection items with respect to the related indexes of the tumor metastasis have been increased and some new indexes have been found successively. The related indexes of the tumor cell metastasis are transferring to clinic from the fundamental experiment to offer the basis to the occurrence of the metastasis of the cancer cells step by step. Taking CK_{19}mRNA as the mark, it can detect CTS_S in the blood circulation around the lung cancer patient and its positive detectable rate can reach up to 50%. Therefore, $keratin_{19}$mRNA (CK_{19}MRNA) in the peripheral blood can be regarded as the mark of hematogenous dissemination of the lung cancer. The positive detectable rate of AFPmRNA in the blood of the patient suffering from micro-metastasis of lung cancer and extrahepatic distant organ metastasis is 100% and AFPmRNA in the peripheral venous blood can be regarded as the mark of the hematogenous metastasis of lung cancer.

II. Xu Ze pioneers the third field of anti-carcinoma-metastasis

The first form of existence of carcinoma in a body is the primary lesion and all the therapies aiming at the primary lesion are called the first field of anti-carcinoma-metastasis; the second form of existence of carcinoma in a body is the metastatic lesion and all the therapies aiming at the carcinoma metastasis (radiotherapy, chemotherapy, intervention and some local therapeutic programs) are called the second field of anti-carcinoma-metastasis. Now it is recognized and put forward by us that the third form of existence of carcinoma in a body is the cancer cell in routing of metastasis, then, all of the therapeutic methods aiming at the cancer cells in routing of metastasis are called the third field (or the third battlefront) of anti-carcinoma-metastasis by us for the moment.

(a) Necessity of putting forward the third field of anti-carcinoma-metastasis

Why is the third field of anti-carcinoma-metastasis put forward and carried out?

It has been mentioned above that the author has found that most patients have met with reoccurrence or metastasis within 2~3 years after operation after follow-up survey of over 3000 patients after carcinoma operation on breast and abdomen. Through detailed analysis, evaluation and reflection of part of the cases suffering from reoccurrence or metastasis, why do the patients meet with reoccurrence or metastasis after standardized radical treatment of the carcinoma? Now that the radical primary carcinoma is removed and the radical regional lymph node is cleaned down, why do the patients meet with the reoccurrence and metastasis after operation in a short time? Where are the residual cancer cells incubated? How many? What is its movement rule? Through repeated meditation, the author has been aware that these cancer cells may be beyond the regional lymph node; or some cancer cells enter the blood circulation through lymph path; or some cancer cells are extruded into the blood circulation in operation. These cancer cells are in routing of metastasis and they are potentially and slowly metastatic, some are monitored, phagocytized and captured by the immunological cells in the blood circulation and some are in dormancy. Some form the metastatic lesion rapidly. The author remembered that in the spring of 1957, a large node just like a mung bean was touched in the upper quadrant out of the left breast on a young patient without any discomfort. It was removed in the clinical operation and it was reported as mammary cancer after 7 days. Then the radical treatment operation was carried out immediately. In the operation, it was found that the metastasis happened in the fifth rib at the left, after the fifth rid was removed, it was reported as metastatic carcinoma. The metastatic lesion of this patient formed so rapidly, just in a week, which was an alert for us. However, some patients' metastatic lesions formed slowly, lasting several months even 1~2 years, the cancer cells in the routing of metastasis were in rest and sleep state. For example, a patient surnamed Li, male, aged 50, was found that he met with effractin of liver cancer at the left in the examination for an emergency treatment of the effractin of liver. It was removed. After the operation, he came to tumor clinic department and took Z-C Medicine orally for treatment. One and a half year passed after operation, it was found that a large node just like a broad bean was protrudent at the incision of the abdominal wall and then it was removed and the abdominal cavity was detected and no abnormity was found in the hepatic skin, gold-beater's skin and omentum of the abdominal cavity. The node was only limited to the incision of the abdominal wall and the pathological section was hepatic cell cancer. He continued to take Z-C Medicine and then got better after 3 years. It was obvious that the node of the incision cancer was implanted by the incision in the first operation and the cancer cells in implantation metastasis in operation had been in the state of dormancy for one and a half year.

The above-mentioned cancer cell in the routing of metastasis is actually the third form of existence of carcinoma in a body and it is absolutely necessary to take measures pioneer the third field for carcinoma therapeutics.

(b) Probability of intercepting the cancer cells in routing of metastasis

The formation of metastatic lesion is the most important turning point. Before metastasis, the carcinoma is only a local problem and good curative effect can be obtained with the local therapeutics. However, when it is metastatic, the local therapeutics cannot cure the patient any more. Therefore, the therapeutics for metastasis is most important. In this stage, there are thousands of cancer cells entering the blood circulation everyday, however, only less than 0.01% of the cancer cells become the metastatic lesions finally. Therefore, it is necessary and possible to carry out the therapeutics for metastasis through intercepting or killing off the cancer cells in routing of metastasis; if appreciate measures are taken to activate the immunological cells in the blood, improve the immunological surveillance of the immunological cells and activate the immunological cell factors, it is possible to intercept the cancer cells in routing of metastasis.

How to intercept and kill off the cancer cells in routing of metastasis?

The patient suffering from carcinoma has low immunologic function, especially the low immunologic function of cells with the development of tumor day by day. The key is how to break through the inhibition of the tumor to the immune system and activate the effective immunological reaction especially the one based on T cell.

The abnormal immune micro-environment, leading to no effective immunological reaction of the organism, is the important factor of immune escape, easy metastasis and reoccurrence of the carcinoma. How to effectively regulate the immunologic function of the host and improve the local immune micro-environment so as to be advantageous to the anti-cancer effect of the host, is an important and effective measure to prevent the metastasis and reoccurrence of the carcinoma after operation and eliminate the residual cancer cells as well as the important content of integrated therapeutics of the carcinoma.

III. Circle system has lots of immune surveillance cells

The cancer cells are intercepted, captured and killed off by the immunological cells in the blood circulation, therefore, it can be said that the blood circulation is the main battlefield of killing off the cancer cells in the routing of metastasis and the immunological cells are the effective strength to kill off the cancer cells.

The circulation system owns lots of immune surveillance cells, which can kill, wound and phagocytize the cancer cells with heterosexual antigen, together with the impact force and the shearing force of the blood stream, the single adrift cancer cell cannot survive. In order to escape from the interception of eth immunological cells, the cancer cells will be adhesive to the blood platelet on the inner wall of the blood vessel and endothelial cells will meet with ameba movement in the inner wall of the blood vessel and it will pass through the blood capillary and settle in the new viscera, gradually forming the new metastatic lesion.

Based on the above-mentioned understanding, XU ZE held it should protect, activate and increase the immunological cells (NK cell, T cell and phagocyte and so on) in the blood circulation. The detailed measures: ① using Z-C Medicine, which can enhance and activate the immunological cells; ② Amidogen alkali can disperse the adhesion of the cancer cells, making the cancer cell group in free state so that the immunological cells phagocytize them one by one. ③ Heparin and medicine for invigorating the circulation of blood and removing blood stasis, preventing the agglutination of the blood platelet, preventing the adhesion of cancer embolus and wall so as to prevent it from passing through the blood vessel and escaping from the immune. Taking the blood circulation as the main battlefield for killing off the cancer cells in routing of metastasis through blood mainly depends on T cell, NK cell, LAK cell and phagocyte; it will prevent the aggregation of blood platelet to prevent the escape of the cancer cells after passing through the blood vessel and the anti-blood fibrin will be used to make T cell identify its antigen.

IV. Xu Ze's new concept and new model of anti-carcinoma-metastasis

a Basic model of anti-carcinoma-metastasis

Among a lot of patients in the clinical practice, it can be found frequently that the assistant chemotherapy cannot prevent the metastasis in some patients after operation. Some patients even meet with metastasis while chemotherapy and re-metastasis while re-chemotherapy. It makes us hold communion with ourselves: why we cannot prevent the metastasis? Whether is the traditional chemotherapy not suitable for the actual condition of the biological properties in the metastasis of cancer cells? With respect to the prevention and curing the cancerous metastasis, whether is it necessary to update the understanding and thinking and whether is it necessary to change the concept and therapeutic mode? XU ZE'S design idea of anti-carcinoma-metastasis is the innovation of the concept, thinking, method and mode of anti-carconoma-metastasis of the traditional therapeutics.

The anti-metastasis drugs refer to the ones interfering or intercepting some link or step of the cancer cells or cancer cell group in the process of metastasis so as to inhibit the formation of metastatic lesion. Although the poison for chemotherapy of cell can kill and wound the tumor cells, postpone the growth of the primary carcinoma and put off the metastasis time, it has no inhibition on the invasion and metastasis process. At present, it lacks of the ideal drugs for killing and wounding the primary carcinoma and inhibiting the invasion and metastasis. Then, we study the measures for interception, prevention and therapy only aiming at the development mechanism of "Eight Steps and Three Stages" of the carcinoma metastasis.

b. Detailed project of anti-carcinoma-metastasis

According to the biological behavior of modern oncology about carcinoma metastasis and the theory of reoccurrence and metastasis, in the past years, this lab has been finding the new drug for anti-carcinoma-metastasis from the natural herbs. In the experimental study of tumor-bearing animal body, the method of traditional Chinese herbs combined with western medicine is adopted by us to interfere and intercept each link of the metastasis steps. Moreover, Z-C immune regulation series anti-metastasis projects and measures are researched and developed.

The carcinoma metastasis is a multi-step and multi-link complicated process, the measures for anti-carcinoma-metastasis shall be comprehensive and they are assorted with each other. Do not rely on one drug or one method, through scientific design, aiming at the metastasis step, we take the different therapeutic methods and countermeasures, see Table 1, which aims at the metastasis step to realize the same goal of anti-metastasis.

Table 1 New Mode of Anti-Carcinoma-Metastasis in XU ZE New Concept (Therapeutic Method and Countermeasures Aiming at Carcinoma Metastasis)

Metastasis step	Therapeutic method	Z-C immune regulation medicine and its role
Hyperplasia of primary cancer	Operation, radiotherapy and chemotherapy	$Z\text{-}C_1$ inhibiting cancer cells $Z\text{-}C_4$ protecting chest and improving immune $Z\text{-}C_8$ protecting bone marrow and hematogenesis
Growth of new blood vessel of tumor	Inhibiting growth of blood vessel	Z-C-TG anti blood vessel formation Z-C-CA anti-adhesion

Invading basement membrance	Anti-adhesion, anti-movement Inhibiting activity of hydrolase	Z-C-K (LWF) anti-adhesion Ind anti PGE2 Z-C-MD anti movement
Passing through blood vessel or lymph	Anti-adhesion, anti-movement Inhibiting activity of hydrolase	Z-CMD anti-invasion blood vessel Z-C-K (LWF) $Z\text{-}C_{1+4}$ immune regulation
In the blood of circulation system	Anti-agglomeration of blood platelet, anti-agglomeration, biological reaction regulation BRM	Z-C-K (LWF) anti adhesion Z-C-N (CZR) anti agglomeration of blood adhesion Z-C-LM Z-C-ASP cancer dissolve plug $Z\text{-}C_{1+4}$ immune regulation
Formation of cancer plug	Anti-thrombus, invigorating the circulation of blood and removing blood stasis	Z-C-K (NSR) anti-cancer plug Z-C-N (CZR)
Passing through blood vessel	Anti-adhesion, anti-movement and anti activity of aminopeptodrate enzyme	Z-C-MD anti out-invasion of blood vessel
Formation of metastatic lesion	Operation, radiotherapy and chemotherapy	$Z\text{-}C_{1+4}$ immune regulation Z-C-TG inhibiting growth of blood vessel
Metastasis of lymph node	Lipide dissolve medicament	Crow gallbladder emulsison fat carrier Entering lymph node

The related factors of invasion of cancer cells include adhesion, enzyme excretion and movement. Inhibition of adhesion, anti movement or inhibition of enzyme excretion can not only prevent the invasion of the primary carcinomas, but also separate the tumor cells from the mother tumor and inhibit the invasion of ground substance and growth of the new tumor blood vessel. In the recent years, the research on blood vessel growth inhibitor to prevent the growth of the new blood vessel has been reported. This lab has found that the traditional Chinese herb TG plays a relatively good role in inhibiting the new blood vessel in the anti-carcinoma and anti-metastasis experiments screened from the tumor-bearing animal experiments. The time when the tumor cells enter the blood of the circulation system is the one when it has worst environment resistance to the host and it is easily killed by the immunological cells of the host. It has been reported by the literature that most cancer cells in circulation will be killed by the immunological cells and only about 0.01% of the cancer cells can survive and may form the metastatic lesion. Besides the mechanical destroy role, most of the cancer cells in the blood are contributed to the damaging effect of eth immunologic function of the host to the tumor cells. The tumor can inhibit the immunological function, the chemotherapy can also inhibit the immunological function, the patient suffering from the tumor meets with the inferior immunological function from time to time. Therefore, we adopt biological regulation regulator, immune regulation regulator and biologic response regulator and traditional Chinese herbs for immune regulation to protect the hematopiesis function of the marrow and stem cells, improve the function of the immunological organ and inhibit the metastasis of the tumor. In the past 10 years, Z-C medicine for immune regulation and anti metastasis has obtained remarkable curative effects in the clinical application of lots of patients of China Anti Cancer Research Cooperation of Chinese Traditional Medicine and Western Medicine.

Reference

1. Xu Ze, New Understanding and New Methods of Treatment of Carcinoma, Wuhan, Hubei Science Press, 2001, 171-173
2. Peng Jirun, Cai Shengli, Leng Xisheng et al, Detecting Peripheral Tumor Cells of Liver Cancer Patients with MAGE Gene mRNA as the Characteristic Sign, Chinese Journal of Surgery, 2002, 40(7): 487-490
3. Lin Guole, Peng Huizhong, Xu Tong. Detection of Perpheral Blood Micro-metastasis of Large Intestine Carcinoma Patients before and after Operation and Its Clinical Significance. Chinese Journal of General Surgery. 2002, 17 (10):605-607

CHAPTER 11

Analysis, Evaluation and Doubt of Systemic Intravenous Chemotherapy on Solid Tumor by Xu Ze

Through reviewing, reflecting, summarizing and analyzing the experience in success and lessons from failure, I have gradually realize that systemic intravenous chemotherapy on solid tumor may be confronted with some important problems, which are worthy of reflection, evaluation and re-discussion.

Why the chemotherapy does not prevent the recurrence and metastasis and get the expected curative effects? Through repeated reflection, we doubt: whether it is reasonable and scientific or not to use route of administration of intravenous chemotherapy to treat the malignant tumor in stomach, intestines, liver, gallbladder, pancreas and pelvic cavity and so on. We think deeply about the route of administration, especially the one for the malignant tumor in the abdomen and find that it is necessary to research and discuss the route of administration over again, the same to calculation of the dose and the evaluation standard of curative effects.

I. Analysis and doubt of the route of administration for systemic intravenous chemotherapy of solid tumor?

The present chemical chemotherapy for tumor is mainly the systemic intravenous chemotherapy, the standard scheme of chemotherapy in the world, the united scheme or the single-agent scheme is mostly the systemic intravenous chemotherapy, the same to the treatment of leukemia, malignant tumor of the blood system, tumor of the lymphatic system, solid tumor, tumor of the abdominal cavity, malignant tumor of stomach, intestines, liver, gallbladder and pancreas and to the assistant chemotherapy after operation or perioperative assistant chemotherapy.

1. Analysis of route of administration and medication of cytotoxic drug for intravenous chemotherapy for solid tumor:

In systemic intravenous chemotherapy, the intravenous drip enters the blood circulation, flows back to the right ventricle via venous blood, and then enters the arteria pulmonalis, after it is oxygenated with blood in lung, it flows into left ventricle via pulmonary vein and then is transfused into the aorta via bender and enters the systemic artery system for systemic circulation. Then it is distributed to the systemic organs with the arterial blood in viscera. At this moment, the chemotherapy drug enters the extracellular tissue fluid via interspace of capillay wall and then comes into play after entering the cancer cells.

As to the systemic intravenous chemotherapy, after the drug is distributed by the systemic blood, only a tiny minority of cytotoxic drug for chemotherapy enters the external organs of tumor cells and a tiny minority of drug enters the cancer cells, with slight curative effects.

Intravenous injection of chemotherapy drug via forearm vein →right ventricle →pulmonary artery→ oxygenation of pulmonary alveoli→ pulmonary vein→ aorta →systemic artery system (the drug is transported to the systemic viscera and is distributed in the whole body) →arteries of viscera→ veins of viscera →venae cavae→ right ventricle→ recirculation as above.

Analysis: as above-mentioned, the drug is spread in the whole body and distributed to all viscera, in this way, the systemic viscera obtain the cytotoxic drug, however, the body surface area or volume of the solid tumor only accounts for a very little ratio of the systemic body surface area or volume, for example, even through one carcinoma of stomach as large as one adult's fist, accounts for a very little ratio of the volume of an adult. Therefore, the carcinoma of stomach as large as one adult's fist obtains a tiny minority of cytotoxic drug in the chemotherapy of systemic intravenous injection, resulting in very little curative effects or roles. Meanwhile, most of the cytotoxic drug for chemotherapy is transported to the normal histiocytes of the viscera (including heart, liver, spleen, lung, kidney, brain, bone marrow, blood, lymph and immune organ), all of which receive the cytotoxic drug for chemotherapy, resulting in side reaction. The more the times of chemotherapy, the larger the dosage, the more the drug combination, the more serious of the accumulative side reaction, even resulting in loss of immunologic function and endangering the life. The patient takes a risk of endangering the life, however, does it have curative effects on the cancerous protuberance? The carcinoma of stomach as large as a fist only can obtain a very tiny minority of dose for chemotherapy entering the cancer cells as per the body surface area, in this way, the curative effects are very little and it is impossible to realize the good curative effects.

Some patients think by mistake that the large side reaction represents the curative effects, the larger the reaction, the better the curative effects, therefore, they mistake that the reaction kills the cancer cell, but they hardly realize that the reaction kills the normal cells: it is the reaction that kills the active normal cells with normal proliferation, such as bone marrow cells, immunological cells and mucous membrane cells of the stomach and intestine and the hair, resulting in decrease of white blood cells and decrease of blood platelets. Meanwhile, no one knows whether the cancer cells are killed by the chemotherapy and how many cancer cells are killed. However, it is known that it kills the normal cells just because the decrease of white blood cells and blood platelets only indicates the completion of the chemotherapy, no one knows whether it has curative effects or not.

Therefore, we analyze the reason why the chemotherapy cannot prevent the recurrence and metastasis is possibly that the route of systemic intravenous chemotherapy does not realize the curative effects you hope and expect, the local cancer lesion is applied with a tiny minority of dose, since a very tiny minority of drug enters the external tissue fluid of the cancer cells and only a minute of dose can enter the cancer cells and takes curative effects.

An example of 5-FU, the common chemotherapy drug: 5-FU intravenous chemotherapy 1000mg/d x 5=5000mg, 85% is catabolized by DPD enzyme in the liver without any therapeutic effects; some of the rest 15% is excreted through the kidney in form of drug prototype, some enters the cells and takes curative effects through anabolism. Given the latter is 8% and the locality with easy recurrence and metastasis of carcinosis accounts for 5% of the volume of the whole body, the effective availability of 5-FU is only:

5000mg x 8% x 5%=20mg (0.4%).

In another word, when intravenous drip is used for systemic chemotherapy, chemotherapy drug 5-FU infused via intravenous drip is 5000mg, after distributed in the whole body by the viscera, the available 5-FU really reaching the cancer lesion is only 20mg, that is to say, only 0.4% of the drug reaches the cancer lesion and is utilized. The drug takes the curative effects in the cancer cells. The rest, namely 99.6% of the chemotherapy drug takes the untoward reaction in the normal cells. In other words, only 0.4% of the chemotherapy drug plays a role in killing the cancer cells while 99.6% of the chemotherapy drug kills the normal cells of the patients with active proliferation, namely bone marrow cells, epith epithelial cells of mucous membrane of the stomach and intestine, hair, white blood cells, blood platelets and immunological cells and so on, resulting in degression of immunologic function, inhibition of hematopiesis of bone marrow cells, emesis, alopecia and obvious decrease of white blood cells and blood platelets.

According to the reports of the literatures, the metabolic pathway of 5-Fu:

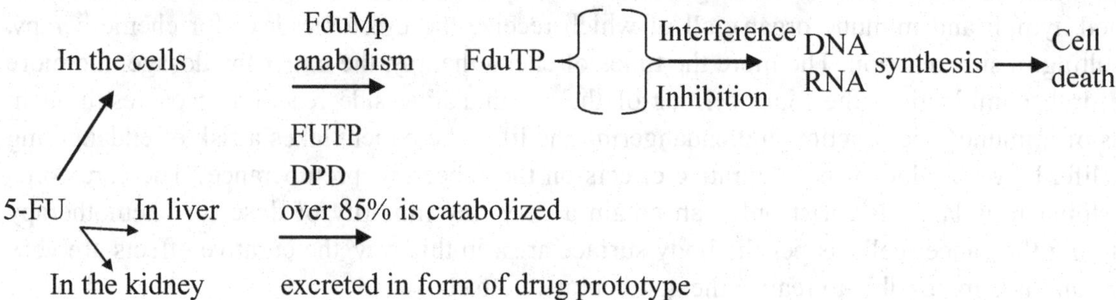

In systemic intravenous chemotherapy, how many chemotherapy drugs can reach the cancer cells and play a role in killing the cancer cells? With an example of the above-mentioned 5-FU, the patient is intravenously injected with 5000mg in 5 days, however, the one really reaching the cancer cells and playing a role is only 20mg, only accounting for 0.4% of the injected chemotherapy drug, the rest of the injected chemotherapy drug, namely 99.6% has the side effects on the normal cells with active proliferation in the whole body in clinical menifetation, namely bone marrow cells, epithelial cells of mucous membrane of the stomach and intestine and immunological cells, the systemic side reactions include arrest of bone marrow, reaction of gstrointestinal tract and toxic reaction of heart, lung and liver; the local toxic reactions include toxic reaction of skin and alopecia and so on.

In systemic intravenous chemotherapy, how does the cytotoxic drug for chemotherapy work from blood to cancer cells intravenously transfused? The chemotherapy drug is distributed and applied in the whole body, finally the chemotherapy drug enters the external tissue fluid of the cells via the interspace of capillay wall and then comes into play after entering the cancer cells.

In systemic intravenous chemotherapy, after the chemotherapy drug enters the vein, the drug is necessarily distributed in the body fluid, among the moisture in the human body, about 5% is blood, 15% is the external tissue fluid of the cells and 40% is intracellular fluid. The chemotherapy drug in blood is circulated and utilized in the whole body and distributed with the blood in the viscera. When the chemotherapy drug is in the external tissue fluid, it is absorbed and metabolized respectively by the viscera. When the chemotherapy drug enters the cells, the drug takes curative effects in the cancer cells while it takes side reaction in a large number of normal cells.

As above mentioned, we should objectively and calmly analyze the advantages, the disadvantages, the gain and the loss of the route of administration of systemic intravenous chemotherapy for the solid tumor? Which are the advantages? And the disadvantages? What the patient gains? And losses? All of which shall be seriously reflected, analyzed and evaluated.

2. It shall be discussed and doubted whether the route of administration of cytotoxic drug to kill the cancer cells of the solid tumor and the systemic intravenous drip are reasonable and scientific or not?

The above-mentioned systemic intravenous chemotherapy is used for all types of leukemia, leucoma and malignant tumor in the blood system, which is reasonable just because the malignant tumor of the blood system and the malignant tumor cells of the malignant leucoma of the lymphatic system are distributed in the systemic blood system or lymphatic system, in this way, they shall be applied with drug through the intravenous drip, which is reasonable and scientific just because there are so many cases and experience in successful treatment.

However, as to the carcinoma for solid tumor, the drug entering the tumor is minute, it plays a minor role in killing the cancer cells, it has obvious side reaction in damaging the systemic proliferative cells. The chemotherapy drug transfused through the route of administration to solid tumor only can kill a tiny minority of cancer cells while most of it kills the normal proliferative cells of the host, resulting in pains from the side reaction of chemotherapy undertaken by the patients.

At present, there are so many solid malignant tumors adopting the systemic intravenous administration route for the assistant chemotherapy after operation or perioperative assistant chemotherapy. Through intravenous drip, the chemotherapy drug enters the right ventricle via the caval vein, enters the lungs via pulmonary artery, enters the left ventricle through the pulmonary vein and then is distributed in the whole body through the aorta, in this way, the chemotherapy drug reaching the cancer lesion is very little, most of the drug is distributed in the whole body and kills the normal cells, especially the immunological cells, hematopoietic cells of bone marrow, causing the patients to be severely damaged; meanwhile, it does not play a remarkable role in the solid tumor. Over half a century, it has been all the same, although it has not taken the expected effects, so many patients have suffered from the pains from the side reaction of the chemotherapy drug widely killing the normal cells. The clinicians should seriously reflect, analyze and evaluate the route of administration, which is unadvisable, unreasonable and unscientific. We shall try to apply the drug to the specific locality instead of applying drug in the whole body and we shall research it and try to correct, reform and innovate it.

II. Analysis and doubt of calculation method of the dose of systemic intravenous chemotherapy drug for solid tumor

1. Based on the above-mentioned systemic intravenous administration route, the medication is calculated as per the calculation method of leukemia, since the leukemic cells are distributed in the systemic circulatory system, the administration must cover the systemic blood system. The malignant lymphocytes of leucoma is also distributed in the systemic lymphatic system, the administration must also cover the systemic lymphatic system, the blood system and the lymphatic system are distributed in all organs, tissues and skin in the whole body, therefore the administration shall be calculated as per body surface area or volume. This kind of route of administration, calculation of dose, pharmacokinetics and bioavailability is reasonable and scientific, which conforms to the distribution of the cancer cells.

2. Since the systemic intravenous chemotherapy has taken good curative effects and experience in all types of leukemia, leucoma, epithelioma of chorion, some malignant moles, blastocytoma Wilms tumor and so on, it has been widely applied to the solid tumor of the viscera in the whole body and the assistant chemotherapy after operation, although we have accumulated much experience and obtained some achievements, we have not had our wish fulfilled just because the death rate has been not reduced, the recurrence and metastasis has been not prevented, indicating it is unreasonable to apply the calculation method to dose of the leukemia and it does not conform to the actual conditions of the solid cancer, therefore, its reasonableness and scientificalness shall be doubted and it shall be further researched for reforming and innovation.
3. Since the carcinoma of the solid tumor is restricted to the viscus before remote metastasis, it is necessary to distribute the drug to the viscus in chemotherapy, however, the drug for systemic intravenous chemotherapy is distributed in the whole body, it necessarily needs relatively more dose. However, the chemotherapy drug is the cytotoxic drug, large dose necessarily leads to large toxicity, which cannot be withstood by the patient, so the calculation of dose for systemic intravenous chemotherapy cannot be calculated as per pharmacodynamics namely how much dose is needed to kill a certain number of cancer cells, but as per the tolerance dose of the patient to the cytotoxic drug just because the patient cannot withstand it if it exceeds the tolerance dose of the cytotoxic drug as the too large toxicity will endanger the life.

In the recent 30-40 years, the systemic intravenous chemotherapy is widely used to the solid tumor or the assistant chemotherapy after operation and there have been various international chemotherapy standard schemes. the schemes and the guides indicate the kind of drug, the dose mg/m^2, from which day to which day, iv or others, indicating how many days are a cycle. The schemes are universal, no matter the side of the solid tumor, no matter whether the solid tumor is ablated or not, the schemes are all the same, the same to the calculation of the dose, which are not individualized. Since the dose determined for each scheme is determined as per the tolerance dose of the cytotoxic drug undertaken by the patient instead of the effective dose. It is calculated as per the distribution of the systemic intravenous chemotherapy in the whole body, therefore, the calculation of the dose for solid tumor and the assistant chemotherapy after operation is not reasonable and scientific just because the normal tissues of the viscera shall not be killed by the cytotoxic drug, which shall be seriously analyzed, individualized, further researched and reformed.

III. Analysis, evaluation and doubt of curative effect evaluation criteria of systemic intravenous chemotherapy for solid tumor

The evaluation criteria of curative effects on solid tumor at present include:

1. Size of tumor: it shall be measured in every examination.
   (1) Shrinkage of measurable volume of tumor and/or metastatic lesion: indicating the degree of shrinkage with the arithmetic product of the max. diameter (cm) and its diameter (cm) of the tumor;
   (2) As to the tumor with immeasurable size, the method for improvement of disease is the calcification of osteolytic tumor again, as to the celiac tumor that cannot be easily measures shall be expressed with the estimated shrinkage value.

2. Remission stage: the remission stage shall begin from the treatment. In both checks in the treatment stage, the tumor grows up once again, the arithmetic product of its orthogonal diameters increases over 25%. The remission stage is calculated in days, weeks or months.
3. Evaluation criteria of size of solid tumor

CR (complete remission; evidently effective): the tumor disappears entirely, lasting over 4 weeks;
PR (partial remission; effective): the arithmetic product of two diameters of the tumor is shrunk to over 50%;
MR (middle remission): the tumor is shrunk to over 25% and below 50%;
NC (or S, stable, unchanged): the tumor is shrunk to below 25% and enlarged to below 25%;
PD (or P, progressive; deteriorative): the tumor is enlarged to over 25% or new lesion appears.

Analysis and discussion

1. **The above-mentioned curative effect criteria of systemic chemotherapy for solid tumor is summarized in three points: size of tumor, remission and remission period.**

Chemotherapy and radiotherapy only kill the differentiated and matured tumor cells rather than the stem cells of the tumor accounting for 0.1%~1.0% of the tumor cells. The remained stem cells of tumor are differentiated and proliferated once again, forming new tumor, with the clinical menifetation of recurrence and metastasis of tumor as well as the failure of treatment, resulting in death of the patient.

At present, although the chemotherapy drug for clinical application can shrink the tumor, the effects are commonly temporary and it cannot obviously prolong the life of the patient. Therefore, the curative effect evaluation criterion is referred to as remission, the remission stage is calculated in days, weeks or months, for example, the complete remission only means the tumor disappears entirely, lasting over 4 weeks, indicating it may recur after 4 weeks. What is meant by remission? I understand it as follows: we rope an animal, then untie it for two hours and then rope it again, in this way, the untying is referred to as remission, the two hours of untying is the remission stage, obviously, remission is not the treatment objective of the patient, the patient is hospitalized for chemotherapy, undertaking the pains and the risks from the side reaction of the cytotoxic drug for chemotherapy, only getting a temporary remission at most, which is apparentlyteh requirements and treatment objective of the patient hospitalized for chemotherapy, which shall not be the objective of clinical treatment.

2. **Why chemotherapy only can play a role in remission? Because:**
   (1) The cytotoxic drug for chemotherapy only can kill the differentiated and matured cancer cells rather than the undifferentiated or immature stem cells or the ones to be differentiated and matured, the chemotherapy drug kills the differentiated and matured cancer cells at this time, however, after a time, the undifferentiated and immature cancer cells are gradually differentiated and matured, the tumor cells are uninterruptedly and progressively divided, proliferated and cloned, one is divided into two, and two into four, in this way, it is multiplied in form of geometric progression, at the same time, the period of effectively killing cancer cells of the patient through chemotherapy drug is only 1~5 days of intravenous drip, that is to say, it only lasts 5-6 days for taking the

effects on killing the cancer cells, the so-called cycle of 3-4 weeks only means that the white blood cells and the blood platelets with bone marrow inhibited can be recovered within 3-4 weeks and withstand the second chemotherapy.

(2) Since the chemotherapy drug only can kill the differentiated and matured cancer cells rather than the undifferentiated stem cells of the tumor or the ones being differentiated, the chemotherapy only can merely alleviate the symptoms, but it cannot treat the root cause, it only can be regarded as the assistant treatment, but not as the radical treatment because the principles of chemotherapy do not conform to the biological characteristics and behaviors of the cancer cells. Although chemotherapy can temporarily shrink the tumor, it cannot obviously prolong the life and one of the reasons why the treat fails is that the tumor cells loss the drug resistance, maybe another reason is the existing therapeutic methods cannot effectively kill the stem cells of the tumor, the treatment of cancer through chemotherapy may be said that "no prairie fire can destroy the grass, it shoots up again with the spring breeze blows". Why? Because the grass is burn, but the root is remained, only some matured cancer cells rather than the stem cells of tumor to be differentiated and matured are killed, the stem cells of tumor will be continually divided and cloned in form of geometrical progression.

(3) The judgment of the curative effects on tumor shall not regard the size of the tumor as the standard: the objective of existing tumor chemotherapy and radiotherapy is mainly to reduce the volume and number of the tumor cells just because they often determine the curative effects by means of the capability of shrinking the tumor, in fact, "the big" does not mean "the bad" and "the small" does not mean "the good". The clinic judgment of chemotherapy at present, no matter the clinic or the sickroom, is mainly based on CT and MRI as well as space occupation, as a matter of fact, the space occupation is not the size of the solid tumor because the peripheric tissue of the solid tumor may affect the space occupation. I am a surgeon and I have been engaged in medicine practice for 54 years and performed over 5000 radical and abscission operations for cancers at breast or abdomen. The size of the tumor seen in the operation has not been always consistent with the one reported in CT and MRI. In addition, although some solid tumors are as large as a fist even larger than a fist, when they are incised, the cancer cells inside is not dense while there are so many interfibrillar interstitial tissues; although some solid tumors are only as large as a table tennis, when then are incised, there are so many highly malignant cancer cells inside, the latter is more malignant than the former. Therefore, I think "the big" does not means "the bad" and "the small" does not means "the good", which cannot be regarded as the standard. We also find from a large batch of tumor-bearing animal models in the lab that although the hypodermically inoculated experimental tumors of some tumor-bearing experimental mice are very large, the cancer cells of the central tissue of the transplanted solid tumor are unlike to the peripheral cancer cells, the mode center is mostly aseptically necrotic or liquefied while its periphery is the active cancer cells, although its volume is increased, the malignancy is low.

(4) The solid tumor has the drug transmission blockage, which in the huge solid tumor results in drug resistance or does not realize the curative effects. Some anti-tumor drugs have very high anti-tumor activity to various tumor cells in culture dish, some even has 100% inhibition rate., which are clinically used to treat malignant tumor in the blood system or the child cancer, with satisfactory curative effects, however, these drug cannot

obviously reduce the rate of death of the adults caused by the most common solid tumor (such as carcinoma of stomach, hepatic carcinoma, carcinoma of large intestine, carcinoma of lung, breast carcinoma, carcinoma of pancreas, prostatic carcinoma, esophageal carcinoma, brain carcinoma and so on).

It can be found through comparison of the malignant tumor in the blood system with the solid tumor that the former can directly contact the single cancer cell in the blood just because it omits the step of districting the drug in the tumor tissue. Therefore, it can be concluded that the drug transmission has some factors in the solid tumor that can cause the drug to produce the drug resistance.

The above-mentioned systemic intravenous administration route, medication, calculation of dose, calculation as per body surface area and curative effect evaluation criteria have been used in the world over half a century, forming the internationalized chemotherapy standard scheme, various guides or idiomatic usages. However, its curative effects cannot be satisfactory, it neither reduces the rate of death from cancer nor prevents the tumor recurrence or metastasis while the patient may undertake the pains and risks of side reactions from chemotherapy.

Through in-depth thinking, review, reflection, analysis and evaluation, Profession Xu Ze summarizes his clinical experience and lessons of treatment of patients over 54 years, puts forward the above-mentioned questions, evaluates, discusses and doubts the route of administration, medication, calculation of dose and curative effect evaluation criteria of systemic intravenous chemotherapy for solid tumor especially the tumor at abdomen and pelvic cavity. Since the above-mentioned questions exist, it is necessary to further research them and improve the traditional therapeutic method based on the traditional approaches as well as update the concept and understanding, make progress in reforming and have the courage to innovate. The innovation must have the challenge to the traditional concept to overcome the disadvantages, correct the defects to make it more perfect. It shall be reformed and innovated.

CHAPTER 12

XU ZE Proposes to Reform the Systemic Intravenous Chemotherapy for Solid Tumor to Intravascular Chemotherapy in Target Organ

Through probing into the route of administration of systemic intravenous chemotherapy for solid tumor, we propose to reform it to the intravascular administration route in target organ and reform the systemic intravenous chemotherapy of solid tumor (especially the tumor of liver, gallbladder, pancreas, spleen, kidney, lung, uterus, ovary, abdominal cavity and pelvic cavity) to intravascular chemotherapy in target organ. Why? Just because we have deeply taken cognizance of its disadvantages. This cognizance has been deepened and strengthened step by step through reviewing, reflecting, analyzing, evaluating and doubting a large number of cases and then the truth has been found gradually. Over the past half a century, million of cancer patients have undertaken the side reaction of chemotherapy once and again after receiving the chemotherapy, only to stilly bear the pains without any other way just because they want to kill off the cancer cells so that they can get well and be full of vim and vigor.

I. Evaluation of Problems and Disadvantages of Systemic Intravenous Chemotherapy for Solid Tumor

(I) Evaluation of the route of administration of systemic intravenous chemotherapy for solid tumor

The route of administration, not the specific targeting administration, distributes the cytotoxic drug in the whole body through the general blood circulation. In this way, it does not have a definite object for administration, but administers drugs in the whole body, resulting in:

1. The diseased cancer lesion area is very small (accounting for very small ratio of the body surface area of the whole body) only can obtain very little cytotoxic drug, resulting in very little action and curative effect.
2. However, the disease-free normal tissue in the whole body is damaged by the reaction of 99.6% of the cytotoxic drug. The normal tissue in the whole body does not need the cytotoxic drug, but it obtains a large number of cytotoxic drugs. However, the cytotoxic anti-cancer drug has relatively toxicity to the tissue with relatively rapid proliferation, such as the toxicity of alimentary canel, hemopoietic system, heart, liver, spleen, lung, kidney, nervous system and endocrine system, in this way, so many patients cannot receive the treatment or have to interrupt the treatment. Killing the tissue with relatively rapid proliferation in the whole body leads to harm to the patients instead of benefits to the patients.
3. The medication of this route of administration, does not have a definite object for administration, but the blind administration, which is non-targeting administration. Without the definite object, it only distributes and administers the drug in the whole body, as a

result, the cancer lesion obtains a minute of cytotoxic drug while the area of the tissue in the whole body damaged by the cytotoxic drug is very large, resulting in bad curative effects, large side reaction and many and heavy complication, so the medication is unreasonable and unscientific.

4. With the above-mentioned medication, the cytotoxic drug administered in chemotherapy does not greatly attack the cancer cells, but only attach the cancer cells slightly (0.4%) while the normal tissue is greatly attacked in an all-round way by the cytotoxic drug (99.6%), at the same time, the cancer patient has low immunologic function by nature, now the cytotoxic drug in chemotherapy kills the hematopoietic cells, immunological cells, T lymphocyte, blood cells and blood platelet of the bone marrow again, resulting in further drop of immunologic function, the cytotoxic drug in chemotherapy attacks and kills the hematopoietic cells and immunological cells of the bone marrow once and again, resulting in the future drop of the immunologic function, in this way, one disaster comes after another, some cytotoxic drugs even urge the breakdown of the immunologic function.

(II) Elevation of calculation of dose for systemic intravenous chemotherapy for solid tumor

1. Since the systemic intravenous chemotherapy for solid tumor is not the specific targeting administration, but blindly distributed in the whole body, it necessarily needs much dose of cytotoxic drug; furthermore, it needs the combination of multiple drugs, in this way, it is possible to make the cancer lesion with very small area obtain the dose for remitting and shrinking the cancer lesion. The reason for large dose is that the 99.6% of the dose is absorbed by the whole body while only 0.4% is absorbed by the local cancer lesion. As a result, the relatively larger the dose, the larger and the more obvious the side reaction, resulting in remarkable drop of white blood cells and blood platelets, sometimes it also needs drug for increasing white cells, so it is unreasonable to calculate the dose.
2. At present, the systemic intravenous chemotherapy for solid tumor is the experience and the method obtained from the treatment of leukemia, however, as to the treatment extended to the solid tumor, its guiding ideology is to administer the drug as per the calculation of the body surface area of the whole body, which is unadvisable. Why? Because the leukemic cells are distributed in the general blood circulation system, in the organs and tissues in the whole body, the target to be treated exists in the general blood circulation system, therefore, it is reasonable and advisable to adopt the systemic intravenous chemotherapy and conforms to the targeting treatment. Because the target cells of the leukaemia are distributed in the general blood circulation system, so it is reasonable and advisable. However, since the solid tumor is limited to a certain organ, its target to be treated is mainly a certain organ suffering from cancer, so it shall adopt the route of intravascular administration in the target organ and specific targeting administration, in this way, it can greatly reduce the dose of cytotoxic drug, as well as greatly reduce and eliminate the side reaction of the cytotoxic drug.
3. The calculation of the dose of systemic intravenous chemotherapy for solid tumor as per the body surface area is not based on therapeutical does by which how many cancer cells can be killed but on the tolerance dose of the organism to the cytotoxic drug. It is unknown whether one chemotherapy and two chemotherapies kill the cancer cells and how many cancer cells are killed by the chemotherapy. It is unknown. Whether there are cancer cells in

the body of the patient? And where? It is unknown. Only one chemotherapy is carried out and only one task is accomplished.

(III) Evaluation of curative effect evaluation criterion of systemic intravenous chemotherapy for solid tumor

1. In a word, the curative effect evaluation criterion of systemic intravenous chemotherapy for solid is mainly embodied in three points: size of tumor, remission and remission time. As to the size of tumor, it is mainly based on CT, MRI or type-B ultrasonic, however, all of the images only reflect the size of occupation. As to the size of occupation, in our opinion, "the big" does not mean "the bad" and "the small" does not mean "the good". In addition, most of the occupations are short-term, the reason has been mentioned above.
2. Remission and remission time. Why the remission is regarded as the curative effect evaluation criterion and why the remission has a certain period? Apparently, the remission is not the objective of treatment or the treatment requirement of the patient or the objective of determination of treatment of the doctor just because the patient pays a certain price after several chemotherapies and only obtains a short-term remission. However, at present, the tumor medicine cannot heal all cancers (namely non-recurrence and non-metastasis) for a long time. Then, to say the latest, remission is better than the failure to remission. It is practical and realistic. Why it only can remit the cancer? Because the cytotoxic drug only harms the cancer cells and destroys their DNA rather than killing all cancer cells, which is only the first order kinetics. In addition, the reaction duration of cytotoxic drug only lasts 24h~48h even 72h after drug injection, after several days, the cancer cells will also be divided, proliferated and cloned in geometric progression, one into two, two into four and four into eight. Since the cytotoxic drug cannot kill the stem cells of the tumor, after administration for chemotherapy, the stem cells of tumor are still divided, proliferated and cloned. So in out opinion, killing the cancer cells does not conform to biological characteristics and behaviors or multi-link and multi-step of the metastasis of cancer cells, it only can regulate and control the cancer cells and prevents their division, proliferation and clone rather than the simple killing.

(IV) Evaluation of side reaction of systemic intravenous chemotherapy for solid tumor

Why the side reaction is so large? Just because this kind of route of administration needs so much dose or has to adopt combined administration. In order to remit and shrink the cancer, it has to determine the tolerance dose of the patient as the dose, in this way, the reaction is necessarily large and the damage is large, the distribution mode of this kind of route of administration leads to large dose or combined administration, otherwise, it is difficult to realize the curative effect criterion of shrinkage, in fact, it is avoidable to administer 99.6% of the cytotoxic drug to the normal tissues, in other words, it is avoidable to reform this route of administration to the specific targeting administration. If it is reformed to intravascular administration in the specific target organ, naturally, the side reaction will become little or be eliminated.

II. We Propose to Reform Systemic Intravenous Chemotherapy for Solid Tumor to Intravascular Chemotherapy in Target Organ

Since the above-mentioned problems are in existence, they shall be further studied. We should continue to improve the traditional curative therapeutic method as per the traditional idea, in the meanwhile, we should update the idea and the understanding, make progress in reforming and have the courage to innovate. Innovation, must challenge the traditional idea instead of replacement, it shall overcome the disadvantages, correct the defects so as to make it more perfect. Innovation, shall open a new path to overcome the cancer. Therefore, we specially propose the new idea, new concept and new principles of anti-cancer as well as new treatment mode and adopt organic integral new treatment mode to reform and innovate the traditional problems based on the biological characteristics and behaviors of cancer as well as the immunologic conditions of the host and the multi-link and multi-step of metastasis.

(I) Necessity, reasonableness and scientificalness of reform the systemic intravenous chemotherapy for solid tumor to intravascular chemotherapy in target organ

1. As above-mentioned, the route of administration of systemic intravenous chemotherapy is not the specific targeting administration but the blind general distribution, which is unreasonable and scientific distribution, so it must be reformed. The cancer lesion is limited to the local of the viscera, so it is necessary to adopt the specific targeting administration with clear target, which is reasonable and scientific. As to the systemic intravenous chemotherapy, since most of the cytotoxic drugs are administered to the general normal tissues, if the drugs are administered to the target organ, it can save the dose administered to the whole body, in this way, the dose can be greatly reduced, thus the side reaction is greatly reduced even eliminated, so the chemotherapy even may have no toxicity.
2. Analyze the source and formation of the side reaction of chemotherapy and probe into the method to eliminate the side reaction. Through review, reflection and analysis, we deeply realize that the source, the blind distribution of the cytotoxic drug in the whole body by the systemic intravenous chemotherapy for solid tumor, is unreasonable. In order to shrink the tumor, it necessarily increases the dose, resulting in unavoidable side reaction.

The increased dose of cytotoxic drug does not entirely react on the cancer lesion, but mainly on the whole body to damage the normal histiocytes while these general normal tissues do not need the cytotoxic drug, however, they get most of the cytotoxic drugs in fact, which is unreasonable. It is necessary to study and reform it.

In view that its source and formation is based on the blindness of the route of administration of systemic intravenous chemotherapy, resulting in increased dose and combined administration and leading to unavoidable side reaction, so the solution is to reform the route of administration.

How to reform the route of administration?

Professor Xu Ze proposes to reform the systemic intravenous chemotherapy for solid tumor (especially the tumor of liver, gallbladder, spleen, pancreas, stomach, intestine, uterus, ovary, pelvic cavity and abdominal cavity) to intravascular chemotherapy in target organ, in this way, the drug is administered to the specific target and then to the cancer lesion of the target organ, necessarily leading in the greatly decreased dose; the reduction of dose of cytotoxic drug necessarily leads to the reduction and elimination of side reaction. The elimination of side reaction of the traditional chemotherapy, makes millions of cancer patients free from the pains and risks of side reaction of chemotherapy and benefits the patients.

Professor Xu Ze holds: the intravascular administration in the specific target organ, reduces the dose, improves the curative effects, eliminates the side reaction, necessarily leading to great reduction of medical charge, saving billions of medical charges and expenditures (in RMB Yuan) for the state and the patients and being advantageous for settling the problems of being difficult and expensive in taking medical treatment.

Over half a century, millions of cancer patients have been deeply damaged by the side reaction of the chemotherapy, therefore, this reform will benefit millions of cancer cells, which is a great pioneering undertaking and an original innovation and promotes the further development of the oncology in the 21st century.

(II) It is necessary to firstly study and make clear where the target is so as to carry out the intravascular chemotherapy in target organ; it is necessary to study and make clear where the cancer cells are so as to kill the cancer cells with cytotoxic drug in chemotherapy? In this way, it can have a definite object.

1. The primary lesion of the solid tumor is in the organ, for example, the stomach cancer lies in the stomach, the liver cancer lies in the liver, the lung cancer lies in the lung, the intestinal cancer lies in intestine, that is to say, the primary cancer lesion lies in the organ, even if it meets with metastasis in the advanced stage, its primary cancer lesion is still in the organ.
2. Where are the cancer cells? The cancer cells of stomach cancer, intestinal cancer, liver cancer, lung cancer and so on are mainly in the portal system and meet with metastasis via the portal system. An example of liver cancer: the main blood supply of liver cancer is from the hepatic artery, the most primary route of the metastasis of liver cancer is the venous system in the liver. The metastasis of liver cancer in liver is the most common metastasis mode, the cancer cells invade the branch of the portal vein, form the cancer embolus in the portal vein, continually extend to the hepatic portal until the left and right branch of the portal vein and its beam are blocked by the cancer embolus, the deciduous cancer cell balls are floating in the portal vein and are spread to the liver through blood.

   The hepatic vein wall is thin and receives the blood flowing back from the cancer lesion, so it is easy to be encroached and the cancer embolus is formed in the hepatic vein, sometimes, the embolus can reach to inferior vena cava and to right atrium and then meet with metastasis via the lung.

   The liver is one of the organs meeting with metastatic carcinoma most commonly. According to information of pathologic anatomy, among the cases of the patients who die of the malignant tumor, about 40% meet with the liver metastasis and its incidence rate is next only to lymphatic system. The liver metastasis of malignant tumor of gstrointestinal tract is the most common.

   The liver receives the dual blood supply from portal vein and hepatic artery, the liver metastasis can come from the portal vein circulation and systemic circulation, that is to say, the cancer cells enters the systemic circulation via pulmonary capilliary station. The blood supply is complicated, about 90%of the blood supply is from the hepatic artery.

3. The administration along the route of hematogenous metastasis of cancer cells for tracking and killing shall follow the flow direction of the tumor vein, the chemotherapy drug follows the flow direction, killing the cancer cells in metastasis with small dose. As to the cancer cells, the cancer cell groups and micro-metastasis cancer embolus in metastasis, it is only necessary to kill $10^{4`5}$ cancer cells with eth cytotoxic drugs for chemotherapy, the rest $10^{4`5}$ cancer cells can be eliminated by the immunological cells and immunological surveillance in the blood circulation of the organism. According to the plan, it is satisfactory for the dose to kill $10^{4`5}$ cancer cells, the dose cannot go so far to kill too many immunological cells. To kill some cancer cells and to protect the immunological cells from being damaged excessively as well, shall be judged with the sign of not affecting the drop of white blood cells and blood platelets. The viscera and organs in the abdomen, such as stomach, rectum, colon, liver, gallbladder, pancreas, uterus and ovary and other tumor-producing vein gather at the portal vein system, therefore, the target organs of tumor at the abdomen shall focus on the portal vein system and hepatic artery.

III. Xu Ze Proposes to Reform the Systemic Intravenous Chemotherapy for Solid Tumor at the Abdomen to the Specific Method and Approach of Intravascular Chemotherapy in Target Organ

(I) Intravascular administration for chemotherapy in target organ

1. Administration via arterial route
   (1) The chemotherapy pump shall be arranged in the hepatic artery;
   (2) Hepatic artery interventional therapy, embolism + chemotherapy;
   (3) Interventional chemotherapy perfusion of bronchial artery;
   (4) Interventional chemotherapy perfusion of internal iliac artery;
   (5) Interventional chemotherapy of arteria pancreatica;
   (6) Interventional chemotherapy perfusion of gastric artery;
   (7) Hepatic artery chemotherapy pump through laparotomy.

2. Administration via portal vein route
   (1) Portal vein chemotherapy pump through laparotomy;
   (2) Omentum venous pump through laparotomy;
   (3) Subcutaneous chemotherapy pump through laparotomy via mesentery vein;
   (4) Subcutaneous deep vein conduit chemotherapy pump: can be used in the treatment of malignant tumor of the intestines and stomach tract.

   Surgical interventional chemotherapy for tumor patient has been widely applied, now the subcutaneous chemotherapy pump for drug delivery system is mostly adopted at present and it is a good route of administration for tumor chemotherapy, which can be divided into three classes: venous duct chemotherapy pump; ductus arteriosus chemotherapy pump and celiac duct chemotherapy pump, compared with the peripheral vein chemotherapy and artery interventional chemotherapy, it has a lot of advantages.

3. Administration via target organ at the abdomen

Oral administration: oral administration→stomach→vena coronaria of stomach (left vein and right vein of stomach)→splenic vein→portal vein, for example, oral administration of Xeloda.

Oral administration: oral administration→stomach→lymphatic vessel under gastric mucosa→lymph node around the stomach→lymph node behind peritoneum→cisterna chyli→thoracic duct, for example, oral administration of Brucea emulsion.

Rectal suppository: rectal suppository (a few of chemotherapy drug)→venae intestinales→vein under mesentery→ portal vein.

A. Route of administration for the target organ of lung cancer: vein of antibrachium→superior vena cava→double lungs
B. Portal vein conduit or pump→liver→hepatic vein→lower caval vein→right ventricle→double lungs
C. Oral administration: oral administration→portal vein→liver→lower caval vein→right ventricle→double lungs

(II) Paying attention to arterial interventional administration

An example of liver cancer: since the onset of liver cancer is insidious, when the patient see a doctor, it is mostly in intermediate and advanced stage, followed by other factors such as high combined hepatocirrhosis rate, relatively low surgical removal rate and high recurrence rate after operation, most of the patients need non-operation therapy. At present, among the non-operation therapies with positively curative effects, interventional therapy is most widely used.

Its indication can be used to the liver cancer in different stages and it is better for the liver cancer in early and intermediate stage. These suffering from serious icterrus, voluminous ascites, serious damage to liver function and widespread metastasia shall be abstained from contraindication.

Generally, the first period of treatment of interventional therapy of liver cancer needs 3-4 times, with the interval of 2-3 months. In principle, the next interventional therapy shall be carried out only after the general condition and liver function of the patient are basically recovered over 3 weeks.

Interventional therapy

Since the interventional therapy will damage the normal tissue especially the liver and the immune system of the organism synchronously, the organism needs a certain time for recovery to understand the second interventional therapy, in the interval of interventional therapy, it shall nourish the liver, improve the immunity and adopt the complex treatment. In Shuguang Tumor Clinic of Shugang Tumor Research Institute, in the past 16 years, all the patients of liver cancer receiving the interventional therapy administer XZ-C medicine after operation and they take oral administration of $XZ\text{-}C_{1+4+5}$ for protecting the chest, improving the immunity, protecting the bone marrow, enhancing hematopiesis, protecting liver and great curative effects have been made. Most of the patients have been in good condition and have had good appetite, their symptoms have been improved, their survival quality has been improved, and most of them have had an obviously prolonged survival period.

(III) Paying attention to the route of administration of chemotherapy pump in portal vein

It is necessary for the specific targeting administration for target organ to understand where the target organ of the cancer cells is. The tumor-bearing vein of stomach cancer, colon and rectal cancer, gallbladder cancer, pancreas cancer, cancer of pelvic cavity and oophoroma flows into the portal vein system, therefore, the cancer cells, and the ones in metastasis are flowing into the portal vein system, therefore, attention shall be paid to the chemotherapy pump in portal vein for targeting tracking and killing the cancer cells.

Chemotherapy pump in portal vein is remained in the portal vein after exploration of laparotomy or remained in the lower omentum vein after laparotomy; or remained in the drug delivery system in the mesentery under the direct vision of the laparotomy.

Chemotherapy pump embedded in portal vein body, also called implanted drug delivery system or subcutaneous embedded drug delivery system, is a kind of drug subcutaneously embedded for local perfusion, which is used for the guiding chemotherapy of cancer and oriented local perfusion chemotherapy for preventing the recurrence after removal of tumor. The drug can directly enter the target organ through drug pump and conduit, improving the lethality and the curative effects to cancer cells and reducing the side reaction of chemotherapy. It is reported by the literature that when the density of the local chemotherapy drug is increased one time, the lethality to the tumor can be increased 6-12 times. This system can increase several times of the density of the local drug. At present, this system is widely used for the clinic at home and abroad and great curative effects have been made.

In a word, as above mentioned, the systemic intravenous chemotherapy for solid tumor, only has a few of drug reaching to the cancer lesion while most of the cytotoxic drugs react on the normal histiocyte in the whole body, especially, they are relatively toxic to the tissue with rapid proliferation such as hemopoietic system of bone marrow, immune system and alimentary system and have the side reaction, however, these normal tissue, not needing the cytotoxic drugs, obtains a large number of cytotoxic drugs, which is unreasonable.

As to the chemotherapy through intravascular administration in the target organ, the drug is directly sent to the target organ via the conduit, the cytotoxic drugs obtained by the cancer lesion are all drugs administered, which is reasonable and scientific, greatly reducing the dose for chemotherapy. The specific targeting administration, reduces the does, improves the curative effects, reduces or eliminates the side reaction. In this way, it improves the curative effects, eliminates the reaction, resulting in the reduction of expenses. It is advantages for settling the problems of being difficult and expensive in taking medical treatment. Since it reduces or eliminates the side reaction, necessarily reducing the medical charge and saving billions of medical expenses and expenditures (in RMB Yuan) for the state.

CHAPTER 13

Opinion on Improving and Perfecting Treatment of Cancer with Traditional Chemotherapy

I. On "gain" and "loss" after taking anti-cancer drugs

The treatment of cancer, no matter in early stage, mid stage or advanced stage, involves the comprehensive multi-discipline treatment.

The operation is a method of local treatment. The surgical oncology scientists hold that the cancer occurs locally at first, then encroaches the peripheral tissues and transfers to other places via lymphatic vessel and blood vessel, as a result, they stress on the local treatment, that is to say, the stress on control over the local growth and diffusion, especially when the cancer meets with metastasis via lymph, the lymph node is cleaned down by operation. For years, although the operative treatment has been improved continually in methodology, the long-term curative effects have not made remarkable progress as yet. The reoccurrence and metastasis after operation seriously threatens the prognosis of the patients, attracting high attention from the medical field, however, there has been no effective prescription up to now.

The radiotherapy is also a method of local treatment, which plays a role in killing off the cells from the local tumor per unit dosage. The radiotherapy effects are mostly affected by the factors including oxygenation of cells, type of tumor and restoration of cells and so on, all these characteristics determine that the radiotherapy is locally inferior to the surgical removal with respect to tumor.

The biological characteristics of cancer are invasion, reoccurrence and metastasis, which are the important reasons why the treatment with operation and radiotherapy fails.

In recent years, some one holds that cancer is a kind of generalized disease, so the generalized treatment should mainly depend on radiotherapy, however, it is a pity, in despite of the emerging new drugs and continually undated therapeutic methods and plans, the radiotherapy effects are not satisfactory. Since the cytotoxic drugs have no selectivity, they kill the cancer cells as well as the normal cells of the host, especially the immunological cells, in addition, they have severe side effects, inhibiting hematopiesis function of the bone marrow and reducing the immunity. Therefore, the traditional radiotherapy does not entirely conform to the well-known actual conditions of the biological behaviors of the cancer at present, for example, the invasion behaviors and metastasis of the cancer cells are of multi-link and multi-step. At present, people have cognized that the anti-tumor drugs do not always prevent the metastasis and reoccurrence.

In 1980s, the tumorous bioremediation emerged, such as immunological therapy, cytokine therapy and gene vaccination therapy. It was proven that some therapies could mediate the immunity of the patients, however, it has not proven that which immunological preparation or method could induce the extinction of tumor.

In the recent 20 years, so many reports on treatment of cancer with traditional Chinese medicine have been made and its outlook has been concerned by the people. Especially, with the further development of the study on medicine and immunology, people have realized that the disorder of the immune system of the organism is closely related to the occurrence and development of tumor and traditional Chinese medicine has its own characteristics and advantages in tumor treatment through mediating the immunologic function of the organism. The immunoregulation of traditional Chinese medicine and development of immunoregulator of traditional Chinese medicine will attract more attention and favor all over the world. With the assistance of operation, radiotherapy and chemotherapy, the traditional Chinese medicine can bring its immunoregulation into full play in the process of treatment and obviously prolong the survival time and improve the survival quality, in this way, the characteristics and advantages of the traditional Chinese medicine are fully embodied, however, it is disadvantageous in unremarkably improving the tumor.

Since the above-mentioned methods have different characteristics in action mechanism and effect with respect to treatment of cancer and different curative effects as well as their own disadvantages, so it is necessary to focus on the advantages and disadvantages of various therapies aiming at the “gain” and the “loss” of the paints, for example, what’s the “advantage” and the “disadvantage” after taking the therapy, what’s the “gain” and the “loss” of the patients? We should learn from the strong points of one therapy to offset the weakness of the other therapies and combine these therapies organically and reasonably to form the comprehensive therapeutic plans for cancer, only in this way, can the side effects from the drugs be obviously reduced, the survival quality of the patients be improved and the total survival time be prolonged. In the past 16 years, Tumor Specialized Clinic of Shuguang Tumor Research Institute has treated over 12000 cancer patients in mid and advanced stage with XZ-C immunoregulation therapy in practice and most of the patients have achieved the effects of improving the survival quality, stabilizing the lesion, controlling the metastasis, keeping survival with tumor and remarkably prolonging the survival time.

II. Actual conditions of chemotherapy in tumor: main cause affecting further improvement of curative effects of chemotherapy

The total effective rate of treatment with anti-tumor drug in clinic is only 14%, the factors impeding chemotherapy’ better curative effects mainly include:

1. **Blindness of current chemotherapy**. Now it is unknown whether the chemical medicine used in the current therapeutic plan for chemotherapy is sensitive to the cancer cells of the patients just because most of the patients are not subject to the drugsensitive test to cancer cells. If the medicine is used by experience, it has blindness, that is to say, it may be beneficial to some patients while harmful to other patients. Based on the drugsensitive test results, remarkable curative effects have been made in treating the infectious diseases with antibiotics, as enlightens us on reasonably and jointly administrating drug through testing the sensitivity of the cancer cells of the patients to the cytotoxic drugs for chemotherapy so as to replace the blind chemotherapy with “individualized” chemotherapy. It is shown by the data that it can double the effective rate of chemotherapy.
2. **Drug resistance of chemotherapy**. Most of the solid tumor, such as stomach cancer, cancer of large intestine, is lowly sensitive or insensitive to the chemotherapy. Some tumor is remitted after chemotherapy, however, it meets with reoccurrence, resulting in ineffective chemotherapy, indicating that the cancer cells has the drug resistance to the

chemotherapy drug. The reasons why the drug resistance appears include many factors such as drug transmission disturbance of solid tumor, cell proliferation, difference in dynamics, immunity and metabolism and so on.

3. Selectivity toxicity of chemotherapy anti-cancer drug. The chemotherapy drug is the cytotoxic drug, killing the cancer cells as well as the normal histiocytes, without selectivity, especially the hemopoietic stem cells of the bone marrow with exuberant proliferation and immunological cells as well as stomach cells and intestinal cells. Compared with the volume of the normal tissue, since the cancerous protuberance only accounts for a minimal proportion, it is possible to "kill one hundred enemies while injuring three thousand soldiers on one's own side". The blindness of chemotherapy and the drug resistance of chemotherapy result in low curative effects, in case that it is expected to improve the curative effects by means of increasing the dosage, increasing the kinds of drugs and shortening the time, the toxic effects will be further aggravated, so the chemotherapy in cancer is still satisfactory in despite of great progress. The drugs shall be selected by testing the sensitivity and drug resistance of the chemotherapy drug so as to have a definite object in view. If the drugsensitive test is made on the chemotherapy patients so as to avoid the damage on the patients from the blind chemotherapy and benefit the chemotherapy patients, the epoch of chemotherapy will be opened up.

III. Suggestion on improving and perfecting the chemotherapy in cancer

Since nitrogen mustard drugs were reported by Gillman and Phillips in 1946 to treat the tumor in hematopiesis function, the chemotherapy has made great progress for 60 years and the great achievements have been made in therapeutics of the malignant tumor, for example, the chemotherapy has cured over 10 kinds of malignant tumor including chorionepithilioma, acute lymphocytic leukemia, Hodgkin disease, seminoma of testis, small-cell carcinoma of the lung and Wilms tumor and so on, and remitted the tumor including breast cancer, children' lymphadenoma, neuroblastoma and osteosarcoman and so on, resulting in prolonged survival time. Thus three principles of treatment including operation, chemotherapy and radiotherapy are established. Since the chemotherapy has made great achievements, especially in the recent 20 years, it has been widely used for various solid tumor, especially in the assistant treatment after operation, so the metastasis and dissemination in some patients has been restrained and improved, giving hope to treatment of solid tumor after operation. However, it is a pity that the reoccurrence and the metastasis happen again after several months and the patients still die of the cancer despite chemotherapy or intensive chemotherapy again. According to the follow-up survey to over 12000 metastasis and reoccurrence patients and the analysis of and experience in treatment summarization in Tumor Specialized Clinic of Shuguang Tumor Research Institute, it is found neither metastasis nor the reoccurrence could not be restrained on thousands of patients receiving the assistant chemotherapy after operation, the survival time and the survival time without cancer are not obviously improved. At present, although the assistant chemotherapy after operation has been made all over the country, there has been no prospective and correlatable scientific data, the assistant chemotherapy after operation is still in study. Of course, there are lots of patients receiving assistant chemotherapy after operation who have been in good condition over 10 years even 20 years, however, due to lack of prospective and correlatable scientific data, what is the comparison result between chemotherapy and non-chemotherapy in the patients after operation? What is the long-term survival rate of the patients not subject to chemotherapy? How to prove the long-term survival results from the chemotherapy after operation? All of these issues shall be further studied. At present, the reports in China lack lots of prospective and correlatable follow-up survey analysis data as well as the prospective and correlatable evaluation data about the assistant chemotherapy after operation just because the case history is kept by the patient instead of the hospital, as a result, the doctors and the hospital cannot make the follow-up survey. Of course, the in-hospital case history is kept for study, however, the in-hospital case history just reflects the short-term curative effects, most of the effects reflected in the in-hospital case history are relatively good because if it is not so good, the patient is not allowed to leave hospital. However, most patients are in good condition temporarily, for example, after the incision heals up, the patient begins to take food again and takes case of itself, the short-term curative effects are good, but it is hardly realized that the cancer cells may be in metastasis and it cannot be tested at present, of course, some tumor markers can be dynamically observed, such as CEA and AFP and so on.

Then, how to make the further study? Start from the existing problems to settle the problems through experiments and clinical study. The treatment of cancer shall be people-oriented and aim at curing the sickness to save the patient.

1. **Actively searching, studying and developing intelligent anti-cancer drugs.** The main contradictions in chemotherapy have been mentioned above and now we should pay attention to how to study and perfect them. The main issue is: the chemotherapy is the cytotoxic drug, without selectivity, so it cannot selectively distinguish the cancer cells from the normal cells, killing off all of them, resulting in some side effects and contradictions. So we should update the thought and actively study, search and develop the "intelligent anti-cancer drug" that only selectively kills the cancer cells instead of the normal cells of the organism, especially the immunological cells. In June 2004, American Society of Clinical Oncology held the annual meeting in New Orleans, with over 20000 oncologists as the attendants and 3700 papers called. Among these 3700 papers, there were 30 papers greatly affecting the treatment of cancer, of which there were 9 papers discussing the intelligent anti-cancer drugs. The intelligent anti-cancer drugs only affect the specific molecules in the cancer cells. The research findings of intelligent anti-drugs come into the world, indicating the treatment of cancer would shift to the epoch of accurate administration with little side effects from the one of chemotherapy with very great side effects. In research and development of the intelligent anti-cancer drugs, the research and development personnel do not spread these drugs at present. I believe that in the coming future, with the wide use of these drugs, people would feel the great effects from them and the patients would benefit from them. **Among the 48 kinds of anti-cancer drugs with relatively good tumor-inhibiting rate screened by this lab from 200 kinds of natural vegetable drugs, there are 3 kinds of vegetable drugs that can entirely inhibit and kill the cancer cells entirely and has no effects on the cultured epithelial cells or fibrous cells in the culture in vitro experiment on cancer cells, including XZ-C1-A, XZ-C1-B and XZ-C1-C. In the in vivo tumor-inhibition experiment on tumor-bearing animals, their tumor-inhibiting rate is 85%-95%. They are a part of XZ-C1, XZ-C immunoregulation anti-cancer medicine.** This experiment takes chemotherapy drug CTX as the control group and CTX obviously inhibits the immunity and the bone marrow. XZ-C anti-cancer medicine has no effects on bone marrow.

2. **Suggestion on immunologic chemotherapy.** Namely immunological treatment + chemotherapy. The immunological drugs can be administered in peri-chemotherapy period so as to reduce the side effects from chemotherapy; after chemotherapy, the immunologic treatment should be continued for a period to enhance the curative effects. The immunological treatment is the most reasonable treatment, it is of 0 order kinetics, however, it ① has relatively small acting force, it acts on 10^{5-6} cancer cells strongly; beyond this range, it acts weakly. ②The immunological drug can improve the immunity of the organism and enhance the immunological surveillance in the organism. ③ It can be continually administered or taken orally. Because the cancer cells are continually divided and proliferated, the treatment shall be also continual. XZ-C immunoregulation medicine can protect the hematopiesis function of the bone marrow, protect the thymus, improve the immunity, improve the symptom and raise the life quality; the action is relatively slowly, little but durably. Since the biological characteristics of the cancer cells are the continual division and proliferation, our countermeasures must be also continual.

   Chemotherapy and immunological treatment currently adopted should learn from other's strong points to offset one's weakness and be comprehensively applied so as to improve the curative effects. The chemotherapy is of intermittent administration while the immunoregulation treatment is of continual treatment. If both of them assist with each other, the curative effects will be improved undoubtedly. If the cancer patient has inferior immunologic function, the operation on cancer will bring down the immunologic function further. In operation, the cancer cells entering the blood circulation by extrusion increase. How to eliminate or control the cancer cells entering the blood circulation in operation? It is held by us that XZ-C medicine should be added before, in and after operation for immunological treatment. XZ-C_4 can protect the thymus and XZ=C_8 can protect the bone marrow. In this way, the central immune organ and immunologic function of the host can be protected, the curative effects of the chemotherapy can be strengthened and the side effects of the chemotherapy inhibiting the immunologic function can be reduced, as a result, it will reduce the opportunity of metastasis of cancer cells, therefore, the improvement of immunologic function of the patient in the peri-operation period or in the period of assistant chemotherapy after operation is an important link of comprehensive treatment.

3. **Making sensitivity test of chemotherapy drugs and implementing "individualized" immunological chemotherapy**. Now the chemotherapy in cancer has stepped into the stage of "individualized" chemotherapy in many hospitals. Previously, the different cancer patients are subject to the same chemotherapy plan, unavoidably resulting in blindness, not conforming to the actual conditions of the patients. It is shown by the study that even though the same kind of tumor with same type of tissue, even the different stages of the same cancer, has different sensitivities to the chemotherapy drugs, therefore, it is necessary to make the drugsensitive test on the individual cancer patients and it is urgent to select the sensitive drugs from various anti-cancer drugs. It is proven by the clinical experience in chemotherapy that the effective rate of administration by experience is very low (14%), if the drug can be selected according to the results measured by drugsensitive test, the effective rate can be raised to 28%-35%.

The effect of chemotherapy in the solid tumor is not as good as the one in malignant tumor in the blood system and the transmission hindrance of drug in the solid tumor is the upmost factor of drug resistance of solid tumor.

It is an important way and one of the current study hotspots to make the sensitive test on chemotherapy drug for tumor and carry out the individualized chemotherapy plan so as to improve the effects of chemotherapy in tumor and reduce the side effects.

Generally, the drugsensitive test on tumor can be made with the method of culture in vitro and culture in vivo, the former includes cell culture method and tissue culture method and the latter refers to the method of culture in vivo in animal. Among the test methods, the method of transplantation in vivo in the nude mice can obtain true and reliable results with respect to drug test or new drug screening, however, the process is long, the operation is complicated and the price is high. The method of cell culture is the most simple, convenient and feasible, however, since the kinetics is not entirely same to the tumor in vivo, the test results often differ from the drug reaction of the tumor in vivo, so it cannot be used to directly guide the administration of the different tumor patients.

Someone makes a study on 3D tissue culture method of tumor, namely Hoffman 3D tissue culture method, which directly uses the clinical samples, avoids the repeated digestion of tumor cells with enzyme or mechanically and features quickness and relatively high success ratio. This method would be helpful to guide the individualized chemotherapy, improve the chemotherapy effects and reduce the drug resistance.

(1) In vitro drugsensitive test: it is very important to establish the reliable anti-cancer in vitro drugsensitive test method so as to help the clinicians select the effective chemotherapy drugs, reasonably design the therapeutic method, improve the curative effects, avoid the side effects from the ineffective drugs and directly screen the new anti-cancer and anti-metastasis drugs with the fresh human tumor samples.

There are so many methods of in vitro sensitive test of anti-cancer drug and they have the common characteristics: simple method, high sensitivity, smaller dose than the in vivo method, quick judgment results, without too many animals; in addition, they also can screen the anti-cancer drugs and most of them are parallel to the in vivo method with respect to the procedures.

(2) in vivo chemotherapy drug sensitive test: at present, as to the chemotherapy drug sensitive test methods, the in vitro method prevails and it has the advantages of quickness, convenience and simple as well as good clinical correlation and good repeatability, however, it also has some disadvantages because it breaks away from the in vivo environment of the tumor and is not consistent with the human tumor in histology and cell kinetics, reducing the coincidence rate of the test results and the clinic.

Various drugs have different concentrations in the body fluid and are affected by the body weight, route of medication, liver and kidney function and so on, in this way, the in vitro method cannot represent the change in drug concentration. Some drugs should be activated and metabolized in vivo before playing a role in anti-cancer, such as CTX; some drugs acting on the cancer cells will bring into play through the immune system. The reaction of the cancer cells to these drugs cannot be tested with in vitro method.

The solid tumor are the spatial structure occupying a certain space. Besides the tumor cells in blood, breast and ascites are directly contact with the drugs, the solid tumor is not so simple. The drugs cannot reach up to the deep part easily; the anoxia caused by ischemia; the uneven blood flow in the tumor; the difference in PH value and osmotic pressure will affect the sensitivity of the solid tumor cells to the chemotherapy drugs.

It is necessary to select the optimal "individualized" joint chemotherapy plan through the drugsensitive test.

CHAPTER 14

A Proposal for Improving Measures for Assistant Chemotherapy after Operation on Cancer

In 1985, I made the follow-up survey of over 3000 patients after operation on cancer in general surgery and thoracic surgery, finding that most of the patients met with reoccurrence and metastasis within 2-3 years after operation, some even met with reoccurrence within several months, which made me realize that the operation was successful and standardized while the long-term curative effects were unsatisfactory or the long-term treatment was unsuccessful.

Since 1990s, in view that the reoccurrence and metastasis rate of cancer after operation was very high, in order to prevent the reoccurrence and metastasis after operation, a series of assistance chemotherapy after operation has been adopted, what's more, the chemotherapy was made before operation (for example, the breast cancer), however, the results had been not so satisfactory. Reoccurrence and metastasis take place in assistant chemotherapy after operation or in the period of treatment or the metastasis takes place synchronously in chemotherapy. It can be seen from so many patients in Wuhan Shuguang Tumor Special Clinic that neither reoccurrence nor metastasis cannot be prevented by the assistant chemotherapy after operation, even in some cases, the intensified chemotherapy promotes the adynamia of immunologic function. All these things should be seriously, calmly, practically and realistically thought and reflected by the clinicians: why the assistant chemotherapy after operation cannot prevent the reoccurrence? Why the assistant chemotherapy after operation cannot prevent the metastasis? Why the assistant chemotherapy after operation on some patients promotes the adynamia of immunologic function? What's the problem and disadvantage of the assistant chemotherapy after operation? What measures should be taken? How to further study and perfect it? How to reform and innovate in the assistant chemotherapy to improve the curative effects?

I. Why to make the assistant chemotherapy after operation on cancer or assistant chemotherapy in peri-operation period?

Currently, the treatment of cancer mainly depends on the operation, however, the reoccurrence and metastasis rate is still relatively high after operation.

1. The potential reason why the local reoccurrence and metastasis after radical operation on cancer takes place may be the following factors viewed from clinic:

(1) Insufficient attention has not been paid to the free-tumor technique, as a result, the operation such as exploration and touch causes the cancer cells on the serosa surface to fall into the intra-abdominal implantation.

(2) The tumor tissue is not thoroughly removed by the operation, as a result, the remained cancer cells are continually proliferating.

(3) The existing metastasis lesion is not found in operation and is not removed, for example, the lymph node in metastasis is not found or is removed incompletely.

(4) As to the clearing of lymph node in operation, traditionally, it adopts the passive separation, in this way, the apocoptic micro-lymphatic vessel may lead to the fluxion, dissemination, residual and transplantation of the cancer cells.
(5) The operation leads to the transplantation of the cancer cells, the cancer cells invading the esophagus, stomach serosa or colon, recta and serosa may easily fall into the abdominal cavity and form the transplantation lesion and the damaged peritoneum in the area of operation may easily meet with transplnation and reoccurrence. The reoccurrence of anastomotic stoma of the colon may be the intracavity exfoliation and transplantation of the enteral cancer cells in the operation.
(6) The metastasis of the lymph node in the patients in the late stage is relatively wide and syzygial, in this way, it is difficult to remove it with operation.
(7) In the operation on gastrointestinal tract cancer, the metastasis of cancer cells in the portal vein takes place, resulting in the metastasis of liver cancer cells after operation. However, it is unseenable in the operation by the naked eyes. For example, when the "radical operation on gastric carcinoma" is made, the cancerous protuberance and the tumid lymph nodes of gastric carcinoma can be seen by us, however, whether the cancer cells exist in the vein and the blood of the portal vein is unknown? How many cancer cells exist? Where do these cancer cells in the vein go? Whether these cancer cells in cluster that can be touched and extruded into the venous blood in operation arrive at the portal vein? Or arrive at the branch of the portal vein in the liver? It is not impossible to touch the cancerous protuberance in exploration and excision of gastric cancerous protuberance and cleaning of lymph node, the operation necessarily makes a large number of cancer cells be extruded and fall down, then they flow into the portal venous blood, resulting in metastasis in liver after operation.
(8) The operation brings about the traumas to the organism, resulting in the inferior immunologic function, in this way, the organism losses the immunological surveillance or is weakened in immunological surveillance, leaving opportunity to the residual cancer cells or the cancer cells in dormancy for reoccurrence and metastasis.
(9) As to the cancer in the progressive stage, the metastasis of cancer cells may take place before operation while these cancer cells in metastasis cannot be seen by the physician in operation. However, it is reported in the pathological section report that the cancer embolus can be seen in the blood capillary and the lymphatic vessel.

Based on the above-mentioned, after the radical operation of the cancer, the residual cancer cells may still exist, resulting in reoccurrence and metastasis of the residual subclinical cancer lesion after operation.

Then, how to make up for the shortage of radical operation with residual cancer cells? Adopt the chemotherapy in peri-operation period to hunt the residual cancer cells in operation with the chemotherapy cytotoxic drug and remove the cancer cells falling off or remained or transplanted in the operation.

However, could the traditional assistant chemotherapy after operation hunt the residual cancer cells in operation? Could it remove the cancer cells falling off, remained or transplanted in operation?

2. **Why the current assistant chemotherapy after operation cannot prevent the reoccurrence and metastasis? It shall be reviewed, analyzed and reflected:**
   (1) The route of administration of assistant chemotherapy after operation shall be further studied and reformed. At present, it mainly adopts the general intravenous chemotherapy after operation, the cytotoxic drug injected is generally distributed, acting on the histiocytes of the viscera in the whole body, in this way, the ones killed are mainly the proliferative cells, immunological cells and bone marrow cells of the normal tissue organs in the whole body. However, the field of operation accounts for a little ratio in the whole body, in this way, the dose obtained is very small, it is difficult to kill the local residual cancer cells or the cancer lesion in the field of operation or the residual cancer lesion of the cancer cells falling off in the operation, therefore, the route of administration shall be reformed.
   (2) The assistant chemotherapy after operation is blinded and the drug administered is not subject to the drugsensitive test. Since the drugsensitive test on the cancer histiocytes of patient is not carried out, the drug is administered by experience, so it is unknown whether the drug is sensitive. If the drug administered is insensitive or drug resistant, it is not only fruitless, without any action on the residual cancer cells, but also kills the proliferative cells, the immunological cells and the bone marrow cells of the normal tissues in the whole body, while these normal tissues in the whole body do not need the cytotoxic drug, resulting in the remarkable side effect, damaging the patient and making the patient suffer from the pain of the side effect. Thus, although the chemotherapy has been made for several times, the expected curative effects cannot be realized, in addition, the cytotoxic drug injected intravenously in the wholly body covers the whole body, kills the general immunological cells and the hematopoietic cells of the bone marrow and makes the immunologic functions of the patient further descend. Actually, the cancer patient is inferior in immunologic function, while the radical operation further brings down the immunologic function, plus the assistant chemotherapy of the cytotoxic drug after operation, the immunological function of the patient is further reduced, like one disaster after another, resulting in metastasis while in chemotherapy. Therefore, as for the assistant chemotherapy after operation, if the drugsensitive test is not made and the drug is administered in form of individualization, the chemotherapy would benefit some patients while damage some patients.
   (3) Assistant chemotherapy after operation. **Since the tumor is removed and the lymph clearing is made, the drug administration plan and the dosage should differ from the ones for the patients without removal by operation,** the dosage in the assistant chemotherapy period after operation would differ from the one before operation, before removal of the tumor, the dosage is calculated as per the body surface area so as to realize the goal of remission and shrinkage, however, after the radical operation, the tumor is removed, so it shall target the potentially residual cancer cells or the micro-metastasis in operation instead of the remission and shrinkage, since both targets differs from each other, in order to remit and shrink the tumor of the patient without operation, the drug must have a certain lethality, as a result, the drug administration plans shall be combined and the dosage shall be up to the one the patient can bear, in this way, the curative effect of remission and shrinkage can be realized. Meanwhile, the assistant chemotherapy after operation, depends on radical operation primarily and the chemotherapy secondarily, only targeted for removal of the potentially residual cancer

cells or the cancer cells falling off in the operation or the cancer cells in metastasis to make some subsidiary treatment to prevent the reoccurrence and metastasis. Therefore, its drug administration plan and dose shall differ from the former and the dosage of the cytotoxic drug shall be greatly reduced.

(4) What determines the indications and the contraindications of the assistant chemotherapy after operation? At present, the indications of assistant chemotherapy after operation are discordant, for example, do the residual cancer cells exist in the patient after this operation on earth? Where? How many? To what extent? All those things should be taken into account and estimated, however, most of the patients receive the "radical operation on cancer" in the general surgery or the specialized surgery, after operation, they come back to the local hospitals or the tumor clinic, the chemotherapy after operation is the general intravenous chemotherapy, the plans selected differ from each other in each place, each hospital by each physician, namely there is no uniform plan, these physicians or nurses responsible for general intravenous injection for the assistant chemotherapy after operation are not always aware of the patient's condition, pathological analysis, the range and the extent of cancer invasion seen in the operation as well as the estimation of the potential residual cancer lesion in operation, the extent of the radical operation and so on. They should know TNM stage and the immunity chemotherapy and estimate the potential residual cancer cells. Who knows it clearly? Only the operation doctor because he can see the range and extent of the cancer invasion through exploration in operation. Therefore, what determines the selection of chemotherapy or radiotherapy after operation? The operation physician shall determine the indications and the contraindications of the assistant chemotherapy after operation as well as the chemotherapy plan, times, dosage and so on to satisfy the actual conditions of the patient.

(5) How to assess the curative effects of the assistant chemotherapy after operation? At present, there is no uniform understanding or standard. The objective curative effects of the chemotherapy on the solid tumor before removal of the tumor shall be assessed according to the area of tumor and the remission of the tumor recognized in the world. However, since the tumor is removed, it shall be assessed according to the improvement of the symptom and the condition instead of area of tumor. At present, what role does the assistant chemotherapy after operation play? Does it kill the cancer cells? How many? Do the residual cancer cells exist in the patient's body? What is the effect? All these things are kept unknown. However, it is well known that it kills the normal cells, the immunological cells and the hematopoietic cells of the bone marrow because the white blood cells fall down, the blood platelets fall down too, but it is the extent of the side effect rather than the effect. As to the tumor sign, it is difficult to determine the definite standard at present and it is necessary to make the fundamental study and clinical study.

II. How to Do well in Assistant Chemotherapy after Operation on Cancer or Assistant Chemotherapy in Peri-operation Period?

XU ZE made a suggestion of reforming and developing the assistant chemotherapy after operation on cancer in abdomen (the malignant tumor such as liver cancer,

gallbladder cancer, pancreatic cancer, gastric cancer, intestinal cancer and abdominal cancer) as follows:

1. Reform the route of administration and change the general intravenous chemotherapy into the chemotherapy through intravascular administration in target organ. All of the operations on cancer in abdomen, no matter the radical operation or palliative excision, or the operation only for exploration instead of removal, shall adopt the built-in pump in ductus venosus in stomach omentum, or built-in pump in portal vein, or arterial pump, or built-in pump in vein of mesentery as much as possible. Why is the chemotherapy pump built in portal system? Firstly, it is necessary to know where the cancer cells after operation on cancer exist. The administration must be targeted for the cancer cell group and the cancer cells of liver cancer, gallbladder cancer, pancreatic cancer, gastric cancer and intestinal cancer are in the tuberiferous veins, which flow towards the portal vein and gather at the portal vein, then flow towards hepatic vein via sinus hepaticus and into the lungs via the right atrium. Therefore, the portal system adopts the targeted intravascular administration targeted through the chemotherapy pump, so it is the direct target and it is reasonable and scientific. It can make the residual cancer cells prowling in the portal vein after operation directly contact the chemotherapy drug to produce the curative effect.
2. Reform the dosage of administration: since the built-pump in portal vein is directly targeted for the cancer cell group in the blood of the portal vein and the chemotherapy drug needed is greatly reduced by contrast with the dosage of general intravenous administration. Since the drug is administered through the target organ of the portal vein, the dosage can be greatly reduced. Because the radical operation on cancer has been made, the cancerous protuberance has been removed and the next thing to be done is to remove the potentially residual cancer cells, generally, the immunological cells in the human body can remove these cancer cells, however, since the immunologic function of the cancer patient comes down, the assistant chemotherapy after operation is used to assist in removal, so only a small quantity of dosage is needed, it shall strive for killing 10^{5-6} cancer cells without damage to the normal cells as much as possible. The rest 10^{5-6} cancer cells will be removed by the immunological cells of the organism. However, as to the tracking and hunting of the potential cancer cells in metastasis in the portal system, although the targeted administration reduces the dosage greatly, the drug concentration in the portal vein will be greatly increased out of question, resulting in the improvement of the curative effect. **Since the dosage is greatly reduced, it will necessarily reduce even eliminate the side effect of the chemotherapy greatly. The elimination of the side effect of the chemotherapy, will benefit millions of cancer patients. Over the past half century, millions of cancer patients have deeply suffered from the pain of the side effect from the chemotherapy and the radiotherapy all over the world, what's more, the lives of some patients have been endangered. Since the side effect of chemotherapy is eliminated, so many cancer patients are secured. The cancer seriously endangers the health of the human beings and makes the medical expenses rapidly increase as well. The direct expenses for cancer treatment in China are approximately RMB one hundred billion Yuan, bringing a heavy economic burden to the patients even the whole society. Now Professor Xu Ze holds: the intravascular administration in the specific target organ, reduces the dose, improves the curative effects, eliminates the side reaction, necessarily leading to great reduction of medical charge, saving billions of medical charges and**

expenditures (in RMB Yuan) for the state and the patients and being advantageous for settling the problems of being difficult and expensive in taking medical treatment.

3. Reform the blindness of the drug administered for assistant chemotherapy after operation. The drug for chemotherapy after operation shall be subject to the drugsensitive test together with the histiocytes of the cancer tissue of the patients for the individualized chemotherapy. All operations on cancer, no matter the radical operations or the palliative operations or the exploratory operations, shall try to obtain the specimen of the cancer tissue, the cancer tissue will be cut up into two halves in aseptic manipulation, one for cultivation of cancer tissue and drugsensitive test and another for pathological section and chemotherapy of immunity group for definite pathological diagnosis.

   Why the specimen of cancer tissue is selected for cultivation of cancer cells and the drugsensitive test? Since the detection of sensitivity and drug resistance of tumor chemotherapy is the foundation of "individualized" chemotherapy. To this day, the tumor chemotherapy has stridden forward to the "individualized" chemotherapy. In the past days, the different tumor patients receive the same chemotherapy mode (plan), resulting in blindness inevitably. It is shown by the study that the same kind of tumor with the same tissue, even the same tumor in different stages has the incompletely consistent sensitivity to the chemotherapy drug. Therefore, it is necessary to make the drugsensitive test on the tumor patient to select the sensitive drug. Especially, with the increase of the anti-tumor drug at present, it is more urgent. It is proven by the clinical experience in tumor chemotherapy that the effective rate of drug administered by experience is very low (14%) while it will be increased to 28%-35% if the results measured with the existing drugsensitive test method is used to guide the selection of the drug, which is a great fruit.

   The detection of the sensitivity and drug resistance of tumor chemotherapy offers an important basis to the foreseeable chemotherapy to reasonably use the anti-tumor drug to reduce the blindness and improve the pertinence, which would undoubtedly improve the level of tumor chemotherapy greatly.

4. The key is to manage and disposal the pump after operation: the drug pump for portal system is in-built in the operation. After operation, it is necessary to continually adopt the long-term light (trace) nontoxic chemotherapy drug and inject the heparin to prevent the embolism, prevent the cancer embolus and prevent the cancer cell group. Where are the cancer cells in the peri-operation period? The cancerous protuberance of liver, gallbladder, pancreas, spleen, stomach and intestine will be carried off by the blood separately after flowing into the blood of the portal vein or many cancer cells meet with homoplasmic adhesion or heterogenetic adhesion with other cells to form the cancer cell group, which floats with the blood and forms the cancer embolus in the blood vessel, then the deciduous cancer cell embolus moves along the direction of the blood of the venous system. The cancer cells continually enter the blood circulation and transfer along the normal direction of the blood. Most of the cancer cells entering the blood circulation will be eliminated by the host and only a few of the cancer cells survive. Within several days after operation, a large number of cancer cells flow over into the portal system via tumorigenic vein in virtue of operation technique and exploratory extrusion. The surviving cancer cells are adhered to the endothelial cells of the wall of the target organ and then enter the target organ after passing through the wall and form the minute metastasis lesion. The cancer cells from gstrointestinal tract can flow into the liver along the portal vein and the liver is the end point

of the blood of the portal vein, therefore, the cancer of gastrointestinal tract often transfers to the liver, forms the cancer cells of the metastasis lesion of the metastasis liver cancer and invades the central vein via the minute branch of the portal vein. The cancer cells can enter the hepatic vein and then flow back to the right atrium via the lower caval vein, then to the lung via the pulmonary artery and form the metastasis lesion of lung.

It can be often seen that the cancer embolus exists in the portal vein branch in the pathological report or the cancer embolus forms in the portal vein branch in CT or MRI report. The cancer embolus is the main factor in the formation of the metastasis lesion. The cancer cells, the fibrin and the blood platelet constitute the embolus and then it is carried to other parts, passes through the wall and forms the secondary tumor around the blood vessel. The formation of cancer embolus is related to the following factors: ① the inherent adhesion and aggregation of the cancer cells; ② the action of Thrombo-Pletinlike substances; ③ action of blood platelet; ④combined action of fibrin.

It is important to do well in management and application of pump after operation. Someone is inbuilt with chemotherapy pump and does not pay a return visit or use the pump after leaving hospital. After operation, the regular return visit shall be paid and the heparin shall be injected via the pump to prevent the blockade and the cancer embolus. A few of chemotherapy drugs shall be injected to hunt the floating cancer cells remaining in the the blood circulation of portal vein.

The surgeons and the nurses shall be responsible for the arrangement, follow-up survey, registration, filling, consultation answer, statistics and summary of the assistant chemotherapy after operation.

5. Reform the single goal of killing cancer cells into the immunological mediation and control therapy in an all-round way. Abandon the goal of only killing the cancer cells, attach importance to the resistance of the organism, reform it into the immunological mediation and control therapy in an all-round way and give attention to both of them, thus, the curative effect will be improved. XZ-C medicine shall be orally taken in the period of assistant chemotherapy after operation and after the treatment course of the assistant chemotherapy to carry out the immunological chemotherapy (immunity + chemotherapy) or immunological chemotherapy radiotherapy (immunity + radiotherapy) so as to reform the unilateral therapeutic outlook of singly killing the cancer cells into an all-round therapeutic outlook of killing the cancer cells as well as improving the immunity of the organism.

III. Why the Assistant Chemotherapy after Operation Cannot Achieve the Expectation

In the past 10 years, the assistant chemotherapy after operation has been widely adopted all over the country, however, most of the assistant chemotherapy after operation is made by experience, the treatment plans differ from each other in different hospitals; the chemotherapy drugs selected differ from each other; the same to the departments and doctors in the same hospital due to the difference experience. The days and the interval of chemotherapy drugs administered differ a little from each other in different hospitals in different places: once per month for someone, once per two months for someone, once per week for someone, 4 times continually for someone, 6 times continually for someone and even 8-10 times continually for someone. The treatment courses are arranged with a certain blindness and differ from each other, without uniform or consistent standard. Because most of the hospitals have not made the drugsensitive test, so the "individualized" chemotherapy cannot be made.

At present, the plans for assistant chemotherapy after operation adopted in different places are basically similar to the ordinary chemotherapy plans, however, the goal or target of the ordinary tumor chemotherapy aims at the primary cancer lesion or the metastasis cancer lesion and the goal of treatment is to shrink, eliminate or remit the primary cancerous protuberance or metastasis cancerous protuberance or the tumid lymph node. These solid cancerous protuberances occupy a relatively large area, so, in order to shrink the cancerous protuberance, it is necessary to take the combined chemotherapy drugs with a relatively large quantity, otherwise, it is difficult to shrink the cancerous protuberance.

However, the assistant chemotherapy after operation is entirely different from this because the radical operation removes and cleans down the primary cancerous protuberance and the tumid lymph node around it, in this way, there is no solid cancerous protuberance. Since the cancerous protuberance is removed, the assistant chemotherapy after operation aims at the potentially residual cancer cells after operation, the potentially remnant micro-metastasis cancer cells or the cancer cells in metastasis and it is targeted for the remnant cancer cells or the potentially metastasis cancer cells instead of the solid cancerous protuberance, so the dosage shall be relatively small, without damage to the immunological cells of the host or with a little damage to the host. So how to assess the curative effect of the assistant chemotherapy after operation shall be measured according to the assessment standard including the improvement of immunity, the improvement of the survival quality, the improvement of the symptom, the elevation of the immunity indexes, the descent of the tumor sign and good mental state and appetite instead of the shrinkage of the tumor.

How to do well in assistant chemotherapy after operation? It is held by us that attention shall be paid to the following:

1. As to the patients receiving the radical operation on the cancerous protuberance, the fresh tumor specimen shall be selected for the chemotherapy drug sensitive test so as to individualize the assistant chemotherapy after operation to avoid the blindness of drug administration.
2. How to judge or estimate whether the remnant cancer cells exist in the body after radical operation so as to determine the indication of the assistant chemotherapy after operation, in this way, the immunity indexes and the tumor signs shall be detected.
3. How to judge the curative effect of the assistant chemotherapy after operation? Are the cancer cells killed or not? Since the tumor is removed, the curative effect cannot be judged as per the existence of the tumor of the volume of the tumor. The immunity indexes, the cytokines and the tumor signs shall be detected to judge the possibility of the reoccurrence and metastasis after operation.
4. The drug administered for the assistant chemotherapy after operation shall differ from the one for primary tumor or the metastasis cancer lesion because the goals are different: the former is to eliminate the primary cancer lesion and the latter is to eliminate the residual cancer cells, as a result, the dosage shall be different and it shall be greatly reduced.
5. The patient receiving the radical operation on cancer is very weak in the body condition and inferior in immunologic function, so the assistant chemotherapy after operation must be accompanied with the immunological mediation and control therapy, namely the immunological therapy + chemotherapy, called immunological chemotherapy. As

above-mentioned, the elimination of the cancer cells in metastasis or the cancer cells or the cancer cell group in the blood circulation after operation mainly depends on the immunological cells in the organism of the host. It is shown by the experimental study that the immunological cells in the organism can eliminate 10^5 cancer cells, so the dosage for the assistant chemotheray after operation shall not be too large under the precondition of not damaging or slihgtly damaging the immunological cells because it is very important to carry out the immunological mediation and control therapy and improve the immunity of the organism to eliminate the cancer cells in metastasis. We deeply realize that in the past 16 years, Wuhan Shuguang Tumor Special Clinic under Wuhan Research Institute of Anti-cancerometastasis and Anti-reoccurrence has diagnosed so many patients like this, some of them are of valetudinarianism or accompanied with other diseases, resulting in failure to chemotherapy and radiotherapy; some of them fail to the chemotherapy again due to the severe response after 1-2 chemotherapy after operation; some of them refuse the chemotherapy after operation; most of the patients meet with the cancer invading serosa and are accompanied by metastasis of lymph node, so they take XZ-C medicine for treatment in the new mode of XU ZE new concept of anti-cancerometastasis treatment and orally take XZ-C medicine for a long term, resulting in a relatively good curative effect.

6. Although the assistant chemotherapy after operation has been widely popularized all over the country at present, there are short of the forward-looking, comparable and appreciable reports on the assistant chemotherapy after operation. According to the report on 5-year's follow-up survey of the assistant chemotherapy or radiotherapy after operation on the patients suffering from the stomach cancer by American Stomach Cancer Group, it was reported by Lence (1994, 3, 3, 1390) that the total survival rate was still low in the patients suffering from the stomach cancer even the patients with the cancer removed through operation, therefore, the people hope to improve the prognosis through the assistant chemotherapy and radiotherapy for the patients with low tumor load after operation. It was shown by the results of the assistant treatment with mitomycin and fluorouracil on the first group of the patients in 1976 by British Stomach Cancer Organization that it had no benefit to the patients after operation, for this reason, the study on the assistant treatment of another group of patients had been made.

The forward-looking, random and contrapositive grouping study had been made on 430 patients suffering from the gastric gland cancer in Stage II and III after operation, accompanied with radiotherapy or the combined chemotherapy of mitomycin, adriamycin and fluorouracil (MAF) plan over 5 years, among which 372 patients died, 7 of which died of the surgical complication and 327 of which died of the reoccurrence of tumor. In the random grouping study, 145 cases only adopted the operation therapy; 153 cases accepted the assistant chemotherapy with the rang of irradiation including hilum of spleen and porta hepatic with the dosage of 4500cGy and the increase in dosage of 500cGy in operative field area; another 138 cases accepted the combined chemotherapy (MPA Plan) with mitomycin 4mg/m^2, adriamycin 30mg/m^2 and fluorouracil 600 mg/m^2, intravenously injected, 3 weeks as a cycle, totaling 6 cycles. The total two-year's survival rate of this group of patients was 33% and the total five-year's survival rate was 17% (13%~21%), compared with the patients with the single operation therapy, as to the patients accepting the assistant chemotherapy, the survival rate was not raised: the five-year's survival rate of the patients with single operation therapy was 20% and the one of the patients accepting the operation plus radiotherapy was 19%.

Therefore, operation is still the standard therapeutic method of the stomach cancer and the assistant therapeutic measures shall be restricted within a certain scope of study.

To sum up, it is held by the author: some large hospitals or medical centers in China should make the forward-looking comparable grouping study to obtain a large number of appreciable scientific data in China. At present, the assistant chemotherapy after operation is still restricted within a certain scope of study.

CHAPTER 15

Xu Ze's New Concept and New Model of Cancer Treatment

I. Strengthening of immunological therapy and improving side effects from chemotherapy

1. Side effects of traditional chemotherapy: when chemotherapy is made on cancer, it usually inhibits immunologic function and hematopoiesis function of the bone marrow, descends WBC and PLT and damages liver and kidney function as well as gastroenteric function, leading to the side effects such as nausea, emesis, abdominal distension, anorexia and so on.

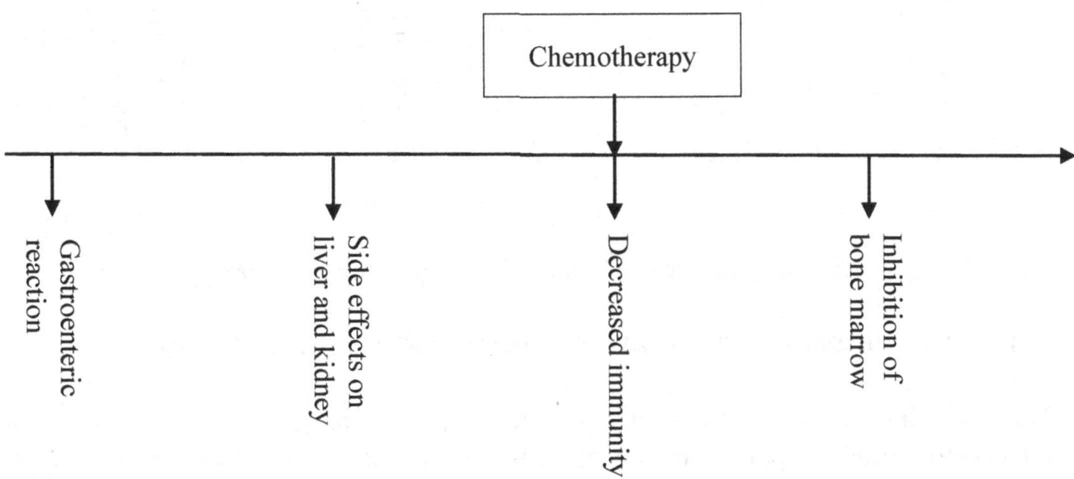

Fig. 1 Side effects of traditional chemotherapy

2. The countermeasures of Xu Ze's new concept: the method to improve the side effects of chemotherapy is to strengthen the supporting therapy and take effective measures to protect the host. Among the traditional Chinese medicine for immunological mediation, XZ-C_4 can protect thymus thus and improve immunity; XZ-C_8 can protect hematopoiesis function of the bone marrow and generate more stem cells; XZ-C medicine for immunity mediation can strengthen physical strength of cancerous patients. See Fig. 2.

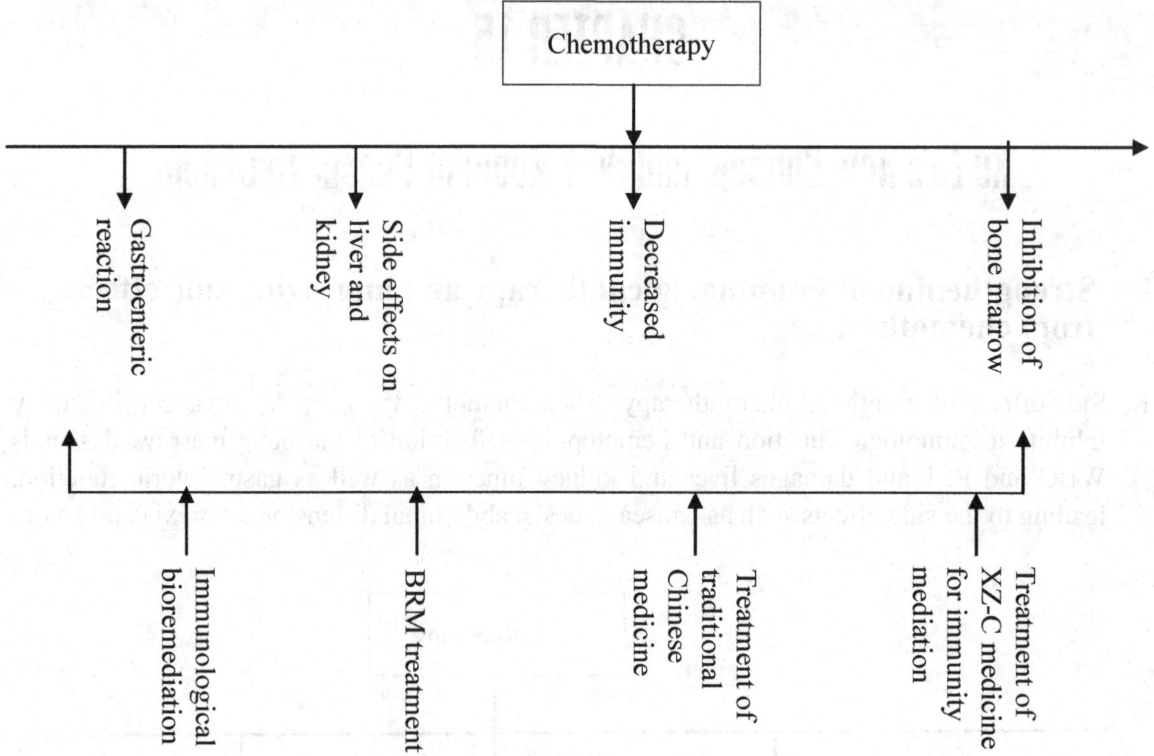

Fig. 2 Countermeasures for side effects of chemotherapy

II. Changing intermittent treatment into continual treatment

1. Traditional intravenous chemotherapy is an intermittent therapy, that is to say, after the drug for chemotherapy is applied for 3-5 days, it is necessary to apply the chemotherapeutic drug for the second course of treatment when WBC and PLT return to normal after 3-4 weeks. The drug for chemotherapy shall not be continually applied during the intermission between the first and the second course of treatment, whereas the cancel cells are still continually and uninterruptedly proliferated and divided in the intermission and increase at the speed of geometrical progression. In addition, because of the inhibition of immunologic function caused by chemotherapeutic drug, the cancel cells escape from or are free of the immunological surveillance, their proliferation and division are quickened during the intermission between these two courses, in other words, the longer the course of treatment of chemotherapeutic drug, the more the combined drug and the more the dose, the more serious of the attack against immunity of the human body, resulting in lack of immunological surveillance, and even resulting in reoccurrence and metastasis in chemotherapy, and shrinkage of tumor firstly before continual enlargement later (see Fig. 3). These cases occur commonly, how to treat them? It is held by us that the following model should be adopted for a continuous immunological therapy in the intermission between two courses of treatment.

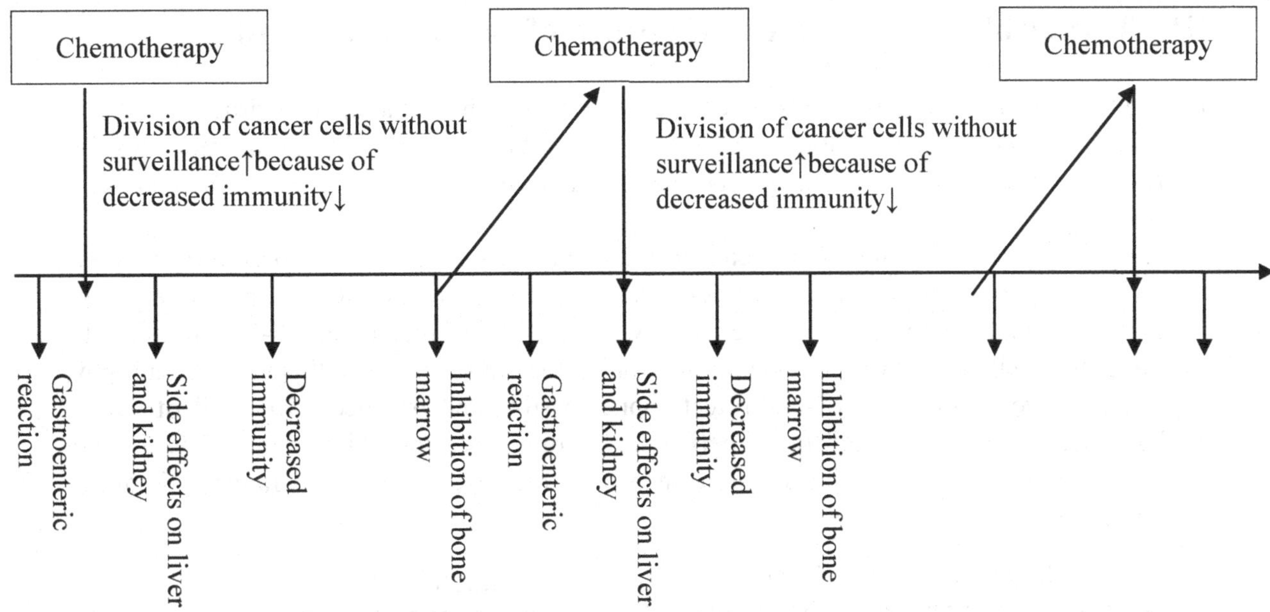

Fig.3 Easy reoccurrence of tumor without treatment in the intermission

2. Xu Ze's new concept and model of cancer treatment is a continuous treatment. It adopts traditional Chinese medicine for immunological mediation, namely XZ-C_1 + XZ-C_4, or BRM for treatment during the intermission. XZ-C_1 was screened through the experimental study on tumor-bearing animals over 7 years and has been proven by a sixteen-year clinical verification that it has only inhibited the cancel cells rather than normal ones and that it can benefit spleen and stomach. XZ-C_4 can protect thymus from atrophy, prevent immunity from decreasing and make it better. Continual treatment in the intermittence with XZ-C medicine can control proliferation of caner cells and also protect the function of immune organs such as thymus.

The combination of chemotherapeutic drug and XZ-C medicine can decrease teh side effects from chemotherapy and strengthen chemotherapy effects against the loss of immunological surveillance as well meanwhile. See Fig. 4.

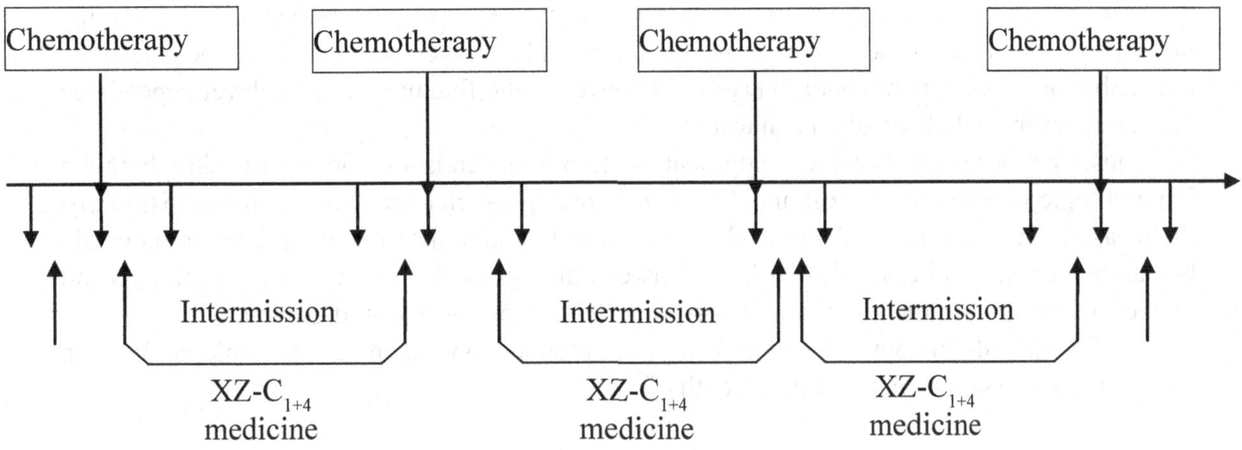

Fig. 4 Continual treatment in the intermission

III. Therapy of protecting the host instead of damaging the host

1. Traditional chemotherapy tends to damage the hosts: chemotherapeutic drugs are the x drugs and function as a double-edged sword, killing both cancer cells and normal ones for the lack of selectivity, inhibiting bone marrow and decreasing peripheral WBC and PLT. See Fig. 5.
2. Xu Ze' new concept and model of cancer treatment tends to protect the hosts: the new-type anticancer drugs only inhibit cancer cells, have no effects on normal cells, protect thymus, improve immunity and protect bone marrow. Among XZ-C medicine, XZ-C_1 only inhibits the cancel cells and have no effects on normal cells; XZ-C_4 protects thymus from atrophy and improves immunity; XZ-C_8 protects bone marrow and produces blood, all of which have been screened through the experiments on tumor-bearing animals over 7 years and have been proven by the clinical data of nearly 10000 cases in the cooperative anti-cancer clinic over 10 years. See Fig. 6.

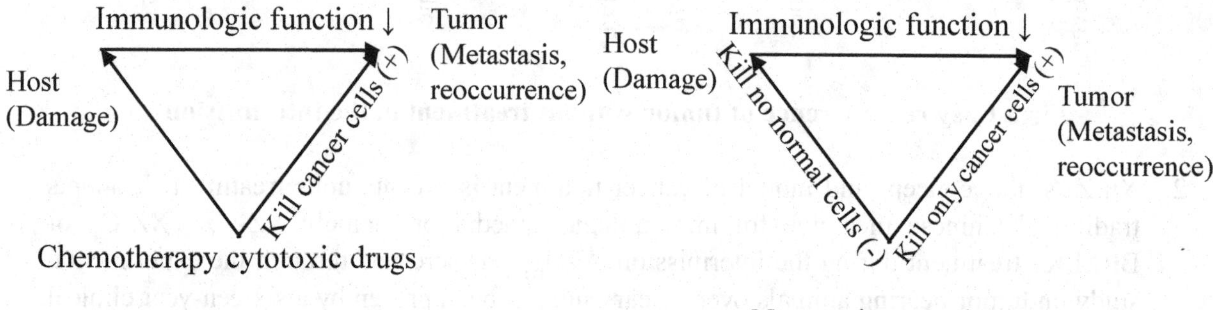

Fig. 5 Effects of traditional chemotherapy Fig. 6 Effects of Xu Ze's new model of cancer treatment

IV. Rebalancing the unbalance between the host and tumor

It has been proven by the abovementioned findings from the experimental study that the positive relationship exists between the occurrence and development of tumor and the structure and immunologic function of immune organs of the host such as thymus and marrow. Enlightened by the seesaws in children's park and the weighing scale in the laboratory, the author took a tumble: if immunologic function was too inferior, tumor would grow up, meanwhile, when the former was improved to a certain level, then the later would be controlled in a stable or improvement condition (Fig. 7). However, the fluctuation of the level depends on further experimental observation and test.

Thus, the occurrence and development of tumor depends on the relationship between immunologic function of the host and the intrinsic biological characteristics of tumor. Similarly, the invasion and metastasis of cancer also rests with the relationship, namely, carcinoma would be put under control in case of the balance between biological characteristics of tumor cells and impacts of the host on the inhibition factors; otherwise, the cancer would grow up.

Traditional radiotherapy and chemotherapy are inclined to weakening immunologic function and lead to a worse unbalance between both of them.

Xu Ze's new model of cancer treatment aims to improve the immunity of patients as much as possible, level off the decreased *immunity* (Fig. 8) and thus inhibit tumor growth and strengthen immunological surveillance.

Immune system is the one composed of immune organs, immunological cell and molecules executing immunologic function, mainly including central lymphatic tissue, peripheral lymphatic tissue and immunological cells. Central lymphatic tissue, the home to immune cells for their occurrence, differentiation and maturation, includes thymus and bone marrow. Peripheral lymphatic tissue includes lymph nodes, spleens and stomachs, in which T cells and B cells settle and these cells make their immune response after the identification of foreign antigen.

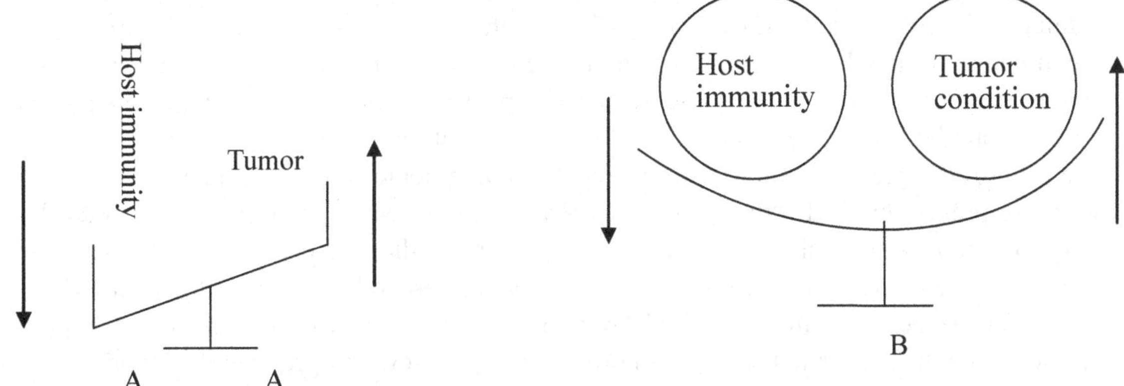

Fig. 7 Schematics of "seesaw" and "weighing scale"

A. tumor grows up in unbalance; B. stabled improvement conditions in balance

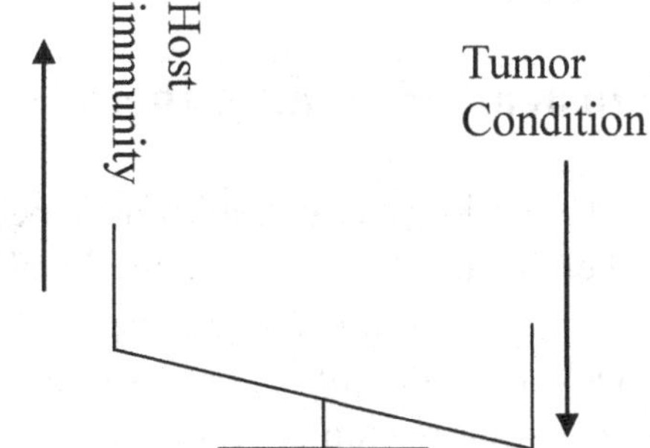

Fig. 8 Improved immunity and controlled tumor

V. Protecting central immune organs instead of damaging it

1. Traditional chemotherapy inhibits immunologic function: when cancer happens, thymus has been inhibited by "cancer-inhibiting thymic factor" and atrophied. Meanwhile, chemotherapy inhibits immunity and bone marrow, damages hemopoietic system and finally lead to the adynamia of the central immune organs as a whole.

   In case of cancerometastasis, a large number of cancer cells are swarming into lymph nodes and destroy their immunologic function. As to the spleen, it could inhibit or destroy cancer cells intruding in the spleen along the blood and provide nowhere for the existence of free cancer cells due to its intrinsic structures and functions. Thus there is generally no primary or secondary malignant tumor in the spleen. However, it is shown by the experiments that the immunologic function of the spleen to tumor is bidirectional, namely, it effectively inhibits tumor in the early stage of cancer but fails in the late stage.

2. Xu Ze's new model of cancer treatment can protect thymus and bone marrow and prevent the immunologic function of the host from damage. According to anatomic experiments on more than 2,000 tumor-bearing animal models, it was found that the growth of tumor is accompanied with the thymus atrophy in form of simultaneously direct proportion. In addition, the death of mice is also proportional to the tumor growth and thymus atrophy. Conclusively, it is necessary to protect thymus and improve immunity. As well as that, in studying the reason why cancer leads to death on thousands of late tumor-bearing animal models, it is found by us that the thymuses apparently atrophied among all grouped dead animals in the final stage of carcinoma, their central immune organ met with atrophy and malfunction. It may be one important reason why the cancer patients died of cancer. It is a common fact that most cancer patients die of cancer in clinic. But further careful analysis and profound consideration would reveal the close relationship between infection bleeding, the failure of organ function and adynamia of immunologic function, which enlightens us to try to prevent or inhibit the thymus atrophy of tumor-bearing animal models in the late stage of tumor. We just aim to find the way to prevent or alleviate thymus atrophy, no matter what measure is taken. After a long-term experimental research, it is found by us that XZ-C_4 and XZ-C_8 screened from the natural herbs, the former can protect thymus and improve immunologic function and the later can protect bone marrow and produce the blood.

XZ-C_4 can protect thymus from atrophy and increase lymphocyte and T cells.

XZ-C_8 can protect hematopoiesis function of the bone marrow, rebuild erythrocyte and leucocyte system and correct anemia.

VI. Non-damage therapy instead of damage therapy

1. For half a century, the traditional anti-cancer therapies have been always the operation, the radiotherapy and the chemotherapy, the first two are the local therapy and the last one is the systematic therapy, all of which would damage the patients to a certain extent. To be specific, operations would attack the ability of the patients to resist disease at a certain level and also cause an implantation, dissemination or residue of exfoliated and free cancer cells, thus resulting in reoccurrence or metastasis after operation. Radiotherapy would cause radioactive inflammatory pathological changes. Chemotherapy has great systemic side effects on the human body. Although currently the traditional therapies have been gradually improved as regional selective local therapy with intubation or catheter on target organs, which aims to increase local concentration and narrow down the damage range of cytotoxic drug, the whole body would still under the effects of medicine disseminated systemically and be subject to obviously toxic effects such as decreased immunity, inhibition of bone marrow, gastroenteric reaction, hair shedding, renal and hepatic injuries and so on. In addition, radioactive rays and chemotherapeutic drugs are two carcinogenic factors despite of the ability of radiotherapy and chemotherapy to kill cancer cells, thus they would be obviously harmful to the patients.
2. The characteristics of the effects of the new non-damage therapy and Xu Ze's new model of cancer treatment: so many new therapies such as biotherapy, immunotherapy, differentiation

and induction therapy, gene therapy, Chinese medicine treatment, combined therapy of traditional Chinese and western medicine and so on, have been emerging in the past 10 years, most of which devote to improving immunity, protecting the host, simulating and inducing the anticancer cell clusters within the anticancer system of the host (including NK cell clusters, K cell clusters, LAK cell clusters, macrophage cell clusters and TK cell clusters) as well as the factor system of anticancer cells (including IFN, IL-2, TNF, LT), regulating and controlling neurohumor system and endocrine system, strengthening the immunologic function and antineoplastic ability of the host and maintaining a balance and sustainability for the host. Z-C medicine was screened from natural herbs on tumor-bearing experimental animals, got a remarkable curative effect by a ten-year follow-up clinical verification with data of approximate 10,000 clinical cases and categorized as non-damage medicine, which could actually constitutes a non damage therapy.

The effects of burgeoning non-damage therapy could be summarized as follows: ① directly improve the anti-tumor ability of the host; ② indirectly improve the anti-cancer ability of the host by diminishing inhibition mechanism; ③ improve the resistance power of the host against oncotherapy; ④ enhance the immunogenicity of tumors.

No matter the traditional therapy or the new concept therapy, operation is the preferred method to treat solid tumor. Radical surgery to resect tumor is the currently best therapeutic method in the range of indication. In 1960s, the author resected huge abdominal tumor more than 6kg for 4 patients, one of which was a female patient, aged 50, with a hysteroma over 18kg. Such a huge solid tumor can't be removed by chemotherapy, immunity, traditional Chinese medicine or BRM. The strategy for treatment of cancerous protuberance is to adopt different methods to eliminate the number of cancer cells to a certain order of magnitude (Someone fixes the order of magnitude at 10^6 mice cells or corresponding 3.5×10^9 human cells and describes it as a spherical nodule with a diameter of 1.5cm) and remediate the human body under this condition. Z-C_{1+4} are verified by the experiments from this laboratory that they could put 10^5 cancer cells under control. Thus if XZ-C medicine is applied in adjuvant therapy after the tumors resection surgery of patients, the body resistance could be strengthened so as to eliminate pathogenic factors and diminish reoccurrence and metastasis.

CHAPTER 16

Xu Ze's Basic Model and Specific Scheme of Anti-cancerometastasis Treatment

Traditional chemotherapy against metastasis mainly aims to kill cancer cells. No matter it is the primary carcinoma, metastatic carcinoma, the postoperative adjuvant chemotherapy preventing reoccurrence and metastasis or when metastasis of lymph nodes is found, intravenous chemotherapy drugs are adopted in all cases. However, because chemotherapy drugs are of no selectivity and kill both cancer cells and normal cells (especially the immunological cells), they act as a double-edged sword. The author holds that various schemes for intravenous chemotherapy are mainly the different combinations of cytotoxic drugs, which are not certainly in line with the multi-link and multi-step biological characteristics of the cancerometastasis process.

I. The basic model of anti-cancerometastasis treatment

Among the innumerable patients in this clinical practice, it is not uncommon to see that some of them are not free from metastasis after the postoperative adjuvant chemotherapy. What is worse is that some of them suffered a simultaneous metastasis in chemotherapy or suffered from the metastasis again after chemotherapy again. All these phenomena make us deeply think about the reason behind the failure to prevent metastasis. Is it the traditional chemotherapy not in line with the biological characteristics of cancerometastasis process? Whether it is necessary to update our knowledge and thinking, or to change our conceptions and treatment model on anti-canceromestasis? Xu Ze's design concept of anti-cancerometastasis countermeasures is just an innovation of the concepts, thinking, methods and models of the traditional anti-metastasis treatment.

Anti-metastasis drugs tend to interfere or blockade a certain link or step of the metastasis process of cancer cells or the cancer cell clusters so as to inhibit the formation of metastasis focus. Although the chemotherapeutic cytotoxic drugs can kill tumor cells, suspend the growth of primary carcinoma and delay the occurrence time of metastasis, they fail to inhibit the process of invasion and metastasis. At present, the ideal drugs killing the primary carcinoma and inhibiting invasion and metastasis are unavailable. Thus, it is necessary to study the strategy of interdiction, prevention and treatment aiming at the development steps and mechanism of the cancerometastasis summarized as "eight steps and three stages".

The invasion and metastasis of carcinoma is a complicated process of many steps and the metastasis process could be generalized as following: proliferation of primary cancerous protuberance→ the formation and growth of newly born micrangium of tumor→ invading and breaking through basement membrance→ cancer cells breaking away from parent tumor and breaking through basement membrance and then perforating micrangiums or micro lymphatic vessels→ the survival and floating of invading blood in the circulatory system→ formation of small cancer embolus from cancer cells clusters wrapped by blood platelet and delivery to remote target organs together with blood stream→ the detention in the micrangium of target organs→ the attachment or adherence of cancer embolus to the wall of micrangium→ breaking through blood vessels and forming micro metastasis focus→formation of newly born micrangium of tumor as the metastasis focus→ the proliferation of the metastasis focus. If we could find the way to blockade one or several links or steps, it is possible to control metastasis, as is the context in which Xu Ze's new model of anti-cancerometastasis treatment is formed and developed.

II. The specific plan of anti-cancerometastasis treatment

According to biological behaviors of modern oncology on cancerometastasis and theory of reoccurrence and metastasis, this libratory has been always searching for new anti-metastasis drugs among traditional Chinese herbs extracted from natural herbs for years. Through experimental study on of tumor-bearing animal bodies with traditional Chinese medicine as well as the combination of traditional Chinese medicine and western medicine, we interfere, obstruct and intercept all the links of the metastasis, and develop an anti-metastasis scheme and countermeasure with XZ-C medicine, including XZ-C-TG against the formation of micrangium, XZ-C-AS dissolving cancer embolus, XZ-C-MD against invading into and breaking through blood vessels, XZ-C-LM with antigenicity, XZ-C-Ind against PGE2; VA and XZ-C-CA as calcium channel blocking drugs against invasion, XZ-C-GB against adherence, XZ-C-TIMP against the resistance to drugs, XZ-C_1 inhibiting cancer cells rather than normal cells; XZ-C_4 protecting thymus and improving immunity; XZ-C_8 protecting bone marrow and improving hematogenesis function and Emulsion of Brucea Javanica into lymph nodes. The comprehensive measures of the above-mentioned treatment schemes have achieved sound curative effects in the clinical practice by our anti-cancer cooperative group.

Because cancerometastasis is a complicated process of multi-step and multi-link, it is necessary to adopt the comprehensive measures in an all-round way to treat the cancerometastasis instead of a certain drug or measure. Thus aiming at the steps of metastasis, we scientifically design and adopt different treatment schemes and countermeasures shown in the following table. Those treatment schemes and countermeasures aiming at the steps of metastasis are to achieve the same goal of anti-metastasis.

The new model of anti-cancerometastasis treatment of Xu Ze's new concept (treatment schemes and countermeasures for the steps of canceromestasis)

Metastasis step	Treatment countermeasures	XZ-C medicine and its role
Proliferation of primary cancerous	Operation, chemotherapy	XZ-C_1 inhibiting cancer cells XZ-C_4 protecting thymus and improving immunity XZ-C_8 protecting bone marrow and improving hematogenesis function
Growth of newly born micrangium of tumor	Inhibiting the formation of micrangium	XZ-C-TG against formation of micrangium XZ-C-CA against adherence

Invasion into basement membrance	Anti-adhesion, anti-kinesalgia and inhibiting the activity of hydrolase	XZ-C-K(LWF) against adhesion Ind against PGE2 XZ-C-MD against kinesalgia
Breaking through blood vessels or lymphatic vessels	Anti-adhesion, anti-kinesalgia and inhibiting the activity of hydrolase	XZ-C-MD against invasion into blood vessels XZ-C-K (LWF) XZ-C_{1+4} mediating immunity
In the blood of circulatory system	Inhibiting the aggregation and coagulation of blood platelet. Biological response modification (BRM)	XZ-C-N (CZR) against the aggregation of blood platelet XZ-C-LM XZ-C-ASP dissolving cancer embolus XZ-C_{1+4} mediating immunity
The formation of cancer embolus	Promoting blood circulation and removing stasis and resisting thrombus	XZ-C-K (NSR) against cancer embolus XZ-C-N (CZR) against aggregation of blood platelet
The breaking out of cancer embolus from blood vessels	Resisting adhesion, kinesalgia, and the activity of hydrolase	XZ-C-MD against the breaking out of cancer embolus
The formation of metastasis focus	Operation, radiotherapy, chemotherapy	XZ-C_{1+4} mediating immunity XZ-C-TG inhibiting the growth of blood vessels
The metastasis of lymph nodes	Liposoluble drugs	The Emulsion of Brucea Javanica as the carrier of lipa entering into the lymph nodes

The correlative factors of the invasion of cancer cells are adherence, enzymatic secretion and kinesalgia. The inhibition of adhesion, kinesalgia and enzymatic secretion is also helpful to inhibit the exfoliation of cancer cells from parent tumor, its break into matrix and the formation of the newly born blood vessels of the tumor besides its contribution to prevent the invasion of primary carcinoma. For years the researches on inhibitors inhibiting the growth of newly born blood vessels are seen in reports. Meanwhile, it is also discovered in the tumor-bearing animal experiment screening the anti-cancerometastasis drugs by this library that traditional Chinese medicine TG is of sound inhibiting effects on newly born blood vessels. Tumor cells are in weakest condition to resist the host environment when entering into the blood of the circulatory system and can be easily eliminated by the immunological cells of the host. It is proved by some literature that a vast majority of cancer cells entering into the circulatory system are killed by immunological cells and only a number of approximately 0.01% thereof could survive and possibly become the focus of metastasis. Except the mechanical damage factors, the cancer cells in blood stream are mainly eliminated by the damaging effects of the immunological function of the hosts against tumor cells. Tumor-bearing patients usually suffer low immunological function inhibited by tumor and chemotherapy. Therefore, it is necessary to adopt immunotherapy, biotherapy and biological response modification and traditional Chinese medicine for immunological mediation to protect the function of immune organs so as to improve the immunity of the host. It is found that XZ-C medicine can protect bone marrow and improve hemogenesis function, protect hemogenesis function of bone marrow as well as stem cells, improve immunologic function and inhibit the metastasis of tumor. According to the clinical application on the innumerable patients in the clinic of Anti-cancer Cooperative Group of Traditional Chinese Medicine Combined with Western Medicine over ten years, XZ-C medicine against cancer and metastasis has achieved significant curative effects.

III. The important role of immunotherapy in anti-cancerometastasis treatment

Among all the current therapeutic methods, operation and radiotherapy are both local therapy while chemotherapy, immunotherapy, biological therapy, therapy with traditional Chinese medicine are systematic therapy. At present, the chemotherapy mainly targets the focus of primary cancer or metastasis focus and the criterion to judge the curative effects is to alleviate and shrink the tumor. In order to fulfill of the above criterion, a significant dose of chemotherapeutic cytotoxic drugs are in need to shrink the lump. Additionally in view of the cell cycle, medicines are necessarily combined in order to achieve a certain level of lethality. If it is a $1cm \times 1cm^2$ lump, it would contain a number of 10^{12} cancer cells and this, requires a considerable dose of chemotherapeutic drugs to shrink it into half. However, it only needs a slight dose if cancer cells are eliminated in the process of metastasis by chemotherapy, because the amount of cancer cells in metastasis process only accounts to 10^7 to 10^8 and most of them could be eliminated. The problem happens as a large amount of immunological cells in blood circulation are destroyed by chemotherapeutic cytotoxic drugs whereas the anti-metastasis mainly depends on the system against cancer cells of the organism itself. Thus it would be a great loss to patients. Chemotherapy could only be conducted with intermission during which time a large amount of cancer cells and immunological cells would be both eliminated. However there still exist a handful of escaped cancer cells during this period which continually split and proliferate or are even more active. More than that, the destroyed immunological cells, decreased immunity and weakened immune surveillance would also lead or contribute to the development and metastasis of cancer cells.

Therefore, the chemotherapeutic drugs should not be overdosed in the anti-metastasis treatment and should not impair a large amount of immunological cells. Meanwhile, chemotherapy should be accompanied by Immunotherapy, Biotherapy, Biological Response Modification (BRM), XZ-C medicine and tonic traditional Chinese medicine so as to give play to each other's advantages and make up each other's imperfections. Because a properly protected and activated immune system of the body could eliminate 10^6 cancer cells and additional chemotherapeutic drugs could destroy most cancer cells in the process of metastasis, it is possible to hold up and cut off the metastasis path and put the diffusion and metastasis under further control.

Xu Ze's new concept of anti-metastasis treatment promotes the application of immunochemotherapy, namely the combination of immunotherapy and chemotherapy. To be specific, immune drugs would be used in the peri-chemotheraputic period, in other words, at the week before the chemotherapy to be implemented, and would not be ceased in the chemotherapy period unless in case of serious chemotherapy response. The immunotherapy will continue for 6 to 9 months after chemotherapy and during intermission for the maintenance of a certain level of immunity and the consolidation of the curative effects. All these above are proved to be reasonable. For 16 years the Dawn Specialist Out-patient of our anti-metastasis laboratory uses XZ-C anti-cancer traditional Chinese medicine for immunological mediation to coordinate chemotherapy, which usually causes less chemotherapy response. Most of the postoperative in our out-patients suffer the liver, gallbladder, pancreas, stomach, intestine, lung and breast cancer. Some suffer a multi-part lymphatic metastasis after radical operations but then meet with serious response after chemotherapy thus come to our out-patient for treatment. Some fail the exploratory operation and some are under palliative operations. Therefore, the author, through combining the small-dosed chemotherapy with XZ-C medicine, usually finds less response and hemogram variation. Because of different conditions of the patients and the absence of comparability, it is impossible to conduct the comparative observation of perspective random allocation. Therefore, the perspective clinical study is conducted by comparatively observing the curative effects of the immunotherapy group and the chemotherapy group with immune indexes (IFN, IL-2 and TNF), the level of tumor marker, the quality of life and the survival time as the evaluative criteria of the two groups.

The immune drugs used in the above-mentioned immunochemotherapy shall increase the immunity indexes of the body. Actually not all traditional Chinese medicine that support healthy energy and eliminate evil are able to improve immunity because some are of bidirectional regulating function, which would improve immunity at a certain dosage range but lower immunity at another dosage range. For example, the glossy privet fruit could significantly increase the spleen and thymus indexes; the bupleurum roots lead to the atrophy of the mice thymus; and the liquid made from the pilose antlers of a young stag could improve the weight of the spleen and thymus of the mice if it is poured into their stomach. Additionally, barrenwort polysaccharide would lead to the atrophy of the thymus but a long-term oral administration turns to increase the weight of thymus. XZ-C_{1+4+8} medicine is proved to be able to increase cytokines like IFN, IL-2, TNF etc and to decrease the level of tumor markers of many terms by many animal experiments and long-term clinical observation. To be specific, XZ-C_4 could protect bone marrow and thymus and improve hematopoiesis functions and immunity thus raises the overall immune level. The test by cultivating cancer cells in vitro reveals that the series of XZ-C1 medicine, including XZ-C_1-A, XZ-C_1-B and XZ-C_1-C, are the three pharmaceutics that 100% kill cancer cells, 100% cause no harm to normal cells and achieve an 85% to 95% tumor-inhibiting rate in tumor-inhibiting experiments on the body of tumor-bearing animals. Cyclophosphane (CTX) as the control group only achieves a tumor-inhibiting rate of 45% and also significantly decreases the immunity.

The removal of focus of primary cancer and metastasis focus depends on local surgical removal or radiation exposure. The focus of primary cancer should be removed by surgical removal if possible and in case of impossibility, it would be helpful to turn to interventional therapy, radiotherapy, radio frequency, focused ultrasound or the injection of absolute ethyl alcohol so as to control the local focus.

The metastasis of tumor is an essential expression of malignancy. The reason why cancer treatment is failed is that the treatment isn't proper and the immunity of the patients isn't sufficiently strong to kill all the cancer cells. Literatures show that a marginally small tumor (1 to 8g) could release millions or even thousand millions of cancer cells in 24 hours into blood. However, a vast majority of these cancel cells would be eliminated by the human body's immune system and only 1% of them are possibly able to survive and evolve into metastasis tumor. The test data of our libratory reveals that the immunity of mice is capable of killing 100,000 cancer cells. The amount could be increased to more than 1,000,000 if XZ-C_1 medicine is used. The question is what destroys them? It is the immunological cells of the body itself. Thus Xu Ze's new concept holds that the immunological cells of body should be protected and not be damaged by any treatments. It is necessary to find ways to protect and activate the immunological function of the host. It would be beneficial for the patients if the immunotherapy and a small-dosed chemotherapy are combined as immunochemotherapy, learning from each other's strong points and offsetting each other's weakness.

CHAPTER 17

Review and Analysis of Clinical Cases of Postoperative Adjuvant Chemotherapy for Carcinoma

People have been struggling with the cancer for hundreds of years. Surgical operation of traditional treatment has been developing for over 100 years, radical treatment for 80 years and chemical treatment for 60 years. But until now, the cancer is still rampant in the crowd, and the three treatments produce little effect. Also its morbidity is increasing year by year and mortality remains high. According to the statistics of 1995, 7 million people around the world have been found with cancerous protuberance every year, and 5 million of them die from cancerous protuberance. In 1996, 1.8 million people had cancer in our country, and 1.28 million of them died from it. In terms of the mortality, tumor ranks first and becomes the most serious illness of threatening the human health. In 1975, U.S. government announced to deploy vast manpower and materials for "the declaration of war on cancer". This was the first time that conquering a disease was treated as the national policy. They attempted to use strong national power to conquer the tumor. But the courses of many events are independent of man's will. In 1993, when American Cancer Society was summarizing research progress since "the declaration of war on cancer", they found that the result of $25 billion financial input for anti-cancer instead was not optimistic, with morbidity rising 7% and survival rate only up 4%. Our academic world and clinicians should calmly, objectively, matter-of-factly and seriously review, analyze, summarize, self-evaluate and rethink our decades of practical cases. We need to sum up experience and lessons of success and failure in the fight against cancer during the half century. We should ask why the traditional treatment does not reduce the mortality obviously. What problem does the traditional treatment have actually? What exactly is the flaw? How should we improve the traditional treatment and correct its shortcomings to make it more perfect?

While continuing to enhance effects of traditional surgical operation, radical treatment and chemical treatment with traditional train of thought, we should open up a new way and look for a new route to conquer the cancer.

According to the writer's analysis of patient history derived from 54 years' medical practices, chemotherapy and radiation must be further practiced on clinical foundation research, and also on analyzing, summarizing, evaluating and rethinking therapeutic effect of verification on clinical cases. The radical or chemical treatment must be tried to eliminate the damage to the host. It is essential to further complete it, improve the treatment of killing off tumor cells but damaging the body, even just damaging the body. Then how to grasp the principle of proportionality is very important. How to evaluate the medical quality for cancer? The writer considers that the medical quality equals the therapeutic effect. The therapeutic effect of tumor for cancer patients should be the good life quality and very long survival time, but not merely the tumor shrinkage or remission. The effect should relieve the patient's pains and prolong the patient's life.

In view of the recurrent relapse and metastasis after surgical radical operation, therefore, postoperative adjuvant chemotherapy has been prevailing universally after the 1980s. While cancer experts have different perspectives whether postoperative adjuvant chemotherapy has arrested relapse, or whether it has prevented metastasis. Specific research report has not yet appeared. According to a group of case reports for five-year follow-up results of postoperative adjuvant chemotherapy or radiation patients by British Stomach Cancer Group, this cancer group adopted mitomycin and fluorouracil to provide adjuvant treatment for the first group patients in 1976. But the result showed that this treatment didn't benefit the postoperative patients. Therefore British Stomach Cancer Group carried out adjuvant treatment research for another group of patients again.

British Stomach Cancer Group adopted prospective, randomized, controlled grouping research for 436 sdenocarcinoma of stomach patients, whose postoperative staging was phase II to phase III. The 436 postoperative patients were respectively treated by radiation or combined chemotherapy of mitomycin, adriamycin and fluorouracil treatment (MAF). During five-year follow-up, 372 patients died, in which 45 patients died from surgical complications and 327 patients died from tumor relapse. In this randomized grouping research, 145 patients adopted surgical operation. 153 patients accepted adjuvant radiation, and the range of irradiation included hilus lienis and porta hepatis region, also the radiation dose was 4500cGy. Another 138 patients accepted combined chemotherapy (MAF Treatment). Mitomycin was 4mg/ ; adriamycin was 30 mg/ ; fluorouracil was 600 mg/ . The three drugs were all intravenous injections, and the treatment cycle was 8 cycles, which three weeks were one cycle. Overall two-year survival rate of this group was 33% (31%~35%), and five-year survival rate was 17% (13%~21%). Compared with the survival rate of patients only adopting surgical operation, the survival rate of patients accepting adjuvant treatment had no increase. The five-year survival rate of patients only adopting surgical operation was 20%, rate of surgery and radiation was 12%, and rate of surgery and chemotherapy was 19%.

Thus, surgical operation remains to be the standard treatment for sdenocarcinoma of stomach. The adjuvant treatment measure should be limited within certain field of research.

The writer of this book sorts, analyzes, evaluates and rethinks the following part of the cases (cases with personal inquiry of medical history, medical examination, diagnosis and treat, complete observation) with nearly ten-year personal clinical diagnosis and treatment.

I. Failure Cases of Postoperative Adjuvant Chemotherapy to Arrest Relapse

Case 1 Patient Wei ××, female, fifty, Changsha Hunan, engineer, patient history number: 3300653

Diagnosis: Cystosarcoma phylloides of left breast had serious malignant change and relapse. In July 1996, the patient was found the enlargement of lump in her left breast. The puncture of the lump diagnosed that the lump was fibroma. In October 1996, the left breast was removed. Pathological examination: cystosarcoma phylloides of left breast, level II. Since December 19, 1996, the patient began to accept VAD treatment for chemotherapy and get chemotherapy once every three weeks. The second chemotherapy was on January 16, 1997. Constantly, the third chemotherapy was on February 24, 1997; and then the fourth chemotherapy on March 6, 1997; the fifth chemotherapy on April 8, 1997; the sixth chemotherapy on April 29, 1997. On July 2, 1997, type-B ultrasonic examined that there was a 15mm×12mm sized lump in the similar 9 o'clock position of the right breast. Considering the relapse and metastasis, the patient came to the anti-cancer coordination group (Hubei Group) for outpatient treatment, adopting traditional Chinese and western medicine combination treatment.

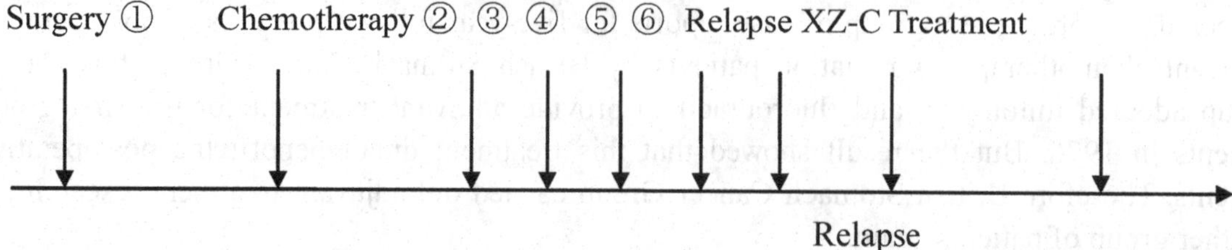

Analysis: This patient had one-year postoperative chemotherapies continuously, defining once every month and five days one time. The treatment was standard systematic chemotherapy. But after stopping chemotherapy for two months, the tumor appeared local relapse. That explained that the chemotherapy failed to arrest relapse. It was speculated that chemotherapy might cause the continuing decline of patient's immunity functions beyond retrieval. The tumor lost the immunoregulation and made rest tumor cells set into the cell cycle. Then the tumor was induced. It prompted that long-time continuous chemotherapy must attach importance to protect the host and confront side effects of chemotherapy drugs to avoid the damage for the host. Although chemotherapy killed off tumor cells, it damaged the body at the same time.

Case 2 Patient Yang ××, female, fifty-four, cadre, Honghu, patient history number: 7201432

Stomach cancer relapsed after surgery. The pain of superior venter had continued for one year. The result of stomachoscopy was stomach cancer. On August 26, 1997, the patient accepted radical operation for stomach cancer. The radical operation was $_2$B1 type. There was a 8mm×5mm sized lump in the lateral side of the lesser curvature of stomach, which caused the pyloric obstruction and enlargement of lymph nodes on the side of the arteria coeliaca. The patient began to accept postoperative chemotherapy after a month. MMC and 5-Fu were seven days one time and the intervals between two times were three weeks. There were total six times in September, October, November, December 1997 and January, February 1998. After that no other treatments were adopted. In January 1999, the patient appeared swallow obstruction and emesis. On February 24, 1999, the patient accepted the stomachoscopy. Front and back of gastric remnant which closed to anastomotic stoma swelled and developed pathological changes. There were mucosal erosion and ulcer. Stomach cancer patient had the postoperative relapse. On March 4, 1999, the patient came to the anti-cancer coordination group (Hubei Group) for XZ-C$_{1+4+2}$ treatment.

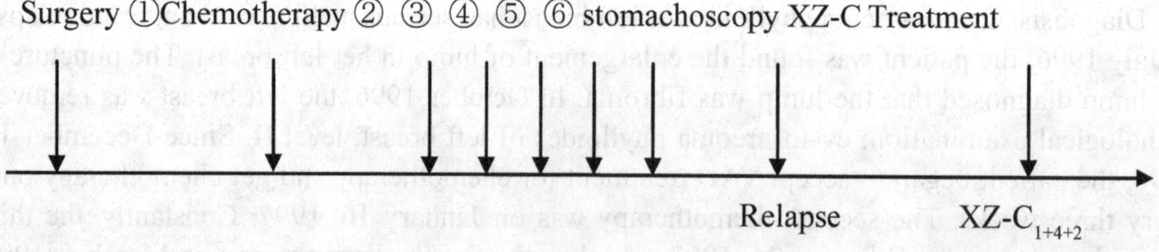

Analysis: This patient had six-time postoperative chemotherapies, defining once every month and seven days one time. The sixth chemotherapy was in February 1998. Until January 1999, the patient appeared swallow obstruction. The result of stomachoscopy was the postoperative relapse of stomach cancer. In this case, the patient had six-time postoperative chemotherapies continuously. It prompted that postoperative adjuvant chemotherapy failed to arrest relapse.

Case 3 Patient Li ××, male, forty-two, Shanxi, cadre, patient history number: 7201427

On November 18, 1997, the patient was found left-liver space occupying lesion through CT in 161 Hospital. On December 2, 1997, the patient accepted the left-liver lateral lobectomy. After 20 days, the patient began to accept postoperative chemotherapy. The chemotherapy drugs were 10mg/dl with intravenous injection and 20mg of hydroxycamptothecine with intravenous injection every other day in two weeks. A course was 15 days. And then the patient needed to repeat the last course after resting 15 days. Before chemotherapy, SGPT was 77μ. After chemotherapy, SGPT was 500μ. In the operation, chemotherapeutic drugs above the chemotherapy pump of portal vein (no chemotherapy pump in the artery) were injected into the organism through the pump. Before the operation, AFP was 200μ. After the operation, AFP was 200μ. In April 1998, the patient accepted the third chemotherapy in the hospital. Chemotherapeutic drugs were injected through the pump. The chemotherapy adopted the high dose pulse therapy, using 6mg of MMC, 200mg of carboplatin and 750mg of 5-Fu. Before chemotherapy, AFP was 180μ. After chemotherapy, AFP was 302μ. On May 19, 1998, the patient accepted the fourth chemotherapy, using the chemotherapy pump as the third time. On June 30, 1998, the patient accepted the fifth chemotherapy with pump. When the AFP was 219μ, it should be detected every other day. On July 28, 1998, the patient accepted the sixth chemotherapy, adopting the high dose pulse therapy through the pump. The reexamination showed that AFP>363. In early August 1998, the examination found that there was a 4cm sized lump under the incision of abdominal wall. On August 27, 1998, the lump was removed in tumor hospital. On September 29, 1998, the patient accepted the seventh chemotherapy with pump. After chemotherapy, the reexamination of type-B ultrasonic, CT and intrahepatic widespread metastasis showed that there were many ball shadows and metastases. In December 1998, the patient accepted hepatic artery embolism and pulmonary intervention in the general hospital of a military region. The examinations found that there were lumps equivalent to the size of an adult fist and infant's head in epigastrium and right abdomen. The lumps were stiff. On March 1, 1999, the patient came to the anti-cancer coordination group (Hubei Group) for outpatient treatment, adopting traditional Chinese and western medicine combination treatment and XZ-C_{1+4+5} series treatment.

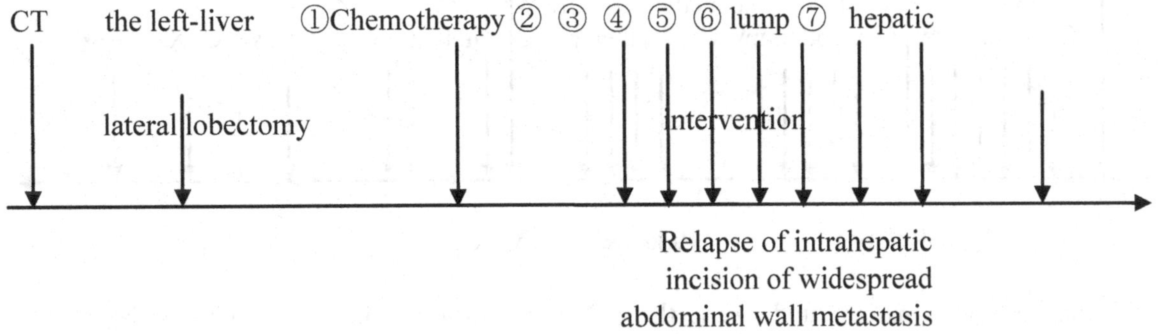

Analysis: This patient suffered from cancer of the liver. After the left-liver lateral lobectomy, the patient had seven-time postoperative chemotherapies continuously, defining once every month. The seventh chemotherapy showed the intrahepatic widespread metastasis and pulmonary metastasis. It prompted that postoperative adjuvant chemotherapy failed to arrest relapse and prevent metastasis.

Case 4 Patient Xiang ××, male, forty-three, cadre, Chongyang, patient history number: 6801345

In June 1994, the disease of this patient was treated as gastroenteritis. Until December, the X-ray examination in city hospital showed that the patient suffered from intestinal obstruction. In early January 1995, the emergency operation explored the disease as a transverse colon tumor. Then the tumor was removed, adopting the end to end anastomosis. Pathological examination showed that the tumor was a malignant tumor. In February, March, April, May, June, July 1995, the patient had six-time postoperative chemotherapies continuously, defining five days one time. In January 1996, the colonic neoplasm of anastomotic stoma was found. The patient accepted the radical excision. At the end of December 1997, the tumor of anastomotic stoma was found again. On March 31, 1998, the patient accepted the palliative excision. In September 1998, another 5.6cm×4.6cm sized lump equivalent to the size of an adult fist was found between stomach and caput pancreatic. On November 24, 1998, the patient underwent an operation again to remove the lump. Those lesser tubercles, such as the omentum, were difficult to be removed completely. And the operation could only remove big ones. In 1996, the patient once accepted four-time postoperative chemotherapies in Tumor Department, defining five days one time. And the patient also took Doxifluridine orally for two months. In April, May 1998, the patient accepted twice chemotherapies. And as well, the patient took two courses of traditional Chinese medicine dispensed by Wang Zhenguo of Shenyang. But the course didn't work. Then the patient took one course of Shijiazhuang Chinese medicine. The course also didn't work. On November 13, 1998, the patient came to the anti-cancer coordination group for outpatient treatment, adopting traditional Chinese and western medicine combination treatment, XZ-C_{1+4} treatment and XZ-C_2 treatment. In November 1999, the patient accepted the reexamination, which showed the stable condition.

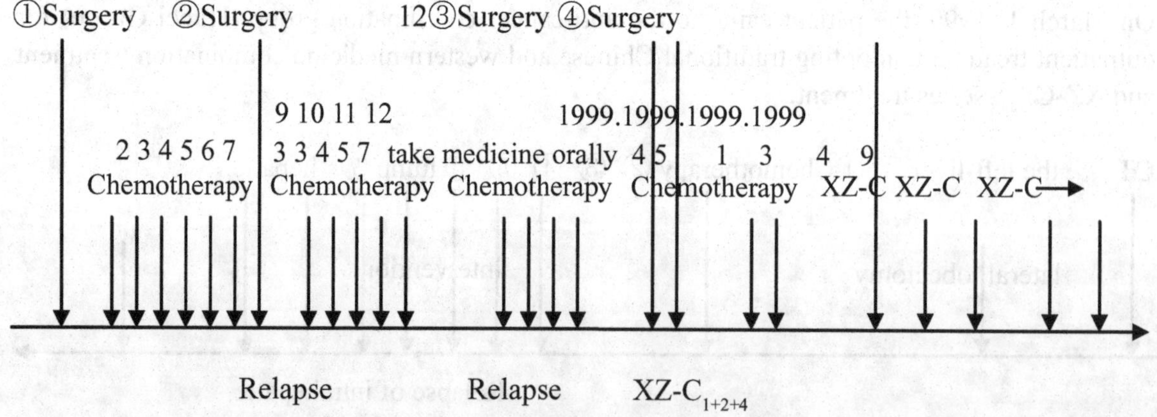

Analysis: This patient underwent the colon cancer operation of removing the tumor. After that, the patient had six-time postoperative chemotherapies continuously, defining once every month and five days one time. Five months later, the colonic neoplasm of anastomotic stoma relapsed and was removed by surgery. During the one year after operation, the patient proceeded with postoperative chemotherapies monthly and continuously. The tumor of anastomotic stoma relapsed and was removed again. The patient proceeded with postoperative chemotherapies. This case prompted that chemotherapy failed to arrest relapse and prevent metastasis. In November 1998, the patient came to the outpatient department for traditional Chinese and western medicine combination treatment, and also took traditional Chinese medicine of $XZ\text{-}C_{1+4+2}$ immunoregulation series chronically and continuously. After taking medicine orally, the patient's condition was improved. In November 1999, the patient accepted the reexamination, which showed the stable condition.

Case 5 Patient Li ××, male, fifty, cadre, Hanchuan, patient history number: 5701131

Diagnosis: Rectum cancer relapsed after surgery.

In December 1994, the patient underwent a radical operation for rectum cancer. The operation was Dixon type. The length of rectum cancer lesion was 12cm. The patient had six-time postoperative chemotherapies continuously, defining once every month and seven days one time. The condition was good after operation. On April 30, 1998, the patient accepted the colonoscopy examination. There was a lump at the area of rectum, having 10cm distances to the anus. The 3cm×3cm sized lump had a rugged surface and swelled towards the intracavity. The biopsy of four living tissues showed that the cell had became allotypic gland cell. On June 25, 1998, the patient suffered from the incomplete intestinal obstruction. Then on July 9, 1998, the patient underwent the Hartmann operation and partial cystectomy. The surgery proved it the recurrent rectum cancer, which had involved the bladder. The patient had five-time postoperative radiotherapies for pelvic cavity with accumulated dose of 5000CGY (from October 12, 1998 to November 13, 1998). The patient also had postoperative chemotherapies for one month. The chemotherapy drugs were 5-Fu and calcium leucovorin (five days, once a day). Since the proctoscopy examined the relapse of rectum cancer in May 1998, the patient came to the anti-cancer coordination group for the traditional Chinese medicine treatment of XZ-C immunoregulation series, which was adopted to control the relapse and metastasis. On November 28, 1999, the patient accepted the reexamination. After taking the medicine orally, the patient regained a high spirit, a good appetite and enough physical strength, which showed the stable condition. The patient continued to live normally without any discomfort.

1994.12 1995.1-1995.6 1998.4 1998.6 1998.7 1998.10-11

Surgery ①②③④⑤⑥ Colonoscopy Intestinal Obstruction Surgery Radiotherapy Chemotherapy

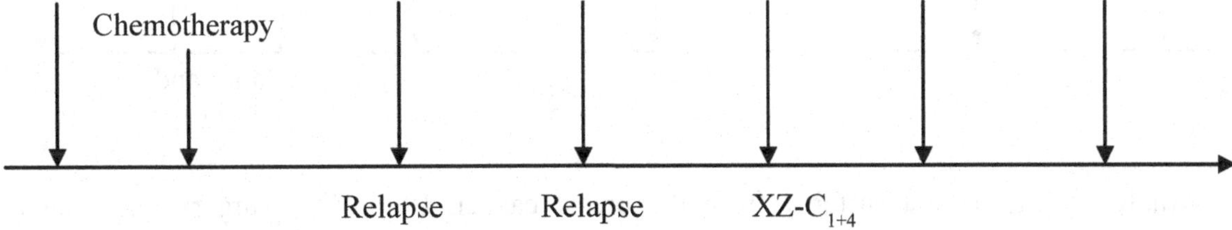

Analysis: After a radical operation for rectum cancer, the patient had six-time postoperative chemotherapies continuously, defining once every month and seven days one time. Two years later, rectum cancer appeared the local recurrence and widespread metastasis. Then the patient continued to accept the chemotherapy, but the rectum cancer relapsed again. It prompted that postoperative adjuvant chemotherapy failed to arrest relapse and prevent metastasis. After the relapse in April 1998, the patient came to the anti-cancer coordination outpatient department for the traditional Chinese medicine treatment of XZ-C_{1+4} immunoregulation series. After taking the medicine orally, the patient's condition was stable and improving. The patient had been persisting in taking the XZ-C medicine for over one year and was being in good health.

Case 6 Patient Luo ××, female, housewife, Gongan county, patient history number: 521020

In September 1994, the patient found a lump in the left breast. The local hospital scanned the lump as a fibroma. In September 1995, because of the enlargement of the lump (5cm×5cm×3cm), the patient underwent a radical operation for breast cancer in the district hospital. Pathology: infiltrating ductal cancer of right breast, ER (+), P.R (+), removal of one subclavicular lymph node and two axillary fusional lymph nodes. After the operation, the patient accepted chemotherapies with CMF treatment for one week. On December 6, 1995, the patient accepted chemotherapies with CAF treatment for one week. On December 26, 1995, the patient accepted chemotherapies with CAF treatment for one week again. From February 5, 1996 to March 30, the patient accepted radiotherapies. In August 1996, the patient continued to accept two courses of chemotherapies, defining three weeks of one course. In September 1997, a lump was found in the right axilla. There were tubercles under the prethoracic skin again. The breast cancer appeared relapse and metastasis. Then the patient came to the anti-cancer coordination outpatient department for the traditional Chinese medicine treatment of XZ-C immunoregulation series. On January 4, 1998, the patient began to take XZ-C medicine during the outpatient treatment. After taking 45-day medicine, the patient's condition kept stable. In October 1998, the patient accepted the reexamination in the outpatient department, which showed the stable condition. There was a tubercle equivalent to the size of the little finger in the top part of right axilla. Above this tubercle, there was another tubercle equivalent to the size of a rice grain. But it had no more growth.

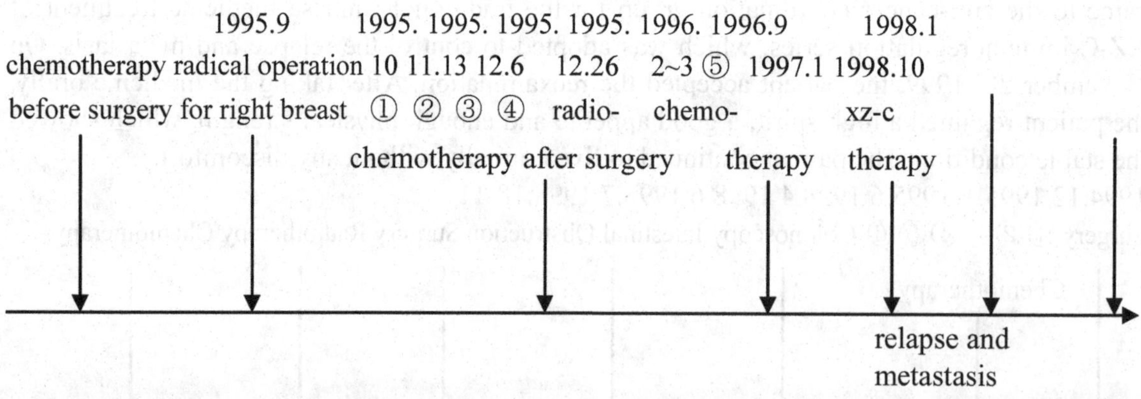

Analysis: The patient suffered from the breast cancer. Before the surgery, the patient accepted one-week chemotherapies. After the surgery, the patient accepted postoperative chemotherapies, defining once every month and one-week one time. But the treatment failed to prevent metastasis, diffusion and progression. In January 1998, the patient came to the outpatient department and took 10-month traditional Chinese medicine of immunoregulation.

The patient's condition was stable. The breast cancer had no more progress. The general condition was improving.

Case 7 Patient Yang ××, female, fifty, Hankou, technical cadre, patient history number: 54001079

Diagnosis: Rectal adenocarcinoma relapsed after surgery.

In June 1996, the patient was diagnosed with rectum cancer for diarrhea. On July 11, 1996, the patient underwent a radical low anterior resection operation for rectum cancer. In the operation, the tumor located under the reflection, which was 5cm×4cm and invaded the muscular layer. The lymph node under the mesentery developed obvious enlargement. The patient recovered well from the operation. Nine days after the operation, the patient accepted chemotherapies of 5-Fu and MMC series. After leaving hospital, the patient took Mifulong orally. On October 4, 1996, the patient accepted chemotherapies in a tumor hospital and then left it. From August 17, 1996 to October 5, the patient accepted three courses of chemotherapies with ELF treatment. From January 14, 1997 to February 3, the patient accepted the third chemotherapies in a tumor hospital of MMC and 5-Fu series. After the chemotherapy, the patient began the attack of diarrhea more than ten times every day. From May 1997 to July 1997, the patient took Mifulong orally. On February 4, 1998, the patient had a return visit for the rectal examination. In the area of the anastomotic stoma, the tubercle could be touched. The rectum cancer relapsed. The patient accepted eight chemotherapies again and 21 radiotherapies. Then the patient had hematuria and diarrhea. It showed that the patient suffered from the radioactive cystitis and radioactive rectitis.

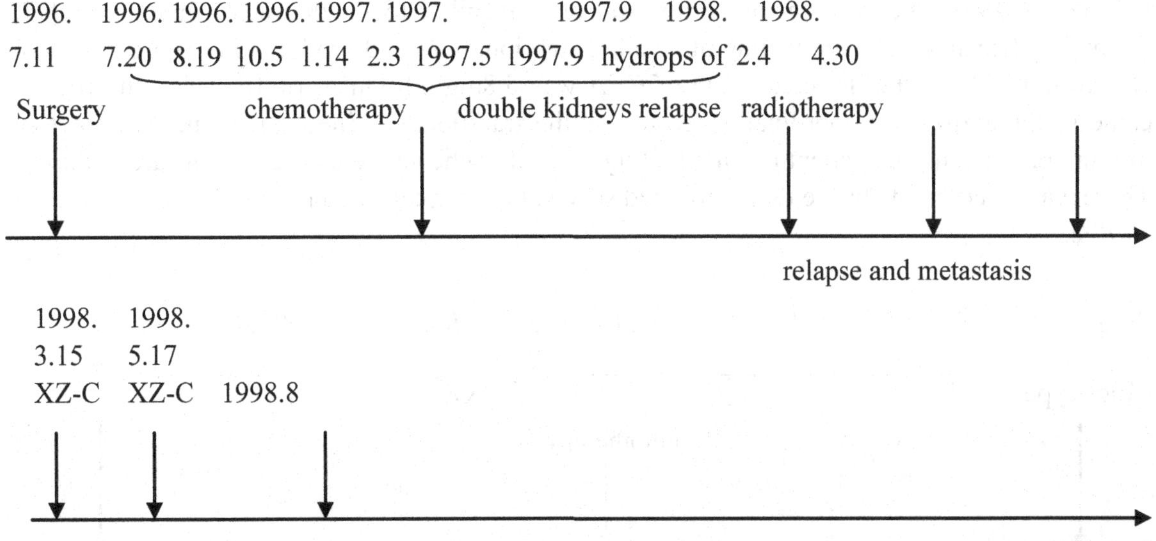

(Afterwards there was no more chemotherapy and radiotherapy. The patient had been accepting XZ-C_{1+4} and brucea fruit latex treatments alone for one year. The patient's condition was stable.)

Analysis: This case was the rectal adenocarcinoma. After the radical operation, the patient accepted chemotherapies continuously. On February 4, 1998, the rectum cancer relapsed in the area of the anastomotic stoma. The patient had accepted continuous and multiple chemotherapies, involving intravenous chemotherapies and oral chemotherapy drugs. But it failed to arrest the relapse of rectum cancer in the area of the anastomotic stoma. After finding the relapse, the patient accepted radiotherapies and chemotherapies continuously again. These treatments also evoked the radioactive cystitis and other complicating diseases. The treatments failed to prevent the progression of recurrent cancer.

On March 15, 1998, the patient came to the anti-cancer coordination group for outpatient treatment, simply adopting the traditional Chinese medicine of XZ-C immunoregulation series and brucea fruit latex for enema. After taking the medicine, the patient's general condition was getting better. And the spirit and appetite were improving. The patient had chronically been taking the traditional Chinese medicine of XZ-C immunoregulation series for eighteen months. The condition of illness was stable. The tumor had been controlled, and it was stable with no more progression. The patient's condition was getting better markedly.

Case 8 Patient Xu ××, female, fifty-six, Macheng, patient history number: 7401472

Diagnosis: Lymph nodes of the left ventral groove metastasized. The adenocarcinoma of anal canal relapsed.

For the blood-stained stool, three blood examinations showed that the patient suffered from the cancer of anus. On February 25, 1997, the patient underwent a Miles-type radical operation for cancer of anal canal. The appendages of ambo-uterus were removed. Lymph nodes of the left perineum and ventral groove were cleaned. The patient had six-time postoperative chemotherapies. The first chemotherapy was on May 24, 1997 with MMC+5-Fu treatment. The second chemotherapy was on July 2, 1997. The third chemotherapy was on August 13, 1997. The fourth chemotherapy was on September 17, 1997. The fifth chemotherapy was on February 8, 1998. The sixth chemotherapy was on November 15, 1998. Since September 1997, the patient began to have the feeling of swell, distention, burn and urodynia in the area of anus. On April 14, 1999, the detected value of CEA was 5.8mg/ml. On April 16, 1999, the patient came to the anti-cancer coordination group for the traditional Chinese medicine treatment of immunoregulation. The patient had the feeling of swell, ache and tenderness in the area of anus. There was a very high chance that exfoliated survival cancer cells had relapsed.
1997.2.25

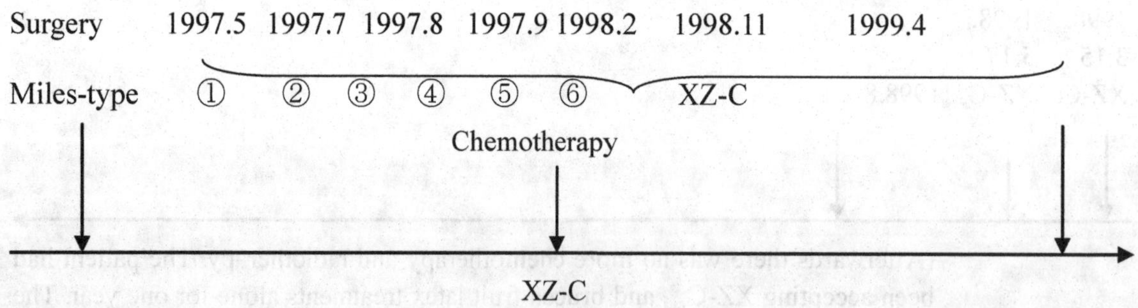

Analysis: After the Miles-type radical operation for cancer of anal canal, the patient accepted chemotherapies of six courses continuously. In September 1997, the patient began to have the feeling of ache and tenderness in the area of anus. And the feeling of pain became doubly intense. It was obvious that exfoliated survival cancer cells were proliferating and relapsing. The poisonous drugs for cancers cells in continuous chemotherapies failed to totally destroy these exfoliated survival cancer cells. Thus, these cancer cells revived again, proliferating and relapsing in partial place.

Case 9 Patient Xiong ××, male, forty-two, worker, Wuhan, patient history number: 6501291

Diagnosis: Rectum cancer relapsed after surgery.

In March 1998, for the blood-stained stool, the disease of this patient was treated as "hemorrhoid". In May 1998, the proctoscop biopsy examination showed that the patient suffered from rectum cancer. On May 29, 1998, the patient underwent a Miles-type radical operation for rectum cancer. The postoperative plug was poorly differentiated rectum cancer. The cancer cells had invaded to the full-thickness of intestinal wall, involving the adipose tissue around the rectum. The lymph nodes around the rectum also had metastases (16/17). The patient accepted the postoperative chemotherapies. The first chemotherapy was in June 1998, adopting the MMC+5-Fu treatment for five days. In July 1998, the patient accepted chemotherapies for twelve days (pelvic cavity, front and back of abdomen) with twenty-four times. And then the second chemotherapy was in September 1998, adopting the MMC+5-Fu treatment for six days. The third chemotherapy was in November 1999, adopting the same drugs as the second chemotherapy for five days. On November 2, 1998, the patient accepted the reexamination of type-B ultrasonic. There was no abnormality in the pelvic cavity. In February 1999, the patient began to feel pain in the area of anus. The examination of type-B ultrasonic still showed no abnormality. In March, the CT examination showed that there was a lump in the deep part of pelvic cavity (the area of anus). On March 15, 1999, the patient accepted the radiotherapies of pelvic cavity for fifteen days. In the following five days, the patient had the chemotherapies. And then the patient proceeded with radiotherapies for six times. During the radiotherapies and chemotherapies, the patient was treated by XZ-C4 to fight against the toxic side effect and protect the chest and marrow for hematopoiesis and immunization. There was no untoward effect in the whole process. Since November 1998, the patient had been using the XZ-C series for the traditional Chinese medicine treatment of immunoregulation. The condition of the illness was stable and getting better.

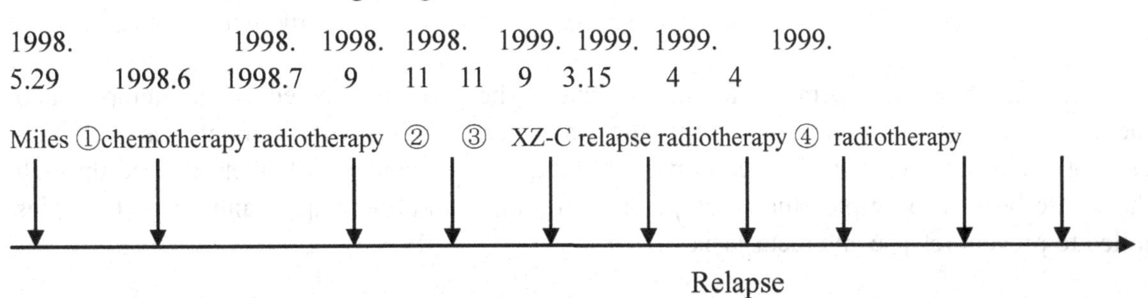

Analysis: After the Miles-type radical operation for rectum cancer, the patient accepted chemotherapies and radiotherapies continuously. Three months later, the CT examination showed that there was a lump in the deep part of pelvic cavity. The patient began to have the feeling of ache in the area of anus. The rectum cancer relapsed in partial place. It prompted that postoperative continuous chemotherapy failed to prevent the local recurrence.

Case 10 Patient Zhang ××, female, forty-four, married, Hankou, patient history number: 7101407

Diagnosis: Infiltrating ductal cancer of right breast relapsed after surgery.

In October 1997, the patient underwent the radical operation of mastocarcinoma for breast cancer (above $5m^2$). Twenty days later, the patient accepted intravenous chemotherapies for eight days with CMF treatment. In December after leaving hospital, the patient accepted radiotherapies for twenty-five times. After that, the patient accepted the chemotherapies again. In February, March, April, May and June 1998, the patient accepted chemotherapies for six times, defining once every month. In April 1998, at the lower end of the incision, a tubercle about the size of a bean could be touched. Since then, the skin tubercles grew more and more. Now eczematoid lesion was diffusing around the skin incision, and the cancer cells had been metastasizing through the whole body. There was a cauliflower-shaped ulcer (3cm×3cm) in the middle part of incisional scar. On February 3, 1999, the patient came to the anti-cancer coordination group for outpatient treatment, adopting the traditional Chinese medicine treatment of XZ-C immunoregulation series and brucea fruit latex treatment. The condition of the illness was stable.

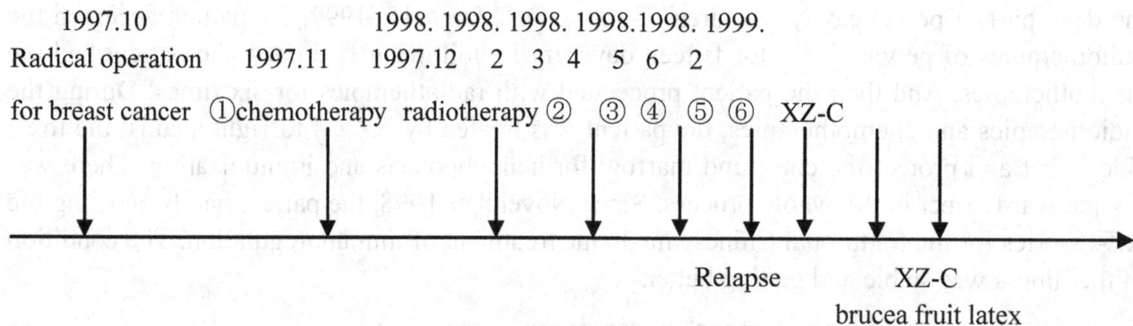

Analysis: After the operation for breast cancer, the patient accepted chemotherapies and radiotherapies continuously. Six months after the operation, when the patient was accepting chemotherapies, the cancer relapsed in partial places and the cancer cells metastasized through the whole body. It prompted that postoperative continuous radiotherapies and chemotherapies failed to prevent relapse and metastasis.

Case 11 Patient Yang ××, female, forty-three, accountant, Henan Luoshan, patient history number: 521024

There was red mucus in the stool for one month. Then on December 23, 1997, the patient accepted the fibercoloscope examination. There was an irregularly shaped new growth (3cm×5cm) at the ascending colon of the blinding end, which had 100cm to the fibercoloscope. The surface of the new growth was rugged and anabrotic. The pathological test proved it villoglandular adenocarcinoma. On December 30, 1997, the patient underwent the radical operation for colon cancer to remove the right hemicolon. In the operation, it could be found that there was a 4cm×4cm sized lump in the juncture between the blind gut and the ascending colon. The lymph nodes of the mesocolic root enlarged. The cancer cells had no metastases to the liver. Pathological test showed that villoglandular adenocarcinoma (part of mucinous adenocarcinoma) had invaded to the full-thickness of intestinal wall. Twenty-two lymph nodes had no metastases. The patient accepted postoperative chemotherapies for six times, defining once every month. The first chemotherapy was on November 26, 1998, continuing for eight days with FAP and hydroxycamptothecine. The second time started from February 12, 1998. A month later, the third time proceeded. The fourth time was on April 25, 1998 with FP treatment. The fifth time was on May 27, 1998. And the sixth time was on June 27, 1998. The chemotherapy continued for eight days. The patient had mild side effects. The white blood cell count (WBC) was 2100. On January 4, 1999, the patient accepted chemotherapies for ten days with MMC and hydroxycamptothecine. From February 1, 1999 to February 10, the patient accepted the tenth chemotherapy. In April 1999, the fibercoloscope reexamination showed the anastomosis ulcer of the colon. And the cancer relapsed in the anastomotic stoma. Then the patient came to the anti-cancer coordination group for outpatient treatment, adopting traditional Chinese and western medicine combination treatment, i.e. XZ-C_{1+4} and brucea fruit latex. The condition of the illness was stable and getting better.

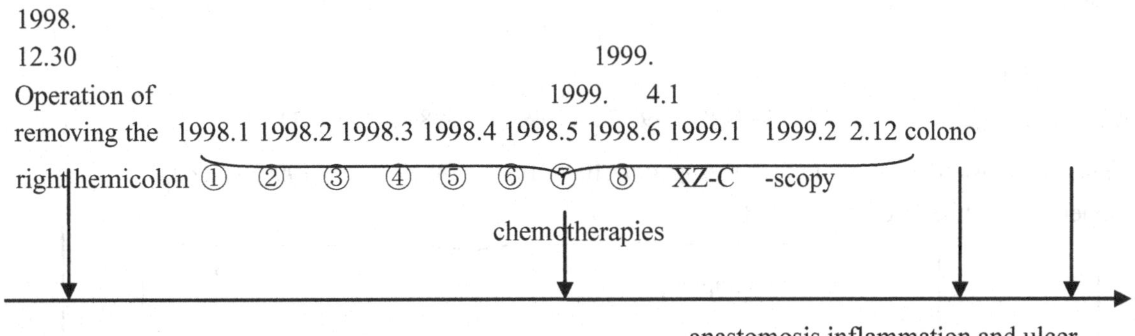

Analysis: After the radical excision for adenocarcinoma of ascending colon, the patient accepted chemotherapies for eight courses, defining one course of one month and eight days of one course. After the eighth course, the fibercoloscope reexamination showed the recurrence of anastomotic stoma. It prompted that postoperative continuous chemotherapies with eight lengthy courses still failed to prevent relapse.

Case 12 Patient Fu ××, male, twenty-four, demobilized soldier, Henan, Hu Aibin. patient history number: 8201626

Diagnosis: The carcinoma of colon relapsed after surgery.

Medical History: In February 1996, the abdominal pain was falsely diagnosed as appendicitis. Then the patient underwent the operation of removing the appendix. Pathological examination of appendicitis showed no inflammation. After the operation, the patient still felt pain in the abdominal region with recurrent paroxysmal pain. And it was treated as the spasmolysis of intestinal adhesion. Until December 1996, the patient underwent the operation of abdominal laparotomy in 153 Hospital of Zhengzhou because of intestinal obstruction. The operation showed that there was a tumor in the right hemicolon. Then the patient underwent the radical excision for right hemicolon. The pathological report was as follows.

The patient suffered from the carcinoma of colon. Half month after the operation, the patient began to accept chemotherapies. The first chemotherapy started from January 1997 and continued for five days with the intravenous injection (iv). And the chemotherapy drugs were 5-Fu+cis-platinum+MMC. The second chemotherapy was in March 1997. The third time was in May. The forth time was in August. The fifth time was in October. The sixth time was in December 1997. In the following year, the patient accepted the chemotherapy every three months. The seventh time was in March 1998. The eighth time was in June 1998. The ninth time was in September 1998. The tenth time was in December 1998. (In 1997, there was one time every two months with a total of six times. In 1998, there was one time every three months with a total of four times.) The eleventh time was in October 1999. In January 1999, the patient began to feel pain and constantly pain in the lumbosacral portion. In August 1999, the patient began to feel pain in the abdominal region and have the abdominal tympania. And there was mucus in the stool. On November 14, 1999, the patient came to the anti-cancer coordination outpatient department for XZ-C_{1+3+4} treatment. On November 15, 1999, the patient underwent a colonoscopy in the general hospital of Chinese People's Liberation Army (301 hospital). The examination showed that there was a recurrent tumor in the region, having 10cm to 30cm distances to the anus. Pathological examination showed that this tumor was the anaplastic adenocarcinoma.

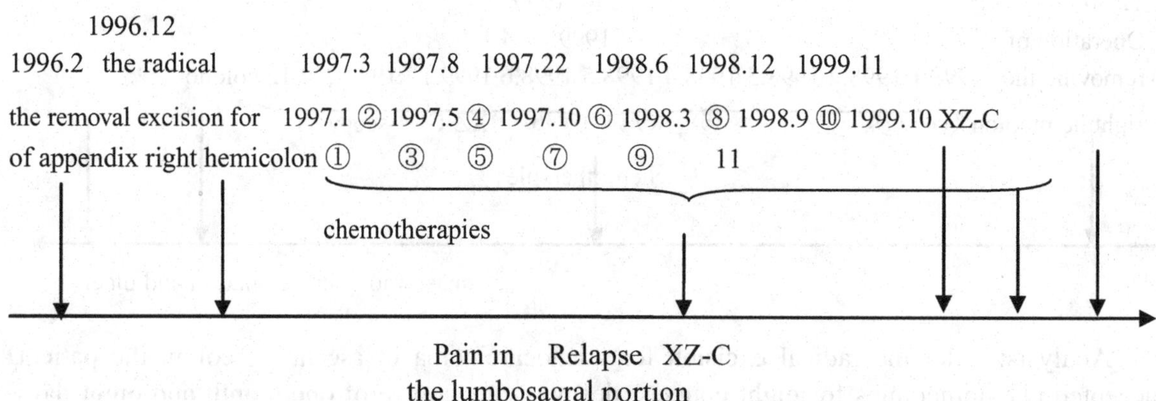

Analysis: This patient suffered from the carcinoma of colon. After undergoing the radical excision for right hemicolon, the patient accepted chemotherapies for eleven times continuously, defining two courses of one month in the first year after the operation and one course of three months in the second year after the operation. Until the tenth chemotherapy, the patient began to feel pain in the abdominal region. Retroperitoneal metastases appeared. The left colorectal cancer relapsed. Relapse and metastasis appeared while the chemotherapies were continuing. It prompted that postoperative adjuvant chemotherapy failed to arrest relapse and prevent metastasis.

II. Failure Cases of Postoperative Adjuvant Chemotherapy to Prevent Metastasis

Case 1 Patient, Xu ××, male, fifty-two, peasant, Xinzhou, patient history number: 6901374

Diagnosis: The hepatic metastases happened after the operation of carcinoma of anal canal.

The patient suffered from the carcinoma of anal canal. On September 23, 1997, the patient underwent the Miles-type radical operation. The tumor had 2cm from the anus, having the size of 3cm×3cm×2cm. The pathology was squamous cell carcinoma of anal canal. The patient accepted the postoperative chemotherapies once a month. There were five days per month for intravenous injection with carboplatin+5-Fu in October and November 1997. There were also five days per month for intravenous injection with MMC+5-Fu in December 1997, January 1998, February 1998 and March 1998. In April and May 1998, the patient switched to the oral route of Ftorafur-207 tablets. In June 1998, the type-B ultrasonic showed no abnormality. But on January 8, 1999, the type-B ultrasonic showed that there were multiple occupying nidi in the liver. The biggest nidus had the size of 8.2cm×8.6cm, diagnosed as intrahepatic metastases and retroperitoneal lymphatic metastases. There were several lymph nodes with the size of 2.1cm×0.5cm.

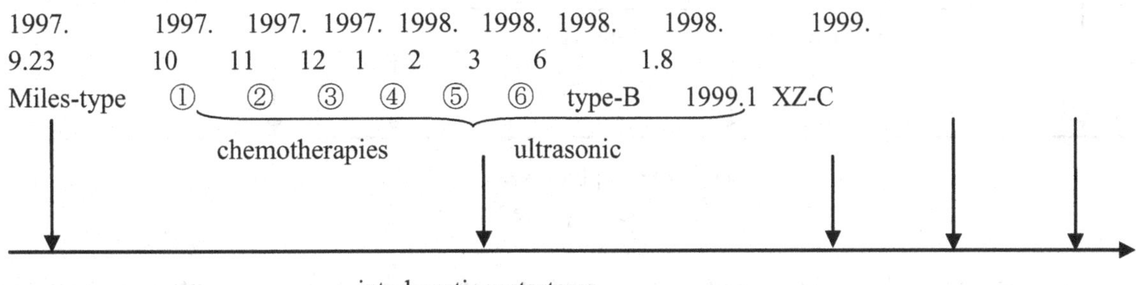

Analysis: This patient underwent the Miles-type operation. And the operation means was right. After the operation, the patient accepted chemotherapies once a month for six times continuously. Then the patient took the chemotherapy drugs orally for two months. The carboplatin, MMC and 5-Fu failed to prevent carcinomatous metastases. The tumor was the carcinoma of anal canal. But the first metastasis was hepatic metastasis. It prompted that continuous and systematical chemotherapies after the operation still failed to prevent hepatic metastases.

Case 2 Patient Yu ××, male, fifty-seven, worker, Nanchang, patient history number: 6901366

On October 22, 1995, the patient underwent the Miles-type radical operation for rectum cancer in a central hospital of Nanchang. After operation, the patient accepted the first chemotherapy was on December 5, 1995 with intravenous injection of 1000mg of 5-Fu once a day ($\mathbf{d_1}$, $\mathbf{d_2}$, $\mathbf{d_3}$, $\mathbf{d_4}$) and intravenous injection of 6mg of MMC ($\mathbf{d_1}$). The second time was on February 2, 1996 with the same FM treatment as the first time. The third time was on March 18, 1996 with the same treatment. The fourth time was on May 24, 1996. The fifth time was on August 14, 1996. The sixth time was on September 14, 1996. All of the chemotherapies adopted the FM treatment. After the chemotherapies, the patient underwent the CT examination. On December 28, 1998, the report showed three points: ①fatty liver and metastatic liver cancer, ②colorectal cancer metastasis, ③polycystic kidney and calculus of kidney. On December 25, 1998, the type-B ultrasonic found the space occupying lesion of liver.

On December 30, 1998, the patient came to the anti-cancer coordination group for outpatient treatment with XZ-$C_{4+5+3.}$ The examination showed that a lump in the form of bar could be touched in the right liver and the lump was hard. On January 20, 1999, the type-B ultrasonic in a central hospital of Nanchang found several tumors of unequal size about 4cm×2.1cm, 2.2cm×1.8cm and 2.0cm×1.7cm in the liver. There was a metastatic liver cancer with the size of 3.0cm×2.9cm in the right liver. On February 20, 1999, after taking the XZ-C_{1+4}, the patient's condition was stable and the patient regained a high spirit, a good appetite. The liver was functioning normally. The patient could walk on the street as a normal people. The symptom had an obvious improvement.

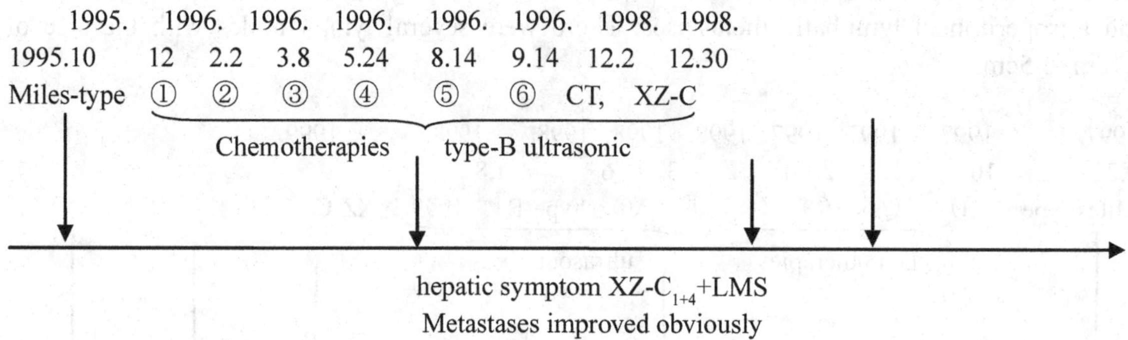

Analysis: After the radical operation of rectum cancer, the patient accepted continuous chemotherapies for six courses. One year later, the hepatic metastases happened. It prompted that systematical chemotherapies failed to prevent metastases.

Case 3 Patient Guo ××, male, thirty-six, teacher, Wuhan, patient history number: 7201425

In October 1996, the patient suffered from gastric bleeding. Then the stomachoscopy showed that the patient suffered from the stomach cancer. The patient underwent the total gastrectomy in a general hospital. Two months after the operation, the chemotherapies started. The patient accepted once every two months, defining ten days of one time. The chemotherapy drugs were MMC and 5Fu with intravenous injection. This course lasted for one year (six times). In the second year, the patient accepted once every half year. The chemotherapies in 1998 were carried out once every three or four months. In September 1998, the patient accepted one time. Every time before the chemotherapy, the patient needed to undergo the examination of type-B ultrasonic. If the type-B ultrasonic showed that there was a problem, the type-B ultrasonic would be switched to CT. The patient underwent the CT examinations for five times successively, and the CT was strengthened. After the last chemotherapy in September 1998, CT showed that the cancer cells were metastasizing to liver and retroperitoneum. Then the patient underwent the photon knife (X-knife) treatment for one time and the interventional chemotherapy for hepatic vessels embolism. In October 1998, the sclera of the patient turned yellow. The CT showed that the nubbly lump of caput pancreatic was oppressing the bile duct. Then the patient underwent the radiotherapies continuously for three times in October, November 1998 and January 1999. The doses at a time were 4000 dela. The patient had an intense reaction with bad physiques and vomiting, and couldn't feed at all. The patient couldn't undergo it and stopped the treatment. On February 28, 1999, the patient came to the outpatient department of anti-cancer coordination group for traditional Chinese and western medicine combination treatment. At that time, the patient had been bedridden. The patient was not able to take in any food for the repeated nausea and vomiting. After taking the XZ-C drugs, the patient was getting better.

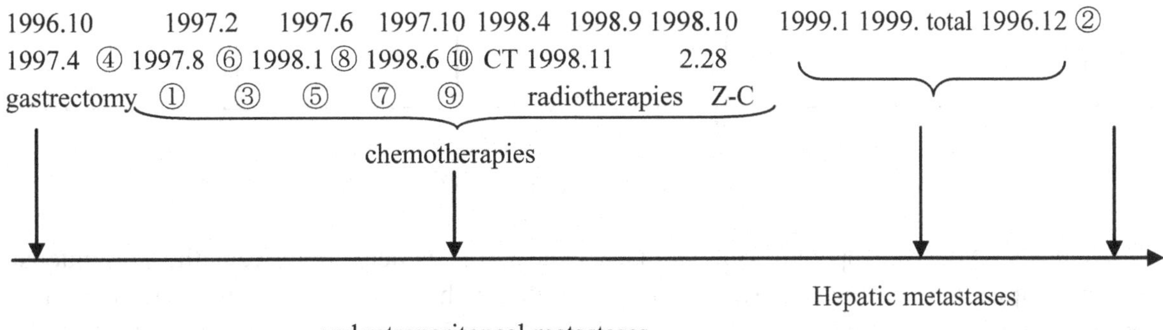

Analysis: After the total gastrectomy, the patient underwent the continuous chemotherapies and radiotherapies for a long time. After the last chemotherapy in September 1998, the CT reexamination showed the hepatic metastases and retroperitoneal metastases. It prompted that continuous and long-term treatments still failed to prevent metastases, even resulting in the failure of immunologic system and threatening the patient's life.

Case 4 Patient Cao ××, male, thirty-five, married, peasant, Hanchuan, patient history number: 470928

Diagnosis: The hepatic metastases happened after the operation of stomach cancer.

On June 28, 1996, the pre-operative diagnosis in the People's Hospital of Hanchuan certified it as the ulcer of gastric angles. The property of the illness was yet to be investigated. The patient underwent the massive resection of the stomach and the resection of great epiploon. The operation was B1-type anastomosis. The postoperative pathological report showed it the sdenocarcinoma of stomach. The cancer cells had invaded the full-thickness of stomach wall with lymphatic metastases of lesser curvature side (4/4). The lymph nodes of greater curvature side had reactive hyperplasia. The patient underwent the postoperative chemotherapies for four times in July, August, September and October 1996, defining once a month and three days every time. The chemotherapy drugs were 5-F and MMC. In September 1997, after the half month of swelling pain in right upper abdomen, the type-B ultrasonic and CT prompted that there were several low-density shadows in the right and left lobe of liver. Those were metastatic hepatic tumors and could be touched below the right costal margin of 3cm with pressing tender. On September 30, 1997, the patient underwent the interventional chemotherapy for hepatic artery. On October 5, 1997, the patient came to the anti-cancer coordination outpatient department, adopting the Z-C series for the traditional Chinese medicine treatment of immunoregulation. After taking the medicine orally, the patient regained a high spirit, a good appetite and enough physical strength. The lump below the right costal margin became soft and narrowing.

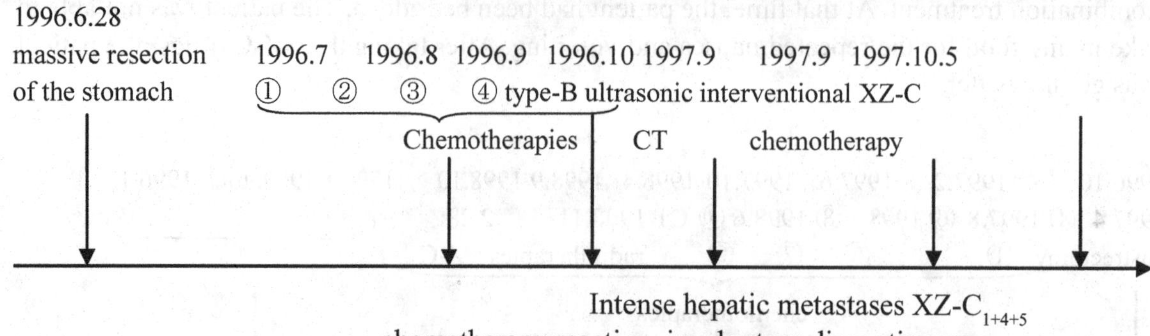

Analysis: After the operation of stomach cancer, the patient underwent the continuous chemotherapies for four times, defining once a month and three days every time. One year after the last chemotherapy, the CT reexamination showed that there were several metastatic lesions in the right and left lobe of liver. It prompted that postoperative adjuvant chemotherapies still failed to prevent metastases.

Case 5 Patient Li ××, male, fifty-five, Huangshi, second-grade actor, patient history number: 2700530

Diagnosis: The cancer cells metastasized to pancreas after the operation of stomach cancer.

In October 1995, the patient suffered from the epigastric discomfort. In November, the stomachoscopy in Huangshi Hospital diagnosed it as the stomach cancer. On November 27, 1995, the patient underwent the massive resection of the stomach. After the operation, the patient accepted five courses of chemotherapies with one course per month. In early May 1996, the last course ended. On June 4, 1996, the CT reexamination showed the space occupying lesion of pancreas. The patient began to have the abdominal distension and bad appetite. Then the patient came to the anti-cancer coordination group for outpatient treatment, adopting the XZ-C_{1+4+2} series for the traditional Chinese medicine treatment of immunoregulation. After taking the medicine orally, the patient regained a high spirit, a good appetite.

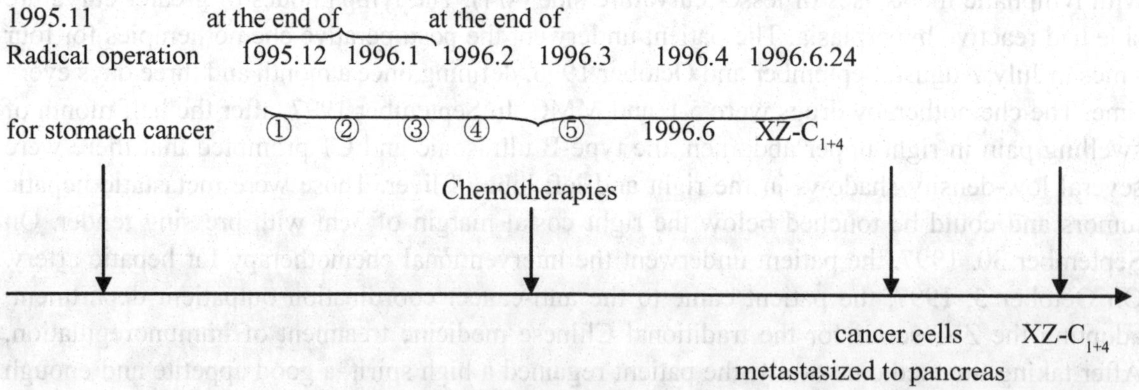

Analysis: After the radical operation of stomach cancer, the patient accepted five courses of chemotherapies with one course per month. After the five courses, the patient underwent the CT reexamination, finding the space occupying lesion of pancreas and metastatic carcinoma of pancreas. It prompted that postoperative chemotherapies still failed to prevent postoperative carcinomatous metastases.

Case 6 Patient Li ××, female, forty-five, Guangshui, teacher, patient history number: 6701324

Diagnosis: The stomach cancer relapsed and metastasized to ovary after the operation. The middle and down section of choledochus had solid space occupying lesions.

In April 1998, the stomachoscopy showed that there was a new growth in the body of stomach with bulb ulcer. On April 20, 1998, the patient underwent the total gastrectomy and lienectomy. Esophagus and empty intestine were connected by the end-to-side anastomosis. The pathological test showed that the patient suffered from the mucinous adenocarcinoma of stomach. The cancer cells had invaded the full-thickness of stomach wall with lymphatic metastases of lesser curvature side. On May 13, 1998, the patient accepted the first chemotherapy, adopting 1000mg of 5-Fu with five-day intravenous injections. On the first day the chemotherapy drugs were added with 10mg of Mitomycin. On June 3, 1998, the patient accepted the second chemotherapy with 10mg of Mitomycin. The third time was on July 1, 1998. The fourth time was on July 29, 1998. The fifth time was on September 9, 1998. The reexamination found the relapse. On December 24, 1998, the type-B ultrasonic showed the cancer of biliary duct and ovarian metastasis. On December 26, 1998, the patient came to the anti-cancer coordination group for outpatient treatment, adopting the XZ-C series for the traditional Chinese medicine treatment of immunoregulation. After taking the medicine orally, the symptom was improving, and the condition of the illness was getting better.

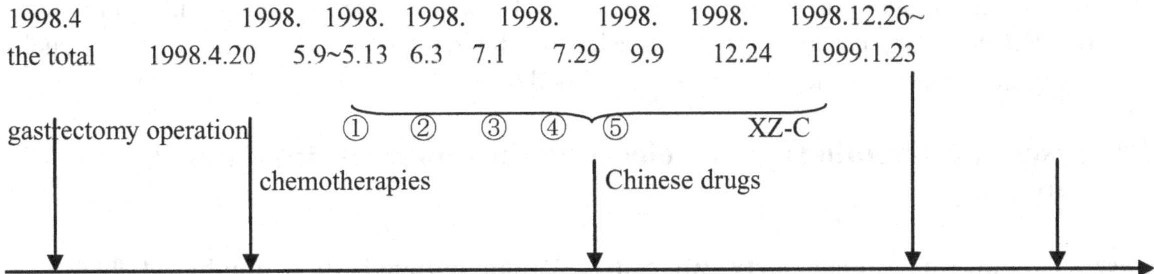

Type-B ultrasonic: relapse of cancer of biliary duct, ovarian metastasis.

Analysis: This patient suffered from the mucinous adenocarcinoma of stomach and underwent the total gastrectomy. After the operation, the patient accepted the chemotherapies once a month with five days per time. After the fifth chemotherapy, the type-B ultrasonic found the relapse of cancer of biliary duct and ovarian metastasis. It prompted that postoperative adjuvant chemotherapies still failed to arrest relapse and prevent metastasis.

Case 7 Patient Li ××, female, thirty-seven, worker, Yingcheng, patient history number: 7401473

Diagnosis: The rectum cancer cells metastasized to ovary after the operation.

Since 1997, the stool had been being with the blood. In June 1998, the colonoscopy showed it as the rectum cancer. On July 9, 1998, the patient underwent the anterior resection of the rectum (Dixon-type, anastomat). There were six-time postoperative chemotherapies. The first time was on July 27, 1998 with carboplatin and 5-Fu. The second time was on September 6, 1998. The third time was on October 2, 1998. The fourth time was on November 19, 1998. The fifth time was on December 25, 1998. The sixth time was on January 31, 1999.

On April 16, 1999, the patient came to the anti-cancer coordination group for outpatient treatment with the XZ-C series. In May 1999, the CT examination showed the rectum cancer cells metastasized to bilateral ovaries.

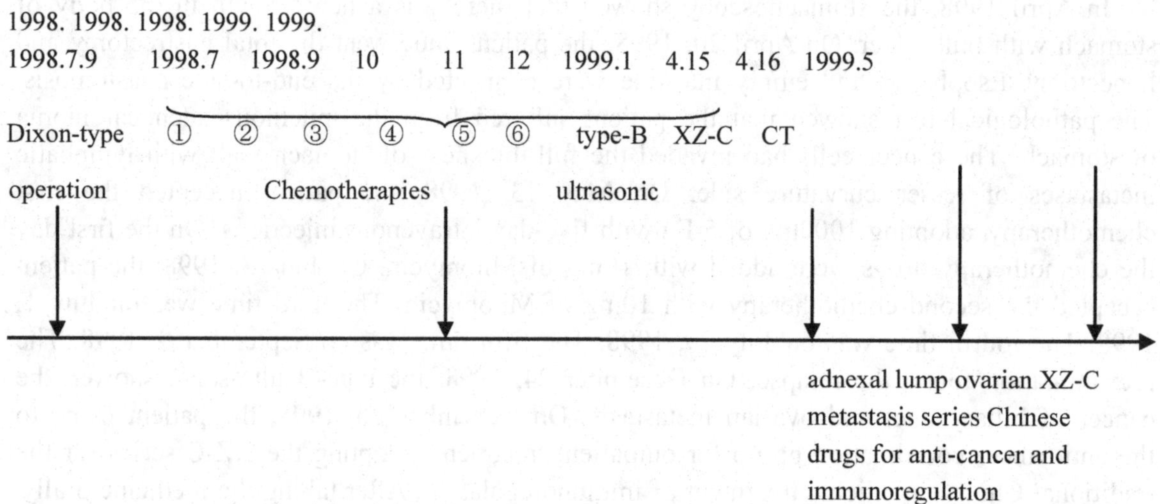

Analysis: After the operation of rectum cancer, the patient accepted continuous chemotherapies for six courses. Three months after the last course, the type-B ultrasonic and CT found that rectum cancer cells metastasized to bilateral ovaries. It prompted that such continuous and long-term chemotherapies still failed to prevent metastases.

III. Cases of Chemotherapy Accelerating the Failure of Immunologic Function

Case 1 Patient, Xu ××, male, forty-two, cadre, Wuhan, patient history number: 420836

Diagnosis: Lung cancer of right middle lobe

In February 1997, fluoroscopy of chest showed no abnormity. Because of the home decorating, the patient had contacted the marble powder bed for about one month. Then this patient began to have a complaint of the chest. On June 1, 1997, X-ray chest film showed the atelectasis of right lung. On June 13, 1997, the CT reported the lung cancer of median lobe and metastases of hilar lymph nodes. The examination of bronchofiberscope showed that each bronchus of the right side became narrower. The brushing biopsy showed it as the adenocarcinoma cell. Right now, the patient had no cough and emptysis. There was a lymph node about the size of fingertip in the right neck region. On June 13, 1997, the patient underwent the interventional therapy for one time. Because of the intense reaction, there was no more interventional therapy. On July 25, 1997, the patient began to accept chemotherapies for two times. The first time adopted the intravenous injection with a large dose of Adriamycin, Cyclophosphane, Cis-platinum and **Xierke**. On August 9, the white blood cell count (WBC) was 1100. Then the patient accepted the blood transfusion, adding with injections of interleukin-2, tumor necrosis factor and interferon. The second time was on August 20. The chemotherapy drugs were same as the first time with intravenous injection. On September 10, X-ray chest film showed no obvious pathological change. On September 11, the patient left the hospital. On October 10, 1997, Emission Computed Tomography (ECT) showed widespread metastatic tumor of bone of the whole body. On October 13, 1997, X-ray chest film showed the lung cancer of double lungs. The lesions increased significantly as compared with the past. After undergoing the reinforced chemotherapies of two courses, the lesions of double lungs spread. The cancer cells quickly metastasized to skeletons of the whole body. The immunologic function broke down. By the end of October 1997, the patient died from the failure of immunologic function.

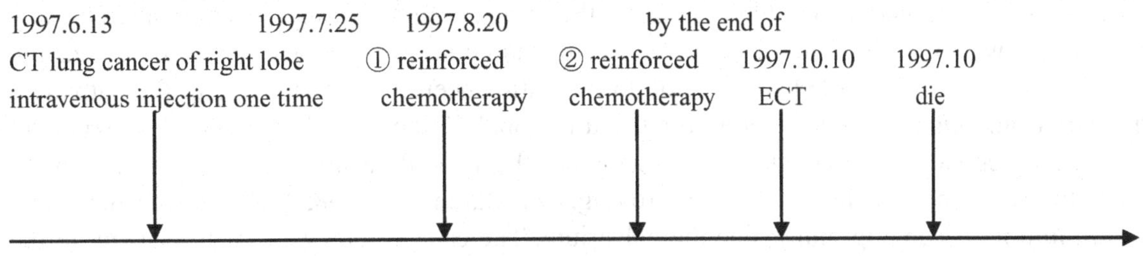

The cancer cells metastasized to skeletons of the whole body. The immunologic function broke down.

Analysis: This patient suffered from lung cancer of right middle lobe. The left lung had carcinomatous metastasis. So the patient couldn't accept the operation. Since July 1997, the patient accepted the reinforced chemotherapies of two courses with four kinds of drugs. The patient began to vomit and couldn't feed at all. After the treatment, the immunologic function of the patient broke down. Emission Computed Tomography (ECT) showed that there were several dozen osseous metastases in the whole body. It prompted: ① the reinforced chemotherapies failed to prevent metastases. ② the reinforced chemotherapies severely suppressed the immunity, which led to the severe failure of immunologic function. The host lost the immune surveillance. The cancer cells immediately spread to the whole body. The osseous metastases resulted in the failure of immunologic function and shortened this patient's life.

Case 2 Patient Feng ××, female, fifty-one, Xiangfan, doctor, patient history number: 4900972

Diagnosis: After the operation of the breast cancer, the cancer cells metastasized to bones, liver and brain.

In February 1995, the patient underwent the modified radical mastectomy for the lump in the right breast. The patient suffered from the metastatic carcinoma of axillary lymph nodes (3/6). Pathology: infiltrating ductal cancer became partly hard. On February 19, 1995, the patient accepted the chemotherapy with the drugs of Adriamycin and Cyclophosphamide. On April 28, 1995, the patient transferred to Wuhan for eleven cycles of chemotherapies with CMF treatment. On May 21, 1996, the CMF treatment was switched to Xierke treatment in the eleventh cycle. The arrest of bone marrow became obvious. The white blood cell count (WBC) dropped to 300! Transfusion of 20g of leucocytes eventually made it come back to the normal value. The doctor gave express order that the patient couldn't accept the treatment after leaving hospital. On June 4, 1996, the Ct reexamination found metastatic carcinoma of the ninth rib. Then the patient accepted the radiotherapies without any chemotherapy. On July 7, 1997, the type-B ultrasonic found the metastatic carcinoma of liver. There was a tumor about the size of 3.2cm×3.9cm in the right anterior lobe of liver. The MRI and CT examinations diagnosed it falsely as radioactive hepatic lesion. On July 17, 1997, the angiography proved it as the metastatic carcinoma of liver. On July 28, 1997, the patient underwent the resection of the right anterior lobe of liver. And the patient was inserted a catheter into the hepatic artery for implantation of the drug pump. The chemotherapy drugs of epirubicin, cis-platinum and 5-Fu had been pumped successively for four times. On November 10, 1997, the type-B ultrasonic found that there were a metastatic carcinoma about the size of 3.4cm×3.3cm in the right lobe of liver and another metastatic carcinoma about the size of 1.7cm×1.9cm in the right anterior lobe of liver. The patient couldn't undergo the surgery, radiotherapy or chemotherapy any more. That was because none of the three treatments could prevent metastasis and extension. On November 16, 1997, the patient came to the anti-cancer coordination group for outpatient treatment, adopting the XZ-C series for the traditional Chinese medicine complex treatment of immunoregulation. After taking the medicine, the patient regained a high spirit, a good appetite. The general condition was improving. On March 17, 1998, MRI showed that there were multiple occupying nidi inside the calvarium. The cancer cells were metastasizing to the brain. Then the patient accepted the reinforced chemotherapies. After a course of reinforced chemotherapies, the patient gradually faded away.

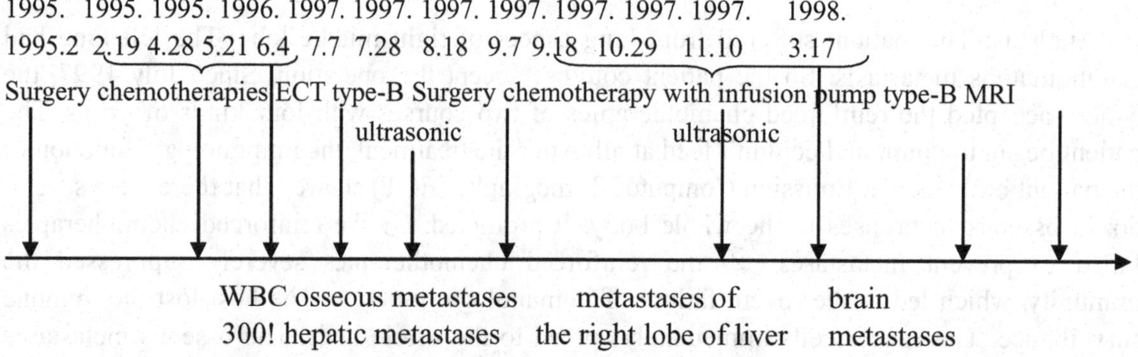

Analysis: (1) After the operation of breast cancer, the patient accepted the continuous chemotherapies, starting with short-course chemotherapies and proceeding with the eleven courses of chemotherapies. And then, the patient was injected with the chemotherapy drugs by the infusion pump. Although the patient continuously accepted the chemotherapies and other treatments without a stop, the cancer still ignored those treatments, slowly and gradually making the distant metastases through the whole body. Why did so many treatments fail to stop metastases and extensions? What kind of role and status did those chemotherapy anti-cancer drugs play and have in this case? The chemotherapies didn't produce the due effect, because after the chemotherapy the cancer cells immediately metastasized to bones, liver.

(2) The chemotherapy suppressed the immunologic function and marrow hematopoietic function. The question was whether the suppression would promote osseous metastases. The reinforced chemotherapies of this case once made WBC reduce to 300. The body's immunological function suffered the severe suppression. The cancer cells lost the immune surveillance and would inevitably have the further multiplications, extensions and metastases.

(3) Why were the chemotherapies of this case useless? The question was whether the chemotherapy drugs had the drug tolerance. If having the tolerance, the chemotherapy drugs of more than one year were totally useless. The drugs didn't produce the due effect on cancer cells. On the contrary, the normal cells of visceral organs in the patient's body, especially the cells of immune organ (Marrow was the central immune organ), ceaselessly suffered form the damage. Then the ability of the body resistance and immunological function severely fell off. It promoted multiplications, extensions and metastases of cancer cells. The chemotherapy not only failed to achieve the therapeutic effect, but also conversely had the adverse effect on attacking the ability of the body resistance and promoting the metastases and multiplications of the cancer cells.

(4) Why were the continuous chemotherapies of this case useless? The question was whether the selected joint chemotherapy drugs were not sensitive to the cancer cells of this patient. (The anti-cancer drugs couldn't accept drug sensitive test as the antibiotic. Thus the drugs were selected according to the experience with certain blindness.) When doctors couldn't get the curative effect, they would increase the dose, intensify the chemotherapy or switch to use the better chemotherapy drugs. In this way, it would produce the more severe immunological suppression, result the failure of immunological function and lead to the further multiplications of the cancer cells, which the cancer cells would present the multiplication like the geometrical logarithm. But the chemotherapy drugs couldn't increase exponentially with the toxic side effect. Thus the increasing speed and quantity of chemotherapy drugs would never be able to catch up those of cancer cells. So the continuous chemotherapies still failed to control metastases and extensions.

Case 3 Patient Lu ××, female, forty-three, shop employee, Changsha, patient history number: 4300857

Diagnosis: The patient suffered from the carcinoma simplex of left breast. The cancer cells had metastasized to the back bone, pelvis and liver.

Medical History: (Omission).

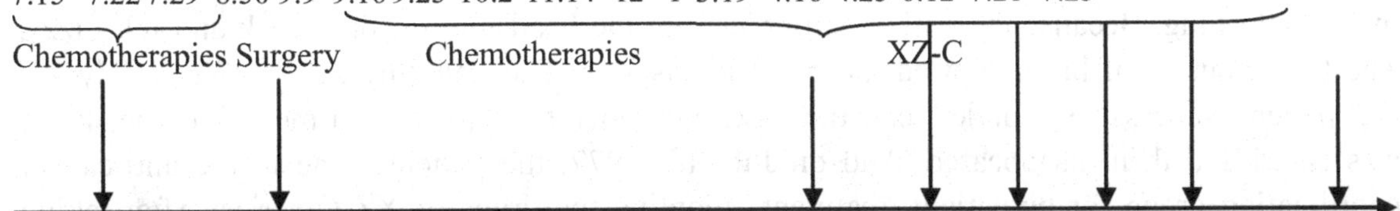

Analysis: This patient accepted the preoperative and postoperative chemotherapies continuously and chronically. After the operation, the patient accepted the chemotherapy once a month, defining five days every time. During the five months after the operation, there were over forty times of radiotherapies and eight times of chemotherapies. The patient underwent continuous multiple CT scans and ceaselessly continuous chemotherapies. But after eight months the cancerous protuberance widely metastasized and spread to skeletons of the whole body. Every time the patient accepted the radiotherapy or chemotherapy, she had to suffer the suppression, bone marrow suppression and the attack to the organisms of the body. The long-term and continuous chemotherapies were essentially the chronic and continuous attack to the immunologic function. The immunologic function of organisms and marrow hematopoietic function suffered such long-term and continuous damage that they couldn't restore the functions. Losing the immune surveillance, the cancer cells were bound to invade and metastasize widely to all of the visceral organs in the whole body.

The real effect of this case was that the treatment killed off tumor cells but damaged the body. It didn't turn out as it should be. In fact, the treatments failed to prevent carcinomatous metastases, essentially damage the function of immunologic and defensive system of the host, attack the ability of the body resistance and promote the invasion and dissemination of cancer cells.

Six months after the operation, metastatic carcinoma of bone appeared. Eight months after the operation, metastatic carcinoma of liver appeared. The radiotherapy and chemotherapy failed to prevent the progression of this disease. How to evaluate the therapeutic effectiveness that the radiotherapy and chemotherapy had on the patient? What kind of role and status did those treatments play and have?

Case 4 Patient Chen ××, male, Thirty-four, counterman, Wuhan, patient history number: 430849

This patient had suffered from the repetitious and irritative dry cough without phlegm for three years. Then this disease was treated as bronchitis. In January 1997, X-ray film of the chest showed large compact shadows in the right upper lung. CT examination reported that there was a compact shadow about the size of 6cm×9cm in the right upper lung. And there was another sarcoidosis behind it about the size of 1.2cm×1.5cm. The sarcoidosis was the central type and had multiple metastases in the lung. On January 11, 1997, the patient underwent the exploratory thoracotomy. In the operation, it could be easily seen that the nidi had widely infiltrated and couldn't be cut off. The tissue slice showed it as the poorly differentiated adenocarcinoma in the right upper lung. Then the chest was closed. In February, March, April and May 1997, the patient accepted postoperative chemotherapies with the drugs of DDP and ADM for one course a month. On July 14, 1997, scanning reexamination showed the enlargement of lump in the right lung. Because the patient suffered from the headache for one week and felt dizzy. The CT scanning of brain showed the brain metastases. Then on July 22, 1997 and July 27, the patient successively underwent the r-scalpel operation for two times. The headache was eased and then disappeared. And on July 13, 1977, the patient came to the anti-cancer coordination group for outpatient treatment, adopting the drugs of XZ-C series. After taking the medicine, the condition of illness was stable. The patient regained a high spirit, a good appetite. The headache and vomit disappeared. The patient walked and talked as the normal people. Three months (one course) after taking the Wuhan Chinese herbal anticancer medicine of XZ-C series, the condition of illness had an obvious improvement. The patient had a rosy cheek, regained the physical strength and walked as the normal people. There was no cough or any kind of discomfort. The breathing sound of right lung faded out. Afterwards the patient accepted the chemotherapy in another hospital, continuously increasing the dose for reinforced chemotherapies. The white blood cell count (WBC) dropped to 300, which was an extremely low value. The immunologic function crocked up.

Analysis: This patient underwent the exploratory thoracotomy for the cancer of right lung. The nidi couldn't be cut off. Then the patient accepted the continuous reinforced chemotherapies. The cancer cells metastasized to the brain. After the r-scalpel operation, the headache disappeared and obtained satisfactory effects. With the immunoregulation treatment of XZ-C series, the general conditions of this patient were getting better obviously and the symptoms improved. But the continuous reinforced chemotherapies resulted in the failure of immunologic function.

CHAPTER 18

Analysis, Evaluation And Reflection Of Clinic Practice

Three traditional therapies of cancel have made great achievements, which have making recognized contributions to cancer prevention and anti-cancer career of human. At the beginning of 21st century, as cancer is still at the top of the death rate, the traditional therapies have failed to inhibit and prevent the occurrence and development of cancer. Though many patients have accepted normal radiotherapies and chemotherapies systematically, the metastasis and recrudesce of cancer cell had been not prevented. The radiotherapies and chemotherapies have made many contributions and achieved a lot, however, they are still far away from the ideal requirements and objective demands in terms of domestic therapies of cancer. Why do the traditional methods fail to prevent the metastasis, diffuse and evolution of cancer? What is the reason for cancer metastasis during chemotherapies? Why can cancer metastasis be examined after chemotherapies? Are these drugs sensitive to cancer cells? Is there any drug resistance or not? What is the theory basis for the period of treatment arranged within 1 to 2years? Is there any cancer cell in patients' bodies after radiotherapies and chemotherapies? Which kind of chemotherapies can be used, local or general? What is the theory and fact basis? What are the curative effects of intensive chemotherapies as well as its influences and complications? Can the curative effects improve the quality of living and prolong the lifetime? Is there any need for chemotherapies? How to make the treatment modality? What are the effects of chemotherapies, positive or negative? Is there any possibility to accelerate the development and metastasis or diffuse of cancer cells?

Therefore, we should conclude the experience and failures of 50-year anti-cancer practice to analyze, reflect and evaluate by ourselves, in order to improve the research and the curative effects.

I. Concept of Cancer Cell Proliferation Dynamics and the Role of Chemotherapy Medicine in Cell Cycle

In this part, we will go on with the analysis, reflection and evaluation through the details of postoperative adjuvant chemotherapies of more the 6000 cases and their records of return visits.

From the point of Cancer Cell Proliferation Dynamics, having one chemotherapy every three or four weeks can hardly prevent cancer recrudesce and metastasis.

1. Basic Concepts of Malignancy Proliferation

As the object that the clinic chemotherapies are faced with is the cancer tissue rather than individual cell, the basic concept of proliferation dynamics should be described using cancer tissue as the representation of the malignant tumor tissue.

1. The collection of proliferative cells, refer to the proportion of the cancer cells that proliferate according to index in the whole cancer cells (meaning growth fraction GF).

Different tumors have different growth fraction. Even one and the same tumor, the growth fraction of the prophase is higher, and different from that of the anaphase. Tumors with higher growth fraction grow rapidly and have higher sensitivity.

2. The collection of resting cells (cells of GO phase), which are the spare cells with proliferating capacity; however they don't enter the cell cycle temporarily. When the proliferative cells are killed by drugs, cells of GO phase enter into proliferating stage. Cells of GO phase have low sensitivity to drugs, which is the root of recrudesce during the treatment.
3. Collection of cells without proliferative capacity which are neither proliferative nor lost. Only a few such cells in the cancer tissue and they are insignificant in the chemotherapies.

The above three kinds of cells are in relative movements instead of standstill as the proliferative cells can change into the cells of GO phase, cells without proliferating capacity or even dead.

2. Cell Cycle

Cells of the collection of proliferative cells in cancer tissue are dividing and proliferating constantly. Cell cycle has been proposed for researching the growing process of individual cell in the collection of proliferative cells. Cell cycle refers to the entire process from the prophase of DNA synthesis to the accomplishment of mitosis. In recent years, with the advanced technologies such as flow cytometry, etc. we have achieved further researches on the proliferating cycle of cancer cells. The proliferating cycle of cancer cells can be mainly divided into four stages:

1. Gl phase meaning the prophase of DNA synthesis, is the stage letting the daughter cells from mitosis go on growing, in which the messengers mRNA and proteins are synthesized. The lengths of G1 phase of different kinds of cancer cells have great differentia from hours to days.
2. S phase meaning the synthesis of DNA, is the stage for duplicating DNA, in which the content of DNA is duplicated. In this phase, some other compounds such as histone, non-histone and enzymes relating to synthesis are also duplicated. It is worthy to note that the synthesis of tubulin has already begun in S phase. The length of S phase fluctuates between 2 and 30 hours, mostly more than 10 hours.
3. G2 phase meaning the anaphase of DNA synthesis or the prophase of division. In this phase, the DNA synthesis has finished and the preparation for cell division is processing, with the synthesis of the proteins and tubulins relating to cancer cell division, which lasts from two to three hours.
4. M phase means the stage of mitosis. Each cancer cell divides into two daughter cells. This phase is very short, only lasting from one to two hours.

The lengths of each phase can be measured by marking thymidines with 3_{HH}. The summation of G_1+S+G_2+M is the cell cycle time (TC). The TC value of acute medullocell is approximately 50~80 hours, in which G_1 phase is 20~60 hours, S phase is about 20 hours, G_2 is almost 3 hours and M is as short as 30 minutes. The TC value of albino rat L_{1210} leucocythemia is some 12.8 hours with M phase being an hour.

Thus during one-time chemotherapy, only making drugs acting on cells and experiencing the entire cycle for 50 to 80 hours, or the drugs for the chemotherapy acting on cancer cell or the cancer cells are soaked in the chemotherapeutant for 50 ~80 hours can kill the cancer cells in some phase. If using disposal catheter to inject drugs or during the chemotherapy, patients only accept 6~8 minute intravenous drip, maybe the drugs can not meet the most sensitive phase, that is to say, the desired curative effects can not be achieved. Just acting on some phase of cell proliferation blindly without selections fails to react on cell cycle.

Antibiotics G_+ or G- kill the bacterium G_+ or G- after contacting. Different from antibiotics, the chemotherapeutants can only react on the sensitive phase and make no effects on other ones. These two are completely different.

In terms of cell dynamics, the chemotherapeutants can be divided into two kinds according to sensitivity to malignant cells of each phase, cell cycle nonspecific agent (CCSNA) and cell cycle specific agent (CCSA)

1. Cell Cycle Nonspecific Agent There is no relationship between cell's sensitivity and its proliferating state. CCNSA can kill the cells of each phase through the entire proliferating cycle. Most alkylating agents and antibiotic drugs belong to this sort.
2. Cell Cycle Specific Agent Cell's sensitivity relates to its proliferating state. CCSA mainly reacts on some phase of the cell cycle, which is classified into two sorts; M phase specific drugs and S phase specific drugs.
   (1) M phase specific drugs mostly acts on mitosis, vegetable drugs like vinblastine and vincristine fall into this sort.
   (2) S phase specific drugs are used to inhibit the synthesis of RNA and proteins, most antimetabolite drugs such as methotrexate, 5—fluorouracil, purinethol and thioguanine and others belong to this sort.

CCNSA can damage tumors cells of each phases including G_0 phase without sensitivity. Cells of S and M phases in proliferation are the most sensitive to the drugs. These drugs include the metabolite(S phase) and the vegetable drugs (M phase) with the characteristic of schedule-dependent when giving drugs. At first, the curative effect of killing the tumor cells is proportional to the dosage, whose dose-effect curve presents exponential decrease. As the amount of cells in S phase or M phase is certain, there are no other benefits to add the dosage; in spite of the cells of S phase and M phase, others are not sensitive to this category of drugs.

For both CCNSA and CCSA, their effects of damaging cancer cells subject to the first order kinetics, that is to say it is impossible to kill all cancer cells but a definite proportion. Though patients accept drugs with high dose for several times, there are always some cells without sensitivity to the drugs. So, cancer cells always exist in the bodies, which can be only relieved rather than healed. This way can only prolong the lifetime instead of charming away (It is difficult to identify whether this therapeutic method can prolong the patients' lifetime or not for it is only considered from the aspect of killing cancer cells by drugs, however in terms of drugs' inhibiting immunity and the toxic side effects to marrow and liver, the living qualities and lifetime of the host cells are still faced with severe challenges).

As that the anticancer drugs damage the cancer cells subjects to the first order kinetics, generally it is difficult to find a perfect chemotherapeutic drugs to cure cancers. However, when the loads of tumors are below 10^6, it is possible to annihilate the cancer cells using XZ-C treatment by Chinese herbs for immunoregulation or immunological therapy.

That is the reasons why the postoperative adjuvant chemotherapies or palliative chemotherapy fail to prevent the recrudesce, the metastasis and the further diffuse of the tumors (Chemotherapies can not achieve the radical cure, so it is only palliative therapy, especially for solid tumors).

The curative effects of postoperative adjuvant chemotherapies for solid tumors are worse, however, we hold the idea that it is possible to gain better curative effects by using chemotherapies added with XZ-C Chinese traditional medicine for immunoregulation against the immunosuppression and toxic side effects to marrow and liver of chemotherapies.

II. Analysis, Reflection and Evaluation from the Angle of Inhibiting Whole Immunity by Chemotherapy

Why has not the quality of living been improved and the lifetime prolonged after postoperative adjuvant chemotherapies? Why does the cancer recrudesce and metastasize after chemotherapies or diffuse from head to foot, osseous metastasis happen immediately after chemotherapies for many patients? In terms of the destructing hosts' immunologic functions, chemotherapies cause the decrease in immunologic functions and immune monitoring capacity of the host cells, thus lead to the further development of cancer.

The immune system consists of immune organs, immune cells and immune molecules. Central immune organs, also called first level immune organs, are the place for the production, differentiation and maturation of immune cells, working as the leader of the circumferential immune organs. Central immune organs include the marrow and the thymus.

1. Thymus is located at the superior part of the mediastinum, back of the breastbone, and separated into two lobes, the right and the left. The size and the structure change with the ages and the state of organisms, with the weight of 10~15g when born. After born, the thymus grows rapidly within 2 years which is the fastigium of the thymus activities. From then on, the thymus augments gradually and reaches the maximum during the adolescence, with the weight of around 30~40g. After the adolescence, the thymus begins to retrogress. On entering the agedness, most thymus tissue is replaced by the adipose tissue, but with some remaining functions. That the thymus is atrophying gradually as the organism is getting older after the adolescence is called physiologic atrophy of thymus, which is usually accompanied with the shrinking of cellular area in the lymph node. The animal experiment has proved that a newborn animal extirpated the thymus, whose lymphocytes in the circumferential immune organs T cellular area are sparse, has apparently reduced lymphocytes in its blood and the damaged humoral immunity function lacking the cellular immune function. The animal has the symptoms of immune deficiency, which may lead to death as the result of consumptive disease as the same as the consumption and exhaustion representations of the animal inoculated cancer. Reviewing the patients with clinic latecancer, their exhaustion deaths also present as the exhaustion of immune function. If embedded with thymus or the extract of thymus, this kind of patients can regain partial immune function.

   The functions of the thymus: thymus is the principle organ that induces the T cells to differentiate and maturate, which has been proved.

(1) Thymus is the place for the differentiation and maturation of T cells. For an adult, the pre-T cells move from the marrow to the thymus, then grow and maturate in the thymus. After maturating, the T cells move out from the thymus with a certain amount (1%~2%) and settle in the circumferential lymphatic organs or tissue. Mature cells can present the antigen receptors and recognize the foreign antigens (pre-T cells cannot). In the anaphase of growth, T cells differentiate further into T cell subsets with different functions, T cell subsets with damage capacity (inhibiting) and adjuvant T cell subsets (inductivity), which explants from the thymus through blood or lympha, then settle in the thymus dependent area of the circumferential immune organs.

(2) Producing thymic hormone: the reticular epithelial cell on the thymus tissue can produce various kinds of thymic hormones, like thymosin, thymopoietin, thymic humoral factor, lymphocyte stimulating factor, etc. The mentioned dissoluble substance is the main component of thymic microenvironment and plays an important role in the differentiation and adjustment of T cells.

2. Marrow is the hematopoietic organ for human, as well as the birthplace of all kinds of immune cells. Though marrow is not lymphatic tissue, it possesses multipotential stem cells with strong differential potential. Marrow can differentiate into myeloid stem cells and lymphatic trunks cells. The former ones grow into erythrocytic series, granulocyte or B cells, and locate in the circumferential immune organs in the end. Moreover, except B and T cells, the lymphocyte cytokines precursors also achieve their proliferation, differentiation and maturations in the marrow, like K cells and NK cells. If the functions of the marrow are defective, it is possible to cause both the cellular immunity and humoral immunity defective. Injecting normal marrow can rebuild the immune functions, which indicates the importance of marrow in executing the immune functions.

The fundamentality of marrow is also regarded as the principle part of producing antibodies. The categories of the antibodies produced are lgG mainly and lgA secondly. As a result, marrow is the main place of immune response. The marrow can produce a large amount of antibodies tardily and continuously.

Circumferential immune organ, also called secondary immune organ, is the residence for T cells and B cells. At the same time it is the part for the immune response after the cells recognize foreign antigens. Lymph nodes, whose amount is about 500~600 in a human body, and spleens as well as other lymphatic tissue make up the secondary lymphatic tissue with complete structure, which locate in the non-mucous membranes mostly and distribute widely in the lymph channels. About 70% of the lymphocytes in lymph nodes are T cells and other 25% are B cells. The superficial cortex of lymph node which B cells settle in is called thymus independent areas, while the deep cortex area for T cells is thymus dependent areas. T cells and B cells in lymph nodes can enter into the blood circulation through postcapillary venules. Sensitized T cell and specific antigens produced by the T cells and B cells in the process of immune response gather in the lymph node medullary sinus and then discharge from the lymph efferents.

As a conclusion, the central immune organs include the thymus and the marrow; while spleen and lymph nodes are the circumferential organs.

We have observed when experimenting with the animal model of albino rat bearing tumor that tumors can excrete some special factor (called cancer-inhibiting-thymus factor temporarily) and act on the thymus, leading to the immune organ's atrophy and the decrease in immune functions. For the patients who are in the cancer procession, or with the metastasis of lymph nodes and the need of chemotherapies, cell poison of chemotherapies will inhibit the marrow severely with the decrease in WBC and the increase in PLT. For the special factor excreted by the tumors has inhibited the central immune organ thymus, the patients suffer the central immune organs' atrophy gradually, weakening and even losing its functions. Now as the cell poison attacks the marrow, patients' central immune organs are totally destroyed. For the circumferential immune organs are bearing the affects and metastases of tumor cells, some of their functions are weakened. Therefore, the patients' thymus, marrow, lymph nodes and other immune organs are damaged in such a way that the immune functions are already inhibited, plus that the chemotherapeutic drugs damage the immune organs, leading a further decrease in immune functions as one disaster after another. What are worse, efficient measures of protecting the host cells, immune organs and the immune functions are not taken, making patients put up with the further decrease in immune functions.

We can get such a conclusion by analyzing and reflecting from this point: chemotherapies must be added with immunotherapies, meaning that chemotherapies should combine with the XZ-C treatment by Chinese herbs for immunoregulation.

As XZ-C4 is used to increase immunity and protect thymus, while XZ-C8 is for hematopoiesis and protecting marrow, during chemotherapies XZ-C drugs must be taken, that is using XZ-C4 to protect thymus and XZ-C8 for marrow functions in order to protect the central immune organs and immune functions of the host cells. The above can help strengthen the chemotherapeutic effects and weaken the side effects of inhibiting immune functions by chemotherapies.

Since patients' immune functions are weak, the surgical operation for cancer may lead further decrease in the functions. While surgery is the principle occasion of forming the nidi of tumors with more cancer cells enter into the blood circulation, so during the peri operation, it is of great importance to improve the patients' immune functions during the complex treatment.

For the question how to control or even eliminate such cancer cells in the blood circulation, we consider that the immunotherapies must be essential in both preoperative and postoperative phases as well as during the operation. Using XZ-C treatment by Chinese herbs can improve immunity and redound to kill the cancer cells in the blood circulation making the lymphocytes immersed surrounding the cancer tissue, thus reducing the opportunities for cancer cells to metastasize.

After operations, immune functions are weakened and further decreased by the postoperative chemotherapies; therefore one of the key problems of taking chemotherapies as soon as possible after operations is to improve patients' immune functions in the prophase. We advocate that before operations or in the prophase after them it is applicable to use immunotherapies and XZ-C Chinese traditional medicine for immunoregulation which has been proved be able to protect central immune organs and strengthen the entire immune functions, to reach the mentioned goals. Making the patients' immune functions on the higher level to make up for the deficiency is benefic for the recovery, preventing the postoperative metastasis and recrudescence as well as the carcinomatosis and cancerometastasis resulting from the further decrease in immune functions.

III. Analysis, Reflection and Evaluation from the Angle of Drug Tolerance

Reviewing, reflecting and evaluating the postoperative adjuvant chemotherapy and curative effects, in many foregoing clinical cases, why does the postoperative chemotherapy fail to arrest relapse of tumor? Why is the postoperative chemotherapy incapable of preventing metastasis? Why do chemotherapeutic drugs injected into the patient have no damaging effect to solid tumor cells? We should reflect and consider whether the solid tumor processes drug tolerance.

Why does the solid tumor become resistant to drugs? One of the reasons is the drug delivery dysfunction in the tumor.

From the clinical standpoint, the drug tolerance means anti-tumor drug therapy causes apparent trauma to host normal histiocytes, but does not avail against the tumor cells. There is a positive correlation between damaging effects of anti-tumor drugs on tumor cells and the product of drug concentration and drug action time. But at the same time, those drugs often cause apparent trauma to normal histiocytes. That is, drugs kill both tumor cells and normal cells, having no selectivity of the two different cells. "Making no distinction between tumor cells and normal cells" or "destruction of good and bad alike", that is the fatal shortage of chemotherapeutic drugs. At the present time, it still has no pleased solution. Therefore the curative effects of most anti-tumor drugs are only in a limited extent which the human body can tolerate the trauma to normal cells.

In recent years, the clinical treatment level of anti-tumor drugs is also improving. Some malignant tumors (e.g. choriocarcinoma, infantile acute lymphatic leukemia and renal matricyte carcinoma, etc.) can individually apply the chemotherapy to cure. However, there are still many common malignant tumors, such as stomach cancer, liver cancer, non-small cell lung cancer and so on, still very resistant to anti-tumor drugs. Curative effects of using chemotherapeutic drugs alone are rather limited. Why do the chemotherapeutic drugs have little curative effects on solid tumor? On this question, it is necessary for us to develop a further study of mechanism of action and anti-tumor drug tolerance.

Currently, chemotherapeutic drugs have better effectiveness on tumor in blood system, but turn relatively poor effectiveness on solid tumor. Besides the reason of chemotherapeutic drugs having no or lower sensitivity to solid tumor cells, drug delivery dysfunction in the tumor is also the main reason:

1. Drug Delivery Dysfunction and Drug Tolerance

Tumor cells directly contacting with sufficient anti-tumor drugs is the prerequisite for chemotherapies to get curative effects. However, anti-tumor drugs must pass through a long way, overcome each obstacle and finally reach the tumor cells. During the drug delivery, a problem of any link is enough to generate drug tolerance.

Oral and Injection Drugs
↓←Absorption obstacle, blood vessel barrier
Absorbed into the bloodstream, near to tumor tissue
↓←Delivery dysfunction in the tumor
Delivery in the tumor (micrangium, stroma, tumor cells)
↓←Membrane transport obstacles
Drugs into the tumor
Delivery dysfunction of anti-tumor drugs in every link

Because of drugs delivery dysfunction in the tumor, the giant solid tumor cells generate drug tolerance, or the drugs cannot reach the curative effects. That is a very important question affecting the curative effects. At the meantime, it is an urgent problem that needs but has not yet been resolved. Some anti-tumor drugs show very high anti-tumor activity to various tumor cells in culture dish, and the suppression ratio of some drugs is up to 100%. With these anti-tumor drugs, Clinical treatment of malignant tumors in blood system and childhood cancer can also achieve satisfactory effects. However these drugs cannot obviously reduce adults' death rates from the most common solid tumors (e.g. stomach cancer, liver cancer, carcinoma of large intestine, lung cancer, breast cancer, prostatic cancer, pancreatic cancer, brain cancer and carcinoma of esophagus, etc.). Comparing the chemotherapeutic process between malignant tumors in blood system and solid tumor, the only difference is the former omits the step of drugs redistributing in the tumor tissues and directly contacts with individual tumor cell in the blood. Thus we can reason out that during drug delivery in the solid tumor, there are some factors which induce tumor cells to generate drug tolerance. Specifically, after anti-tumor drugs having been injected or taken by mouth, drugs deliver through blood to whole-body organs and tissues, some of which deliver to the targeted object—tumor tissues. If eliminating such a big solid tumor (abdominal surgery solid tumor, with hundreds or thousands of grams, even tens of kilograms), drugs have to be of high concentration, which is sufficient to eliminate each tumor cell of such a big solid tumor, to diffuse and distribute in the whole tumor. Then the drugs delivering through blood to tumor can contact with each tumor cell, which enable the chemotherapy to achieve curative effects. Nevertheless, the solid tumor often utilizes advantaged barrier to tackle against this diffusion process, which results in uneven and/or low concentration, even no drug distribution in the tumor. That leads to the drug tolerance of tumor.

There are mainly three mechanisms that the solid tumor applies to obstruct drugs to deliver in the tumor: ① Blood vessels of tumor have non-balanced distribution. Areas with fewer blood vessels cannot directly take drugs from the blood circulation. Thus some tumor cells fail to contact drugs directly. In other words, drugs cannot work on this part of cells; ② The pressure of tumor stroma rises abnormally, disturbing the diffuse, permeation and distribution of drugs in the tumor. ③ The structural anomaly of tumor vessels and high blood viscosity also affect the drug delivery in the tumor.

The penetrating power of some drugs to the tumor mainly depends on their structures. The malignant tumor generally consists of the following portions: ① Proliferative cells or tumor cells commonly account for less than half volume of tumor. ② Blood vessels zigzag back and forth through the tumor tissue, making up about 1% to 10% of the tumor's volume. ③ Collagens efficient matrixes fill up most space of the tumor tissue, which is much larger than extracellular matrixes in the volume of healthy tissue, and enclose the tumor cells to divide them from vascular structures. To determine the trace of drugs in the tumor, Kakesh K and the other people choose tumor cells which are singly into the artery and out of the vein to implant into the body of rodent (a), or optionally obtain this kind of tumor from patients, utilizing artificial circulation to maintain blood flow (b). The two models are used to measure the sum of drugs into and out of the tumor, and also calculate the absorptive amount. Later they adopt Sandison-Algire Tumor "Window Technique" to implant the tumor into the rabbit ear (c), mouse brain (d) or mouse skin of back, and place into the transparent apparatus. Then they use the microscope to directly observe new vascular development of the tumor tissue and the diffusion and distribution process of drugs in the tumor. The result displays that after twenty days of implanting the tumor into mouse skin of back, tumor peripheral regions have overgrown a labyrinth of vessels. But the tumor center loses the blood supply plentifully and appears white. Therefore the tumor is deprived blood vessels which deliver drugs directly to the central region.

On this account, if drugs are to approach toward each cell, they should firstly access to the blood vessels in the tumor, and then through the vessel wall enter in the stroma. Finally they have to difficultly pass through matrixes. But there are significant differences between vascular system in the tumor tissue and blood vessels in the normal tissue and organ. At the very start, tumor use existing blood vessels in this region to obtain blood. As tumors grow, eventually they produce "their own" minute vessels, which quickly branch, wind into curved shapes and gradually vary their growth directions. Consequently, some regions of the tumor present favorable blood vessels to supply rich blood, but others may be supplied with little or no blood. Such non-balanced distribution of blood vessels affects drugs distribution in the tumor. Regions which lack blood vessels cannot directly take drugs from the blood circulation. Therefore, in this region drug concentration is so low that it cannot produce the anti-tumor effect. Moreover, abnormal distorted branches of the vascular structure often slowdown the blood flow. High viscosity of blood in the tumor also slower the blood flow. Slow micro-circulating blood obstructs drugs delivery to regions where tumor vessels lack. These regions cannot (or seldom) obtain anti-tumor drugs. Thus, it's hard to produce anti-tumor effect.

The above non-balanced blood supply is the main reason for obstructing drugs diffusing in the tumor. And abnormal rise of interstitial pressure is also an important reason. The increasing pressures disturb drugs to flow among vessel wall, stroma and inside stroma, leading to the reduced concentration of drugs in the stroma.

The internal pressure distribution of tumor tissue is different from that of healthy tissue. The pressure of capillary network of healthy tissue is higher than that of stroma. The latter is about zero. However average internal pressures of the whole tumor stromata are almost equivalent to those of capillary network. The reason may be that the tumor grows in normal tissue, uses existing blood vessels and depends on the present lymphatic system to discharge excess liquid from stromata. As the tumor grows, its new blood vessels cannot produce their own lymphatic system. Moreover for inordinate hyperplasia of the tumor, its press causes abnormal vessels to vary in geometrical shape, reducing the blood flow rate and further increasing pressure in the capillary. Thus large amounts of liquid soak into stromata from blood vessels. Due to the lack of functional lymphatic system, exosmic liquid cannot be removed effectively. The liquid is piling up until the internal pressure in stromata is equivalent to that in blood vessels. The internal pressure in the tumor is impressively high, exerting obvious influences on drugs infiltration and distribution in the tumor.

2. Membrane Transport Obstacles

Transport obstacle method of drugs entering to tumor cells is not entirely clear. It may have a close correlation with drug structures and physicochemical properties. Such drugs include methotrexate, phenylpropionic acid chlormethine, chlormethine, cisplatin, cytosine arabinoside, anthracene nucleus, vincristine, and son on. In addition, Drugs into the tumor cells need mediated transport by carriers. Therefore, affinity degree for carriers can influence transportation. In belief, drugs transport obstacle is the main reason for chemotherapeutic drugs tolerance of the tumor. To make the application effect of chemotherapeutic drugs in vivo equal to that of experiment in vitro, we have to surmount these obstacles.

3. Immunity and Drug Tolerance

The immune state before tumor patient accepts any treatment is of influence to drugs curative effects. Generally, the more complete the body's immunologic function, the better the patient's response to medication. Among patients who accept cytotoxic drugs therapies, the complete immunologic function before therapy is relevant to the better prognosis.

The animal experiments prove that elspar can kill most tumor cells in animals' bodies with suppressed immunologic function. But drug-resistant tumor cells survive, proliferate and finally kill the animals. In animals' bodies with better immunologic function, drug-resistant or surviving tumor cells will be destroyed by the immunologic system. When the host suffers from sensitization, the mouse fleshy tumor induced by chemicals can strengthen the anti-tumor action of cyclophosphane, but doesn't work for the host without sensitization. For patients suffering from acute granulocytic leukemia, chemotherapies combined with immunotherapies show better effects than those of single chemotherapies. Meanwhile, it's reported when the patient accepts non-small cell lung cancer chemotherapies, effects of chemotherapies combined with thymic peptides are better than those of single chemotherapies.

When some experienced doctors adopt medications to treat cancer patients, they also examine patients' immunologic function in detail. Facts prove that it has some values for designing chemotherapies. We have found that choriocarcinoma's "antagonizing against" chemotherapies is related to the gradual decline in immunologic function. If the immunologic function can restore, reusing the drugs which have been subject to the obvious antagonism is still in effect.

4. Metabolism and Drug Tolerance

Anti-metabolic drugs are a kind of drugs interfering with cell metabolism. Their chemical structures are often similar to required substances of nucleic acid metabolism, such as folic acid, purine and pyrimidine, etc. These drugs can utilize specific antagonism to interfere with nucleic acid metabolism, especially DNA synthesis. They also prevent cell division and reproduction, and then produce the anti-tumor effect.

All the clinical common anti-metabolic drugs except MTX, need to be converted to active structures by metabolizing, then they can really possess the anti-tumor effect. If the coloboma of activating enzyme leads to insufficient activation of anti-metabolic drugs, the drugs lose the ability of anti-tumor and anti-metabolism.

5. Dynamics of Cell Proliferation and Drug Tolerance

Tumor dynamics of cell proliferation has three fundamental concepts, i.e. ① Grouping theory of tumor cells; ② Cell cycle theory; ③ Heterogeneity theory of tumor cells.

1. Grouping theory of tumor cells It is represented based on the motion law of cell growth, proliferation and death, i.e. all the tumor cells are made up of three colonies, proliferative cell colony, resting cell colony and cell colony with non-proliferative capacity. Tumor cells of different colonies have different responsivity to chemotherapeutic drugs. ① Proliferative cell colony refers to continuous exponential proliferation of tumor cells. The tumor body grows quickly. Its chemotherapeutic drug susceptibility is also higher.

② Resting cell colony includes auxiliary cells, i.e. G_0 phase cells, which are temporarily not into cell cycle. When cells of proliferative phase are killed by drugs, resting cells can enter into proliferative phase. During this stage, internal drug tolerance of tumor cells is the recurrent root in the tumor therapy. ③ Cell colony with non-proliferative capacity has little significance in chemotherapies.

Understanding the grouping theory of tumor cells can help to design the optimal therapeutic schedule. In recent years, progresses in tumor chemotherapies are not some newfound effective chemotherapeutic drugs but are precisely the applications of dynamics of cell proliferation therapy that have designed plenty of high-level chemotherapies.

2. Cell cycle theory It is another fundamental concept of tumor dynamics of cell proliferation, which is represented based on studying individual cell growth in the proliferative cell colony. The relevant information has been stated in above paragraphs. Proliferative cycle of tumor cells can be broadly divided into four phases: DNA pre-synthesis phase (G_1), DNA synthesis phase (S phase), DNA post-synthesis phase or division phase (G_2), mitotic phase (M phase).

   According to anti-tumor drugs' selective acting on different phases of tumor cell cycle, in terms of the cell cycle theory, anti-tumor drugs can be divided into phase-specific and phase nonspecific chemotherapeutic drugs.

   Cell cycle nonspecific chemotherapeutic drugs can only kill off cells in certain sensitive phase of cell cycle (usually as S phase). This is because that during the administration, some cells do not pass through the sensitive phase, so cells are insensitive to drugs. As to cell cycle phase nonspecific chemotherapeutic drugs, they can kill off cells in all phases of cell cycle, especially the rapid proliferative cells. For the rapid proliferative tumor, it has high growth ratio, short interphase and is sensitive to chemotherapies. For the slow-growing tumor, its growth ratio is low and interphase is long, which inevitably engender unbearable toxic side effect. By this time, the tumor often becomes resistant to chemotherapeutic drugs.

   Facts have proved that for nidi of tumor cells below 10^6, their cells are totally in division cycle. While for nidi of tumor cells above 10^6, a certain proportion of tumor cells are often outside the division cycle. The "optimal" therapeutic schedule can either not treat the tumor. For there reasons, it can be concluded generally that S phase-specific chemotherapeutic drugs can effectively fight against the leukemia, and cell cycle nonspecific chemotherapeutic drugs are available to battle the solid tumor. Clinical trials have confirmed the above conclusion. Compared with leukemia and lymphoma, the solid tumor's resistance to chemotherapies is because its multiplication and division time is long, proliferative quantity is small and label index is low.

3. Heterogeneity theory of tumor cells It is another fundamental concept of tumor dynamics of cell proliferation proposed in recent years. It means that a primary tumor is composed of different cell subsets, which have varying drug susceptibility. Especially the different cell subsets between primary and infiltrative nidus (or metastatic nidus) remain far more diverse in the drug susceptibility. In the same host tumor, some cell subsets may be sensitive to a drug; while others possess internal drug tolerance. This theory has some values for clinical applications. At present, combined chemotherapeutic drug types have an increasing trend. It might be closely related to that theory.

Drug tolerance is a clinical question of vital importance. If one patient is resistant to this chemotherapeutic drug, but the clinician has no idea whether this patient has drug tolerance, then this clinician relies on the experimentalism and continuously adopts this drug to complete each course by intravenous administration or infusion through catheter and drug pump. Afterwards, the patient suffers from serious damage. Because of the drug tolerance, the chemotherapeutic drugs have no effect on the patient's cancer cells, but cause extremely serious damage to immunologic system, marrow hematopoietic system and toxic side effects of liver and kidney. The drugs even result in immunologic and marrow hematopoietic function failures, which lead to infection, bleeding, organ failure and finally cause death. So the clinician must seriously and prudently treat the multidrug resistance (MDR) question, and place great emphasis on patient's safety.

The fundamental goal of drug tolerance studies is to find the method or drug for overcoming the drug tolerance. So far it has made certain progress, and some drugs and methods have been developed in the clinic. But more methods are still in the preclinical study, even the contemplation stage.

China has the traditional Chinese medicine and herbalism. And the effective component in herbs, i.e. TTMP has been confirmed to reverse the adriamycin tolerance of mouse Ehrlich's ascites carcinoma. We have observed from the laboratory experiment: TTMP has certain anti-metastasis effects to the mouse's liver cancer cells metastases. Our developed medicine $XZ-C_4$ also contains a small quantity of TTMP. We believe that Traditional Chinese Medicine could find the highly original method to reverse the drug tolerance of clinical tumor.

CHAPTER 19

Chemotherapy To Be Further Studied And Improved

I. Some Wrong Ways in Current Chemotherapy

1. Current chemotherapy emphasizes on only killing cancer cells and neglects to protect or even damage host cells

It is essential to attach importance to the interrelation and the interaction among host cells, tumors and drugs. Here chemotherapy is cytotoxic drug without selectivity, so it can not distinguish tumor cells and the normal with killing them together. The initial target of chemotherapy is to kill cancer cells; however, actually it also kills the proliferative cells of host cells that are damaged as a result. Especially, chemotherapy inhibits the immune system and medullary hemopoietic system of the host cells, which leads to the general decline in immune function. Consequently, that tumors are not monitored by immunity promotes the evolution of tumors. That is the reason why tumors are constringed or relieved temporary, but continue to increase and evolve after a while or even metastasize and relapse during the period of treatment. Therefore, there is one problem about chemotherapy that has not been paid much attention, namely taking no actions to protect host cells and their immune organs and immune function. The strategy of curing cancer is to destroy cancer cells protect autologous functions at the most.

2. Chemotherapy as cytotoxic drug can aggravate the inhibition on central immune organic

It is well known that consist of central immune organs and peripheral immune organs, the former ones are thymus and marrow, the later are spleen and lymph node.

When patients are in chemotherapy, their three immune organs suffer damage (see Fig. 19-1), which leads to the decrease in immune function. Literature and the experimental results by the author have proved that when cancer emerges, tumors can produce a kind of immunorepressive factor (called factor of inhibiting thymus by cancer temporarily) and make thymus atrophied gradually. At the same time, chemotherapy also inhibits marrow. For the patients with cancer, the inhibition of both thymus and marrow by the chemotherapeutic cytotoxic drug make the function of the entire central immune organs inhibited, which reduces the holistic immune function as one disaster after disaster.

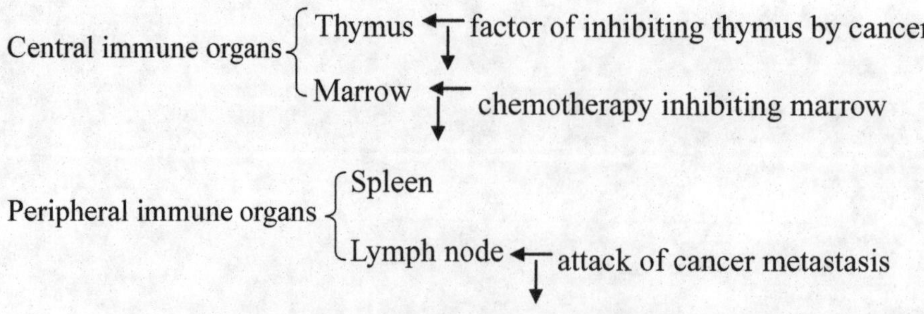

Fig. 19-1 the damage of immune organs during chemotherapy

Lymph nodes in peripheral immune organs as well as the areas around the focus, and lymph nodes in the process of metastasis are invaded by cancer metastasis and lost partial function, which lead to further decrease in immune function consequently. It is inevitable that tumors will evolve further, relapse and metastasize with weak immune monitor or even without it.

Due to the decline in the holistic immune function, the anti-infection ability is weakened, so chemotherapy can not continue. There may be serious complications during the process of chemotherapy, such as mycotic superinfection, viral and infectious infection. However, the antibiotics can not control them efficiently. As a result, the patients die of immune function prostration.

3. During chemotherapy general untoward reaction may occur due to the effect of cytotoxic

During chemotherapy, general untoward reaction can bring down immune function, and lead to arrest of bone marrow, hepatic and nephric toxic reaction, gastrointestinal response dysfunction, phalacrosis, etc. However, there is no positive and effective protection currently.

Inhibition of marrow is a usual clinic toxic reaction as marrow is the organ to store hematopoietic stem cells. It is mainly the dynamic effect of antineoplastics to the specific stem cells that chemotherapeutic drugs destroy the specific stem cells in marrow, which can reduce the number of mature and functional blood corpuscles in peripheral blood. The degree of reduction is related to the lifetime of cell components in peripheral blood, for instance, the lifetime of hematid is long, so the number of hematid in the peripheral does not change apparently; while the lifetimes of blood platelet and granular cell groups are shorter with 3 days and 67 hours respectively, so the numbers of peripheral blood platelet and granular cell groups reduce rapidly if the groups of megakaryocytic stem cells and granular cell groups are destroyed. After administering drugs, stem cells increase the time of division to make up for the amount in the process of restoration.

Most antineoplastics can result in the gastrointestinal mucosa reaction by inhibiting gastrointestinal mucosa epithelial cells.

Many kinds of antineoplastics can lead to renal toxic reaction and also affect the excretion of drugs through the kidney. It must be noticed that the damage of renal function can aggravate the general toxic symptoms or worsen the inhibition of marrow. Many kinds of antineoplastics can damage liver in different degree and affect liver function.

Such serious geneal toxic reaction of chemotherapy can lead to nausea, vomit as well as anorexia, even being unable to take food. Consequently, the general anticancer ability declines obviously and the function of anticancer system of host cells is weakened apparently. The anticancer ability of organism and evolution of cancer are locked in a “zero-sum” game, which conduce to the further development of tumors.

4. Theoretic foundation of choosing chemotherapeutic drugs

Choosing chemotherapeutic is based on cell generation cycle and pathology and physiology of cancer, or accords to the principle of pharmacokinetics. The current chemotherapeutic scheme does not always accord with the theory of cell generation cycle. During the period of treatment (3~5d), cytotoxic drugs will inhibit cancer cells. After the treatment, these cancer cells continue to proliferate and divide. Currently, the use of chemotherapeutic drugs differs in different medical institution, in which some use the treatment of 5 days, others are 3 days;

some of the used drugs aim at S stage and some are for M_1 stage. No matter the treatment is 3 to 5 days or 5 days, the effective period of cytotoxic drugs on cancer cells is less than 120 hours with cell generation cycle of 50 to 80 hours, so the treatment can only act on one and a half cell generation cycles. However, the proliferating cycle of cell mass continue for years, while the effect of chemotherapeutic drugs can only last from 3 to 5 days, so the effect of killing cancer cells can just happen at the stage of proliferating cycle when the drugs take effect, such as S stage, and then disappear. After the treatment of 3 or 5 days, cancer cells continue to proliferate and divide. As a result, tumors and the metastasized lymph nodes may shrink in volume, but they are likely to augment soon.

5. Failure to take actions to control cancer cells continuously and consolidate the effect at the interval of two times of chemotherapies

The treatment between two times of chemotherapies is blank, and the actions to continuous killing or control on cancer cells are not taken to consolidate the curative effect. What have been done is waiting the restoration of leucocytes and blood platelets to achieve the aim of stand chemotherapy next time. Actually, the treatment at the interval is very important, for cancer cells are out of control and proliferate and divide further positively and potentially at intervals due to the heavy decline in immune function. The more times of chemotherapies and the larger dosage of drugs, the more cytotoxic drugs will be used correspondently, so that the general immune function is worse and worse and the immunity of organism is less and less able to control the proliferation of oncocytes and prevent the metastasis leading to relapse and metastasize after continuous chemotherapies. Therefore, it is necessary to adopt immunological therapy or Chinese traditional medicine for regulating immunity to avoid relapse.

6. Theoretical foundation of postoperative auxiliary chemotherapy, the length of the intervals between two times of chemotherapies and the time of chemotherapy

The arrangements of chemotherapy differ in different locations and medical institutions, among which some use once a month or once every two months, some adopt six times in a row, or continuous four or eight times. The treatment is much blinder, especially postoperative auxiliary chemotherapy. The current arrangement of chemotherapeutic period is that only when leucocyte and blood platelet restore, can the next chemotherapy be taken. In fact, it is more helpless instead of meeting the pathological and physical demands (since the time of restoration is longer for some patients, when cancer cells have been in the process of division and proliferation continuously). What is the aim of auxiliary chemotherapy? How to achieve the aim? Are there any residual cancer cells in the body although the aim of chemotherapy is to kill cancer cells? Where do the cancer cells hide after surgeons, in the local of the surgeon, lymph nodes or in the blood? Taking gastrointestinal surgeon for instance, do the residual cancer cells hide in portal vein blood, or in celiac lymph nodes, or even in the local area of the surgeon? How long can the residual cancer cells lurk after surgeons before devastated by host cells? How to arrange the period of postoperative auxiliary chemotherapy? Knowing the location of cancer cells may be good for controlling the residual cancer cells in the area of surgeons and portal vein.

In a word, the current choice of postoperative auxiliary chemotherapy and the arrangement of chemotherapeutic period are very blind. It is essential to do further clinic research to ensure the indication, contraindication, medication and route of administration as well as a more uniform scheme so as to conclude analysis and evaluate.

7. Blindness of current chemotherapy

It may be helpful for some patients to take on chemotherapy blindly just according to experience, but it is harmful for a considerable number of patients. For instance, if some patient was resistant to this kind of drug, it would be harmful, rather than fruitless, for the cytotoxic drugs of chemotherapy can not act on cancer cells, instead of killing normal histiocyte, especially immunocyte, myeloid cell, which will lead to the prostration of immune function.

Drugsensitive test is a must to verify whether the patient is allergic to the used drugs. Only doing like this can ensure the accuracy of administering drugs. Currently, it is common that clinical administrate of drugs depends on experience blindly. Such blind administrate is potentially dangerous. If the drug is really sensitive to the patient's cancer cells, it will be effective (CR, PR). But if the drug is not sensitive to the cancer cells, it will only kill the normal cells and inhibit the marrow hematopiesis leading to the reduction in leucocyte and blood platelet as well as the decline in immune function without any damage on cancer cells, which will definitely promote the evolution of tumors and result in the prostration of immune function and hematopiesis. The decrease in immune function makes tumors be beyond the immune monitor and develop further, and then promote the relapse and metastasis. Therefore, it is necessary to take on individual drugsensitive test and drug resistant test.

8. Cure of cancer aims to kill tumors, reserve organism and regain health

The cure of cancer should always run through both strengthening health and wiping evil off, in which wiping evil off means inhibiting and killing cancer cells, clearing up lumps; strengthening health means protecting organismal ability to recognize dissidents, exciting the organismal positive factors of anti-cancer and improve the organismal ability to resist cancer. These two are dialectic and united. However, the current treatment on cancer only emphasizes killing cancer cells and ignores the protection of host cells, which damages the immune system and the system of marrow hematopiesis resulting in wiping both evil and health away. If tumors are drug resistant to this chemotherapeutic drug, it is likely to be harmful to health without wiping evil away. The treatment on cancer needs a scientific designed scheme, for cancer results from losing the balance between the organismal immune capacity of anti-cancer and the development of tumors, and from losing immune monitor, which leads to the further development of tumors. So it is necessary to try to restore the balance. Taking teeterboard in a children's playground for instance, tumor and the immunity of host cells represent the two ends of a teeterboard respectively. The comparison of the two parties' power decides the direction of tilt and the final result. Besides, the example of "scale" can be explained in the same way. However, chemotherapy does not emphasize the protection of host cells but promotes the diffuse and evolution of tumors.

9. Standards for the curative effects of chemotherapy should be good quality of life and prolonged lifetime

How to evaluate the curative effect of postoperative auxiliary chemotherapy? As the tumor has been ablated, it is unable to evaluate the effect in terms of its shrink.

Most patients only regard untoward reactions after chemotherapy, like decline in leucocyte and blood platelet, nausea and disgorge, anorexia, hypodynamia and abdominal distention as the curative effects, but they hardly realize that these symptoms are not the effects at all. It is unable to evaluate the postoperative curative effects until now. The current diagnostic methods are still laggard, as when tumors are detected, they have been very serious. Therefore, molecular biology is the only way to solve this problem.

Generally speaking, the standard for curative effects is remission. In terms of remission, the efficiency is defined as the shrink of the tumor, however, the quality of life is not improved and the lifetime is not prolonged, which is not the aim of handling diseases for the patients with cancer.

10. Anti-Carcinomatous drugs used currently can not always resist metastasis and relapse and the drugs for anti-carcinomatous metastasis and anti-cancer should be different

For many cases, postoperative auxiliary can not prevent relapse and metastasis, which relates to the fact that the current anti-carcinomatous drugs are not always able to resist metastasis and relapse besides other various possible factors mentioned above. Drugs for anti-metastasis should be different from anti-carcinomatous drugs as generally anti-cancer drugs have cytotoxicity and aim at killing cancer cells, destroying and inhibiting cell division and proliferation, whereas drugs for resisting metastasis are mainly used to resist the invasion of tumor cells, to antagonize the adherence of cancer cells inside the blood vessels, to inhibit the nascent micrangium and strengthen the organismal immunity to kill cancer cells. Most of anti-carcinomatous metastasis drugs have no cytotoxicity.

Research on anti-cancer drugs has stepped into a new stage. It is confronted with theoretical and technical renovations and the change in the train of thoughts when the field of research on anti-cancer drugs is not restricted to the traditional thoughts based on cytotoxic and the working method of cytotoxic drugs. New methods like inducement of differentiate, regulator of biological reaction, immunoregulation, genetherapy, combination of Chinese and western medicine, etc. have been taken into consideration in succession.

Although chemotherapy has been applied for sixty years, it is not satisfactory that many problems still exist reflected by the statistic, analysis and evaluation of applied information from a large number of clinical suffers. It is pitiful that cancer may metastasize and relapse after or during the process of chemotherapy.

In conclusion, the possible reasons that postoperative auxiliary chemotherapy is unable to prevent relapse and metastasis are, ①chemotherapeutant can promote the decline in immune function and inhibit hematopoiesis of marrow; ②failure to continue aftertreatment at the intervals of chemotherapies; ③chemotherapeutic drugs can not protect host cells; ④lumps may has drug resistance; ⑤chemotherapeutic drugs may be not sensitive; ⑥chemotherapeutic drugs for solid tumor may be not infiltrate into tumors; ⑦the arrangement of chemotherapeutic period is not reasonable; ⑧drugs may not act on the sensitive period of cell proliferation; ⑨it is difficult to restore immune function and hematopoiesis probably.

II. Main Contradictions in Traditional Chemotherapy

So far, the aim of chemotherapy has been still focusing on killing cancer cells. The majority of chemotherapeutic drugs are cytotoxic drugs without selectivity, so both cancer cells and normal ones will be damaged. Besides, chemotherapy has serious untoward reaction, suffers will have intensive feeling and have to give up the treatment at last. In the last ten years, the author has helped nearly ten thousand cancer cases in Wuchang Shuguang Tumorous Clinic, many of whom have tried chemotherapy. They came to anti-carcinomatous clinic for treatment as there were no curative effects after several periods of treatment. It can be implicated that auxiliary treatment does not prevent carcinomatous invasion, relapse and metastasis, and it also can not improve the quality of life and prolong lifetime obviously. Through the feedback of those cases, analysis, evaluation and reflection, the author have recognized that there are the following contradictions in traditional chemotherapy.

1. The contradiction between chemotherapeutic cytotoxic and the damage to host cells

The aim of curing tumor is to eliminate tumors and preserve the organism as well as regain health. However, currently the chemotherapeutic cytotoxic kills both cancer cells and the normal with internecine result of damaging host cells, which is the heavily unreasonable contradiction between cytotoxic and suffers (or host cells). What should be done is to try to eliminate or resist the effect of killing normal cells and to research positively on intelligent anti-carcinomatous drugs with selectivity.

2. The contradiction between succession and discontinuity

It means the contradiction between the continuous divisions of cancer cells and the discontinuous chemotherapeutic period of treatment. The division and proliferation of cancer cells are continuous according to cell cycle, but chemotherapeutic drugs can be used with intervals for they inhibit the hematopoiesis of marrow and the blood corpuscle in the peripheral, which results in the severe contradiction between continuous divisions and proliferation of cancer cells and the discontinuous chemotherapies. Cancer cells divide successively, whereas chemotherapies are of interval, so cancer cells continue to divide during the intervals. Even a large dosage of chemotherapeutic drugs can only kill limited number of cancer cells, but can not destroy the whole. Even the majority of the cancer cells can be killed during the 3 to 5 days with chemotherapeutic drugs, the residual tumorous stem cells will continue to divide, to proliferate, to clone, and then metastasize and relapse when the effects of medicine fade away after several days. Therefore, killing cancer cells simply does not accord with the biological traits and behavior of cancer cells.

3. The contradiction between increase and decrease in immunity

That chemotherapeutic drugs usually can reduce the immunity contradicts the fact that the treatment on cancer should improve the immunity. As chemotherapeutic drugs can weaken the immunity, the longer the period of treatment, the more decrease in immunity, which promotes the decline in immunity, and even leads to lose monitor and the further development of tumors. This unreasonable contradiction between chemotherapy and immunity can weaken the curative effects heavily and even lead to diffuse. Therefore, treatment on tumors must aim at improving immunity and restoring immune monitor so as to stabilize the cancer, to make it and regain health.

4. The contradiction between periods of treatment and curative effects

That chemotherapy can inhibit marrow forces the peripheral leucocytes and blood platelets decline, so it is necessary to design the time of administering with intervals, which means the next time of chemotherapy should be taken on after restoration. Currently the intervals are just for waiting, instead of taking any measure to control cell division. On one hand cancer cells proliferate successively, on the other hand the chemotherapy stops. Due to this contradiction, it is difficult to gain the curative effects though chemotherapy. The more times of chemotherapy, the more serious immune inhibition will be, the more actively cancer cells proliferate during intervals, which results in evolution and metastasis during the process of chemotherapy.

5. The contradiction between the period when drugs act and the cell cycle during the period of administer through intravenous drip

It is only effective when the time of administer meets the sensitive cycle of cancer cells. If not, it is of no effect. Chemotherapeutic administer aims at cell cycles. During the period of administer, the cell cycles of most cancer cells in the crowds are not simultaneous but much different from each other, for instance, administer via intravenous drip from 8 am to 10 am when some of the cancer cells are in S stage, others are in G_1 or M stage. Thus, if the drug aims at S stage, it is effective to the cancer cells in S stage, but the drug given at this period (8 am to 10 am) is of no effect to the cancer cells in other stages, that is to say the sensitivity of chemotherapeutic drugs to cancer cells in different stages are differential. So during the period of administer through intravenous drip, it is effective to some sensitive cancer cells but not to those in insensitive periods.

6. The contradiction between inhibition and protection of marrow

Chemotherapy is cytotoxic and can inhibit the hematopiesis of marrow where hematopoietic stem cells are stored. Inhibition of marrow is a common clinical toxic reaction, which is the kinetic effect of chemotherapeutic drugs on specific stem cells. Chemotherapeutic cytotoxic drugs can damage the specific crowd of stem cells in marrow and will definitely reduce the number of mature and functional blood corpuscles in the peripheral blood. The degree of reduction relates to the lifetime of the cell components in the peripheral blood, for instance, the lifetime of hematid is longer, so the degree of reduction in the amount of blood corpuscles in the peripheral blood and the number of blood corpuscles in the peripheral blood during the treatment do not change obviously. However, the lifetimes of blood platelet and granular leucocytes are shorter with 3 days and 67 hours respectively, so the numbers of peripheral blood platelet and granular leucocytes reduce rapidly if the groups of megakaryocytic stem cells and granular cell groups are destroyed. If the amount of leucocytes and blood platelets decline to a very low level, it is extremely easy to cause subsequent serious infection or haemorrhage. In some cases, using large amount of broadspectrum antibiotic to resist the serious infection may lead to double infection or mycotic ingection, even endangers the life.

To sum up, in order to solve the contradictions in the current chemotherapy, to ameliorate its disadvantages and make it better, the author thinks that it is necessary to update thoughts and to research on new drugs and new principles to resist cancer and metastasis as well as relapse, except improving chemotherapy further in traditional thoughts, only the changes in the opinions on curing cancer and the creativities and reforms of technologies can bring further development into the treatment of cancer.

CHAPTER 20

Review And Prospect Of Surgical Treatment Of Tumor

Surgical operation is a definite and effective cure for malignant tumor therapy. Even though today's cancer treatment has developed to the multi-discipline and multimodality treatment, surgical operation is still one of the most central and common means for malignant tumor therapy, and makes itself an integral part of multi-discipline and multimodality treatment.

In the 18th century, therapists held that the early cancer was a local disease, which could be cured by surgical treatment. In 1881, Bill-roth first carried out the surgical removal of tumor—subtotal gastrectomy. In 1890, Halsted actualized the radical resection of breast. He first elucidated the principle of en bloc resection, which meant resections of lymphatic vessel and lymph node in the chosen zone of primary tumor. This resection laid a good foundation for most modern surgical operations of tumors. The surgical technique of tumor resection has been developing along with surgery. After the middle of the 20th century, it gradually developed into an independent subject—tumor surgery. Since the 1950s, due to the improvement and development of surgical technique, preoperative (postoperative) care and operative supporting measures, such as blood transfusion, anesthesia, aseptic technique and antibiotics, the surgical risk, complications and fatality rate have reduced greatly; the range of tumor surgical technique tends to expand; a series of super radical operations arise, such as expansive radical mastectomy. But many years' practice proves that expanding the range of surgical resection cannot improve the survival time without tumor and total survival time of most tumors, such as lung cancer, liver cancer and pancreatic cancer.

Since the 1970s, people's understanding of tumor biology has changed a lot. At present, people hold that most tumors are not local diseases and may have been systemic diseases since the clinical examination. The hematogenous spread is common. When finally diagnosed, many patients may have suffered from micro-metastases. Whether obvious metastases have happened since the clinical examination, depends upon biological characteristics of tumor cells and interactions between tumors and hosts. Neither the more extensive regional surgery nor the share of surgery and radiotherapy can affect metastases.

1. Great Achievements in Surgical Removal of Tumor in 20th Century

In the 20th century, great achievements mainly focus on researching various methods of tumor surgical resections, operation procedures, preoperative (postoperative) care and cleaning range of lymph nodes; studying, understanding and getting familiar with regional anatomy and pathophysiology of bearing cancer organs, such as resection technique and organ reconstruction technique of liver cancer, pancreatic cancer, stomach cancer, esophageal cancer, colorectal cancer, lung cancer, breast cancer, cervical cancer, brain cancer and so on; taking measures to raise resection rate, reduce complications, lower operative mortality rate and improve perioperative care. In terms of esophageal cancer surgery, how to raise the resection rate? How to reduce anastomotic leakage? How to improve Esophagogastrostomy upon (down) Aortic Arch? How to carry out the cervical anastomosis? How to improve anastomose technique, such as scarf-type anastomosis? And in the case of liver cancer, how to perform regular or irregular hepatectomy? How to conduct (expanding) lobectomy of liver? How to carry out combined segmentum hepatis resection, second resection of intrahepatic recurrent cancer after resection, and liver cancer resection of special regions? How to retain residual liver functions? For the breast cancer, how to perform radical or super radical operation? Then how to conduct conservative operation procedures? In the case of stomach cancer, how to carry out D2 and D3 operations? How many groups of lymph nodes are needed to clear? For the operation procedure of rectal cancer, select Mile or Dixon procedure? Retain anus or not? Use anastomat or not? In terms of pancreatic cancer, select Whipple or Child procedure? How to conduct anastomose procedure of gall bladder and bowel? How to perform the resection of hepatic hilar cholangiocarcinoma? For the lung cancer, how to carry out the resection of pulmonary segments, lung lobes or the whole lung? In conclusion, researches are about how to resect the tumor en bloc and completely? How to increase operative resection rate? How to reduce or avoid complications? How to lower operative mortality rate? And how to help patients recover? By the 1990s, cancer resections of esophagus, stomach, bowel, liver, gall bladder, pancreas, lung, mammary gland and thyroid gland fully pass the test. All the operative routine techniques are already mature. Operative mortality rates have dropped to a very low level. Operations are basically safe. Many cancer radical operations have been widely diffused among county hospitals and basic hospitals. But how to prevent recurrence and metastasis has not yet generally attracted people's attention.

In some large hospitals, doctors have perceived that though operations are performed very thoroughly and canonically, postoperative recurrence and metastasis in the short (long) term still puzzle some specialists. Then in the 1990s, some experts have followed suit, announcing the study that disposes cast-off cells caused by operative wound. Chen Junqing in Shenyang has spent over ten years on researching and processing cast-off cells of stomach cancer, finally making brilliant achievements. The study conducted by South Hospital, which heats, washes and processes cast-off cells after the operation of rectum cancer, has got satisfactory efficacy. Yang Chuanyong at Tongji Hospital has always been devoting himself to exploring the pharmacokinetics of intraperitoneal chemotherapy of hepatic portal venous blood. At present, the technique of surgical excision of the tumor is basically successful, which is an honorable achievement in the 20th century. But these difficulties that cancer patients suffer from postoperative recurrences and metastases with no good countermeasure, and frequently come back to the clinic for further consultation, still bother vast numbers of medical workers.

2. The Objectives of Surgery in 21st Century Should Be the Study on Prevention and Control of Recurrence and Metastasis after Radical Operation of Carcinoma

In 1985, the writer himself made follow-up to more than 3,000 patients who had accepted surgical radical excisions of tumors. The results show that 2~3 years after the operation, most patients suffer from recurrences or metastases. While some patients even bear it after six months, less than a year or just over one year. These patients do not always come back to the previous surgery physician for further consultation but go to Tumor Hospital or Tumor Department for medical treatment. Once recurrences appear, however, only a few patients can accept the second operation. But most patients cannot receive effective therapies and soon pass away. It has made the writer more aware that though the operation at that time was successful and standard, the long-term follow-up result is dissatisfactory. That is, the late result is a failure (Certainly tens of patients can survive for 10, 20 or 30 years after the operation, but it is only a very few cases.). Therefore, the study must be done to prevent postoperative recurrence and metastasis. Follow-up results present an important problem that postoperative recurrence or metastasis is the key factor for long-term postoperative effectiveness. While researching method and measure of preventing postoperative recurrence or metastasis plays the key role in improving long-term effectiveness and lengthening survival time. Therefore, the clinical fundamental research must be done for preventing cancer recurrence and metastasis. If no breakthrough in the field of fundamental research, it will be hard to improve clinical effectiveness. Then the writer as well as his colleagues has established the Institute of Experimental Surgery, where they have carried out experimental tumor research, implemented transplantation of cancer cells to animals, constructed tumor animals' models. They have also developed a series of experimental tumor researches: ① Explore mechanism and rule of cancer recurrence and metastasis; ② Probe into the relationship between tumor and immunity, and that between tumor and immune organ; ③ Research into the method of arresting progressive atrophy of immune organs with the growth of tumor and the way of immunologic reconstitution; ④ Seek effective measures to adjust and control cancer invasion, recurrence and metastasis; ⑤ Conduct inhibition rates experiments of tumor-bearing animals to respectively filter 200 literature-approved traditional Chinese medicines which are commonly used for anti-cancer; ⑥ Carry out experimental researches to seek new drugs from natural drugs with resistances to cancer, recurrence and metastasis.

The writer has gone through a complete review of almost 54-year practical cases of clinical treatment and also made the follow-up. Then he analyzes and rethinks the lessons of success and failure, from which he comes to understand a truth. That is, conquering cancer needs to break with the conventional ideas and update the thought; conduct investigations, researches and analyses with patients; carry out self-reflection and self-evaluation. Renew ideas, innovate methods, look for an opening in urgent problems of tumor researches and weak links of modern medicine. The writer has also realized that techniques of surgical resections of tumors in the 20th century have made brilliant achievements. The next researching objective and task of surgeons are not only to have further studies on seeking for greater perfection of radical operation, but also to prevent postoperative recurrence and metastasis. Experiments and clinical researches on preventing recurrence and metastasis after cancer radical operation should be done to further improve postoperative long-term effectiveness. Because the operation is just a regional treatment, if the tumor is limited in a certain visceral organ, the surgical effect may be very good; but if the tumor is not just limited in this visceral organ but has invaded the serosa outside the organ, no matter how thorough the operation is, the possibility of recurrence and metastasis is still in existence. Especially for stomach cancer and rectum cancer, though lymph nodes are cleared completely, many cancer cells still remain in venous blood vessels. A lot of research materials have identified that clearance of lymph nodes is only to prevent lymphatic metastasis but that is just one side. The involved lymph nodes should be cleared, but excising lymph nodes cannot prevent hematogenous metastasis. Therefore, hepatic metastases rates in the short/long term are both high after operations of stomach cancer and intestinal cancer. At present, surgical excision of the tumor as well as regional lymphatic vessels and lymph nodes cannot prevent hematogenous metastasis and spread, implantation and dissemination of cast-off cells. Consequently, the next objective of tumor surgeons' research work should focus on experiments and clinical researches for preventing cancer recurrence and metastasis after radical operation.

That is, in the early 20th century, researchers should make great achievements on studies of preventing cancer recurrence and metastasis. If postoperative recurrence and metastasis cannot be solved, short/long-term effectiveness of surgical cancer treatment will fail to get satisfactory result.

3. Design of Surgical Radical Operation of Tumor to be Further Studied and Perfected

Since recurrence and metastasis happens after the radical operation, it is necessary to analyze whether the radical operation itself has connection with postoperative recurrence and metastasis, and carry out retrospective analysis and reflection. Among the present radical operations, some have been used for over 100 years, such as the radical operation of breast cancer. Over a century, thousands of cancer patients have accepted different kinds of radical operations, the majority of which have got satisfied short-term effectiveness. But long-term recurrence and metastasis rates are still very high. As the name implies, "radical cure" means thorough or eradicating treatment; but if it is "radical operation", why the purpose of radical cure fails to achieve and the recurrence still happens? Now that lymph nodes have been cleared, why the metastasis still appears? The question is whether those recurrences and metastases are due to cast-off cells left by operation or operative techniques, related to procedure design, concept foundation of operative design or not entirely consistent with the present known Biological characteristics and biological behaviors of cancer cells. The present radical operation refers to the en bloc resection of primary tumor and regional lymph nodes. Logically, it is not the radical cure, and cannot approach the purpose of radical cure. That is because the malignant tumor has four routes of metastasis, which are lymphatic channel metastasis, hematogenous metastasis, implantation metastasis and direct spreading. While the surgical operation just completely clears lymph nodes and radically cures the route of lymphatic channel metastasis, it has no specific technical measure to prevent hematogenous metastasis, and also do nothing to bring forward definite and effective countermeasures to implantation of cast-off cancer cells as well as implantation and dissemination of chest and peritoneal cavity. Lymph nodes having been thoroughly cleared off cannot prevent hematogenous metastasis, and moreover, only the clearance of lymph nodes can't prevent peritoneal implantation and dissemination of peritoneal cavity by cast-off cancer cells, either. Surgical operation belongs to a regional treatment. Experts in tumor surgery hold that cancer develops in a local area of the body, invades the surrounding tissues and metastasizes to other areas through lymphatic vessels, etc. Accordingly, the main point of treatment is often put on the local area, controlling local growth and diffusion, especially lymph nodes metastasis, such as the clearance of lymph nodes. For years surgical treatment has been updating on the operation method and type, but its long-term effectiveness—5-year survival rate still has no obvious improvement. The postoperative recurrence and metastasis seriously threaten patients' postoperative survival. Therefore, the present radical operation is just a relative one, which is on a quote. Young doctors should know that the present type design still has weak links, which need the further experimental and clinical studies to explore new techniques and methods to definitely and effectively prevent routes of metastases. Accordingly, in recent years the writer's laboratory has always been doing experimental exploration in this respect, such as experimental study of free-tumor technique in radical operation (Fig. 20-1), free-tumor technique study in radical operation of cancer-bearing animal models, counting of intraoperative cast-off cancer cells as well as detection and counting of cancer cells in venous angioma, experimental observation of dyeing tracking of gastric lymph nodes. Preventing postoperative cancer metastasis and recurrence must be started from the radical operation.

In order to study why cancer cells can dissociate and cast off from the tumor body, cast-off cancer cells still have the vitality and can implant to other areas, the writer's laboratory use electronic microscope to observe and study cancer cells' ultrastructural organization of cancer-bearing animal models (Fig. 20-2, 20-3).

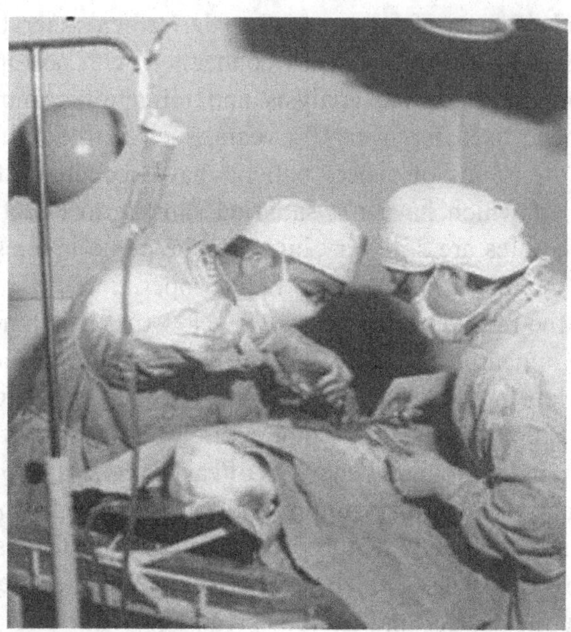

Fig. 20-1 Experimental study of free-tumor technique in radical operation

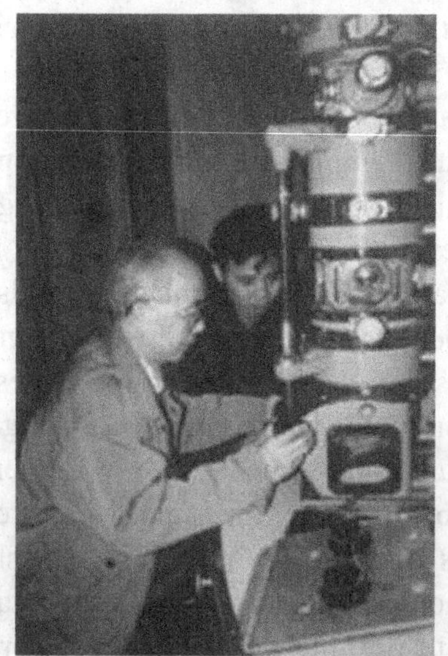

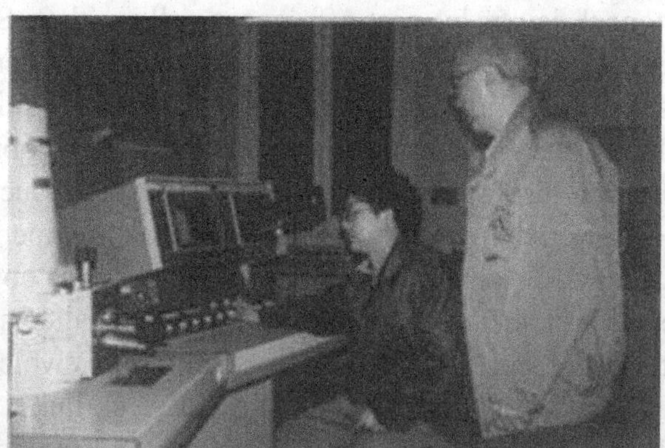

Fig. 20-2 Observation of ultrastructural organization of experimental model's cancer cells with electronic microscope

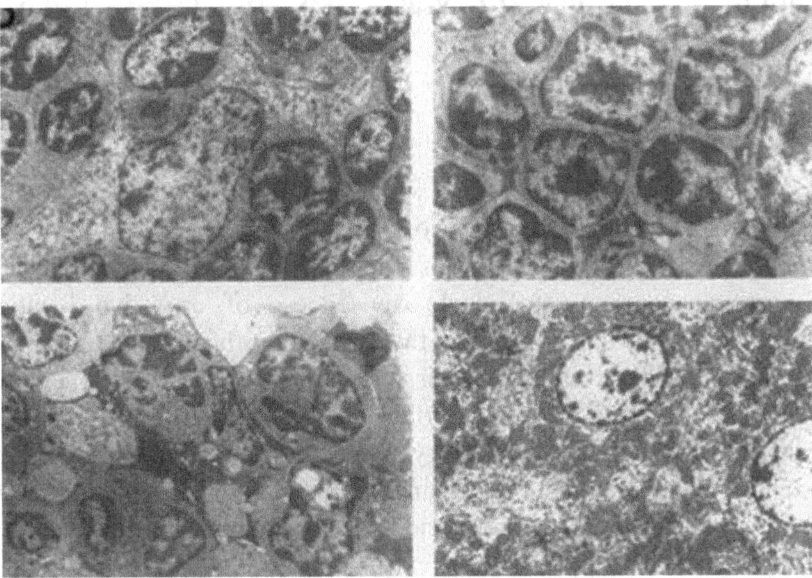

Fig. 20-3 Ultrastructural organization of hepatic cancer cells of cancer-bearing mouse H_{22}

4. Strengthening Fundamental and Clinical Study on Molecular Biology of Radical Operation of Recurrence and Metastasis after Operation

Inhibiting angiogenesis factors to induce the formation of blood vessels and preventing endothelial cells to construct new blood vessels are both new ways to explore preventions from recurrence and metastasis. In the experimental study of inhibiting actions of ethyl acetate extractives (TG) of traditional Chinese medicine—Common Threewingnut Root with different dosages on new blood vessels of transplanted tumor of mice peritoneum, the writer's laboratory observe influences of TG on the form and number of new-born micro-vessels in and around transplanted tumor of mice peritoneum, and on the diameter and flow rate of tumor arterioles and venules. They have made the preliminary confirmation that TG has certain inhibiting actions on new-born blood vessels of metastatic carcinoma focus and has been taken on clinical trials.

Study of preventing postoperative recurrence and metastasis of cancers must base on establishing animal models of recurrence and metastasis, and also proceed on levels of Molecular Biology and Gene. In the past decade and more, due to the rapid development of Molecular Biology, experts have found that the generation, progress, invasion, metastasis and recurrence of tumor are all in connection with cancer genes, cancer suppressor genes, metastatic genes and suppressor metastatic genes. To research related genes and seek control methods to prevent recurrence and metastasis as well as clinical measures of preventing recurrence, such as biological therapy, gene therapy, biological reaction control agent therapy, may be an important research aim in the future. In the 21st century, gene therapy will provide new efficient way for tumor therapy, and Molecular Biological Immunology will also stimulate the development of tumor therapy.

5. Prevention of Recurrence and Metastasis after Operation Should Be Established in Operation

(1) Surgical techniques of cancer surgery

Free-tumor technique is vitally important, which should prevent operation techniques from causing or actuating hematogenous metastasis of cancer cells.

Surgical principles of general surgery also applies to tumor surgery, such as operation techniques of aseptic operation, sufficient exposedness of operative location, the least intraoperative damage of normal tissues for the early-stage healing, etc. In addition, tumor surgery should take note of preventing the dissemination of cancer cells in the operation, in which the free-tumor technique is vitally important.

Ever since the end of the nineteenth century, people have realized that operation techniques may cause or actuate the dissemination of cancer cells. Therefore, the free-tumor technique of tumor surgery has been attracting more and more attention in recent years. For instance, intraoperative procedures of preserved skin, extrusion and anatomy can directly lead to the dissemination of tumor cells, stimulate formations of tumor embolism and metastasis which are near to or far away from blood vessels and lymphatic vessel. And tumor cells cast off and pollute surgical wounds, which results in local implantation recurrence, etc. Along with the development of Cell Pathology and inspection technology of tumor cells in blood stream, the phenomenon of tumor dissemination has been confirmed in clinical trials and animal experiments. For example, active cancer cells and cancer tissue masses can be found in vessel douche and surgical wounds douche of tumor operative specimen; cancer cells can be easier found in the output venous blood flow of tumor during the operation. Therefore, it is important that in the operation surgeons should first ligate and cut off output vena of tumor.

It should be noted in surgical operation that all the techniques are favorable toward preventing cancer cells' metastases. Do not stimulate or increase chances of cancer cells' metastases to cause iatrogenic metastasis and dissemination. For the surgical resection of tumor, all the operations must stress and observe free-tumor concept and technique, no matter big or small. Surgeons should give equal emphasis on free-tumor concept and aseptic concept, free-tumor technique and aseptic technique. The free-tumor technique is even stricter than aseptic technique. The surgical knife, scissors, needle and thread in the surgical operation, even every procedure is possible to cause metastasis of cancer cells. Such a possibility may increase with excessive extrusion, needle punching through the skin, knife cutting and other negative operative procedures by surgeons on tumor body or tissues. At present, applied molecular biology or immunohistochemistry method has proved that the operation technique itself can cause iatrogenic implantations, diffusions and metastases of cancer cells. Cancer cells can be found in surrounding blood circulations when many patients are undergoing the surgical operation; or cancer cells convert from the preoperative negative result to the postoperative positive result. The above evidences indicate that operation techniques are possible to induce the diffusion of cancer cells. It also suggests that some patients' postoperative recurrence and metastasis may be caused by improper operation techniques, such as the incision implantation.

Therefore, preventing postoperative recurrence and metastasis must start out from all the techniques in the surgical operation.

The route and type of tumor dissemination vary according to different pathologic types of tumor. Whether or not the metastasis can come into being is also related to the body's immune state. Consequently during the therapeutic process, the modern tumor surgeons should both prevent tumor dissemination and be careful to maintain the body's resistibility or immunity.

(2) Prevention from the dissemination of cancer cells

It is well-known but always overlooked that tumor's localized examination and operation techniques should be gentle and skillful to prevent the dissemination of cancer cells. Therefore, the following points should be noted: ① Preoperative tumor palpation should be gentle, and the number of times ought to be minimized. ② Preserved skin for operation should be gentle and skillful, or more cancer cells will invade small veins by the over friction. ③ operation techniques should be gentle and skillful, incision must be sufficient to expose, dissect and resect. Avoid pressing the tumor. ④ Adopt sharp dissection (dissecting knife or scissor); Strictly avoid blunt dissection to reduce dissemination. ⑤ Deal with the output vein before the artery. ⑥ Dispose the farther lymph nodes before the nearby lymph nodes to resect them wholly with the tumor.

(3) Prevention from the implantation of cancer cells

Cast-off cancer cells easily implant and grow on the traumatic tissue wounds, so: ① Use the gauze pad to protect cutting shoulder and wound surface. ② if the tumor is unwittingly incised or cracks, it should be covered and bound up with gauze pads. Replace timely polluted gloves and surgical instruments. ③ Adequate excision extent, involving enough normal tissues around the pathological changes. ④ Avoid the blood out-flowing from polluted wounds when anatomizing tissues near the tumor. Therefore, when two blood vessel forceps are used to clamp blood vessels, they should stick close to each other. Ligate immediately after being cut off. Replace timely gauze pads that are contaminated with blood.

Postoperative local recurrence (cover about 10%) of colon and rectum cancers often occurs in anastomotic stoma, incision of abdominal wall or outside of intestinal wall. This kind of recurrence is usually caused by the implantation of cancer cells. In recent years, a strip of cloth is used to ligate intestinal canals belonging to the upper and lower segment of tumor before the excision of intestinal loop, in order to stop cast-off cancer cells from continuing to diffuse along the intestinal cavity in the surgical operation. Use 1:500 corrosive sublimate or fluorouracil solution to douche intestinal cavities of both ends before the anastomosis, which can obviously improve the long-term effectiveness and may be relevant to the before-mentioned reduction of recurrence.

After all, to review significant achievements of 20-century techniques of surgical tumor excision; to preview glary prospects of 21-century tumor surgery study of prevention from recurrence and metastasis. In the coming period, the highlight of anti-cancer work should be anti-invasion, anti-metastasis and anti-recurrence. Anti-recurrence is the key of operative effectiveness; and anti-metastasis is the core question of cancer treatment. Cancer invasion and metastasis depend on specific potentials of two factors: biological characteristics of tumor cell itself and the host's influence on its restraining factors. To keep a balance is to control; to lose a balance is to progress

CHAPTER 21

The experiment research of searching etiology of cancer factor and pathogenesis and pathological physiology to seek for the effective control methods

In 1985 the author visited 3000 of his patients who had general surgical procedures for their different types of cancers. He found that most of the patients had cancer recurrence and metastasis during two or three years after their operation. Some of them recurred and died several months after the operation. Therefore, the author found that even if the operation is successful, the long-term therapy isn't satisfied or is failure. The patients had a big surgery and only were alive for one or two years or three years. Apparently this is not the patient's goals and not our aim. Generally, we only pay attention to five year surviving rate, but five year death rate. For example, the five year survival rate of stomach cancer is 20%; in another side, the five year death rate of stomach cancer is 80% which made the patients' family surprised. After following up many patients we found that the key factors for long-term therapy are recurrence and metastasis. Meanwhile, wc found that important questions: to look for the method and ways of preventing cancer from recurrence and metastasis is the key to improve the survival rate after surgery.

Currently there are very high metastasis rate which is related to many factors such as cancer's stage, grade, and differentiation, and the host immunology function. Now there are high recurrence rate in outpatient setting. Fo instance, during one week the author treated forty cancer patients including fifteen recurred patients after the operations so that in order to prevent the recurrence and metastasis after the surgery, we must start to do something since the operation time. Because the cancer removal operation can easily leave some remaining cancer cells, the tissue cells will seed and metastased easily. Once there are remaining, the cancer cells wil recur and metastasis, which cause terrible results. Therefore, Oncology surgery must follow the basic oncology rules. To remove the tumor during the surgery is the same important and strict thing as the sterilized rules during the general surgery, even more strict. There are two goals of performing no-tumor rules: 1. Preventing spread ; 2. Preventing planation. The key to the surgical long-term results is recurrence and metastasis. During 20 century the oncology surgery has made extremely success. The task during 21 century is to prevent recurrence and metastasis to improve the long-term surgical results.

If there is no out break on basic research, the clinical efficiency will not be improved. If there questions are resolved, the oncology surgery will have significantly success. There fore, in 1985 the author built his own experimental research laboratory to conduct the cancer research. First, to make the experiment tumor model, then to start the basic research from the clinical practice.

To look for the tumor pathogenic factors, pathogenesis and metastasis mechanism to search the preventive an treating methods through many steps of cancer cells metastasis. After seven years tudy, the research projects are all the clinical questions which got explanation from the basic research. After seven years animal research, the author finished the following research work by steps and steps.

1. The experimental research of making cancer animal models

   Why can human being get cancer? Under what condition can cancer happen? Why can some get cancer, others can not get cancer under the same condition can the same environment? Are there intrinis or extrinis factors or both of them? Therefore, we should make the animal cancer models to study?

   a. To make the cancer animal models in order to do tumor experimental research

      The author was the chairman in Department of surgery in the affility hospital of Hubei traditional medical University so that he could do clinical work and do animal experimental together such as the tumor samples from the patient in Operation room to place to the animal bodies after 30 minutes xxxx, however there were no tumor growth after 100 times experiment(more than 400 animals). After removing the thymus, then transplant the tumor again, the animal models were built up(210 animals models). Some of tumor animal models were set up by injection of steroid to reduce small animal immune function, then transplant the tumor.

      After removing thymus five days, the tumor were transplant to the body, then during 5 or 6 days the lump which size is yellow been-size will grow, during 12-21 days the lump size will become thumb-size. The tumor can be alive three or four weeks, however it cannot be passed from generation to generation.

      1. It was found that after removing thymus, the tumor animal model can be set up. The steroid injection can assist to make the animal tumor models set up.
      2. The result showed that tumor growth and development are related to the host's immune response and has significant relation to host immune organs and immune tissue functions
      3. The result showed that thymus and immune system have certain/sure relations to the cancer growth. After removing host's thymus, the cancer animal models can be set up.

         If the thymus didn't be removed, the animal model cannot be built. Alsoinjection steroid can decrease the host immune response, which is helpful to set up the animal model. If the immune system doesn't reduce, the animal models will not set up.

         The research result showed that the correlation between the immune response and cancer cell growth is negative. When the immune response difficiency or decrease, the tumor can grow, which will not be get rid of by hosts' immune response.

   b. Which is the first happen: immune decrease caused the cancer or the cancer cause the immune response decrease ?

      There are 320 Quanming mice which are separated into A, B, C, D group. Each group has 80 mice. The methods of removing thymus and injection of tumor cells are the same as before.

      In group A, first remove thymus, then five days later injection of 106 cancer cells;in group B, first inject the steroid, then seven day later injecting cancer cells; in group

C, first inject the cancer cells, then 10 days later removing thymus; in group D, first injecting cancer cells, then 10days later inject steroid. The result showed: the tumor growed in group A, B; There are only 18 mice which grew the green pea-size tumor in the 14day. This experiment implied that first the host's immune function decreased, or immune organ thymus has difficiency, then tumor can grow. If the host has good immune function, the tumors will not grow so that we get the conclusion: first immune function decrease, then cancer can develop and grow. If the immune system doesn't decrease, we can not built the cancer model successful. From this research, to improve and to maintain good immune function and to keep the good immune organ function are the most important methods to prevent from cancer growth.

c. The research animal model of tumor metastasis:

In 1985 the author built his tumor metastasis animal models, which he injected human cancer cells into the mice whose thymus is removed. Later he built up tumor metastasis model through lymph system. In 60 mice0.2 ml / 106 /ml H22 cells fuild was injected into animals' claw skin. After seven or eight days, an xxxxsize tumor grew up and the whole foot and ankle started to swell. After 16 days there are 8 mice which the right inguinal lymph nodes started to enlarge so that the lymphatic drainage metastasis animal models were built. Later the author built blood metastasis animal models which 0.4ml 106/ml of H22 cell were injected into the vein, then caused multiple tumors growth in lungs. After that, the liver metastasis animal models were built. 80 Quanming mice are divided into two groups A, B. In A group, there 40 mice. First inject steroid, seven days later 10% 75mg/kg xxxx

Was injected into abdominal cavity, then open it through cutting in with 0.5cm opening, expose spleen. 10ul H22 liver cells were injected into it and pressure 3-5min to prevent cells from flow out so that cells can flow into lymphatic system and blood system. After 11 days

These animal were sacrified to get the liver and to count the tumor nodes in liver. The result show that in A, B groups, the tumors grew, however, the tumor number in A group are much more than those in B group. In A group there are 3-5 nodule which sizes are around 1mm. In Bgroup there are 1-3 nodules.

The result showed us that metastasis is significantly related to immune syterm. When the immune system decrease s or when the medicine inhibits the immune system, the tumors will grow up.

2. The experimental research of searching the relation between tumors and immune organ to seek the methods of immune organ control

Removing thymus, decreasing immune or immune deficiency can build the liver meatatasis animal models so that thymus and tumors growth have certain relation. Thymus is the central immune organ and spleen is the biggest peripheral immune system. What is the relation between spleen and tumors? In order to find the relation between immune system function and the tumor growth and development, the experimental research were done:

a. The experimental research of the effects of spleen on tumor growth:

Spleen is peripheral immune organ which is very important during the anticancer. In order to seek the effect of spleen on the tumor growth and development, the following experiments were done.

270 quanming white mice were divided into spleen group and no spleen group. In no spleen group, the first cancer cells injection and them removing spleen; the first removing spleen and them cancer cells injection and then injecting the cells again. All of the results showed that : spleen inhibit the tumor growth in the early stages by 25%. In the late stage, spleen shrinkles and lost it inhabitation. After implanation of the spleen, the spleen anticancer function was recovered by 54%.

We found that spleen has two stages: in the early stage, it inhibit the tumor growth. In the late stages, it lost the inhibitaion, after implanation of the spleen, the inhibition function will be recovered.

b. The experimental research of seeking the effects of tumors on thymus and spleen:

As we discussed before, the centrol immune organ thymus and peripheral organ spleen can influence the cancer cells growth. However, do tumors affect the host thymus and spleen? The following research are done:40 Quanming white mice were divided into four groups, then measured the lymphocyte transferation rate before injecting the cancer cells and on the third, seventh and fourteen days after injection of the cancer cells, then sacrified the mice to observe the weight of thymus and spleen and to make the histological slides.

The result showed : in the early stages of the tumor growth, the spleen filled blood and enlargement, and the cells proliferation increases; in the late stages the spleen started to shrinkle and the cell proliferation was inhibited. The thymus started to shrinkle immediately after injection of the cancer cells and the cell proliferation was inhibited and the volume was significantly decreases and the weigh significantly decreased which showed the organ immune functions were inhibited.

This experimental results showed that the tumors will inhibit the thymus function significantly and also canuse the thymus shrinkle.

c. The experimental research of searching the anticancer function of the tranditional Chinese medicine of enhancing the spleen function soup

As the above the spleen has certain effect on tumor growth and spleen implanation can increase the the inhibition rate of the spleen on the tumor growth. The spleen in the trandition Chinese medicine is different from thespleen in western medicine. They are different in the theory, pathogenesis and clinical. However both of them are the same names "spleen", even if they have different functions, whether can we use the enhancing the spleen methods and combined with the above model medicine experimental research results to build the tranditional enhancing spleen function medicine and to do animal experiments to observe whether these medicine can inhibit the tumor growth or not. 40 Quanming white mice are divided into experimental groug(n=30) and control groug(n=10) both of which were injected 0.1x107 cancer cells. In the experimental group the enhancing spleen soup were given for 14 days to observe the tumor growth, mice live quality and the mice survival time.

The result showed that these enhancing medicine can delay the occurrent time of the tumor lump after the injection of the tumor cells and inhibit the tumor growth and increase the survival time and have certain anticancer function.

3. The experimental research of searching the methods of inhibition of thymus shrinkle during the tumor growth and reconstruction of thehost immune function

When the author made the tumor animal models, he found that the animal models were set up only after removing the thymus and after repeating the same experiments three times, the results are the same, which showed that thymus and the tumor growth have the relation. The above experiment of the relation between the immune organ and tumor growth showed that the tumor growth can inhibit thymus and caused the thymus shrinkle so that tumors not only inhibit the function of thymus but also cause thymus shrinkles.

Because of these, we have to search the ways to stop the thymus shrinkle and to recover the thymus function to rebuild the immune system function. Therefore, we must designe some ways to implant immune organs to rebuild the immune function such as implanation of the embryo liver, spleen, thymus. 200 Quanming white mice which were made into xxx tumor models were divided into six experimental groups and two contral groups which were implanted embryo spleen, thymus, liver to record the tumor growth, disappear, survival time, the immune function and the tissue pathology change and compared each experimental group number. The results showed that in three experimental groups the rate which the tumors were completely disappeared is 40% in the early stages and the rate which the tumors were completely disappeared in the later stage is 46.67%. After the tumors completely disappeared, the animals can survive for a long time. The partial disappeared rate is 26.67% in the early group and is 13.33% in the long-term group. In the partial group the average survival time is above one month which the immune function increase and immune organ enlarge. The immune organ histology slides showed that the organ cells proliferation increased. This result showed that the reconstitution of immunce system organ completely and partially can help the host to fight the tumor and to improve the treatment effects.

4. Searching the medicine of inhibiting the new vascular formation from nanetural drug

In 1986 when the author cultured the cancer cells, he found that cancer cells can proliferate, however cann't form the tumor mass, occasionally found that if one to two chicken soup drops was added in the tubes, the tumor cells form the cells masses. If one or two drops of xxxbasic was added, this mass will be dissolved. Currently, it is known that ther are several steps which the cancer cells metastase: 1. Cancer cells escape from the primary sites into blood through the vesscle then flow into microvascular, then into the organs, then stay in the organ as tumor mass without the vascular system which can not grow big. Later the new vascular system will form soon and the tumor will grow big. If any step can be stopped, the tumor metastasis will be stopped. Because the author considered that forming microvascular system is the key of metastasis and tumor growth and tumor nodes formation so that the experimental research of searching the medicine which can inhibit the formation of tumor vascular system from the natural herbs are designed as the following:

1. The observation of forming mice vascular after injection of tumors into abdominal muscle's

   20 Quanming white mice were injected EAC cells fluid to form the tumor microvascular models, then use Olymphus microscopy to observe the microvascular formation and count the microvascular flow rate and flow amounts. In the first day of implanation, we found that there is no vascular formation. On the second day, the host's microvascular system will grow out the thin and curve new vascule into the tumor masses. On three or four days, the density of the new microvascules ourtside the tumor will increase.

2. The effects of different TG dose on mice immune function:

   40 Quanming white mice were divided into TG1, TG2,TG3 and TG4 for different doses groups. After 12 days feed, the mice were sarastified on the 13th day to weigh thymus, spleen, body weight. The result showed that the different doses of TG has different effects on immune organ. A small dose 20mg/kg can increase the thymus weight and a big dose 80mg/kg can cause the thymus shrinkle.

3. The experimental research of TG inhibition of the growth of tumor microvascules in abdominal muscles

40 Quanming white mice which was injected with EAC in abdomen muscle was put on the observation table. The observation table put on the microscope in the temperation machine to observe the microvascular system growth such as the shapes, numbers in the tumor masse or around the tumor masses and took the pictures and measures the dentisy of the microvascular which come into and go out from the tumor masses and the average dimaster of the tumor vascule of the artery and vien and blood flow rates.

The results showed that TG(20mg/kg) significantly inhibit the growth of tumor new vessels in the early stages.

This experimental result showed that TG can significantly inhibit the new microvascular growth inside the tumor and around the tumors and decreases the density of the microvascule which entrance and extrance the tumors.

Currently many scientist from our country and other counties pay attention to inhibiting the formation of tumor new microvascules to control the tumor growth and metastasis masses formation. In May 1998 American Folkman reported that two of his medication such as Angiostation and Endostatin can inhibit the formation of the tumor new microvascules. In the tumor animal models, they can decrease the tumors significantily, which these medicine will inhibit the growth of vascules and shrinkle microvascule and the supply for the tumor will cut off so as to kill the cancer cells. He was planning to use these medicine in the human being in 1999.

The author finished TG experimental research in July 1997 because TG is trandition medication for more than hundreds years in Chinese medicine and is used in the clinical for a long time, however in the past TG is never used in inhibiting the growth of the microvascules. Since September 1998 the author started to use it as anticancer medication to use in the clinical patients. Until December 1999 more than 80 cases which had stage II, III cancers used it, which showed the good results of controlling the reccurence and metastasis. Now TG is in clinical trail stage.

CHAPTER 22

Experimental Study on Effects on the growth of tumor from spleen

In recent years, effects of spleen on the anti-tumor immunity are receiving more and more attentions from people. Its anti-tumor effects are extremely complicated. At present there are many differences and doubts. For further investigating effects of spleen on the growth of tumor and understanding the relation between spleen and tumor immunity, the experimental surgical method is adopted to prepare Ehrlich ascites tumor model. Group without spleen should respectively remove spleen before and after the inoculation of cancer cells. Then by contrasting it to the group with spleen, we perform the following experiment to observe whether the splenectomy will affect tumor immune state.

[Material and Method]

1. Experimental Animal Grouping Kunming mice, no gender classification, mice age 50~60d, weight 15~20g, and quantity of 300. According to the group with or without spleen, different sequence of splenectomy and inoculation of cancer cells, they are divided into 5 groups. Then on the basis of various amounts of inoculated cells (1×10^4 ml or 1×10^7 ml) and different inoculated regions (abdominal cavity or subcutaneous), each group is further separated into subgroups A and B. The specific grouping is shown in the following table 22-1.

Table 22-1 Summary table of experimental animal grouping

Group \ Inoculation Method	cancer cells concentration 1×10^4/ml		cancer cells concentration 1×10^7/ml	
	percutaneous	transabdominal	percutaneous	transabdominal
Group I simulating spleen removal	I A_1 (15)	I A_2 (15)	I B_1 (15)	I B_2 (15)
Group II (spleen removal before inoculation)	II A_1 (15)	II A_2 (15)	II B_1 (15)	II B_2(15)
Group III (inoculation before spleen removal)	III A (30)		III B (30)	
Group IV (spleen removal before inoculation+ splenic cells)	IV A_1 (15)	II A_2 (15)	IV B_1 (15)	IV B_2 (15)
Group V (administration of Chinese medicine)	V A (15)		V B (15)	

The Fourth Section Experimental Study

Group I: Control group with spleen. Firstly simulating spleen removal, after 7d transabdominal or percutaneous inoculation of Ehrlich ascites cancer cells 0.1ml, the number of cancer cells is 1×10^4 or 1×10^7 (table 22-2).

Table 22-2 Control group of simulating spleen removal (Group I)

Group I	Inoculated Cancer Cell Number	Inoculated Regions	Mice Number
I A_1	0.1×10^4	right armpit subcutaneousness	15
I A_2	0.1×10^4	abdominal cavity	15
I B_1	0.1×10^7	right armpit subcutaneousness	15
I B_2	0.1×10^7	abdominal cavity	15

Group II: Group of spleen removal before inoculation. Firstly spleen removal, after 7d percutaneous or transabdominal inoculation of Ehrlich ascites cancer cells 0.1ml, the number of cancer cells is 1×10^4 or 1×10^7 (table 22-3).

Table 22-3 Group of spleen removal before inoculation

Group II	Inoculated Cancer Cell Number	Inoculated Regions	Mice Number
II A_1	0.1×10^4	right armpit subcutaneousness	15
II A_2	0.1×10^4	abdominal cavity	15
II B_1	0.1×10^7	right armpit subcutaneousness	15
II B_2	0.1×10^7	abdominal cavity	15

Group III: Group without spleen, i.e. group of inoculation before spleen removal. Firstly inoculation of cancer cells, after 7d spleen removal. Both are right armpit subcutaneous inoculations. The number of cancer cells is 1×10^4ml or 1×10^7ml (table 22-4).

Table 22-4 Group of inoculation before spleen removal

Group III	Inoculated Cancer Cell Number	Inoculated Regions	Mice Number
III A	0.1×10^4	right armpit subcutaneousness	15
III B	0.1×10^7	right armpit subcutaneousness	15

Group IV: Group of spleen removal before inoculation, and further transabdominal transplantation of splenic cells or clear liquid of splenic tissue. Firstly remove spleen, after 7d inoculate cancer cells. In another 1d, transabdominal injection of living spleen cell suspension or supernatant liquid of splenic tissue (table 22-5).

Table 22-5 Group of spleen removal before transplantation of splenic cells or clear liquid of splenic tissue

Group IV	Inoculated Cancer Cell Number	Inoculated Regions	Processing Factor	Mice Number
IV A_1	0.1×10^4	trans-sub right armpit	injection of supernatant liquid of splenic tissue	15
IV A_2	0.1×10^4	transabdominal	injection of supernatant liquid of splenic tissue	15
IV B_1	0.1×10^7	right armpit subcutaneousness	transplantation of splenic cells of newborn mice	15
IV B_2	0.1×10^7	abdominal cavity	transplantation of splenic cells of adult mice	15

Group V: Group of taking Traditional Chinese Medicine (TCM) complex prescription with efficacy of strengthening the spleen and replenishing qi (table 22-6).

Table 22-6 Group of taking Traditional Chinese Medicine (TCM) complex prescription with efficacy of strengthening the spleen and replenishing qi

Group V	Inoculated Cancer Cell Number	Inoculated Regions	Processing Factor	Mice Number
V A	$10^7\times0.1$	right armpit subcutaneousness	firstly take TCM for 10d, after inoculation continue to take medication for 3 weeks	15
V B	$10^7\times0.1$	right armpit subcutaneousness	after inoculation take medication for 3 weeks	15

2. Instruments and Materials
   (1) An animal sterile operating room and a set of sterile surgical instruments.
   (2) Hank liquid, improved Hank liquid, calf serum, PRH, triple-distilled water, 0.9% sodium chloride solution for injection, ketamine, soluble phenobarbital, heparin sodium, trypan blue stain, Giemsa stain, Wright's stain, hydrochloric acid baking soda, L-glutamic acid, sensitization and non-sensitization zymosan.
   (3) Centrifugal machine with 400 rounds per minute, glass homogenizer, medicine vibrator, filtering metal gauze (size 1000), funnel, thermostat, baker, low temperature water tank, microscope, relative sterile workbench.
   (4) Animal feed are refined pellet feed. The drinking water is tap water. Rearing cage is plastic mouse cage.

3. Tumor Inoculation and Model Preparation Ehrlich ascites tumor cell strain is introduced from Wuhan Biological Research Institute Cell Room. Ascites containing cancer cells are extracted from ascetic-type tumor animal abdominal cavity of mice Ehrlich ascites tumor. Firstly use improved Hank liquid to clean and centrifugate ascites for 3 times with 800 rounds per minute of centrifugal speed and five minutes. Remove supernatant liquid, and respectively combine deposited cancer cells with Hank liquid to make up the cancer cell

suspensions, containing 1×10^4 ml or 1×10^7 ml inoculated cells. The trypan blue dead cells exclusion test proves that the living cell rate is above 95%. Then inoculate cancer cells to experimental mice through right armpit subcutaneousness and abdominal cavity. Each mouse is inoculated with cancer cell suspension of 0.1ml, i.e. amounts of containing cancer cells are 1×10^4 ml or 1×10^7 ml.

4. Splenectomy Combine ketamine with soluble phenobarbital to execute intraperitoneal anesthesia. Dosages are 0.4mg/10g and 0.2mg/10g. After anesthesia, fix the mouse on surgery board. Shear the belly fur. Use iodine (2.5%) and ethanol (75%) to disinfect the belly. Bespread the sterile cloth on it. An incision is made into each layer of abdominal wall tissue through left lower abdomen. Then enter into abdominal cavity. Expose and dissociate the spleen. Use silk thread of size 0 to ligate the splenic stalk. Excise the spleen. Ensure the strict sterile operation, gentle action and thorough hemostases. During the operation, notice whether there is a splenulus. In case there is, excise it together. For simulating spleen removal of control group, only open the abdominal cavity; pull but do not excise the spleen. Antibiotics are not used in and after the operation. Infection of incisional wound is 1.0%. After operation, continue to feed the mouse with refined pellet feed.
5. Preparations of Splenic Cell Suspension and Supernatant Liquid of Splenic Tissue
   (1) Preparation of splenic cell suspension: Execute newborn Kunming mice of 24~48h or adult mice. An incision is made into abdominal wall to take out the spleen. Cut off peripheral envelope and adipose tissue of spleen. Use Hank liquid to irrigate them in sterile glass culture dish for 3 times. Then put spleen into the glass homogenizer. Add in Hank liquid for 5ml. Grind up the splenic tissue. Filter it with stainless silk net of size 100. Centrifugate the filtering medium (1000 rounds per minute, 10 min). Remove supernatant liquid. Use Hank liquid to dilute deposited cells and make up the splenic cell suspensions of 5×10^7/ml. Suspensions are dyed by trypan blue stain and proved that the living cell rate is above 97%. Then transplant splenic cell suspensions into abdominal cavity of experimental mouse. Each mouse can only accept splenic cell suspensions of 2ml which belong to one receptor.
   (2) Preparation of splenic cell homogenate: After excising the spleen, use quick freezing (-20 centi degree) and rapid rewarming to induce the cracking of dead splenic cells proved by trypan blue stain and microscopic examination. Then centrifugate the filtering medium (1000 rounds per minute, 10 min). Reserve supernatant liquid and remove deposits. Inject supernatant liquid through abdomen into the experimental mouse.

6. Observation Item
   (1) Observe success ratio of cancer cell inoculation, occurrence time of subcutaneous tumor nodi and speed of tumor enlargement.
   (2) Every day use vernier caliper to measure diameter and size of subcutaneous tumor nodi; measure mouse' weight; observe metastasis condition and moving degree.
   (3) Observe the quality of life, fur color, vitality, state of nutrition, breath, mental state of tumor-bearing mice and survival time of bearing tumor.
   (4) Observe abdominal shape and prohection of ascetic-type tumor-bearing mice. Also according to prohection state, divide ascites content into 5 grades.
   Grade 0: the abdomen is not of fullness, without ascites, note as (-).
   Grade 1: slight prohection of abdomen, with a little ascites, note as (+).
   Grade 2: prohection of abdomen, with medium content of ascites, note as (++).

Grade 3: obvious prohection of abdomen, with more ascites, note as (+++).
Grade 4: shape of frog abdomen, with plentiful ascites, note as (++++).

During necropsy, measure the content of ascites, microscopic examination of cancer cell shape, count living cell rate and content.

(5) Determine immunologic functional condition of red blood cells of tumor-bearing mice: test for measuring C_3b receptor garland with semi quantitative method.
(6) Necropsy and pathological section: dissect each dead experimental mouse. Observe tumor's size and weight, infiltrating and metastatic condition, morphological structure and involvement condition of visceral organs; measure the content of ascites; extract tumor tissue, liver, spleen, thymus gland, lung and other visceral organs to carry out the examination of pathological section.

[Experimental Result]

1. Resulting comparison and analysis on different groups with right armpit subcutaneous inoculation of small dose of 0.1×10^4 ml Ehrlich ascites tumor cells.
   (1) Comparison on occurrence time of tumor nodi with different processing method (T test), see table 22-7.

Table 22-7 Comparison on occurrence time (d) of tumor nodi with different processing method (T test)

Group	Group I A_1 (Control group with spleen)	Group II A_1 (Group of spleen removal before inoculation)	Group IIIA (Group of inoculation before spleen removal)	Group IVA_1 (Spleen removal before inoculation+supernatant liquid of splenic tissue)
Occurrence time (d)	8	7*	9	9*

Note: ① *. Compared with Group I A_1, $P<0.05$ has remarkable significance; ② In Group I A_1 (control group with spleen), one experimental mouse (accounts for 7.6%) suffers no tumor nodi after inoculation of cancer cells. It survives for a long term (i.e. survival time is above 90d). No tumor is found during dissection. Treat it as inoculation failure. Not for statistical treatment; also in Group IVA (group with transabdominal injection of supernatant liquid of splenic tissue), 3 experimental mice (accounts for 25%) fail to be inoculated.

According to table 22-7, the earliest occurrence time of tumor nodi in above groups belongs to group of spleen removal before inoculation (Group II A_1). Control group and group with injection of supernatant liquid of splenic tissue have the later occurrence time.

(2) For different processing methods, maximum diameter comparison of each group's tumor nodi on the seventh, fourteenth and twentieth day, see table 22-8.

Table 22-8 Size comparison of each group's tumor nodi on the seventh, fourteenth and twentieth day after subcutaneous inoculation of 0.1×10^4 ml cancer cells (maximum diameter mm)

Group	Group I A_1 (Control group with spleen)	Group II A_1 (Group of spleen removal before inoculation)	Group III A (Group of inoculation before spleen removal)	Group IVA_1 (Spleen removal before inoculation+supernatant liquid of splenic tissue)	*P*
seventh	0	3.3±0.48	0	0	<0.01
fourteenth	11.43±5.99	14.4±6.2	11.8±7.45	8±4.33	<0.01
twentieth	18.92±9.98	21.12±8.28	19.7±5.98	13.89±7.63	<0.01

Note: Values *P* in the table are gained through analysis of diameter variance (*F* test).

From above results in the table, the tumor which belongs to group of spleen removal before inoculation (Group II A_1) appears first and grows fast. Before the fourteenth day, its tumor volume reaches biggest. On the twentieth day after inoculation, tumors' sizes of control group (Group I A_1), group II A_1 (group of spleen removal before inoculation), group of inoculation before spleen removal (Group III A) reach unanimity. While tumors which belong to group of injecting supernatant liquid of splenic tissue (Group IV A_1) have the smallest volume. That explains that during early growing stage of tumor (before the seventh day), spleen has tumor inhibitory action. But during medium and advanced stages (experimental group sets: medium stage is from eighth day to fourteenth day since the inoculation; since the fourteenth day, it is tumor advanced stage), the inhibitory action of spleen weakens or disappears. Furthermore, it can be observed that after cancer cells inoculation of spleen removal group, since the fourteenth day, tumor nodi often bear liquefaction, necrosis and ablation, which result in the shrinkage of tumor volume. Even some incisions have healed. Why does such phenomenon appear? That needs to have a further observation.

(3) Comparison of mean survival time (MST) for groups of subcutaneous inoculation with 0.1×10^4 ml cancer cells, see table 22-9.

Table 22-9 Comparison of each group's mean survival time (MST)

Group	Group I A_1 (Control group with spleen)	Group II A_1 (Group of spleen removal before inoculation)	Group III A (Group of inoculation before spleen removal)	Group IVA_1 (Spleen removal before inoculation+supernatant liquid of splenic tissue)	*P*
MST (d)	41.61±12.24	38.73±19.63	44.8±15.95	50±27.21	<0.05

Note: Values *P* in the table are gained through *F* test.

From table 22-9, mean survival times of groups I A_1, II A_1, III A are close to each other. T test shows there is no difference among these three groups, $P > 0.05$. While for injection of supernatant liquid of splenic tissue, mean survival time of this group is obviously longer than those of other groups, $P < 0.05$. The significant difference exists.

2. Resulting analysis of each group's transabdominal inoculation with 0.1×10^4 ml cancer cells
   After inoculation of cancer cells, experimental mice can survive above 90d without any ascite or tumor nodus. Also a dissection of corpse shows no tumor. The above results are treated as inoculation failures. It explains the fact that vaccinal cancer cells are rejected by the organism and no tumor forms.
   (1) Comparison of inoculation failure rate for each group's transabdominal inoculation of 0.1×10^4 ml cancer cells without ascites, see table 22-10.

Table 22-10 Comparison of each group's inoculation failure rate (T test)

Group	Group I A_2 (Control group with spleen)	Group II A_2 (Group of spleen removal before inoculation)	Group II A_2 (Spleen removal before inoculation+supernatant liquid of splenic tissue)
failure rate	26%	0**	54%*

Note: **. indicates the comparison with control group, T test $P<0.01$, with high degree of significant difference; *. indicates $P<0.05$, with significant difference.

Results of table 22-10 show that all experimental mice in the group of spleen removal before inoculation form ascites, and failure rate is zero. The inoculation failure rates of control group with spleen and injection group of supernatant liquid of splenic tissue are 26% and 54% respectively. It process that tumor is easy to grow in the mouse without spleen after inoculation of tumor. That is, the removal of spleen promotes the growth of tumor. On the contrary, injection of supernatant liquid of splenic cells will suppress the growth of tumor.

(2) Comparison of survival time for each group's transabdominal inoculation of 0.1×10^4 ml cancer cells, see table 22-11.

Table 22-11 Comparison of each group's survival time (F test)

Group	Group I A_2 (Control group with spleen)	Group II A_2 (Group of spleen removal before inoculation)	Group IVA_2 (Spleen removal before inoculation+supernatant liquid of splenic tissue)	*P*
survival time (d)	51.46±29.35	35.6±18.93	57.6±14.85	<0.05

From table 22-11, the mean survival time of group with spleen removal before inoculation is 35.6±18.93 days. While mean survival times of control group with spleen and injection group of supernatant liquid of splenic tissue are 51.46±29.35 days and 57.6±14.85 days respectively, and P<0.05. Significant differences exist among these three groups. In three groups, group of spleen removal before inoculation has the shortest survival time. Group with spleen owns long survival time; while group without spleen owns short survival time. That shows the removal of spleen promotes the growth of tumor and shortens survival times of tumor-bearing mice. On the contrary, injection of supernatant liquid of splenic cells will suppress the growth of tumor and prolong survival times of tumor-bearing mice.

3. Results of each group's subcutaneous inoculation with 0.1×10^{7} ml cancer cells
   (1) Comparison on occurrence time of each group's subcutaneous tumor nodi, see table 22-12.

Table 22-12 Comparison on occurrence time of each group's subcutaneous tumor nodi

Group	Group I B_1 (Control group with spleen)	Group II B_1 (Group of spleen removal before inoculation)	Group III B (Group of inoculation before spleen removal)	Group IV B_1 (Spleen removal before inoculation+transplantation of fetal mouse's splenic cells)	*P*
Occurrence time (d)	5.5	5	7.5	9	<0.05

Mice of group IIIB are removed spleens on the seventh day after inoculations. So after seven days group IIIB and control group with spleen (Group I B_1) are in the same condition. The table shows that for the group with spleen removal first, occurrence times of subcutaneous tumor nodi are slightly earlier than these of other groups. While for group IVB_1 (transplantation of fetal mouse's splenic cells), occurrence times of tumor nodi are obviously later than these of other groups. It proves that the removal of spleen promotes the growth of tumor. While transplantation of splenic cells intensively suppresses the growth of tumor.

(2) Comparison of maximum diameter average on each group's subcutaneous tumor nodi on the seventh, fourteenth and twentieth day after inoculation, see table 22-13.

Table 22-13 Comparison of maximum diameter on each group's tumor nodi on the seventh, fourteenth and twentieth day (mm)

Group	Group I B_1 (Control group with spleen)	Group II B_1 (Group of spleen removal before inoculation)	Group III B (Group of inoculation before spleen removal)	Group IV B_1 (Spleen removal before inoculation+transplantation of fetal mouse's splenic cells)	*P*
seventh	5.07±1.847	10.88±5.278	2.83±1.948	3.0±1.56	<0.01
fourteenth	19.85±4.598	21.12±5.3	20.3±6.07	11±5.69	<0.01
twentieth	30.9±7.87	24±7.86	25.25±4.77	16±4.95	<0.01

Note: Values *P* in the table are gained through *F* test.

(3) Comparison of each group's mean survival time (MST), see table 22-14.

Table 22-14 Comparison of each group's mean survival time (subcutaneous inoculation of 0.1×10^7 ml cancer cells)

Group	Group I B_1 (Control group with spleen)	Group II B_1 (Group of spleen removal before inoculation)	Group III B	Group IV B_1 (Spleen removal before inoculation+transplantation of fetal mouse's splenic cells)	*P*
MST (d)	33.1±13.15	49.56±24.39	38.7±14.45	50.75±19.30	<0.01

From table 22-13 and 22-14, on the seventh day after inoculation, for the three groups-control group with spleen (Group IB_1), group of spleen removal before inoculation (Group IIB_1) and group of inoculation before spleen removal (Group IIIB), their maximum diameter averages of tumor nodi are $\overline{X}(IB_1)$ = (5.07±1.847) mm, $\overline{X}$ (IIB_1) = (10.88±5.278) mm, $\overline{X}$(IIIB) = (2.83±1.948) mm respectively. $P<0.01$. Significant differences exist among these three groups. Tumors which belong to the group of spleen removal before inoculation (IIB_1) have the maximum volumes. Now on the seventh day, in fact groups IB_1 and IIIB have the spleen, which is in proliferative active phase. While group IIB_1 has no spleen. The tumor volume of group with spleen is smaller, and the tumor volume of group without spleen is larger. It indicates that the spleen can suppress tumor during early stage or the removal of spleen can promote the growth of tumor. While on the fourteenth day after inoculation, their average maximum diameters of tumor nodi are $\overline{X}(IB_1)$ = (19.85±4.598) mm, $\overline{X}(IIB_1)$ = (21.12±5.3) mm, $\overline{X}$(IIIB) = (20.3±6.07) mm respectively. $P>0.05$. Significant differences disappear among these three groups. On the twentieth day after inoculation, the tumor volume of control group with spleen is larger than that of other groups. The maximum diameter $\overline{X}$ = (30.9±7.87) mm. At this time, the spleen of tumor-bearing mouse has extremely shrank, and lost the tumor inhibitory action. From the experiment, since the fourteenth day after inoculation, most mice tumors of group with spleen removal begin to bear liquefaction and necrosis. Some lumps ulcerate and ablate, whose volumes shrink. The reason that tumors in this period suffer from liquefaction, necrosis and ulceration is not clear at present. That needs to have a further observation.

Therefore, during the early stage of tumor, spleen can suppress the growth of tumor. For the group with spleen, the tumor growth rate is slower. Tumor volume is smaller. While on the advanced stage of tumor, the inhibitory action of spleen weakens or disappears. The tumor size of all groups reaches unanimity.

Furthermore, it can be seen from the stable that tumors of the group (IVB_1), which removes spleen before inoculation and transplants splenic cells of fetal mice, have obviously slower growth rate than that of other groups. The tumor volume is smaller. Its survival time is longer that that of other groups. These conditions prove that splenic cells of homogeneous variant fetus have obvious tumor-inhibitory action.

4. Results of each group's transabdominal inoculation with 0.1×10^7 ml cancer cells
   (1) Comparison on occurrence time of ascites for each group, see table 22-15.

Table 22-15 Comparison on occurrence time of ascites for each group of transabdominal inoculation with 0.1×10^7 ml cancer cells

Group	Group I B_2 (Control group with spleen)	Group II B_2 (Group of spleen removal before inoculation)	Group IV B_2 (Spleen removal before inoculation+transplantation of splenic cells)
Occurrence time (median, d)	5	3*	4*

Note: **. indicates the comparison with control group, T test $P<0.05$, with significant difference.

(2) Occupying percentages of ascites content greater than (++) for groups on the fifth, seventh and fourteenth day after transabdominal inoculation of 0.1×10^7 ml cancer cells, see table 22-16.

Table 22-16 Comparison on ascites content of transabdominal inoculation with 0.1×10^7 ml cancer cells

Days after inoculation (d)	Group I B_2 (Control group with spleen)	Group II B_2 (Group of spleen removal before inoculation)	Group IV B_2 (Spleen removal before inoculation+transplantation of splenic cells)
2	0%	75% **	10% *
7	28%	100% **	70% *
14	100%	100%	100% *

Note: **. indicates the comparison with IB_2 (control group), T test $P<0.01$; *. indicates $P<0.05$; no *. indicates $P>0.05$.

(3) Comparison of survival time (d) for each group's transabdominal inoculation of 0.1×10^7 ml cancer cells, see table 22-17.

Table 22-17 Comparison of each group's survival time

Group	Group I B_2 (Control group with spleen)	Group II B_2 (Group of spleen removal before inoculation)	Group IV B_2 (Spleen removal before inoculation+transplantation of splenic cells)
survival time (d)	20.15±4.59	15.56±10.94*	16.67±8.34

Note: *. indicates the comparison with IB_2, $P<0.05$, with significant difference; no *. indicates the comparison with IB_2, $P>0.05$, without significant difference.

Integrating tables 22-15, 22-16 and 22-17, results show that for the group with spleen removal first (IIB_2), tumor growth rate is faster. Amounts of ascites are more. Survival time is shorter. Also visceral organs are easier to metastasize. Those explain that removal of spleen can promote the growth of tumor. Transabdominal transplantation of splenic cells of homogeneous variant adult mice can partially suppress the growth of tumor. But its inhibitory action is weaker than that of control group with spleen and group with transplantation of fetal mouse's splenic cells.

5. Results of necropsy and pathological examination Each mouse accepts the postmortem necropsy. Visually observe tumor shape, involved visceral organs and diffusion condition. And extract tissues for pathological section examination. The result shows that Ehrlich ascites tumor cell strain owns features of stable proliferation, strong invasiveness and so on. Subcutaneous inoculation is easy to induce the form of solid tumor. Necropsy proves that after inoculation tumors or ascites are easy to form in some regions, easily infiltrating to surrounding tissues. The metastases of cancer cells rarely happen to mice with subcutaneous inoculation. While for mice with transabdominal inoculation, cancer cells easily metastasize to liver, kidney and lymph node in advanced stage. Only two of two hundred and seventy experimental mice suffer from splenic metastases, proving the weak affinity of spleen to cancer cells. This group of experiments has also found phenomena that for the group of spleen removal before transabdominal inoculation, multiple carcinomatous metastases appear in visceral organs of abdominal cavity. Metastatic ratio is up to 50%. These metastases invade liver, kidney, pancreas and mesenteric lymph nodes, always implicating more than two visceral organs. While for control group with spleen and group with transplantation of homogeneous variant splenic cells, carcinomatous metastases rarely occur. Metastatic ratios are 20% and 25%, which are obviously lower than those of the group without spleen. It shows that spleen can suppress the growth of tumor. While the group without spleens lose the inhibitory action, consequently leading to easy diffusion and metastasis of tumor.

   Furthermore, dynamic observation of this group of experimental mice shows that thymus and spleen of tumor-bearing mice present a series of changes with the process of illness, which own certain regularity. About seven days after inoculation, the thymus presents acute and progressive atrophy. Its volume shrinks; the diameter of each normal lobule shortens from 5~8cm to about 1mm; the weight reduces from (70±10) mg to (20±5) mg. While soon after the inoculation of cancer cells, spleen becomes congested and tumid. The volume enlarges; weight increases; texture becomes fragile. Microscopic examination shows the increase of germinal centers and active cell proliferation. On the fourteenth day after inoculation, the spleen also quickly presents progressive atrophy. Its volume shrinks; the weight reduces from (140±15) mg to (50±10) mg. Germinal centers obviously decrease; cell proliferation is suffocated. The spleen also suffers from hyperplasia of fibrous tissues, fibrosis with gray color and rigid texture.

6. Testing results of erythrocytic immune function This group of experiments choose 100 mice to carry out the erythrocytic C_3b receptor garland test. The result shows that after the removal of spleen, bonding ratio of C_3b receptor garland of tumor-bearing mice is on a progressive declining tendency. That explains that after the removal of spleen, immunological adhesive competence of red blood cells drops to some extent.

[Discussion]

1. As seen from experimental results, spleen can suppress the growth of tumor. After the removal of spleen, compared with the control group, the growth rate is faster; the

occurrence time and volume of subcutaneous tumor nodi is earlier and larger in the same period. For group with transabdominal inoculation of cancer cells and group with the removal of spleen, occurrence time of ascites is earlier; ascites content is greater; cells content is also higher. Survival time is shorter than that of control group. Necropsy finds that cancer metastatic rate of the group with the removal of spleen is 30% above that of control group (metastases to liver, kidney, pancreas and mesenteric lymph nodes). From table 22-13, group IIB_1 (spleen removal before inoculation) and group IIIB (inoculation before spleen removal) accept splenectomy in different time. On the seventh day after inoculation, maximum diameter averages of their subcutaneous tumor nodi are $\overline{X}(IIB_1) = (10.8\pm5.28)$ mm and $\overline{X}(IIIB) = (2.83\pm1.948)$ mm respectively. The former is obviously longer than the latter one. But on the fourteenth day after inoculation, the tumor of group IIIB quickly proliferates after the removal of spleen. The difference between them almost disappears. $\overline{X}(IIB_1) = (21.2\pm5.3)$ mm, $\overline{X}(IIIB) = (20.3\pm6.07)$, $P>0.05$, without significant difference. It prompts that the removal of spleen promotes the growth of tumor, i.e. spleen can suppress the growth of tumor.

In recent two decades, people find that spleen not only performs a great role in anti-infection, but also has the all-important influence on anti-tumor immunity. The active mechanism may be by producing Natural Killer cell, macrophage (Mϕ), Lympholine-Activated Killer cell, TH/Ti cell, B cell, Ts cell, etc. to realize the cellular immunity; and by secreting lymphokines of Tufisn factor, TNF factor, IL-2, interferon, addiment, antibody, etc. to kill tumor cells. Ge Yigong once used rat Lw56 pulmonary sarcoma model to the effect of removing spleen on tumor growth. Mr Ge holds that success ratio of tumor inoculation after the removal of spleen is higher than that of group with spleen. The metastatic ratio increases. Results are similar to this group of experimental results.

This group of experimental results also prompts that after the removal of spleen, bonding ratio of C_3b receptor garland of organism peripheral blood is 40% below that of healthy group with spleen. It explains that erythrocytic immune function of organism reduces after the removal of spleen.

2. Spleen's inhibiting action on tumor growth mainly occurs in the early stage of tumor course. While in the advanced stage of tumor, spleen's inhibiting action on tumor growth weakens and disappears. As seen from tables 22-8 and 22-13, in the early stage of tumor (within 7d), the tumor of group without spleen has a faster tumor growth rate than that of control group with spleen. The volume of subcutaneous tumor nodi is large and ascites content is great. While in the advanced stage (after 14d) of tumor, tumor nodi of control group with spleen and group with the removal of spleen basically have the same volume. No significant comparability. No obvious difference between survival times. Necropsy and pathological examination of three hundred experimental mice find that spleen of tumor-bearing mice present a series of regular changes with the process of illness. In the early stage of tumor (within 7d after inoculation), due to the cytostimulation, the spleen becomes congested and tumid. The volume enlarges; cell proliferation accelerates; germinal centers increases. While in the advanced stage (since 14d after inoculation) of tumor, the spleen presents progressive atrophy. Its volume shrinks; germinal centers fall sharply. The spleen also suffers from hyperplasia of fibrous tissues. The fibrosis of spleen occurs; therefore, its anticancer immunization weakens or disappears. Even it can pass through the suppressor T

cell. Macrophage and immune inhibiting factor can suppress the anticancer immunization of organism and promote the growth of tumor. That explains that spleen's effect on tumor immune state is bidirectional, has obvious time phase and is relevant to stadium. In early stage, the spleen owns the anti-tumor action. In advanced stage, the spleen owns immune inhibiting action. But the basic reason that leads to the immune inhibiting state of organism is the tumor itself. Spleen just plays a certain part in the forming process of this state.

Transabdominal injection of supernatant liquid of healthy splenic cells and transplantation of homogeneous variant splenic cells can suppress tumor growth. For group of injection with supernatant liquid of splenic cells or transplantation of splenic cells (Group IV), comparative results with other groups show that the tumor growth rate is slower; the occurrence time of tumor nodi is later; the volume is smaller; ascites content is less. After the inoculation of small dose of 0.1×10^4 ml cancer cells, success ratio of inoculation for tumor-bearing mice is obviously lower than that of other groups. Moreover, after a little ascites or subcutaneous lesser tubercle firstly appearing in several mice, the tumor can disappear naturally. The survival time is above 90d (as long-term survivors). Especially splenic cells of homogeneous variant fetal mouse (group IVB_1) have obvious tumor-inhibitory action. The tumor inhibition rate is 54%. The survival time is 17d longer than that of control group. Pathological examinations of this group of tumor-bearing mice find that after transplantation of homogeneous variant fetal splenic cells, splenic islands grow on the abdominal cavity and (or) mesentery of seven mice (account for 50%). Pathological examination proves it as living splenic tissues. Fetal splenic cells have features of weak antigenicity, deficient quantity and strong cell proliferation, etc. After the transplantation of splenic cells of homogeneous variant mice, there is no sharp rejection. And moreover, it is not subject to blood group ABO. Do not need the cross test of different blood groups. Here in China some people use traumatic splenic cells to prepare LAK cells for treating advanced malignant tumors, which achieves better curative effects on inhibiting tumor growth and prolonging mouse's lifespan.

At present, adoptive immunotherapy of tumors with transplantation of fetal splenic cells has not yet been reported in the literature. This group of experiments needs to have a further observation.

3. Negative correlation between anti-tumor immunological action of the organism and the quantity of cancer cells This group of experiments finds that anti-tumor immunological action of the organism is obviously affected by the quantity of inoculated cancer cells. The less the quantity of cancer cells, the stronger and more significant the anti-tumor effect; on the contrary, the weaker the anti-tumor effect. As for 0.1×10^7 ml inoculated cancer cells, immunological action of the organism is obviously suppressed. The tumor growth rates of group without spleen and group with spleen have bigger difference in the early stage. While after medium stage (after 7d), the difference will quickly disappear. There is also no significant difference in survival time. But for 0.1×10^4 ml inoculated cancer cells, anti-tumor action of the organism is relatively significant. The inoculated failure rate of group with spleen is obviously higher than that of group without spleen. The growth rate of tumor is slow; the volume of tumor nodi is small; and the survival time is long. Furthermore, after the transplantation of homogeneous variant splenic cells for small dose of inoculated cancer cells group, anti-tumor immunological action goes up remarkably. The growth rate of tumor decreases obviously. Some tumor nodi even can naturally

disappear after its formation. Also the survival time is long. These results show the negative correlation between anti-tumor action of the organism and the quantity of inoculated cancer cells. While there is a positive correlation between cancer's immunological inhibiting action on the organism and the quantity of inoculated cancer cells. The spleen participates in tumor immunoregulation, which has double influences on immune state of tumor-bearing mice. In early stage, the spleen shows a certain anti-cancer action. As the development of tumor, the number of tumor cells is increasing. The spleen is shrinking gradually. Then the anti-cancer action is converted into immunological inhibiting action. But the basic reason of immune inhibiting state is the tumor itself. The progress of cancer, an increase in the number of cancer cells and the reinforcement of inhibiting action lead to the atrophia of spleen, thymus gland and other immune organs.

4. Experimental result prompts of this group
   (1) The spleen has certain anti-tumor effects. In tumor's early stage, spleen can suppress the growth of tumor. While in advanced stage of the course of disease, the anti-tumor action of spleen weakens or disappears. The spleen even can promote the growth of spleen.
   (2) Adoptive immunotherapy of tumors with transplantation of homogeneous variant splenic cells of fetal mice can reinforce anti-tumor immunological action of the organism, and suppress the growth of tumor.
   (3) There is a negative correlation between anti-tumor action of the organism and the quantity of inoculated cancer cells. The more the quantity of cancer cells, the more easily the immunological action of the organism is suppressed or damaged. The faster the growth rate of tumor, the worse the prognosis.

CHAPTER 23

Experimental Observation of Effects on Thymus and Spleen from Tumor

It is usually considered that the immune functions of organisms affect the occurrence, development and prognosis, however at the same time tumors can inhibit the immune state of organisms. These two are mutually causal and intricate and complicated. When doing the animal experiments on the influences of spleen on the tumorous growth, the author have observed that the immune organs thymus, spleen of the cancer-bearing mice have changed a lot. It seems that this process presents a certain law. In order to study further on the relationship and laws between tumors and spleens or thymus, the following experiments are designed to observe dynamically the changes of conversion rates of thymus, spleen and lymphocyte of cancer-bearing mice in different phases and probe into the relationship between them.

[Material and Methods]

I. Experimental animal and grouping

Use 40 Kunming mice and divide into four groups at random with the age of 40~50days and the weight of 15~18g, ignoring the sexes.

Group I: Control group of healthy mice which are not inoculated with cancer cells. After executing them, take away their thymus, spleens and circumferential blood to do the experiment.

Group II:Inoculate the mice with $0.1*10^7$ ehrlich ascites carcinoma through abdominal cavity, execute them after 3 days and observe.

Group III: Inoculate the mice with cancer cells (as the above) execute them after 7 days and observe.

Group IV: Inoculate the mice with cancer cells, execute them after 14 days and observe.

Use the results of anatomizing 100 cancer-bearing mice after natural death as the alterant results of thymus and spleen in terminal period. In this period the average diameter of thymus of cancer-bearing mice is 1.2±0.3mm, average weight is 20±5 mg with a bit hard texture. While spleens are extremely easy to atrophy, whose average weight is 60±12mm, texture is hard, and its color is gray, with the germinal center reducing and fibrosing.

II. Experimental methods

Execute the mice of each group by digging out their eyes and blooding them at the preconcerted time. Reserve the whole blood of each mouse (using heparin for anti-coagulation) to do the experiment of lymphocyte conversion and then anatomize them immediately; observe the range of soakage, volume of ascites and the situation of all viscera; emphasize on observing the anatomical shape of thymus, spleens and lymph nodes and take out the thymus and spleen integrally, then measure their volume with a vernier caliper; weigh them respectively using analytical balance and send them to the department of defection.

III. Measuring the conversion rate of peripheral blood lymphocytes of mice in each group

Measure by
Dig out their eyes and blood with heparin for anti-coagulation.

IV. Making tumor model

As same as the experimental part in Chapter 22.

[Experimental Result]

1. Thymic weights of mice in each group after inoculated with cancer cells in different phases (see table 23-1)

Do analysis of variance with the statistical data in table 23-1, see table 23-2. Using a curve to present the results of table23-1 and table 23-2, draw the curve of change in the thymic weights (chart 23-1); the thymic weights of the 25th day and 30th day in the chart are quoted from the results of the experimental part in chapter 22.

Table 23-1 Comparison of thymic weights of mice in each group (mg)

Group	Group I healthy	Group II on the 3rd after inoculated	Group III on the 7th after inoculated	Group IV on the 14th after inoculated		
X_i	72.8	78.2	90.0	40.0		
	50.0	83.4	66.0	32.2		
	56.4	89	85.4	39.8		
	96.4	68	106.5	23.5		
	77.4	74.8	51.7	38.0		
	100.7	95.4	77.8	36.0		
	87.5	115.0	73.0	16.0		
	76.8	56.4	60.0	20.0		
	112.7	43.0	49.6	55		
	51.0			20		
ΣX	781.07	703.2	736.3	350.5	ΣX	2 571.7
N_i	10	9	10	10	N	39
$\bar{X}$	78.17	78.13	73.63	35.05	$\bar{X}$	65.94
ΣX^2	6 6261.79	58 566.66	57 033.75	18 467.25	ΣX^2	191 324.75

Table 23-2 Analysis of variance of table 23-1

Resources of variation	SS	V	MS	F	P
Between groups	12967.10	3	4322.36	12.85	<0.01
Within groups	11777.12	35	336.48		
Total	24744.22	38			

It can be noticed that thymuses of the cancer-bearing mice present the regular change from table 23-1, table 23-2 and chart 23-1. Within 7 days after inoculation, thymuses have no obvious change observed by eyes; however their weights begin to lose weight. After 7 days, they present acute progressive atrophy; in the later period, the diameter of the thymuses reduce from the normal level 5~8 mm to about 1mm and the weights decrease from 76.1mg to 20mg with the texture becoming hard and the functions declining even lost, which indicates that the cellular immune functions are operated and inhibited increasingly with the development of tumors, and the immune functions are declined to a lower level with tumors growing more and more rapidly.

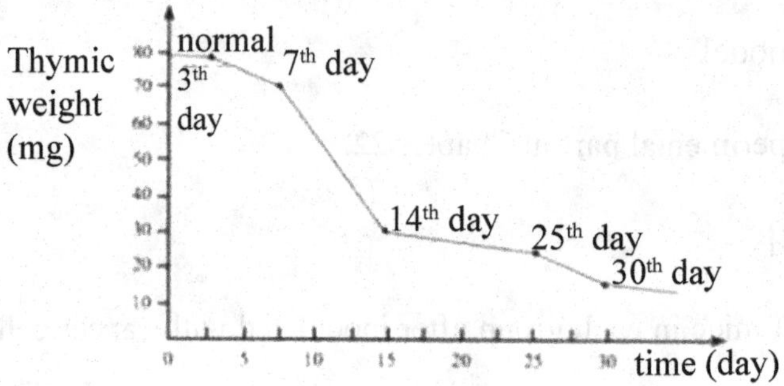

Chart 23-1 the curve of variation on the thymic weights

2. Splenic weights of mice in each group after inoculated with cancer cells in different phases (see table 23-3 and 23-4)

Table 23-3 splenic weights of cancer-bearing mice in each group in different phases

Group	Group I healthy	Group II on the 3rd after inoculated	Group III on the 7th after inoculated	Group VI on the 14th after inoculated		
	98.4	103.0	152.8	120.7		
	86.0	110.3	175.8	96.9		
	139.0	153.2	154.5	103.0		
	126.0	96.7	154.0	102.0		
	194.4	206.0	290.4	91.0		
X_i	130	137.0	156.0	122.3		
	107.4	174.0	184.0	88.6		
	82.8	143.0	232.0	109.0		
	86.0	160	86.3	102.4		
	82.0			119.0		
ΣX	1 258.4	1 209.0	1 720.9	1 021	ΣX	5 210.2
N_i	10	9	9	10	N	38
$\bar{X}_i$	125.84	134.43	172.09	102.1	$\bar{X}$	133.59
$\Sigma_i X^2$	169 020.88	175 088.97	322 834.65	106.41	ΣX^2	773.385

Table 23-4 Analysis of variance of table 23-3

Resources of variation	SS	V	MS	F	P
Between groups	25345.12	3	8448	5.68	<0.01
Within groups	51983	35	1485.24		
Total	77328.12	38			

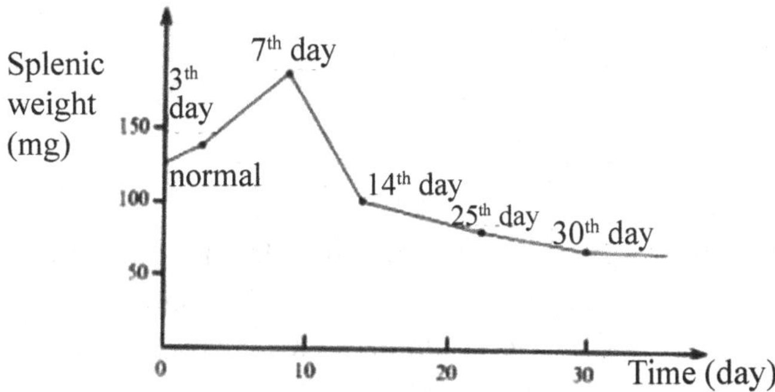

Chart 23-2 the curve of variation on the splenic weights

Inspect the 100 corpses in the experimental group in chapter 22 and get the average splenic weight is 60±12 mg. Use a curve to describe the change in splenic weights (chart 23-2).

From the statistical data in table 23-3, 23-4 and chart 23-2, it can be found that spleens of cancer—bearing mice in the early stage the volume is enlarging gradually and the weight is increasing, while in the later stage, the spleens present progressive atrophy. The above indicates that in the early period, cellular proliferation is active and the effects of immune response are reinforced as well as the inhibition on tumors due to the tumor simulation so as to react on inhibiting the growth of tumors; while in the latter period, as the number has enlarged plentifully, a great of inhibitory factors are produced to inhibit cells and immunity to stop the proliferation of splenic immune cells and consume effector cells, which results in atrophy and fabric tissue hyperplasia, the inhibition on tumors is weakened even promote the growth of tumors.

3. Comparison of experimental results of peripheral blood lymphocytes of the cancer-bearing mice conversion at different time (see table 23-5 and 23-6)

Table 23-5 Comparison of the conversion rate of peripheral blood lymphocytes in each group at different time (%)

Group I healthy	Group II on the 3rd after inoculated	Group III on the 7th after inoculated	Group VI on the 14th after inoculated
45	53	43	31
40	62	32	28
51	48	26	19
42	43	45	21
60	52	30	22
39	51	32	23
	50		

ΣX	277	359	208	144	ΣX	988
N_i	6	7	6	6	N	25
$\bar{X}_i$	46.17	51.29	24		$\bar{X}$	39.52
$\Sigma_i X$	13 111	18 611	7 498	3 560	ΣX^2	42 780

Table 23-6 Analysis of variance of table 23-5

Resources of variation	SS	V	MS	F	P
Between groups	2820.64	3	940.21	21.614	<0.01
Within groups	913.59	21	43.51		
Total	3734.23	24			

Using a curve to present the results of table23-5 and table 23-6, draw the curve of lymphocyte conversion rate of the cancer-bearing mice at different time (chart 23-3).

Chart 23-3 curve of lymphocyte conversion rate

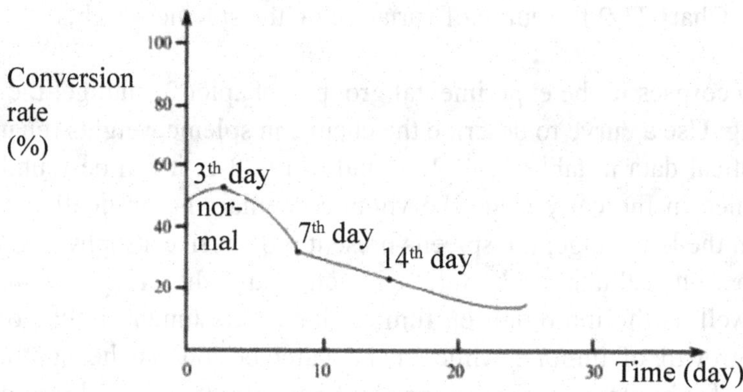

From table 23-5, 23-6 and chart 23-3, it can be seen that the change in lymphocyte conversion rate of the cancer-bearing mice presents certain regularity: after inoculation the conversion rate increase slightly and then presents an acute progressive decrease. Until 14th day (later period), it declines to normal level about 50% and continue declining after that, which indicates that in the whole course of diseases, tumors produce inhibitory effect on the cellular immunity; what's more, with the course of diseased this effect becomes more intensive and the immune functions are damaged.

From chart 23-1, 23-2 and 23-3 it can be known that the changes in thymic volume and weight are extremely similar to the curve of lymphocyte conversion rate presented as synchronism. By contrast, the changes in splenic volume and weight are different from them with increase in the early period and the decrease, which indicates that during the middle and later period, both the organismal humoral immunity and cellular immunity are damaged and inhibited.

4. Changes of thymic and splenic pathology
   (1) Thymus presents progressive atrophy during the whole course of disease; on the 3rd day after inoculated with cancer cells, thymus shrinks slightly and the color is gray; on the 7th day, thymic volume shrinks obviously and the cellular proliferation is stopped with reduced mature cells; during the later period of tumors, thymus shrinks extremely and its volume is as big as a sesame with the diameter of 1 mm and hard texture.
   (2) Spleen is congested and tumefied; the volume is augmenting with being black red and crisp. The number of germinal centers increase and mature decrease; while from the 14th day after inoculation, spleen also presents progressive atrophy.

CHAPTER 24

Experimental Study On Treatment Of Malignant Tumor By Adoptive Immunologic Reconstitution Through Combined Transplantation Of Fetal Cells

I. Experiment on Adoptive Immunologic Reconstitution of Fetal Liver, Spleen and Thymus Cells through Combined Transplantation

In this paper, the author introduces the experiment on the systematic adoptive immunologic reconstitution with the mice bearing Ehrlich ascites cancer (EAC) subcutaneous solid tumor through combined transplantation using the same kind of fetal liver, spleen and thymus cells. In this experiment, set up groups of monomial transplantations of fetal liver, spleen and thymus respectively; the groups of bigeminal transplantation of fetal liver and spleen cells, fetal liver and thymus cells as well as fetal spleen and thymus cells, and then observe the time of the growth, regression and survival, index of cellular immunity as well as all items of pathological examination in each group respectively; compare the curative effects of each groups. The research results show that the curative effect of trigeminal group is better than that of the bigeminal group which is better than the individual groups in turn. For the experimental group of trigeminal cell transplantation, the complete regression rates of the tumor in near and forward future are 40% (n=15) and 46.67% (n=15) respectively, and the partial regression rates (the percentage of the tumor regression is more than 50%) are 26.67% and 13.33% respectively. Those whose tumors regress completely can survive for a long time and the lifetimes of those whose tumors regress partially are prolonged for more than a month on average, and their immune index improves obviously and the immune organs are of hypertrophy. The sections of immune organ tissue reveal the active cell proliferation. Moreover, the pathological sections of tumor tissue show that a large amount of lymphocytes soak around the tumor tissue and in stroma, and then form parcel; flaky concretion, liquefaction necrosis, karyorrhexis and other pathologic phenomena emerge in the central tumor tissue. For the experimental groups of bigeminal cell transplantation, except a few cases of partial regression, there is no complete one. All the improvement of the immune indexes, the prolonged lifetime, and the soakage of lymphocytes in tumor tissue are less obvious than those of the experimental trigeminal group. As to monomial groups of cell transplantation, the results of regression, lifetime and immune indexes as well as the pathological examination results are less apparent than the former two groups, but better than the control group of the tumor-bearing mice. It can be implied that compared with partial reconstitution, systematic adoptive immunologic reconstitution can develop the anti-carcinomatous immunologic function and improve the curative effects though overall systematic synergism.

Thanks to the theory of biological response modifier (BRM), treatment of tumor has been experiencing a profound reform. The fourth generation of the modality of tumor therapy, biological treatment of tumor has become the focus in the field of tumor therapy after surgeons, chemotherapy and radiotherapy. According to a large number of clinical and experimental researches, it can be found that the organismal immune state exhibits progressive inhibition with the evolution of the stadium. Therefore, how to restore and reconstitute the anti-carcinomatous immunologic function is the core of the research of tumor biological treatment. The adoptive immunotherapy developed by Rosenberg who is the representative has got outstanding achievement in this field. Except transferring the active factors amplified in vitro and various kinds of artificial immunologic factors, fetal immune organs and cell transplantation are promising researches. Although the technique of biotherapy is expensive, it possesses several advantages like economy, convenient technique and easy popularization in that the sources of embryo are broad in China, which is worthy of thorough research and exploration. In recent years, many scholars at home have developed the research on transplantation of fetal liver, spleen and thymus from the level of cells to tissue and then to the level of organs for curing advanced malignant tumors and they have achieved some curative effects. The thorough researches can explain the source, proliferation, differentiation and the function of lymphocytes as well as the function and effects of reconstituting immune organs and peripheral immune organs clearly. Currently, in many cases of adoptive immunologic treatment with transplanting fetal immune organs, only single fetal organs is utilized, cell transplantation of fetal liver, spleen and thymus cells as well as tissue transplantation, etc. there is no similar literature or reports on the question that it is possible to carry out adoptive reconstitution systematically and integrally. The combined transplantation of fetal liver, spleen and thymus cells, in which the transplantation of fetal liver cells has analogous function of marrow transplantation and is combined with the transplantation of fetal thymus and spleen cells, can make the adoptive reconstitution approach to the systematical and integral level. But it is worthy of researches and exploration that whether it can bring synergism into play and improve curative effects.

[Material and Methods]

1. Animals and tumor model
   (1) Experimental animals: 200 cross bred Kunming mice in closed flock, 5 to 6 weeks old, 18±2.1g in weight, no gender limitation.
   (2) Facilities for model of planting tumors: prepare mice of ascitic type after the anabiosis of the root of Ehrlich ascites tumor; when the ascites are formed, draw out the ascites of the cancer cells and centrifuge washing with Hank for three times(800r/min), five minutes for one time; remove the supernatant liquid, then dilute the liquid with the precipitated cancer cells to the concentration of 10^7/ml; use eosin exclusion teat to verify that the percentage of living cells is above 95%; inoculate the experimental mice under the skin of the right hollow viscera, 1ml for each mouse; after a week, all the mice have tumor nodes with the diameter of 9.5±1.5mm in the point of inoculation to make the subcutaneous solid tumor model bearing Ehrlich Ascites tumor.
2. Grouping
   Group the experimental animals with random into control group bearing tumors (Group B, n=9), observation group for combined transplantation of fetal liver, spleen and thymus cells in forward future (Group CI, n=15), observation group in near future (Group CII, n=15, carry on combined transplantation to this group once a week for successive 5 weeks and then execute the mice), treatment group with transplantation of fetal liver cells

(Group F), treatment group with transplantation of fetal spleen cells (Group G), treatment group with transplantation of fetal thymus cells (Group H), treatment group with combined transplantation of fetal liver and spleen cells (Group I), treatment group with combined transplantation of fetal liver and thymus cells (Group K), $n_F=n_G=n_H=n_I=n_J=n_{K=}$ 12. When the model is prepared, carry out correspondent cell transplantation once a week for each group respectively for five times in a row. As to the control group, use Hank as comparison.

3. Preparing of the suspension of fetal liver, spleen and thymus

   Use the female mice that copulate naturally by stages and have been pregnant for 15 to 18 days; paunch them aseptically to take out the fetal mouse, liver, spleen and thymus; rinse them through the Hank individually under 4℃, then individually mix them with aseptic homogenate to the full; dilute the mixture with Hank under 4℃ and filter them to collect the suspension with adequate cells; Sample the suspension and do bacterial culture and pyrogen experiment; if the experimental results are negative, divide them and package as standby.

4. The approach and method for cell transplantation
   (1) Transplantation of fetal liver cells: use the prepared suspension of fetal liver cells for caudal vein injection, 0.2ml for each mouse at a time.
   (2) Transplantation of fetal spleen cells: use the prepared suspension of fetal spleen cells for intraperitoneal injection, 0.2ml for each mouse at a time.
   (3) Transplantation of fetal thymus cells: use the prepared suspension of fetal thymus cells for intramuscular injection in the back leg, 0.2ml for each mouse at a time.

   The treatments for the experimental mice mentioned above begin after a week from cancer cell inoculation, once a week for successive five weeks. As to the control group, use the same amount of Hank as comparison.

5. Observation item
   (1) General items: after cancer cell inoculation, observe the time when tumor emerges; measure the size of the tumor nude with a vernier caliper every two days (the average vertical diameter, mm), the quality of life, the situation of the tumors and the lifetime (d).
   (2) Dynamic observation on T cells in peripheral blood: in this experiment, use Alpha Naphthyl Acetate Esterase (ANAE) staining method to take count of the T cells in peripheral blood. Prepare six pairs of nitrogen magenta solution and 2% ANAE solution respectively, store them in the shade under 4℃; before using the prepared solution, add 89ml, 1/15mol/L, pH=7.6 phosphate buffer into the 6ml nitrogen magenta solution gradually and mix up fully, then add 2.5ml, 2% ANAE solution gradually, then mix up to the full. The final sample is amber with pH being 6.4 as solution for incubation. Put this into the water bath of 37℃ for warm-up. Cut the tip of the mouse's tail, and get the section. After the section has dried by natural wind, soak it into the solution for incubation for 1 to 3 hours, then wash it clear by tap water and air it. Use 1% methyl green to dye for 1 to 3 minutes, wash with tap water. After airing, observe the section under microscope. There are black red granules, namely ANAE positive cells in different size and quantity (the amount generally is 2 to 5). Count 200 lymphocytes and then calculate the percentage of T lymphocytes. Observe the percentage dynamically

after a week from having built the model and from treatment respectively and measure it every two weeks.

(3) Dynamic observation on the conversion rate of lymphocytes: Measure the conversion rate with the morphologic method of microdose whole blood culture in vitro. Prepare RPMI 1640 complete medium (1640 is the product of Japanese Juchheim, containing 10.4g dry powder in each bag), which consists of 1ml, 20%, 30.0g/L L—glutamine of killed calf blood serum, 3ml 60.0g/L aseptic $NaHCO_3$, 10000U penicillin and 10000μg streptomycin. Sanitize the tail strictly and cut the tip for 0.2mm; collect blood aseptically for 0.1ml with heparinization microdose sampler; add 1.8ml complete medium and then o, 1ml PHA; cultivate the sample in the water-jacket incubator under constant temperature of 37℃ for 72 hours and stir it once a day. After the cultivation, draw most of the supernatant liquid out and add 4ml 8.5g/L NH_4Cl to mix up; place the mixture in the water-bath of 37℃ for 10 minutes, then centrifugalize it in 2500r/min, discard the supernatant liquid; Add 5ml fixation fluid (9 units of methanol and an unit of glacialaceticacid; place the sample under ambient temperature for 10 minutes and centrifugalize it in 1500r/min for 5 minutes, discard the supernatant liquid and reserve the precipitate. Add Hank to the precipitate to the volume of 0.2ml, mix the precipitate and Hank and drop on a clean glass to stretch uniformly. After natural airing, dye it with Giemsa for 5 minutes, then wash with tap water. After drying, observe 200 lymphocytes under the microscope and calculate the percentage of the conversion rate of the metrocyte. As same as T cells, observe the percentage dynamically after a week from having built the model and from treatment respectively and measure it every two weeks.

(4) Measuring the green weights of immune organs: do comprehensive autopsy in detail for each dead or the executed mouse, cut the thymus and spleen and observe their sizes, then weight them with a torsion balance; calculate the ratio of the green weight of the immune organs to the body weight for each mouse.

(5) Pathological examination: do systematic pathological autopsy to each dead and the executed mouse, observe the tumor soakage and tumor metastasis; reserve tumor tissue, thymus, spleen, lung, liver, kidney, etc. for tissue pathological section ant attach importance to observe the lymphocyte soakage in tumor tissue and the pathologic changes in the immune organs.

[Experimental Results]

1. Comparison of the average lifetime of the mouse in each group (geometrical average) and the persistence in different ages of tumors

According to Table24-1, the lifetimes of all treatment groups are prolonged obviously compared with the control group with P being less than 0.05. Especially, the effect of the treatment group of trigeminal cell transplantation is most obvious, with P being less than 0.01. Other treatment groups have significant difference compared with the trigeminal treatment group with P being less than 0.5. In Group CI, the tumors in 7 cases regress completely, which gain a long-term survival and no tumor relapse. The rate of tumor regression in 2 cases is more than 50%, in which the two mice survive for 2 months and die of tumor relapse. Regarding the persistence in different ages of tumor, in the third week after bearing tumor, all treatment groups have significant differences compared with the control group. With the extent of the stadium and observation period, compared with the control group, Group CI shows notable differential all along, but other treatment groups lose the difference from the control group gradually and show the significant difference from that of Group CI.

Table 24-1 comparison of the average lifetime of the mouse in each group and the persistence in different ages of tumors

Group	N	Lifetime(d) $\overline{X}$+S	The persistence in different ages of tumor							
			1week	2week	3week	4week	5week	6week	2weeks	3months
GroupB	9	13.3±1.2	100	55.6	11.1	11.1	0	0	0	0
GroupF	12	22.5±1.6△*	100	83.3	58.3*	50	33.3	33.3	0△	0△
GroupG	12	21.4±1.9△*	100	75	75*	50	33.3	16.7△	0△	0△
GroupH	12	26.2±1.4△*	100	100	100*	58.3*	41.7	33.3	0△	0△
GroupI	12	27.4±1.7△*	100	91.7	91.7*	50	33.3	33.3	8.3△	0△
GroupJ	12	28.3±1.8△*	100	83.3	83.3*	66.7*	41.7	41.7	16.7	0△
GroupK	12	23.5±1.5△*	100	100	100*	58.3*	33.3	25	16.7	0△
Group CI	15	47.2±2.0**	100	93.3	93.3*	73.3*	66.7*	60*	46.7*	46.7*

Note: ①in Table 24-1, Group B is the control one bearing cancer; Group F is the treatment group with fetal liver cells; Group G is the treatment group with fetal spleen cells; Group H is the treatment group with fetal thymus cells; Group I is the group of combined treatment of fetal liver and spleen cells; Group J is the group of combined treatment of fetal liver and thymus cells; Group K is the group of combined treatment of fetal spleen and thymus cells; Group CI is the group of combined treatment of fetal liver, spleen and thymus cells; ②*means that comparing the each treatment groups with the control group, $P < 0.05$; **means $P < 0.01$; △ means comparing the treatment groups with Group CI, $P < 0.01$.

2. The curative effect and the analysis on the effect

Table 24-2 the analysis on the curative effect

Group	N	Curative rate	The rate of apparent effect	Effective rate	Rate of inefficiency	Total effective rate
GroupB	9	0△△	0	0	100	0
GroupF	12	0△△	0	34.4(4)	66.4(8)	33.4(4)△△
GroupG	12	0△△	0	25(3)	75(9)	25(3)△△
GroupH	12	0△△	8.3(1)	33.4(4)	58.3(7)	41.7(5)△*
GroupI	12	0△△	8.3(1)	33.4(4)	58.3(7)	41.7(5)△*
GroupJ	12	0△△	26.67(2)	41.7(5)	41.7(5)	58.3(7)*
GroupK	12	0△△	26.67(2)	33.4(4)	50(6)	50(6)*
GroupCI	15	46.7**	13.3(2)	20(3)	20(3)	80(12)**

Note: *means P <0.05 compared with the control group, ** means P <0.01 compared with the control group; △ means P <0.05 compared with Group CI, △△ means P <0.01 compared with Group CI

The standards of curative effects:

① Cure: The tumors regress completely, the suffers regain long-term survival without relapse;

② Apparent effects: The tumors regress partially (the regression rate is more than 50%), and the survival time is more than 2 months;

③ Being effective: The lifetime is prolonged for more than one time without obvious tumor regression.

④ Inefficiency: The tumors grow progressively leading to death in short term (3 to 4 weeks).

According to Table 24-2, the curative effect of Group CI reaches 46.67%, and is obviously different from other groups with P <0.01. There is no obvious difference among each group as to the rates of apparent effect and being effective respectively. The comparison of the total effective rate shows that except the treatment groups of unitary fetal liver or spleen cells, the total effective rate of all other treatment groups have visible distinction from the control group, with their curative effects being in the rank that the trigeminal is better than the bigeminal which is above the monomial. Moreover, in the groups of monomial cell transplantation, the curative effect of TH cells treatment group is the best, and in the groups of bigeminal cell transplantation, the curative effect of the group containing TH cells is better than that of the groups without TH cells, which indicates that thymus cells play an important role in the course of treatment, but sole liver or spleen cell transplantation have little effects. However, if two of liver, spleen or thymus cells are combined, the curative effect can be improved. And the combination of the three can improve the curative effect significantly.

3. Observing and comparing the growth rate of tumors, the regression and prognosis

In this experiment, the mimic clinical method is used to file case history for all the experimental mice in each groups to record their growth rate of tumors, regression and the prognosis. Measure the average vertical diameter every two days. For the cases of death, all the terminal measured values are regarded as effective sample parameter in the following measures within the same group. After a week from the establishment of the model, tumors grow rapidly with the average vertical diameter being 9.5±1.5mm. After a week from beginning the treatment, tumors continue to grow. Until the second week, the results of each group become differential that the mice bearing tumors have progressive exhaustion with the tumors growing rapidly in the control group; within four weeks, all mice are dead. In the group of sole cell transplantation, the life quality of the experimental mice are improved apparently with their tumors growing slowly, but all the mice bearing cancer die within two months. In the groups of bigeminal cell transplantation, the growths of the tumors are inhibited obviously. Five cases have partial regression but all the mice die with three months. In the group of trigeminal cell transplantation, there are nine cases with apparent tumor putrescence, fall off and ulcer, then scab. In other seven cases, the tumors regress completely, and then canker, scab. In two cases, the regression rate of tumors is more than 50%. As to other cases, except the mice in two cases die in the second and the third week respectively, tumors in the residual cases are in dead state until the death from exhaustion. The sufferers whose tumors regress completely regain long-term survival without relapse for more than six months, and they have normal capacities to become pregnant and give birth. From the above observation, it can be found that the sole or bigeminal cell transplantation is able to inhibit the growth of tumors, improve the life quality and prolong the lifetime; the trigeminal cell transplantation can not only inhibit the growth of tumors, but also result in apparent complete or partial regression and prolong the lifetime.

4. Dynamic observation on the number of T lymphocytes in peripheral blood and the conversion rate of lymphocytes

From table 24-3 and 24-4, after a week from the establishment of the model, the cellular immune indexes of the experimental groups decline obviously with the average decrease being more than 50% compared with that of the control group (the number of T cells in the normal group X is 62.5±1.7 and that of lymphocyte transformed X is 66.8±4.8), indicating that the development of tumors does inhibit immune function. After a week from beginning treatment, all immune indexes are improved ($P < 0.05$) and there are no apparent differential among all treatment groups from the comparison between the treatment groups and the control group as well as the comparison of the indexes before and after the treatment. Seen from the growth of tumors, the immune indexes are improves, but the inhibition of tumors is not apparent. The continuous dynamic observation shows in the groups of sole and bigeminal cell transplantation, the inhibition of tumors and the improvement of immune indexes last for a certain period (3 to 4 weeks), after that period the immune indexes tent to decline, so that the state of the mice bearing cancer deteriorates, which is consistent with the reports on the clinical monitor of immunologic functionand the prognosis. In the group of trigeminal cell transplantation, the immune indexes have persistent improvement, especially the tumors regress obviously. For those who regain long-term survival, the above indexes measured two months later are still close to the indexes of normal mouse. By contrast, for those suffering deterioration, the indexes measured before their deaths have declined below the level before treatment. The above indicates that the cellular immune indexes do reflect the curative effects and can be regarded as a good prove for prognosis; at the same time it can indirectly prove that immunocyte transplantation is able to achieve the aim of immunologic reconstitution for cancer-bearing organisms.

Table 24-3 dynamic observation on the number of T lymphocytes in peripheral blood (ANAE)

Group	N	The number of T lymphocytes ($\overline{X}$±S)							
		n	1 week	n	2 weeks	n	4 weeks	n	6 weeks
GroupB	9	9	3.42±4.8	5	29.1±2.9	1	32	0	
GroupF	12	12	31.4±3.6	10	54.6±5.12△*	6	48.7±2.2△	4	36.7±4.9
GroupG	12	12	35.5±3.9	9	52.5±4.7△*	6	46.6±3.3*	2	33.4±5.1
GroupH	12	12	32.6±4.1	12	56.6±4.1△*	7	50.9±2.1△	4	40.7±3.8△
GroupI	12	12	36.2±2.7	11	53.4±3.5△*	6	55.3±3.6△	4	39.3±4.2△
GroupJ	12	12	30.8±4.3	10	55.8±3.8△*	8	56.4±1.9△	5	42.6±2.7△
GroupK	12	12	33.7±3.4	12	57.3±4.4△*	7	55.8±2.8△	3	41.3±4.5△

GroupCI	15	15	31.8±3.1	14	59.6±2.6△*	11	62.5±1.7△	9	67.8±3.4△

Note: * means P<0.05 compared with the control group; △ means P<0.05 in the comparison before and after the treatment

Table 24-4 the dynamic observation of the conversion rate of the lymphocytes in peripheral blood

Group	N	The conversion rate of lymphocytes ($\overline{X}$±S)							
		n	1 week	n	2 weeks	n	4 weeks	n	6 weeks
GroupB	9	9	3.25±5.4	5	25.51±3.6	1	28	0	
GroupF	12	12	31.6±3.7	10	51.2±2.7△*	6	54.2±6.1△	4	36.1±5.4
GroupG	12	12	29.8±4.3	9	48.4±4.6△*	6	52.8±1.8*	2	33.5±2.5
GroupH	12	12	34.1±4.1	12	56.5±2.1△*	7	52.4±3.7△	4	40.7±1.9△
GroupI	12	12	28.5±5.1	11	53.4±3.5△*	6	50.5±2.9△	4	37.3±3.2△
GroupJ	12	12	29.4±2.9	10	58.1±3.5△*	8	60.6±3.4△	5	46.5±4.5△
GroupK	12	12	30.7±1.8	12	54.9±5.2△*	7	57.5±4.3△	3	45.8±3.9△
GroupCI	15	15	31.5±3.2	14	55.8±2.8△*	11	63.9±3.2△	9	66.8±4.8△

Note: * means P<0.05 compared with the control group; △ means P<0.05 in the comparison before and after the treatment

5. Anatomic observation of immune organ and comparative analysis of immune organ's green weight

The observation results are seen in table 24-5 and table 24-6. In this experiment, in order to see the changes in immune organs of cancer-bearing organisms and the relevance to the curative effects, another near-future observation group of trigeminal cell transplantation is set up (Group CII, n=15, the tumors in six cases regress completely and the regression rates in four cases are more than 50%). After building the model, give the treatment to the mice in Group CII for five times and then execute them. At the same time, set a normal group for comparison, using Hank to simulate the model and execute the mice in the sixth week. Anatomize the mice and observe the changes in their immune organs; measure the green weight of the immune organs and calculate the ratio of immune organs to the body weight; compare the values in Group CII with those of the other groups. From the results, it can be found that in all the cases that in all experimental groups, the tumors develop progressively and lead to death, the thymus shrink apparently and the degree of atrophy is relevant positively to the tumor development. The atrophied thymus is dull-colored and of crisp texture. As to spleen, its change is not as obvious as that of the thymus. In most cases, the spleens are congested and swelling. Only in a few cases the spleens are atrophied. However, in Group CII in all the cases that the tumors regress completely and partially, the thymus and spleens are hypertrophied, so as the indexes of thymus and spleen increase. Through statistical disposition, these indexes are not only differential apparently from the death cases in each group (or the cases without tumor regression), but also different from the normal control group.

Table 24-5 the comparison of the green weight of the immune organs between the death cases and the normal control group.

Group	N	Thymus(mg)/body weight(g) $\overline{X}\pm S$	spleen(mg)/body weight(g) $\overline{X}\pm S$
Normal	10	2.97±0.38	3.80±0.23
Group B	9	1.02±0.32**	4.01±1.32
Group F	8	1.21±0.41**	4.213±0.87
Group G	10	1.18±0.46**	4.45±1.63
Group H	8	1.28±0.25**	4.47±1.24
Group I	8	1.34±0.43**	4.67±0.48
Group J	7	1.47±0.28**	4.56±0.62
Group J	9	1.43±0.35**	4.89±1.47
Group CII	5	1.96±0.37**	5.12±1.56

Note: * means P＜0.05 compared with the control group; ** means P＜0.01 compared with the normal control group

Table 24-6 the comparison of the green weight between the cases of complete or partial tumor regression and the cases without apparent regression in Group CII

Immune organ(mg/g)	Normal group (N=10, $\overline{X}\pm S$)	Group with tumor regression (N=10, $\overline{X}\pm S$)	Group without tumor regression (N=10, $\overline{X}\pm S$)
thymus	2.79±0.38	4.65±2.21**△△	1.96±0.37
spleen	3.80±0.23	10.15±2.29**△△	5.12±1.56

Note: ** means P＜0.01 compared with the normal control group; △△means P＜0.01 in the comparison between the group with tumor regression and the group without tumor regression.

6. The comparison of pathological examination

In this experiment, anatomize the mice in each group and observe the pathologic section. Observe the tumor soakage and metastasis as well as the changes in immune organs like thymus, spleen, etc. Reserve the viscera like tumor tissue, lung, kidney, thymus and spleen as tissue pathological section for observation. The results show that with the course developing, the range of local tumor soakage expends and the tumor becomes hypertrophied without apparent remote organ metastasis. The thymus shrinks obviously, which has positive relevance to the evolution of the tumor. As to the spleen, it is congested and swelling. In the near-future observation group of trigeminal cell transplantation, the thymus, spleen and liver in the cases of complete or apparent partial regression do not become hypertrophied obviously, which exhibits significant differences from the normal group. When the mice in the cases of complete regression are anatomized, no residual cancer cells can be found in the part of tumor inoculation with both naked eyes and microscope. At the 3rd or 4th week when the tumor putrescence is the most apparent, reserve the tumor tissue as pathological section for observation. It can be found that there are large amount of lymphocytes soakage around the tumor tissue and in the stroma which wrap the tumor tissue resulting a wide range of tumor cells are liquefied and solidified to be dead. The sections of immune organs show that the thickness of the thymus cortical area and the denseness of lymphocytes as well as the increase in epithelial reticular cell, phagocytotic phenomenon and thymus corpuscles. In the spleen, the white pulp area enlarges and the lymph nodes increases, also the lymphocytes become dense. In the control group, the sections of tumor tissue show that the tumor cells soak into the deep-layered muscular tissue and there are cancer embolus formed by tumor cell transplantation in the blood vessels but no lymphocytes soakage. As to the thymus, the cortex atrophy and the cells are sparse, the blood vessels are congested. In the spleen, the amount of lymphocytes decreases significantly and the cells are sparse. In other treatment groups, the tumor sections show that the boundary of the tumor are clear with a little lymphocyte soakage and the changes in thymus and spleen is between the group of trigeminal cell transplantation and the control group. Moreover, the arrangement of the cells is dense with light atrophy.

[Discussion]

1. Therapeutic evaluation

It can be found from the results of the above experiment that the adoptive immunological therapy through transplantation of immunocyte with the origin of embryo can inhibit the growth of tumor and improve the life quality in different extend and force the tumor to regress completely or partially, and then improve the immune indexes apparently and prolong the lifetime, which indicates that immunocyte transplantation with the origin of embryo can reconstitute the anti-carcinomatous immunologic functionfor cancer-bearing organisms. The combined reconstitution of central immunity and the peripheral immunity at the same time is the best and better than the partial reconstitution of bigeminal and monomial cell transplantation.

2. Possible mechanism

The possible mechanisms to take effect are mainly the following: ①After the cancer-bearing organisms accept the same kind of xenogenous embryo cell transplantation, the immune system of the organism gets non-specific simulation to produce immune hyperplasia so as to improve the immunologic function to resist tumors. ②Cell transplantation belongs to organ transplantation, which can keep active for a certain period of time in the acceptor. By immunocyte transplantation with the origin of embryo, fetal liver cells can provide stem lymphocytes, which is combined with thymus and spleen cell transplantation so as to achieve the combined reconstitution of central immunity and peripheral immunity and enable the organism to gain adoptive immunity. A large number of researches home and abroad on the proliferation, differentiation and function of fetal immune organs and histiocytes show that when fetal immune organs are in their 16 weeks, they put up obvious proliferation to the original simulation of division, which becomes more intensive in the 24th week. In the 8th week of pregnancy, lymph tissue begins to emerge in the fetal thymus and lymph nodes as well as the cells with secretion in the 20th week. All these researches indicate that fetal immunocytes are able to bring immunoreaction into play. ③Some researches show that both the supernatant liquid from fetal thymus tissue cultivated outside the body and thymus extractive have the ability to promote the formation rate of the acceptor's E—wreath and the transformation of lymphocytes obviously. Therefore, fetal immunocyte transplantation can strengthen the cellular immunity of the cancer-bearing organism for cancer-bearing organism. ④ low immunogen of the fetal organs and the homology between the transplanted fetal organs and the acceptor's immune organs are in favor of forming immunologic tolerance to the transplanted for the acceptor, which can not only avoid rejection or have light rejection, but also simulate each other to achieve synergetic effects so as to reconstitute immunity. Moreover, as the curative effects of the trigeminal cell transplantation group are much better than those of the other groups, it is be believed that the effects result from the relatively complete reconstitution of central immunity and peripheral immunity at the same time which lead to the synergetic effects. In a word, the mechanism is much more complex than the above mentioned. It will be useful to step further to make the mechanism clear if the level of the immune factors that are closely relevant to anti-tumor immunity like IL-2, TNF, INF, etc. and the activity of the immunocytes that relate directly to anti-tumor immunity like NK, LAK, TIL, etc. in peripheral blood can be detected and the transplanted cells can be marked to make clear their distribution and survival inside the acceptor.

1. Problems about the barrier of transplantation

   Although fetal organs have low immunogen, it is still impossible to avoid rejection, just in different degree. Therefore, the problem about the barrier of transplantation exists and directly relate to the success of transplantation and that whether the transplant can continue to act inside the acceptor. In this experiment, the animals used belong to the hybrid species in closed flock, which ensures largely that the mice in each experimental group have relatively close genetic background. It is probably the important reason for the success of transplantation with tissue matching except the low immunogen of embryonic tissue. Apart from those, it is possible that the mismatch of histocompatibility leads to the cases with inconspicuous curative effects in Group CI and Group CII. Thus, the key of improving curative effects may lie in studying and solving the barrier of transplantation.

2. The choice of the approach and method of transplantation

   The transplantations of fetal immune organs from the level of cells, to tissue, then to the level of entire organ belong to adoptive immunity. In terms of the current repots, for fetal liver and spleen, blood cell transplantation is the best; for thymus, spleen and tissue, omentum embedding is the best. Although the technique of cell transplantation is simple and easy to be successful, it can only last for a short time. Therefore, the best approach of transplantation needs further observation and research.

II. Progress of Study on Treatment of Tumor by Adoptive Immunity through Transplantation of Immunocyte with the Origin of Embryo

According to a large amount of clinical and experimental researches, the immunity of the tumor-bearing organisms tent to be in progressive inhibition with the course the disease. So how to reconstitute the anti-tumor immunity is the core of the research on immunological therapy. In 1980s, the fourth generation of tumor treatment mode, namely biological treatment of tumor, brought tumor therapeutics into a new era, when the adoptive immunotherapy was the most outstanding achievement. For those whose tumors were in the advanced stage, several kinds of the conventional therapies were of no effects. However, adoptive immunotherapy of LAK, TIL and gene-modified TIL, which is represented by Rosenberg gained prominent curative effects, attracting the attention all over the world. In this technique, it is needed to gain a great amount of artificial synthesized IL-2 with high purity by biotechnology and plentiful immune competent cells through cultivate and proliferation in vitro in a long term to reach the aim, so the cost was very expensive. Currently, this project is still in depth research. As only a few institutes at home have developed the research in this area, there is no doubt that the above mentioned therapy is an extremely prominent research direction in treatment of tumor, however it is some difficult to become popularized in China. Besides, treatment of tumor by adoptive immunity through transplantation of immune cells, tissue and organs with the origin of embryo is another prominent research in the treatment of tumor by adoptive immunity, which is featured by simple technique, low cost and popularity. In recent years, some researchers have used embryonic liver, spleen and thymus to do transplantation from the level of cellular tissue to organs with vessel pedicles, which has been applied in the treatment of advanced malignant tumor gaining some curative effects, and paid much attention gradually.

i. Research status of fetal liver cell transplantation (FLT)

In 1958, Uphoff was the first one to fetal liver cells into the mice who died from ray of fatal dose with the remarkable effects of regaining hematopiesis. From then on, that fetal cell transplantation can be applied in curing the diseases in hemopoietic system and in the therapy of regaining hematopiesis after chemotherapy and radiotherapy for those with malignant tumors is researched extensively. In the following researches it has been found that FLT can not only reconstitute hematopiesis, but also reconstitute immunity. Wu Zuze and other researchers have found that FLT is able to reconstitute T and B lmphyocytes. They have also found that founder cells in fetal liver and spleen nodes are possessed with the basic features of several kinds of hematopoietic stem cells or lymph myeloid stem cells through the comparative research on the proliferation and differentiation between fetal liver cells and myeloid hematopoietic stem cell. Fetal liver cells contain a small amount of macrophages and lymphocytes. After 5 months from being pregnant, the amount of T lymphocytes begins to increase gradually, which is thought to be the substantial foundation of applying FLT to cure hematopoietic disorders immunologic deficiency disease to reconstitute hematopiesis and immunity. These features of fetal liver cells, especially the ability to reconstitute immunity make FLT play an important role in improving immunity. In recent years, there have been more and more researches on applying FLT to treatment of tumor.

ii. Research status of treatment of tumor through fetal spleen cell transplantation

1. Research on the relationship between spleen and the growth of tumor

   It has been thirty years since Old and others began to study the influence of spleen to the growth of tumor. During this period, many scholars have done a large number of experiments and clinical researches on the effect of spleen in anti-tumor immunity, but they can not get a consistent conclusion as they hold that spleen has both positive and negative effects on anti-tumor immunity. With more deep researches on splenic surgery and its function, most scholars tent to confirm the anti-tumor immune function. As spleen is the biggest immune organ in bodies, it is the place where Th and Ts cells become mature. The antibodies, Fibronetin, Tufftsinr-1NF and IL-2, etc. immune factors secreted by Th and Ts cells as well as killer cells like LAK and NK, etc. play an crucial role in anti-tumor immunity. Ge Yigong, etc. have found when researching the effect of ablating spleen to the growth of W256 rat's sarcoma that in the group of spleen ablation, the survival rate of the tumor inoculation and the diameter of tumor are higher apparently than those of the control group. Meanwhile, in the former group, the postoperative changes of T cell subgroup in peripheral blood are manifested by the reduction in T and Th cells and slight increase in Ts cells which is on the low level continuously after inoculation and have remarkable differential from the group without tumor and the tumor-bearing control group($P < 0.001$). That is consistent with the research on the effects of spleen to the growth of tumor that was done before. They have also found that after ablating spleen, there was positive correlation between the decline in the ratio of Th/Ts in T cell subgroup and the diffuse and metastasis of tumor. Lersch has reported that lymphocytes inside the spleen of tumor-bearing mice decline progressively with the growth of tumor, which is consistent with the experimental results mentioned above. All these researches can indicate that spleen plays an important role in anti-tumor immunity.

2. Researches on treatment of tumor through fetal spleen cell transplantation

   Based on the understanding of the action of spleen in anti-tumor immunity, many scholars have begun to develop the experimental and clinical researches on treatment of tumor through fetal spleen cell or tissue transplantation. Ma Xuxian, etc. report that fetal spleen cell transplantation has been used in nine cases of advanced malignant tumor. All sufferers in these cases feel better after the treatment. The author also has found that fetal spleen cell transplantation can inhibit the growth of tumor apparently when studying the effects of spleen to the growth of tumor. What's more, some scholar has studied the feature and approach of fetal spleen transplantation and found that transplantation through vein is the best, intramuscular injection and celiac injection follow. For tissue transplantation, omentum embedding is the best; both HVGR and GVHR are few. The mechanism of spleen cell transplantation is still in research.

iii. Research status of treatment of tumor through fetal thymus transplantation

Among immune organs, thymus has the closest relation to anti-tumor immunity and the researches on thymus are the most profound. Thymus plays a decisive role in cellular immunity and even the entire immunoregulation as thymus is the central immune organ where T cells develop and grow up.

1. Research on the relationship between thymus and the growth of tumor

   The function of thymus has close connection with the occurrence of tumor that can lead to thymus atrophy, low level of thymosin or lack of analogous thymic factor. For those experimental animals, that the thymus are ablated or irradiated by dead dose ray can promote the tumor metastasis. Therefore, fetal thymus transplantation or thymic epithelial cell transplantation as well as injection of thymosin can put off thymus atrophy and reconstitute immune function. The above researches indicate that thymus plays an extremely important role in anti-tumor immunity.

2. The application of fetal thymus transplantation in treatment of tumor

   Many scholars have done plentiful researches on treatment of tumor through fetal thymus transplantation. Zhou Shifu, etc. have performed the treatment of tumor through fetal thymus transplantation for 14 tumor cases. After 46 hours, the immune indexes have been improved and the conditions of the sufferers have been remitted and improved. Song Ruze, etc. have used the treatment of advanced malignant tumor through fetal thymus tissue omentum transplantation and gained the same curative effects. Liu Dungui, etc. have used cell transplantation, tissue transplantation and transplantation of thymus with vessel pedicle to treat advanced liver cancer resulting in that tumors in some cases shrunk significantly and the lifetime was prolonged for six months. All these can indicate that fetal thymus transplantation is an effective approach of immunotherapy of tumor.

Moreover, some scholars have studied on the features of the immune organs in different ages with the origin of embryo like the activity and the saving time, etc. They have found that the activity of fetal organs after five months' pregnancy is best. The researches on the approach of transplantation show that fetal liver and spleen cell transplantation through vein is the best, and omentum embedding is best for spleen and thymus tissue transplantation.

All these researches provide precious theoretic and experimental basis for treatment of tumor by adoptive immunity through immune organ transplantation with the origin of embryo and contribute to further studies.

CHAPTER 25

Tg's Inhibition On Angiogenesis Of Transplantation Tumor Of Mice

Since Folkman presented the concept that the growth of tumor depends on vascularization in 1971, the following researches further confirm that angiogenesis is a key factor for the growth of tumor. Thereafter researchers have brought forth the concept of anti-angiogenic therapy, that is, by preventing neovascularization and (or) spread of new-born rete vasculosum and (or) destroying new-born blood vessels to stop the production or establishment of small solid tumor, and finally to prevent the growth, evolution and metastasis of tumor. At present, foreign experts have done a lot of studies in this respect and made gratifying progress. Therefore anti-angiogenic therapy is expected to be an effective means to cure tumor. But domestic relative studies start fairly late; and very few reports are given to it except some counts about capillary density of tumor tissues.

Along with the deepening research of Common Threewingnut Root, its new pharmacological actions are constantly to be found, such as anti-tumor action and two-way regulating action on immune system. Especially the recently discovered Common Threewingnut Root, which inhibits in vitro the formation of lumen that induced by the migration, proliferation and differentiation of vascular endothelium cells, has a better inhibiting action on neovascularization. In order to further explore the inhibiting action of Common Threewingnut Root on new-born blood vessels of tumor in vivo, the writer adopts transplantation tumor model of mouse's abdominal muscles. Based on the observation of formation characteristics of tumor blood vessel and its relation with tumor, researchers' new findings in recent years and the writer's experimental results both prove that Common Threewingnut Root has the two-way regulating action with dose dependent on immune system. Choose adequate doses of TG with no effect on the body's immune function to carry out the experimental study of TG's inhibiting action on new-born blood vessels of transplantation tumor of mouse's abdominal muscles. The study is to know about TG's inhibiting capability on tumor angiogenesis, which can provide experimental references for further anti-tumor study in terms of blood vessels.

I. Experimental Study on Observation of Angiogenesis of Transplantation Tumor at Mouse's Abdominal Muscle

This experiment depends on the anatomical position and structural features of mouse's abdominal muscle, adopts EAC transplantation tumor model of abdominal muscle, fixes and displays blood vessels with transparent specimen, which are all for finding out the formation characteristics of tumor blood vessel and its relation with tumor.

[Material and Method]

1. Materials
   (1) Animals: 20 Kunming mice, 18~22g, a 50:50 proportion of male and female.

(2) Cancer-bearing mouse: Kunming mouse with the intraperitoneal inoculation of EAC cells.

(3) Instrument and apparatus: mouse retaining plate, 1ml injector, test tube and heparin tube, glass slide, ophthalmic scissors, microsurgery scissors and surgical clamps, small cutting needle, 1-0 silk thread, ophthalmic needle holder, glass petri dish, light microscope, Olympus Japanese microscopic observation and photographic system of type BH-2.

(4) Reagent: Wright stain, 0.2% physiological saline of trypan blue, Hank solution, depilatory, 1% pentobarbitale sodium solution, 10% formaldehyde solution, tertiary butyl alcohol solution of 70%, 80%, 90%, 95% and 100%, methyl salicylate.

2. Method

(1) Prepare EAC cell suspension (6.0×10^7/ml): Aseptically draw ascites of cancer-bearing mouse with the inoculation for 7~9d; put ascites in a sterile tube; draw another little ascites in a heparin tube for cell count; store tubes in ice blocks. Drop remaining ascites in the empty needle on a glass slide, cover with another slide and stain the specimen with Wright stain, finally use it for differential counting of cells, the proportion of cancer cells ≧ 95% (if insufficient, choose another cancer-bearing mouse). Dilute ascites in the heparin tube with physiological saline to 10 times and 100 times; respectively take 0.95ml blending with 0.1ml trypan blue physiological saline of 0.2%; use the counting method of white blood cells to count the total number of tumor cells and dead tumor cells, calculate the survival rate, which should be ≧ 95% (if insufficient, choose another cancer-bearing mouse). Finally dilute ascites in the tube with sterile pre-cooling Hank solution to 6.0×10^7/ml and use it for the inoculation.

(2) Inoculation in the area of peritoneum: Use depilatory in advance to clean a mouse's ventral seta two days ago; anaesthetize it injecting with 1% pentobarbitale sodium (0.3mg/10g weight) into the abdominal cavity; lie on its back and fix it on mouse retaining plate; sterilize the abdominal skin; cut open the skin about 1.2cm long from the middlemost place about 1cm below the processus xiphoideus; conduct the blunt separation to one side gently and carefully, then find an area on this side with few blood vessels in the abdominal muscle; inoculate 0.04ml EAC cell suspension with the concentration of 6.0×10^7/ml, then present a full small "swelling" without any collapse, which explains the correct inoculation location without penetrating the peritoneum. Finally stitch the skin and isolate this mouse for protection until it regains consciousness safely.

Note: During the process of inoculation, always store the test tube with cancer cell suspension in ice blocks so as to ensure the constant survival rate. And also require a fast and stable manipulation.

(3) Group and make transparent specimen: 20 inoculated mice, randomly divide into 10 groups with 2 mice of each group. Since the first day after the inoculation, pull off the cervical vertebra to execute one group each day for making transparent specimen. The specific making procedures are as follows.

Submerge and fix the execute mice in formaldehyde solution with the concentration of 10% for 24h. Take out the mice, cut open their skin, peel off the whole abdominal muscle membrane, rinse it with distilled water for 1 min, and submerge it orderly in the tertiary butyl alcohol with different concentration (70%, 80%, 90%, 95% and 100%) to dehydrate for 6~8h. Finally submerge it directly into the methyl salicylate until the tissue is completely transparent.

(4) Observe and shoot tumor vessels: Use Olympus microscope of type BH-2 to observe the transparent specimen in the small petri dish with methyl salicylate. Note the shape, quantity and distribution of new born capillary around tumor tissues and in the tumor. Then take microscopic photos and use Olympus microcirculation microscopic photographic system to observe the flow rate of new born capillaries.

[Experimental Result]

On the first day after the inoculation, there is no new born vessel in the inoculation area, around which the original host's capillaries slightly exude. On the second day, tumor cell mass swells. It is clear that original host's capillaries put forth slim but crooked new vessels, which invade into the tumor. There is no continued vessel segment. On the third and fourth day, the tumor tissue has a further growth. The density of new vessels outside the tumor increases; the caliber is irregular; vessels array in disorder. In the tumor, incontinuous and imperfect new vessels with maldistribution and various thicknesses are obviously in the direction of muscle fiber. Some vessels are comma-shaped or bud-shaped, and irregular bud-shaped vessels connect each vessel. On the fifth and sixth day, the tumor presents the progressive growth. Capillaries outside the tumor twist or distend or cluster to distribute with various thicknesses; vessels in the tumor start to interlace with each other or show irregular sinusoid dilatation. On the seventh and eighth day, the color in the tumor becomes red. Capillaries outside the tumor distend, twist and come in different shape and size; in the tumor only a few incontinuous and short vessels present an irregular distribution, most vessels have no any figure and fuse in the shape of flake or mass. On the ninth and tenth day, there is only a red mass-shaped zone in the tumor, which is fused by vessels. Brown area of hemorrhage and necrosis appears in the centre of the tumor. Vessels with extreme dilatation and distortional appearance can be made out in some areas.

Transplantation tumor model of mouse's abdominal muscles helps to have a more intuitional observation, from inflammation changes of stimulating the angiogenesis since the first day after inoculation to tumor vessels that gradually appear later. It reflects the formation characteristics of tumor's new-born capillaries and their relations with the tumor. That is, new-born capillaries generally register as the abnormal route, irregular arrangement, irregular diameter, the lack of continuity and integrity, and even comma-shaped or bud-shaped immature differentiation and growth. The relation between capillaries and tumor is the continued proliferation and enlargement of tumor cell cluster along with the formation and growth of new-born capillaries in the inoculation area. Simultaneously, the tumor mass characterized by progressive growth causes the blood vessels in the central part to bear the rise in blood pressure, dilatation, and necrosis, which appear as a red fused mass.

II. Experimental Study on Effects of TG with Different Dosages on Immunologic Function of Mice

In recent years, reports about Common Threewingnut Root having the two-way regulating action with dose dependent on immune system have continued to arise. TG is a refined product that separated and abstracted repeatedly from the crude drug—Common Threewingnut Root. In order to have a better understanding of the two-way regulating action, this experiment chooses three different doses of TG to act on the phagocytic function of mice celiac macrophages (M ϕ) and immune organs. Their drug reactions can basically reflect TG's effect on the immune function of mice.

i. TG's effect on the phagocytic function of mice celiac macrophages (M ϕ)

[Material and Method]

1. Materials
   (1) Animals: 40 Kunming mice, 18~22g, a 50:50 proportion of male and female.
   (2) Drugs and reagents: ① TG turbid liquor: Pulverize TG tablets; use 0.5% Carboxythmethyl Cellulose (CMC) to respectively prepare turbid liquors of three different concentrations, TG_1 10mg/10ml, TG_2 10mg/20ml and TG_3 40mg/10ml; ② 0.5% CMC solution; ③ 2% chicken red blood cell (CRBC) suspension: Sterile venous sampling of 2ml under the chicken wing; put the blood sample in a heparin tube; clean it for three times with physiological saline; after centrifugation, abandon the supernatant fluid and white blood cell layer at the interface; when the specific volume of blood cells keeps stable, use physiological saline to prepare 2% (V/V) red cell suspension; ④ Sterile calf serum; ⑤ 1:1 acetone-methanol solution; ⑥ 4% (V/V) Giemsa-phosphate buffer.
   (3) Instrument and apparatus: Gastric lavage needle, thermotank, and for the rest, please sees "Experimental Study on Observation of Angiogenesis of Transplantation Tumor at Mouse's Abdominal Muscle".

2. Method
   (1) Grouping: 40 mice are randomly divided into 4 groups with 10 mice of each group, group TG_1, TG_2, TG_3 and control group.
   (2) Gastric lavage: According to the proportion of 0.2ml/10g (weight), respectively inject TG suspension into the stomach with corresponding concentrations (group TG_1 20mg/kg, TG_2 40mg/kg and TG_3 80mg/kg) and 0.5% CMC solution for 12 days.
   (3) Induction and functional examination of celiac M ϕ : On the tenth day after gastric lavage, sterile injection of 0.5ml calf serum into each mouse's abdominal cavity. On the thirteenth day, inject 1ml CRBC suspension with the concentration of 2% into each mouse's abdominal cavity. 30min later pull off the cervical vertebra to execute the mouse. Cut open the abdominal wall skin from the middlemost place. Inject 2ml physiological saline into the abdominal cavity and turn the mouse's body. Aspirate 1ml celiac lotion, averagely drop it on two glass slides and put slides into an enamel box with wet paper cloth. 30 min after moving the box into 37°C thermotank for warm cultivation, rinse the two glass slides with celiac lotion in physiological saline, dry

by airing, fix in 1:1 acetone-methanol solution, dye them with 4% Giemsa-phosphate buffer, rinse with distilled water and dry by airing. Finally conduct the count of M ϕ (200 M ϕ on each slide) under the oil immersion lens of microscope. See the following mathematical equation to calculate the phagocytose percentage.

$$\text{Phagocytose Percentage} = \frac{\text{Amounts of M}\,\phi\text{ that phagocytizes CRBC}}{200\text{ M}\,\phi} \times 100\%$$

(4) Statistical treatment: The data is represented by average ± standard error ($\overline{X}$ ±S), and analyzed by *t* test.

[Experimental Result]

Determination result about TG's effect on the phagocytic function of mice celiac M ϕ can be seen in table 25-1.

Table 25-1 TG's effect on the phagocytic function of mice celiac M ϕ ($\overline{X}$ ±S)

Group	Dosage(mg/kg)	Case load	Amounts of M ϕ that phagocytizes CRBC (%)
Control group	-	10	44.83±0.41
TG_1	20	10	47.20±0.35*
TG_2	40	10	45.72±0.25
TG_3	80	10	44.40±0.45*

Note: Compare to the control group, **P*<0.05

As seen from the table 25-1, in low doses of 20mg/kg, TG can obviously activate the phagocytic function of M ϕ ($P<0.05$); in median doses of 40mg/kg, TG has no obvious effect on the phagocytic function of M ϕ ($P>0.05$); in high doses of 80mg/kg, TG will inhibit the phagocytic function of M ϕ ($P<0.05$). The above results indicate that TG can affect the phagocytic function of mice celiac M ϕ and have the obvious characteristic of dose dependent, that is along with the gradual increase of TG dosage, the phagocytic function of mice celiac M ϕ can respectively present three different effects of being activated, no obvious effect and inhibition.

ii. TG's effect on immune organs of young mice

[Material and Method]

1. Materials
   (1) Animals: 40 three-aged Kunming mice, 10~12g, a 50:50 proportion of male and female.
   (2) Drugs and reagents: TG suspension and 0.5% CMC solution: Preparation is same as stated before.

(3) Instrument and apparatus: Analytical balance and for the rest, please sees "Experimental Study on Observation of Angiogenesis of Transplantation Tumor at Mouse's Abdominal Muscle".

2. Method
   (1) Grouping and gastric lavage: see "Experimental Study on Observation of Angiogenesis of Transplantation Tumor at Mouse's Abdominal Muscle".
   (2) Weighing of thymus gland and spleen: On the thirteenth day after the experiment, pull off the cervical vertebra to execute the young mouse. Cut open its skin, chest cavity and abdominal cavity. Excise the whole thymus gland and spleen. Use filter papers to suck dry the blood and finally weigh thymus gland and spleen on an analytical balance.
   (3) Statistical treatment: The data is represented by average ± standard error ($\overline{X}$±S), and analyzed by *t* test.

[Experimental Result]

Weighing results of thymus gland and spleen can be seen in table 25-2. As seen from the table 25-2, TG at different dosages has different effect on immune organs of young mice. In low doses of 20mg/kg, TG can stimulate the weight gain of young mouse's thymus gland ($P<0.05$); in median doses of 40mg/kg, though there is a trend in weight loss, no obvious difference exists when compared with control group ($P>0.05$); in high doses of 80mg/kg, thymus gland appears as obvious atrophia compared with control group ($P<0.01$). Only in high doses, TG can inhibit the growth of young mouse's spleen ($P<0.05$); while in median and low doses, there is no obvious effect ($P>0.05$).

Table 25-2 TG's effect on immune organs of young mice ($\overline{X}$±S)

Group	Dosage(mg/kg)	Case load	Thymic weight (mg/10g weight)	Spleen weight (mg/10g weight)
Control group	-	10	26.38±1.22	70.43±0.76
TG_1	20	10	30.20±0.74*	72.65±0.83
TG_2	40	10	23.48±0.88	69.88±0.56
TG_3	80	10	21.12±0.76**	68.44±0.42*

Note: Compare to the control group, *$P<0.05$, ** $P<0.01$

Experiments about TG's effect on the phagocytic function of mice celiac Mϕ and weight of young mice's immune organs can basically reflect TG's two-way regulating action with dose dependent on mice's immune function. That is, along with the gradual increase of TG dosage, there are three different immune effects of enhancement, no obvious effect and inhibition. It prompts that the application range of TG can be expanded by different effects of choosing different dosages of TG on immune system.

III. Experimental Study on Inhibition of TG of Different Dosages on Angiogenesis of Transplantation Tumor at Mouse's Abdominal Muscle

i. Observation on new-born capillaries of transplantation tumor at mouse's abdominal muscle

Researches in recent years have found that Common Threewingnut Root has the characteristic of inhibiting migration and proliferation of endothelial cell to suppress angiogenesis. In order to have a further exploration of its inhibiting action on tumor angiogenesis, this experiment bases on the previous experiment and chooses adequate doses of TG (40mg/kg) that have no effect on mice's immune function. Through observation in vivo by microcirculation microscope, experts can carry out an experimental study on angiogenesis of transplantation tumor at mouse's abdominal muscle.

[Material and Method]

1. Materials
   (1) Animals: 40 Kunming mice, 18~22g, a 50:50 proportion of male and female.
   (2) 6.0×10^7/ml EAC cell suspension; see [Experiment 1] for preparation.
   (3) 20mg/10mg TG suspension and 0.5% CMC solution; see [Experiment 2] for preparation.
   (4) HH-1 microcirculation detection system (microcirculation microscope, photomicrography system and display system, video light mark blood flow meter, etc.), other required reagents and instruments are same as those mentioned in the previous experiment.

2. Method
   (1) Inoculation: see this chapter "Experimental Study on Observation of Angiogenesis of Transplantation Tumor at Mouse's Abdominal Muscle".
   (2) Grouping: 40 inoculated tumor-bearing mice are randomly divided into medication administration group and control group with 20 mice of each group. Then each group is also randomly divided into four groups with 5mice of each group, which is the third day, sixth day, ninth day and twelfth day.
   (3) Gastric lavage: Since the first day after inoculation, medication administration group and control group begin to undergo the gastric lavage of 20mg/ml TG suspension and 0.5% CMC solution according as the proportion of 0.2ml/10g (weight).
   (4) Observation of new-born tumor capillaries: Respectively on the third day, sixth day, ninth day and twelfth day, observe new-born capillaries of tumor at mouse's abdominal muscle among the proper group of medication administration group and control group (groups of the third day, sixth day, ninth day and twelfth day). Specific method and procedure are as follows: ① Carry out the anesthesia with the injection of 1% sodium pentobarbital (0.3mg/10g weight) in abdominal cavity before operation, carefully cut open the skin below the processus xiphoideus to the lower abdomen, conduct blunt separation of skin to the middle axillary line of one side, and then cut open the abdominal muscle along the white line. This operation should be careful and gentle.

If there is a little oozing of blood, use small gauze dipped in tepid physiological saline to stanch the bleeding. ② Make the mouse lie on side on the self-made observation platform, overturn the abdominal muscle that is detached from one side of the skin, and fix incision edge on the outer margin of the window of observation platform, which lets the half-side abdominal muscle cover the whole window and makes the tumor mass be located in the middle of the window. ③ Put the observation platform with mouse on the microscope carrier that is in a thermotank (Refer to the preparation of Tian Niu and make an improvement), and drop 37°C Ringer-Locke liquor in the overturned abdominal muscle to moisten it. ④ Start the cold light source and bring into focus for observation.

(5) Observation project: Use HH-1 microcirculation detection system to observe the shape and quantity of new-born capillaries in and around the tumor, and take microscopic photos. Measure the density of new-born capillaries which enter and leave the tumor, as well as the average diameter and flow rate of tumor arterioles and venules. Use a vernier caliper to measure the maximum diameter and transverse diameter of tumor, and calculate its maximum transverse section.

(6) Statistical treatment: The data is represented by average ± standard error ($\overline{X}$ ±S), and analyzed by *t* test.

[Experimental Result]

1. Changes in the shape and quantity of new-born capillaries in and around the tumor. See table 25-3.
2. The density of new-born capillaries which enter and leave the tumor (the number of new-born capillaries around tumor cell cluster/mm^2). See table 25-4.

The above results indicate that the density of new-born tumor capillaries of group TG is obviously lower than that of control group (P<0.05), which shows that TG has an inhibiting action on tumor vascularization. Especially on the third and sixth day, this manifestation is more apparent (P<0.05). The angiogenesis speed of control group is faster during the previous six days, but then it gradually slows down. While the angiogenesis speed of group TG during the previous six days is slower than that during the next six days and capillaries are obviously smaller that those of control group, indicating that TG significantly slows down angiogenesis speed during the previous six days and suppresses the angiogenesis. During the next six days, the angiogenesis speed of group TG gradually increases to that of control group on the tenth day to twelfth day. It shows that during the next six days TG's inhibiting action on tumor vascularization begins to remit. But as seen from table 25-4, on the twelfth day the density of new-born tumor capillaries of group TG is still obviously below that of control group, indicating that the comprehensive effect of drugs still appears as the inhibition of tumor vascularization up to now.

Table 25-3 TG's effect on the shape and quantity of new-born capillaries in and around the tumor

Observation Date	Control Group	Medication Administration Group of TG
The Third Day	Obvious, unbalanced and new-born capillaries in the tumor; unbalanced and crooked capillaries around the tumor; capillaries unevenly enter and leave the tumor. The whole tumor body is light red.	No crooked new-born capillaries enter and leave the tumor; capillaries around the tumor grow straight in the original direction; no obvious, unbalanced and new-born capillaries in the tumor. The whole tumor body is milky white.
The Sixth Day	Abundant capillaries with various thicknesses around the tumor branch from minute blood vessels of the host, twist into the tumor and form a nodular capillary network, which make the whole tumor body become light red.	Slender earthworm-shaped capillaries grow around the tumor; there are new-born capillaries without dilatation and distortion in the tumor. The whole tumor body is light red.
The Ninth Day	Abundant twisty and spreading capillaries grow around the tumor; abundant unbalanced and new-born capillaries appear in the tumor and intertwine with each other to form the shape of fasciculation and twist. There are new-born vascular buds resembling a pointed cone or cyst. The whole tumor is flesh-colored.	A small quantity of new-born circuitous capillaries start to grow around the tumor; capillaries in tumor grow in number and begin the irregular dilatation. The whole tumor body is light red.
The Twelfth Day	Abundant capillaries around the tumor look like a string of beads, or intertwine with each other to cause an irregular arrangement, or penetrate the tumor and form into concentrated clumps; capillaries in the tumor extremely distend and fuse into the shape of mass or anal sinus, which form a vast light-tight area of hemorrhage and necrosis in the centre of the tumor. The whole tumor body is maroon.	New-born slender capillaries around the tumor grow in number without interlaced phenomenon. Capillaries in the tumor distend and fuse, but there is no the area of hemorrhage and necrosis. The whole tumor is flesh-colored.

Table 25-4 TG's effect on the density (the amount of capillaries/mm²) of new-born tumor capillaries ($\overline{X}$±S)

Group	Case load	The Third Day	The Sixth Day	The Ninth Day	The Twelfth Day
Control Group	5	3.40±0.14	8.34±1.05	11.26±1.28	13.1±0.90
TG Group	5	1.84±0.12**	3.64±0.64**	6.58±1.20*	9.90±0.92

Note: Compare to the control group, *P<0.05, ** P<0.01

3. The average diameter and flow rate of tumor arterioles and venules
Results can be seen in the table 25-5, 25-6, 25-7 and 25-8.

Table 25-5 TG's effect on the diameter (μm) of tumor arterioles ($\overline{X}$±S)

Group	Case load	The Third Day	The Sixth Day	The Ninth Day	The Twelfth Day
Control Group	5	15.0±0.71	18.8±1.07	20.8±0.84	21.4±0.75
TG Group	5	14.2±0.97	19.0±1.14	18.0±0.71*	19.2±0.58*

Table 25-6 TG's effect on the diameter (μm) of tumor venules ($\overline{X}$±S)

Group	Case load	The Third Day	The Sixth Day	The Ninth Day	The Twelfth Day
Control Group	5	22.6±0.68	24.0±0.71	25.6±0.51	26.8±0.58
TG Group	5	22.4±0.93	23.2±0.86	23.4±0.75*	19.2±0.68*

Table 25-7 TG's effect on the flow rate (mm/s) of tumor arterioles ($\overline{X}$±S)

Group	Case load	The Third Day	The Sixth Day	The Ninth Day	The Twelfth Day
Control Group	5	0.42±0.014	0.45±0.022	0.39±0.011	0.36±0.015
TG Group	5	0.43±0.018	0.47±0.013	0.42±0.012	0.41±0.013*

Table 25-8 TG's effect on the flow rate (mm/s) of tumor venules ($\overline{X}$±S)

Group	Case load	The Third Day	The Sixth Day	The Ninth Day	The Twelfth Day
Control Group	5	0.35±0.016	0.32±0.014	0.28±0.014	0.23±0.016
TG Group	5	0.34±0.014	0.35±0.013	0.32±0.012	0.29±0.015*

Note: Compare to the control group, *P<0.05

As seen from the above tables, on the ninth and twelfth day, diameters of tumor arterioles and venules of TG group are obviously thinner than those of the control group ($P<0.05$); on the third and sixth day, there is no significant difference between the two groups ($P>0.05$). On the twelfth day, flow rates of tumor arterioles and venules of TG group are faster than those of the control group ($P<0.05$); on the third, sixth and ninth day, there is no significant difference between the two groups ($P>0.05$). It indicates that TG also has an influence on minute blood vessels (feeding the tumor) of the original host. Especially during an advanced stage, narrowing the diameter and quickening the flow rate can affect the amount of tumor blood supply.

4. The maximum cross section of tumor
   Results can be seen in the table 25-9.

Table 25-9 TG's effect on the tumor size ($\overline{X}$ ±S, mm)

Group	Case load	The Third Day	The Sixth Day	The Ninth Day	The Twelfth Day
Control Group	5	9.46±0.65	21.78±1.90	34.11±1.62	65.99±2.21
TG Group	5	4.91±0.76**	14.01±1.27**	27.09±2.16*	62.64±2.45

Note: Compare to the control group, *$P<0.05$, ** $P<0.01$

The above results indicate that in the previous nine days TG inhibits the growth of tumor ($P<0.05$); especially in the previous six days, this effect is more obvious ($P<0.06$). On the twelfth day, there is no significant difference between the tumor size of TG group and that of control group ($P>0.05$). It prompts that TG can obviously inhibit the growth of tumor in an early stage. While in the middle-late stage, this effect decreases. Finally in the advance stage, there is no significant inhibiting action.

ii. Determination of plasma endothelin (ET) in mice with transplantation tumor at abdominal muscle

ET is a kind of biologically active peptide synthesized by epidermic cells with extensive biological effects. Recently, increasing researches indicate that ET has an intimate relation with the growth and development of tumor, and also can participate in and promote the vascularization. In order to have a further understanding of tumor, ET and TG's effect on ET of tumor mice, experts carry out the following experiments.

[Material and Method]

1. Materials
   (1) Animals: 60 Kunming mice, 18~22g, a 50:50 proportion of male and female.
   (2) EAC cell suspension of 6.0×10^7/ml, 20mg/10ml TG suspension and 0.5% CMC solution: Preparation is same as stated before.
   (3) Endothelin radioimmunoassay kit.
   (4) The gamma (γ) radioimmunoassay counter of SN-682.

   Other required reagents are same as those mentioned in the previous experiment.

2. Method

(1) Grouping and gastric lavage according to the table 25-10.

Table 25-10 Grouping and gastric lavage of experimental mice

Animals (mice)	Grouping	Gastric lavage (0.2ml/10g)
20 uninoculated mice	Normal group ① 10 mice	physiological saline×6d
	Normal group ② 10 mice	physiological saline×12d
40 inoculated mice	Control group ① 10 mice	0.5% CMC×6d
	Control group ② 10 mice	0.5% CMC×12d
	Administration group ① 10 mice	20mg/10ml TG×6d
	Administration group ② 10 mice	20mg/10ml TG×12d

*. The inoculation method refers to "Experimental Study on Observation of Angiogenesis of Transplantation Tumor at Mouse's Abdominal Muscle".

(2) ET determination: Six days after gastric lavage, collect specimens of blood from the eye socket of mice with 2ml of each mouse in normal group ①, administration group ① and control group ①. Put the blood sample in the tube with 10% EDTA · Na 230μl and 40μl aprotinin. Lightly shake the mixture well. Centrifuge for 10min with 3000 revolutions per minute at 4°C. Separate plasma and store it at—20°C for determination. Twelve days after gastric lavage, for the mice of remaining groups to adopt the same method to collect specimens of blood, separate plasma. Use the specific radioimmunoassay and gamma (γ) radioimmunoassay counter of SN-682 to measure both the present and previous plasma. Operating procedures should be seriously carried out according to instructions of radioimmunoassay kit.

(3) Statistical treatment: The data is represented by average ± standard error ($\overline{X}$ ±S), and adopt analysis of variance—*F* test to carry out the comparison among groups.

[Experimental Result]

Determination results of plasma endothelin (ET) in mice can be seen in the table 25-11.

Table 25-11 TG's effect on the plasma endothelin (ET) in mice with transplantation tumor at abdominal muscle ($\overline{X}$ ±S, pg/ml)

Group	Case load	The Sixth Day	The Twelfth Day
Normal group	10	93.6±4.72	93.4±4.83
Control group	10	126.4±3.87**	132.8±4.02**
Administration group	10	106.4±4.49*	114.6±5.41*

Note: Compare to the normal group, *P<0.05, ** P<0.01; while compare to the control group, Δ P<0.05, Δ Δ P<0.01

The above results indicate that ET of administration group and control group is obviously higher than that of normal group (P<0.05), which shows that the tumor can increase the plasma endothelin (ET) of mice. While ET of administration group is apparently lower than that of control group, and this phenomenon is significant during the previous six days ($P<0.01$), which shows that TG can reduce the increase of plasma endothelin (ET) caused by the tumor and effects in the early stage are stronger.

Results of observation on new-born capillaries of transplantation tumor at mouse's abdominal muscle with microcirculation detection system indicate that TG can inhibit the growth of new-born capillaries in and around the tumor, reduce the density of new-born capillaries which enter and leave the tumor and suppress the growth of tumor. Furthermore, those effects of TG are significant in the early stage, and TG can change the diameter and flow rate of tumor arterioles and venules in the advanced stage to narrow the diameter and quicken the flow rate. Determination results of plasma endothelin (ET) show that the tumor can increase the plasma endothelin (ET) of mice. But TG can reduce the increase of plasma endothelin (ET) caused by the tumor with stronger effects in the early stage.

[Discussion]

1. Analysis and evaluation on the observation method of new-born capillaries by building the transplantation tumor model of mouse's abdominal muscles

At present, the methodology of tumor capillaries research is still in the process of constant exploration and improvement. Generally choose the rabbit cornea, chorioallantoic membrane (CAM) and yolk sac of chick embryo, and hamster cheek pouch for in vivo techniques; and also insert manual apparatus into rabbit ear chamber and subcutaneous air pouch of rat's back, which are called "sandwich" observation room, as the location of transplantation tumor for viviperception. In recent years, corrosion casting and immunohistochemistry are also used to display and identify vascular composition. Each of the above methods has its merits and drawbacks. At present, experts are still exploring to find a kind of simple, economical model and method with high quantitative feature and repeatability for the angiogenesis research. Therefore, combining concrete conditions of this laboratory, the writer has studied and designed the transplantation tumor model of mouse's abdominal muscles, applying improved microcirculation observation techniques to observe new-born capillaries of tumor. This method is easy, convenient and intuitional, and finally becomes a new approach for the tumor capillaries research on the methodology.

(1) Model evaluation: The approach of transplanting tumor at mouse's abdominal muscles is adopted to study and observe the relation between tumor and capillaries, as well as the drug effect on tumor capillaries, which has the reliable theoretical and practical basis.

The abdominal muscle layer of mouse is thinner. A thin layer of aponeurosis lies between the exterior of abdominal muscle layer and skin. The interior of abdominal muscle layer links closely with the abdominal membrane. The Hunter's line divides the abdominal muscle layer along the centre position into right and left halves, which are provided blood circulation by inferior epigastric arteries and veins. The right and left halves diverge one more into tiny branches (arterioles and venules) and capillary branches, which form rich anastomoses around the abdominal muscle of each side. The center position has fewer vascular branches and ramus anastomoticus and becomes an area with rare vessels, where is convenient for the observation of new-born capillaries.

When EAC cell suspension is injected into the abdominal muscle layer, tumor cells will quickly begin the infiltrative growth and expand along the flat surface of abdominal muscle without any adhesion of skin and organs in the abdomen. When the tumor grows up to a certain extent, it will gradually break through the abdominal muscle layer, penetrate inward through the abdominal membrane, move into organs in the abdominal cavity through implantation metastasis and finally produce ascites.

Consequently, the better choice is to inoculate in the area with rare vessels and observe tumor capillaries during the period of the tumor not yet penetrating through the abdominal membrane, which can both make a clearer observation of the emergence and change of new-born capillaries and avoid many factors' combined effects on new-born capillaries, such as ascites and tumor diffusion caused by the tumor's penetration through the abdominal membrane.

Combined with this experiment content, in order to have a better reflection and observation of the transplanted tumor in abdominal muscle and the whole growing and developing process of new-born capillaries, the writer has carried out repeated trials and finally chosen EAC cell suspension with the concentration of 6.0×10^7/ml for inoculation. According to the growth status of tumor, the writer arranges 10 days' observation and 12 days' treatment. Divide four time spans of the third day, sixth day, ninth day and twelfth day to reflect the tumor's reaction to drugs in the early, intermediate and advanced stages.

The transplantation tumor model of mouse's abdominal muscles can intuitively and clearly reflect the formation and change of new-born tumor capillaries, and it also provides new idea and method for studying new-born tumor capillaries' selection of transplantable parts and preparation of animal model. There are a few points that should be remembered when preparing the model: ① Inoculation site should be chosen in the abdominal muscle with rare vessels, not penetrating the peritoneum. The mark is a full small "swelling" without any collapse on the inoculation site. ② The experimental operation should be gentle and careful. Try to keep away from the tiny venous tributary (generally only 1~2 vessels) that links skin and abdominal muscle, so that no local hemorrhage is caused. Then the inoculation effect and the growth of new-born tumor capillaries after inoculation will be unaffected. ③ Appropriately increase the number of experimental mice to reduce errors of different location of rare vessels of abdominal muscle caused by individual difference.

(2) Evaluation of observation method

① Observation of transparent specimen: The tissue of abdominal muscle membrane is thinner. After transparent treatment, other sites are all transparent except vessels are red. Naked eyes can clearly see vessels' routes. Microscope observation can show the shape, distribution and interrelation of capillaries. The transparent specimen is not only convenient and intuitive but also preserves the natural form of vessels and associative perception. When preparing the transparent specimen, do not inject with Chinese ink or other pigments, but directly display vessels through natural color of blood, which prevent particle size, dispersion degree and viscosity of perfusate from affecting the specimen quality and changing the shape of vessels due to improper injection pressure. The transparent specimen must completely reflect the condition in vivo so as to make displayed vessels be closer to the reality.

The transparent specimen of abdominal muscle—membrane can clearly display various vessels in the abdominal muscle, involving the route, shape and distribution of capillaries around and in the tumor as well as localized congestion, oozing of blood and bleeding, which make it more convenient for observing new-born capillaries inside and outside of the tumor. The transparent specimen can only show the change of capillary form after animals have died, but it cannot reflect their blood flow state. Therefore, combined with the dynamic state of vital blood flow and functional parameters to have observation, it will be more favorable to have a complete understanding of new-born tumor capillaries' features.

② In vivo observation with microcirculation microscope: The mouse's abdominal muscle membrane is thinner with the shape of film and is easy to transmit light, whose vascular form and fluid state can be clearly seen through the microcirculation microscope. Inoculated tumor cells begin the infiltrative spreading growth in the abdominal muscle. In the early stage, the abdominal muscle membrane still can transmit light and display the vascular form in tumor tissue due to unobvious increase in thickness. In the advanced stage, the tumor tissue grows and thickens; the pressure of central part increases; necrosis and hemorrhage arise, which appear as a light-tight solid mass; vessels in this part cannot be seen, but the form of vessels in other transparent parts of tumor can be seen at present. The microcirculation microscope is used to observe new-born capillaries inside and outside of transplantation tumor at abdominal muscle and those which enter and leave the tumor as well as tumor arterioles and venules, which can completely reflect the relation between tumor and vessels as well as drugs' effect on new-born tumor capillaries in the respect of vascular form and fluid state.

The above two observation methods can complement each other with joint application. Observation of transparent specimen can cover the shortage of not observing vessels in a light-tight part of tumor in vivo; while in vivo observation makes up for the observation of dynamic state of blood flow. The above methods can only make one-off observation and cannot have a continuing dynamic monitoring in a long term, so they also remain inadequate. In order to have a more accurate and deeper research, the methodology needs the further improvement and completeness.

2. Evaluation of experimental drugs Common Threewingnut Root generally refers to the plant belonging to Tripterygium of Celastraceae. There are three varieties in China, which are Common Threewingnut Root, Tripterygium Hypoglaucum and Common Threewingnut Root of North-East (Tripterygium regelii Sprague et Take). This kind of drug has an acrid-bitter flavor and medicinal properties of cold and hot. The drug passes through main channels of liver and spleen as well as twelve regular channels, which has efficacies of clearing away heat and toxic material, expelling wind and removing dampness, relaxing the muscles, stimulating the blood circulation and removing obstruction in channels, reducing swelling and alleviating pain, destroying parasites and relieving itching. This drug, which contains about 70 components, is recorded in *Sheng Nong's herbal classic* at the earliest. Since the 1970s, it has been used in treating rheumatoid arthritis, which results in certain curative effect. In recent twenty years, it has been widely used in treating chronic nephritis, hepatitis, purpura haemorrhagica and all kinds of skin diseases. At the same time, the research of pharmacological action also becomes deeper, widely covering adrenal gland, immunity, generation, micturition, central nerve and blood system. Experts all agree that this drug can enhance adrenal cortex function, relieve inflammation and alleviate pain, resist fertility and

prevent tumor activity. Only as to its effect on immune system, experts each sticks to their own viewpoint. There were many controversies and inferences. In an early period, experts embarked on the research of its effect on immune system because of its unique effect on treating rheumatoid arthritis. The earliest result indicates that this drug can suppress immunity. As more and more researches are done deeperly, most researchers gradually tend to the viewpoint of "two-way regulation". They hold that Common Threewingnut Root has the two-way regulating action with dose dependent on immune system. For instance, Zheng jiarun, Yan Biyu, Luo Dan, Lei Yi and Fan Yongyi respectively report that Common Threewingnut Root has the two-way regulating action on mouse's thymic weight, human thymocyte hyperplasia, NK activity of mouse's spleen cells, T and B cell function of mouse's spleen and proliferation of T cells in vitro. Through the experiment of the effect of TG with different dosages on M ϕ function of mice abdominal cavity and immune organs by the writer, it reflects that Common Threewingnut Root has the two-way regulating action on immune system. The above results indicate that Common Threewingnut Root does not have the only effect of immunological suppression. Many experiments have proved that a small dosage of Common Threewingnut Root can enhance the immunization to some extent. While within a certain limits, there will be a reversible manifestation between enhancement and inhibition. It can also show nearly no appreciable effect on immunologic function. When further increasing the dosage, this drug will show the complete inhibiting action on immunization. The inhibiting action of Common Threewingnut Root is obviously related to its dosage.

Given the above conclusions, the writer chooses the dosage of TG, which has no appreciable effect on immunologic function, to carry out the experiment. It can avoid drugs' influence on immunologic function, which may complicate the research of TG's inhibiting action on tumor capillaries. At the same time, it can provide experimental considerations and exploring foundations for experiments and clinical researches of TG's anti-tumor action on the premise that Common Threewingnut Root will not damage the body's immunological function.

The drug of this experimental research is a kind of prepared product after repeated separation and abstraction. The amount of active principle is higher and the untoward effect is less. In order to have a further exploration of angiogenesis inhibition of active principle in this drug, various chemical compositions and monomers after the second separation and purification still need further study.

3. Features of tumor angiogenesis Under normal conditions, the angiogenesis only limits in embryonic development, repair in trauma and endometrial regeneration. Furthermore, the host can strictly control its growth with various mechanisms. But in the recent twenty years, experts haven't found any mechanism which can suppress tumor angiogenesis. It indicates that tumor angiogenesis has its own features.

Through the observation on new-born capillaries of transplantation tumor at mouse's abdominal muscle, it is easy to find that as the formation and growth of capillaries in the inoculation area, tumor cell cluster constantly proliferates and its volume continually expands. It starts with the exudation of original host's capillaries, and then slender and crooked new-born capillaries gradually come out with the characteristics of disorganized arrangement, uneven distribution and irregular diameter. Especially these capillaries, which enter into the tumor, have incontinuous routes, lack completeness and present the shape of comma or bud. The above signs indicate that those capillaries are not fully mature and cannot form complete and continuous basilar membrane. Furthermore, they are not blocked and packed by well-differentiated vascular walls with multilayered structure, which make vessels expand irregularly in the shape of nodositas or sinus. Along with the progressive growth of tumor, dust-color area of hemorrhage and necrosis appears in the centre of the tumor. Capillaries in adjacent sites are hard to be seen because of extreme dilatation, which may be due to the constantly rising pressure within tumor caused by the continuous proliferation of tumor cells. The pressure of central part in tumor is relatively highest, and the central part is far away from new-born capillaries that penetrate from the outside of tumor, so the central part is easy to suffer from necrosis because of ischemia, involving the necrosis and hemorrhage of vessels. But there still are different-shaped tumor capillaries with active proliferation at the margin of tumor, which can ensure the required nutrition for the further infiltrative growth. This phenomenon also indicates that the tumor grows indefinitely and cannot be adjusted and controlled.

At present, experts have been adopting various methods to study tumor vessels. The existing achievements have proved that the formation of tumor vessels is different from the angiogenesis in a normal physiological state. It has its own special uniqueness, such as infantile differentiation, incomplete vascular wall and out of the body's control, etc. While the whole process and regulatory mechanism of tumor angiogenesis remains obscure and are still in further exploration. This experiment just superficially reflects the relation between tumor and vessels, as well as some features of tumor vessels. The deeper study also needs the breakthrough of methodology, and the continued clarification of biological characteristics of tumor vessels in terms of the physiology and pathology of angiogenesis, biochemistry and molecular biology.

4. Exploration of TG's inhibiting action on new-born tumor capillaries Since Common Threewingnut Root is explored and applied, domestic and foreign medicine circles have been starting to pay great interest and attention to it and carrying out multi-disciplinary study and exploration one by one for broadening the application range. The recent researches show that Common Threewingnut Root can inhibit the migration and proliferation of vascular endothelial cells (EC). Zhu Jinbo and another two Japanese scholars utilize self-made F-2 and F-2C of EC strain to study the effect of Common Threewingnut Root on the process of angiogenesis. The result shows that Common Threewingnut Root can directly act on EC and inhibit its migration, proliferation, differentiation and the formation of lumen, which prompts that Common Threewingnut Root has a better inhibiting action on angiogenesis. The experimental study of TG's inhibiting action on new-born capillaries of transplantation tumor at mouse's abdominal muscle finds that TG can suppress tumor angiogenesis with stronger effects in the early stage. Presumably TG's active mechanisms may include the following respects.
   (1) Directly act on new-born tumor capillaries: The experimental results indicate that TG can obviously suppress the growth of capillaries in and around the tumor and reduce the density of new-born capillaries which enter and leave the tumor. Thus it can be inferred that TG may directly act on endothelial cells of tumor vessels, suppress the migration and proliferation of cells and reduce the formation, differentiation and growth rate of tumor vessels.

(2) Directly act on tumor cells: TG's direct damaging effect on tumor cells has been proved in an early period. It is generally acknowledged that TG comes into the effect of cell toxicant by directly interfering with DNA replication of tumor cells and suppressing RNA and protein synthesis. During the process of angiogenesis, the tumor cell itself can produce multiple angiogenesis factors, such as fibrocyte growth factor (FGF), angiogenine, transfer growth factor (TGF) and tumor necrosis factor (TNF-2), etc. Furthermore, the tumor cell can release some chemical mediators to induce the angiogenesis of host and tumor. The above substances that are released by tumor cells and can induce angiogenesis are collectively called "tumor angiogenesis factor (TAF)" by Folkman. TG can reduce the production of TAF by directly killing tumor cells, which indirectly inhibits the angiogenesis.

(3) Change of tumor blood flow: Determination result of the average diameter and flow rate of host's tumor arterioles and venules shows that TG can change the blood flow in the tumor and affect the growth and change of tumor and its new-born capillaries by acting on the blood supply of tumor.

(4) Reduction of plasma ET content: The recent researches indicate that ET has the effect of growth factor on promoting cell proliferation, which can stimulate the growth of endothelial cell and the proliferation of vascular smooth muscle cells. ET has an intimate relation with the tumor, which can promote the transcription and expression of proto-oncogene and the growth and differentiation of tumor, increase the blood flow of tumor tissue and stimulate the angiogenesis. The determination result of mouse's plasma ET indicates that ET of inoculated group is obviously higher than that of normal group. It proves that ET has an intimate relation with tumor and the tumor can increase mouse's plasma ET content. While ET of TG group is apparently lower that that of control group, which indicates that TG can obviously lower mouse's plasma ET content and reduce the growth effect on promoting tumor and angiogenesis caused by ET.

Furthermore, TG has a feature in this experiment that its inhibiting action on tumor angiogenesis in the advanced stage is weaker than that in the early stage. In addition to TG's pharmacological characteristic of suppressing angiogenesis, its inhibiting power is also related to drugs' accumulative action. It is conjectured that TG accumulates in vivo and plays an extensive pharmacological effect with prolongation of medication time, and thus affects its inhibiting action on tumor angiogenesis.

This research result indicates that TG can suppress tumor growth by inhibiting tumor angiogenesis with no significant effect on the immune system, and moreover, TG's effect in the early stage is significant. This study provides references for the further multi-field and multi-angle TG researches, and also new ideas for the research of TG anti-tumor mechanisms. Without doubt, this conclusion still needs extensive repeated experiments to be verified. At the same time, drug purification and methodology improvement are necessary for the further deeper study.

Inhibiting the formation of new-born tumor capillaries to suppress the tumor growth is a new idea on oncology that emerges in recent years.

This topic is on the basis study of formation features of new-born capillaries of transplantation tumor at mouse's abdominal muscle as well as capillaries' relation with tumor and TG's two-way regulating action with dose dependent on the immune system of mouse, and thus by choosing the TG dosage (40mg/kg weight) of no obvious effect on mouse's immune function to carry out experiments of TG's effect on the shape and quantity of new-born capillaries of transplantation tumor at mouse's abdominal muscle, the density of new-born capillaries which enter and leave the tumor, the average diameter and flow rate of tumor arterioles and venules, tumor size and plasma ET. The above experiments find that TG can inhibit tumor angiogenesis through various mechanisms of direct action on new-born tumor capillaries as well as tumor cells, the change of tumor blood flow and the reduction of plasma ET content, and moreover, TG's effect in the early stage is significant. This research result shows that the anti-tumor study of TG from the angle of vessels has certain significance and needs the further study confirmation and deepening.

IV. The Significance of Inhibition of Angiogenesis in Treatment

Tumorigensis is a complicated process and is affected by many factors, involving the foundation of tumor vascular net. Many researches have proved that tumor growth must depend on angiogenesis. By inhibiting certain steps or the whole process of tumor angiogenesis to control tumor growth is of great importance to tumor therapy and prevention of tumor's distant metastasis.

i. The relation between tumor angiogenesis and the generation and growth of tumor

At present, the question about tumor generation mainly focuses on the study of oncogene; nevertheless, malignant change of tissues, tumor formation and tumor gene activity are just necessary conditions instead of the whole. Folkman Judah and other scholars in Children's Hospital of Harvard Medical School do a series of studies about the generation of pancreatic islet B cell tumor of mutant mice. The study result finds that tumor gene activity is related to the proliferation of B cells, and moreover, angiogenesis plays an important role during the generation of B cell tumor. The generation of tumor is caused by getting angiogenic ability of hyperplastic tissue. The research proves that one of evident characteristics of most precancerous lesions is the lack of obvious neovascularization. Compared with the tumor with abundant new-born vessels, the transition from precancerous condition and lesion to blood vessel phase may be the "switch" for tumor generation. It indicates that the induction of angiogenesis and the consequent neovascularization are both ahead of the tumor generation. Once the tumor is found, its further growth must depend on the continuous generation of vessels. This concept has been put forward by Folkman in 1971. He holds that tumor cells and vessels combine into a highly integrated ecological system. If there is no angiogenesis, the tumor will not swell. Many experimental research evidences in recent years further support the above views.

The growing period of solid tumor cells can be divided into invading prophase without vessels and invading growth phase of vascularization. During the invading prophase, the growth of tumor cells mainly depends on diffusion to gain nutrition. When the diameter of solid tumor exceeds 1~3cm and cell number is up to about 10^7, tumor's central part and its continued growth must be provided with oxygen and nutrient substance by vessels. ① Observe the black tumor cell cluster of mouse that is cultured in agar. When the cluster grows to 1mm^3, the proliferation of its peripheral cells and the necrosis of central cells are equivalent. When the tumor body continues to swell, the proliferation and necrosis achieve a dynamic equilibrium. If the tumor grows in the organism, then this phase can also be called the blood vessel phase of tumor growth. Breaking this state needs the growth of new and functional capillaries so as to provide adequate oxygen and nutrient substance. ② Observe the growth rate of transplantable tumor in the subcutaneous transparent cavity of mouse. The tumor shows a slow linear growth before angiogenesis. While after angiogenesis, the tumor shows a rapid exponential rise. ③ Implant tumor tissue masses into the rabbit cornea. The tumor stands back from the host's vascular bed. The new-born capillaries around the cornea are found to gather toward the tumor. The growth rate averages 0.2mm/d. After new-born capillaries grow into the tumor, the tumor mass begins to grow rapidly and exceeds $1cm^3$. ④ The tumor grows in the isolated perfused organ of mouse. Because there is no vascular proliferation, the tumor limits in $1mm^3$. If this tumor is transplanted into the mouse, it will rapidly grow to $1\sim2cm^3$ after angiogenesis. ⑤ Suspend tumor cells in the aqueous humor of anterior chamber of rabbit eyes. Because there is no vessel, the tumor size is less than $1mm^3$. If this tumor is transplanted into iris vessels, it will grow rapidly with 1.6 times of its original volume in two weeks. ⑥ When the human retina blastoma is transplanted into the vitreous body or anterior chamber, the growth of this tumor will be limited due to the lack of vessels. ⑦ Use ^3H—thymine to label tumor cells of fixed cancer. The label index of tumor cells reduces with the increase of distance between the nearest open capillaries and tumor cells. The mean value of label index of tumor cells is the function of label index of tumor vascular endothelial cells. ⑧ Transplanted tumor in CAM. During the avascular period (≥72h), the growth of tumor is restricted. A set of experiments show that the tumor diameter is no more than (0.93±0.29) mm. In 24 hours after the vascularization, the tumor starts growing rapidly. On the seventh day, the average diameter of tumor is (8.0±2.5) mm. ⑨ Oophoroma metastasizes to the abdominal membrane. Before the vascularization, this tumor grows slowly and its size seldom exceeds $1mm^3$. ⑩ If the tumor diameter is less than 1mm, there will be no vascularization in the metastatic cancer of rabbit cornea. All other metastatic cancers, whose diameter is greater than 1mm, have the formation of vessels.

All these above can indirectly or directly prove that tumor growth must depend on vascularization and the vascularization is a key factor for tumor development.

ii. The anti-tumor action of angiogenesis inhibitors

In the early 1970s, along with the presentation and research of the concept that tumor growth depends on vascularization, researchers also bring forth the relevant concept of anti-angiogenic therapy. That is to say, by preventing neovascularization and (or) the expansion of new-born vascular net and (or) destroying new-born vessels to stop the generation or establishment of small solid tumor and also arrest the growth, development and metastasis of tumor. Ways of adopting anti-angiogenic therapy: ① Suppress tumor to release tumor angiogenic factors (TAF); ② Neutralize the tumor angiogenic factors (TAF) that have already been released; ③ Inhibit the reaction of vascular endothelial cells (EC) on angiogenic factors; ④ Disturb the synthesis of basilar membrane; ⑤ Destroy the formed new-born tumor vessels, etc. In conclusion, ideal tumor angiogenesis inhibitors must be able to suppress one or more procedures or the whole process of tumor angiogenesis.

At present, people have done a lot of researches in this respect. Experimental results indicate that angiogenesis inhibitors (AI) can inhibit the growth of tumor. ① According to more domestic reports, the combination of heparin and hydrocortisone is acknowledged as an effective angiogenesis inhibitor. Experiments prove that their combined application can suppress the angiogenesis in CAM, promote tumor regression, prevent metastasis and inhibit the neovascularization of rabbit cornea that caused by tumor. That this kind of inhibitor is used to cure some mice tumors can bring about a striking effect. For instance, after the oral administration of heparin (200U/ml) and subcutaneous injection of hydrocortisone (250mg), 100% reticulum cell sarcoma, 100% Leuis lung cancer and 80% B16 melanoma can have a complete regression. What's more, 80% tumors will not suffer from the relapse after regression. ② Fumagillin is a kind of antibiotic which is naturally secreted by aspergillin. For the in vitro experiment, Fumagillin can inhibit the proliferation of endothelial cells. For the in vivo experiment, Fumagillin can inhibit the angiogenesis caused by tumor and also suppress the tumor growth of mice. For example, 30mg/kg of Fumagillin can inhibit the growth of Lewis lung cancer and B16 melanoma. ③ 1μg/ml TNP-470 (a kind of Fumagillin synthetic analogue) can inhibit the growth of cultural endothelial cells of human umbilical vein. 3~10mg/kg TNP-470 can suppress the growth of nude mice's transplanted tumor of human oophoroma. ④ Platelet factor 4 (PF_4) is a kind of 28kDa protein that is released by the dense body when blood platelets aggregate together. There is a great affinity between PF_4 and heparin. Taylor and other scholars have found that PF_4 can effectively inhibit the growth of CAM vessels. Recently Maione and others have discovered that recombination of human PF_4 ($rHuPF_4$) can suppress the reproduction and migration of human endothelial cells, and also produce an avascular area in chick embryo CAM. Sharpe has carried out the research about mice melanoma and human colon cancer, which proves that human PF_4 ($rHuPF_4$) has an inhibiting action on the growth of solid tumor. ⑤ α-Difluoromethylornithine (DFMO) is a kind of nonreversible ornithine decarboxylase inhibitor. It can inhibit the angiogenesis caused by melanoma in chick embryo CAM, and then inhibit the tumor growth in CAM. ⑥ The latest approved angiogenesis inhibitor—Angio stain is a kind of 38kDa protein, which can inhibit the generation of endothelial cells and angiogenesis in the Lewis mice tumor. When Folkman injects Angio stain into the mouse with transplanted tumor, this new type of inhibitor can keep this transplanted tumor in a state of dormancy, that is to say, the multiplication rate of tumor is equal to the death rate of cells. In addition, Angio stain can suppress the growth of human tumor.

At present, people have realized that the anti-tumor effects of many anti-tumor methods directly or indirectly act on the structure or function of tumor vessels, such as anti-tumor angiogenesis, the change of tumor blood flow and its regulation, etc. That by inhibiting the angiogenesis of malignant tumor to suppress the growth and metastasis of tumor is a new way to fight against cancer, and meanwhile adopting angiogenesis inhibitors to cure tumors will open up a new and promising therapeutic area clinically. For instance, cooperating operation, chemotherapy, radiotherapy and immunological therapy will certainly improve the overall tumor treatment level.

Tumor cells produce multiple tumor angiogenesis factors (TAF), such as basic fibroblast growth factor (bFGF), acid fibroblast growth factor (aFGF), endothelial cell growth factor (ECGF), vascular endothelial cell growth factor (VEGF), platelet derivation endothelial cell growth factor (PDECGF), epidermal cell growth factor (EGF), transforming growth factor (TGFα, TGFβ), tumor necrosis factor (TGF-α), granulocyte colony stimulating factor (G-CSF) and granulocyte macrophage colony stimulating factor (GM-CSF), etc. TAF has the promotional effects on tumor generation, development and metastasis. Exploring the generative mechanism of tumor capillaries and the inhibition of capillaries' formation and growth is one of the effective measures to prevent and cure tumors, and may also become a new promising anti-cancer therapy after the surgical treatment, radiotherapy, chemotherapy and biological therapy

CHAPTER 26

Survey of Study on XZ-C Medicine for Immunologic Regulation and Control

I. Experimental Study

In 1985, the writer made system follow-up statistics to more than 3,000 patients who had accepted cancer operations of chest and abdomen performed by the writer himself. The results show that 2~3 years after the operation, most patients suffer from relapses or metastases. To reduce the relapse rate and increase the curative rate, the clinical fundamental research is a must. If there is no breakthrough of fundamental research, the clinical effect is hard to improve.

Current anti-cancer drugs are cell toxicants that kill both cancer cells and normal cells. The untoward reaction is intense. Now a kind of anti-cancer drug is extracted from traditional Chinese medicine, such as vinblastine, which is extracted from vinca rosea as alkaloid, has been used as anti-cancer drugs for clinical practice. But it will also kill normal cells. So the untoward reaction is intense too. While we hope that anti-cancer drugs have fewer untoward reactions, may be taken by mouth and can build up patient's strength and resistance. Then scientific research is being designed. The plan is to adopt animal experiments of tumor-inhibition in tumor-bearing mice, and from natural drugs to find new anti-cancer drugs, anti-metastasis and anti-relapse drugs, traditional Chinese medicine that only inhibit cancer cells but not normal cells, and new drugs that can adjust the regulation and control relation between host and tumor.

According to cell proliferation cycle theory, anti-cancer drugs must maintain long-term application and make cancer nidi chronically and continuously immerse in drugs. Only in this way can the cell division be inhibited and relapse and metastasis be prevented. Drugs have to be used for a long term, which is the only way to control existing cancer nidi and prevent the formation of nascent cancer cells. But current used anti-cancer drugs induce intense untoward reaction, and therefore they cannot be used chronically and continuously but only be applied as per the treatment course for a minor cycle. All the current anti-cancer drugs have a series of untoward reactions, such as suppressions of immunologic function, bone marrow hematopoietic function and thymus gland, etc. the formation and development of cancer is due to the loss of immune monitoring caused by the reduction of patient's immunity. Therefore, all the anti-cancer drugs must improve immunity and protect immune organs, but should not suppress immunity.

To this end, our laboratory has carried on the following experimental studies for screening of new anti-cancer and anti-metastasis drugs from traditional Chinese medicine.

1. Adopt the method of cancer cells cultured in vitro to carry on the screening experimental study of tumor inhibition rate of traditional Chinese medicine

Screening test in vitro: adopt the method of tumor cells cultured in vitro; observe drugs' direct damage to tumor cells.

1. Method
   (1) Preparation of crude drugs' agentia: dry crude drugs; add sixty times of water; heat and extract filtering liquid; decompress filtering liquid; distill it to dryness; form coarse dust; then it can be applied.
   (2) Screening test in culture dish: 1×10^5/ml cells of Ehrlich ascites tumor (FAC), or fleshy tumor 180 (S-180), or ascites liver cancer (H_{22}), or carcinoma of uterine cervix, fetal calf serum 10%, coarse crude drugs 500μg/ml, based on the above proportion to inject 20ml solution in culture dish of 10cm×15cm. Place it at 37 centi-degree for a given time. Then compare the quantity of surviving cells with those of control group. Measure suppression ratio of cell proliferation caused by cytotoxicity.
   (3) Drug screening: put crude drugs respectively into test tubes that used for culturing human cancer cells. Observe them whether crude drugs have inhibiting action on cancer cells. For 200 kinds of anti-cancer traditional Chinese medicines identified by traditional Chinese doctors, the writer carries on the in vitro screening test in sequence. Also under the same condition, use those medicines to carry on fibrocytes culture of normal person. Measure this medicine's cytotoxicity to fibrocytes, and then compare it with that of control group.

2. Experimental Result after animal screening tests by the writer in laboratory, 48 kinds of crude drugs (totally 200) certainly have and even hold sovereign inhibiting action on cancer cells proliferation. Tumor inhibition rate is above 90%. But some commonly used traditional Chinese medicines, which are generally considered to have anti-cancer effects, are verified by experiments to have no or little anti-cancer effects. The suppression ratio of another 50 kinds of traditional Chinese medicines is below 30%, such as Chinese clematis, selfheal, earth worm, akebia stem, cortex lycii, rosa multiflora and so on.

2. Make animal model, carry on the experimental study of tumor inhibition rate of traditional Chinese medicine in cancer-bearing animals

1. Screening test of tumor-inhibition in vivo tumor-bearing animal model: each batch of experiment needs 240 Kunming mice, divided into 8 groups. Each group has 30 mice. For the first, second, third, fourth, fifth and sixth experimental group, each group chooses one kind of traditional Chinese medicine. The seventh group is set as the blank control group. The eighth group selects fluorouracil or cyclophosphamide as control group. All the mice are inoculated with 1×10^7/ml EAC or S-180 or H_{22} cancer cells through right front axillary subcutaneous injection. After three days, green gram-sized subcutaneous tumor nidi grow. 24 hours after inoculation, each mouse is fed orally with coarse dust of crude drugs, as per the weight 1000mg/kg. The feeding time is once a day for eight weeks. Mice's weights and sizes of tumor nidi need to be measured daily. After eight weeks, 20 mice of each group are executed. Measure their weights of body, tumor, liver, spleen, lung, thymus gland and other organs. Make pathological section to observe tissue condition and know metastatic condition. Another 10 tumor-bearing experimental mice are chronically fed with the screening traditional Chinese medicine. Observe the surviving time and untoward reaction. Calculate prolonged survival rate and tumor inhibition rate. Each batch (i.e. screen each kinds of traditional Chinese medicine) of experimental cycle is three months. Each batch of experiments can simultaneously screen and study six kinds of traditional Chinese medicines

or prescriptions. One group of experiments can simultaneously get screening results of six kinds of traditional Chinese medicines.

This research institute can test three experimental groups over the corresponding period. Three master or doctor postgraduates manage one experimental group. In this way can tumor inhibition experiments with eighteen single traditional Chinese medicines or prescriptions be simultaneously studied. In this year, 72 kinds of single traditional Chinese medicines screening experiments which are used for in vivo tumor-inhibition of tumor-bearing mice can be carried on and completed. Thus the writer has continuously carried on four-year experimental studies and another three-year study on pathogenesis and metastatic compound mechanism of tumor-bearing mice and exploration of reasons that why cancerous protuberance can cause the death of host. 1000 tumor-bearing animal models are used every year. A total of about 6,000 tumor-bearing animal models have been done during four years. Each experimental mouse is performed with pathological anatomy on liver, spleen, lung, thymus gland and kidney after death. More than twenty thousand pathological sections have been accomplished to explore and seek cancerogenic micro-pathogens. Use microscopes to observe tumor micrangium establishing and microcirculation condition of 100 tumor-bearing mice. Through experimental studies, the writer firstly finds in China that traditional Chinese medicine TG has obvious effects on suppressing the formation of tumor micrangium. Now this medicine has been used for clinical anti-metastasis treatments on over 200 patients. Curative effects are being observed.

2. Discussion
   (1) Through experimental studies, put forward new thought, new knowledge, new concept and new strategy for resisting against cancer: over a period of seven years; over 6,000 tumor-bearing animal models; in vivo tumor-inhibition experiments for anti-cancer, anti-metastasis and anti-relapse in sequence with 200 kinds of natural traditional Chinese medicines; have cognizance of train of thought, knowledge and experience to renew concept, thought, traditional principle and method for traditional anti-cancer work.

   Use tumor-bearing animal models to carry on scientific, objective and strict experimental screening, analysis and evaluation on 200 kinds of traditional Chinese medicines in sequence with so called anti-cancer curative effects by Chinese Medicine Literature. Results show that only 48 kinds of medicines have better anti-cancer effects. Although another 152 kinds of medicines are the commonly used anti-cancer medicines by veteran practioner of TCM, they have been verified by this group of experimental screenings to have no anti-cancer effects or little tumor inhibition rate. These 200 kinds of traditional Chinese medicines used for experimental screening are chosen from over ten books with TCM anti-cancer famous prescriptions. They are also common medicines with anti-cancer effects described in Journal of Traditional Chinese Medicine and literature reports. While the experimental study results prove that 152 kinds of medicines have no tumor inhibition rate or low anti-cancer effects. The reason might be that Chinese Medicine Literature has no distinction between lump, abdominal mass of Chinese medicine and cancer of modern medicine. 48 kinds of medicines in this group, which are screened through animal experiments, really have better tumor inhibition rate. Through optimization grouping and repeated trials, different medicines are composed to XZ-$C_{1\sim10}$ immunoregulation anti-cancer Chinese materia medica preparation. It has been verified clinically for sixteen years. Over 12,000 cancer patients have used this preparation and obtained better curative effects.

Through experimental screening study results of this group, we have realized that TCM prescriptions are gained from prolonged experience. The prescription matches symptoms of disease and is the synthesis composed with various kinds of crude drugs. As seen from Chinese Medicine Literature, symptoms of abdominal mass and accumulation seem similar to those of cancer. Traditional Chinese medicines are used to treat abdominal mass. Sometimes symptoms can be improved, but not all abdominal mass are cancers. In general, TCM has no effect on cancer. So we should adopt modern scientific methods to verify, observe and reevaluate cancer resistance and carcinogenicity of various crude drugs in prescriptions of traditional Chinese medicine, and avoid unscientific parts of traditional Chinese medicine and pharmacology.

In medicine screening experiments, it's found that single crude drugs have worse tumor-inhibition effects than optimization grouping compound of many kinds of crude drugs. The reason may be that single crude drugs can only suppress tumor proliferation. While optimization grouping compound of many kinds of crude drugs not only can suppress tumor proliferation of tumor-bearing mice, but also can build up strength, improve immunity, promote to produce cancer-inhibition cytokines and protect normal cells.

Since 1992, over seven-year scientific experiments, different medicines are screened and composed to XZ-$C_{1\sim10}$ immunoregulation anti-cancer Chinese materia medica preparation. This medicine owns curative effects on anti-cancer, supporting healthy energy to eliminate evils, clearing away heat and toxic materials and activating blood circulation to dissipate blood stasis.

From experimental study to clinical verification, and then from clinic to experiment again, the writer has organized to set up the joint breakthrough research coordination group for cancer prevention and resistance. This coordination group has experimental study base and verification base of clinical application. The former is in medical college and medical university laboratory; the latter is in clinical medical department of nationwide coordination group for cancer prevention and resistance studies combined with traditional Chinese and western medicine. From experimental study to clinical verification means the clinical application on the basis of successful experimental study. Then new problems are found during the clinical application, which need fundamental experimental studies. Afterwards new experimental results are applied to clinical verification. Experiments → clinic → experiments once more → clinic once more, recurrent ascent continuously; through eight-year clinical practical experiences, knowledge also continues to improve. Summation, analysis, reflection and evaluation ascend to theory, putting forward new knowledge, new concept, new thought, new strategy and new therapeutic route and scheme.

Breakthrough research experience of coordination group includes: ① Choose the way that professors, experts and postgraduates of universities and colleges coordinate to carry on scientific researches and joint breakthrough; advocate large-scale coordination of scientific researches; give prominence to concentrate scientific research and technology strength of all parties; enrich anti-cancer strength. ② Cancer prevention and resistance should make use of nation-wide advantages; give full play to the advantage of traditional Chinese medicine; conform to actual conditions in China.

③ Fundamental studies are important, but application and development research are more important. It should be observed that fundamental research → applied research →development research. Emphases are application and curative effects. Focus on increasing life quality of cancer patients, improving symptoms and prolonging survival time. ④ Restore the conservation of outpatient records (since 1976, Hubei province cancels conservation system of outpatient records and sends them to patients.); fill in full and detailed outpatient records. Therefore, full information of clinical verification is obtained to be convenient for analysis, statistics and follow-up survey (Generally, 80%~90% patients accept outpatient service, 10%~20% patients receive hospital treatment. At present hospital records are reserved to analyze and study clinical data. That 80%~90% patients accept outpatient service leads to the inexistence of outpatient records. Analysis, statistics and follow-up survey of patients' curative effects in out-patient department, and follow-up statistics of scientific researches may become impossible. Hospital records can only observe short-term curative effects; while the conservation of outpatient records can observe long-term curative effects.) Restoring and reserving outpatient records data is favorable toward outpatient clinical research to improve medical quality.

(2) Experimental work of finding new anti-cancer drugs, anti-metastasis and anti-relapse drugs from natural drugs: it's aimed at screening new anti-cancer drugs with non-tolerance, no untoward effect and high selectivity that can chronically be taken by mouth. As known to all, although current anti-cancer drugs can suppress cancer cells proliferation, due to their severe untoward effect, while using many patients have to stop administration. Afterwards cancer cells proliferate again and begin to have drug tolerance. Such as the famous anti-cancer drug formyli sarcolysine quinine, as seen from ongoing cancer cells tissue cultures, drug tolerance is up to 20,000 times. Before the appearance of drug tolerance, the dosage is usually only several milligrams. While when drug tolerance is produced, such dosage cannot meet the demand. Then it is necessary to increase the dosage. But when its dosage increases to ten times, it will cause the death of patient. Therefore, drug tolerance of cancer cells on anti-cancer drug and untoward effect of anti-cancer drug on host are long-standing problems that puzzle tumor treatment researchers. Our purpose of finding new drugs is to avoid those disadvantages and screen anti-cancer drugs with non-tolerance, no untoward effect and high selectivity that best can chronically be taken by mouth. Western anti-cancer drugs have single ingredient. Micro dosage is effective, but it will suppress normal cells. Its toxic reaction is quite strong. Some current anti-cancer drugs are extracted from traditional Chinese medicine, such as vincristine, camptothecin and colchicine; these alkaloids are similar to traditional anti-cancer drugs, i.e. micro drug is effective, but toxicity is very high.

The question is whether anti-cancer traditional Chinese medicine, which can suppress the growth of cancer cells but not kill normal cells, can be extracted from TCM. Through several years' experimental screening, the writer finally finds such kind of TCM with rather ideal anti-cancer effects. Usually when the dosage reaches 500μg/ml, it has inhibiting action on cancer cells. The writer also finds XZ-C_1 and XZ-C_4 drugs that can 100% suppress cancer cells and never kill normal cells. XZ-C_1, XZ-C_4

and XZ-C_8 also can improve the immunologic function of host, which is a superior feature of anti-cancer TCM.

As seen XZ-C series of TCM, its anti-cancer effect changes as the change of dosage. When the dosage is 250μg/ml, it can only suppress 60% cancer cells; when the dosage is 125μg/ml, suppression ratio is zero. Micro A-type drugs will be effective, such as vinblastine, berberine in Chinese goldthread, and myrobalan fruit in alkaloid, etc. But they can also suppress normal cell proliferation, which is same to traditional anti-cancer drugs. B-type drugs are other anti-cancer TCM. Only high concentration is effective. That is, micro dosage has no inhibiting action on cancer cells. Effect is directly proportional to dosage. If the dosage is larger, curative effects will be better, such as XZ-C_{1A} and XZ-C_{1B}.

3. Verification of clinical effects over the past ten years, the writer has applied experimental crude drugs to clinical medicine. XZ-C series drugs have distinctive clinical effects. That is, a certain period after the administration of B-type drugs, cancer cells neither proliferate nor shrink, while the patient begins to restore vigorous energy. Several months later, the physical strength recovers gradually. The tumor starts to shrink slowly. That is probably not toxic effect on cancer cells, but the result of creating a circumstance that is adverse to cancer cells proliferation in organisms. The long-term administration has no toxic cumulative effect on normal cells. Many patients have taken XZ-C_1 and XZ-C_4 drugs for 3~5 years, there is still no relapse, metastasis and untoward effect. The long-term plentiful administration can obtain unexpected good results.

Different types of XZ-C preparation match with various kinds of cancers, such as cancer of alimentary canal, lung cancer and cancer of uterus, etc. Compound prescriptions must be made from symptoms. Only in this way can good results be obtained.

Different from traditional medicinal broth, what the writer chooses is the mixture with every kind of single crude drug through 100 mesh screening. These crude drugs are composed as compound prescription, which is not the decoction of combined preparation, but is the mixed preparation. This kind of mixture can preserve pharmacological characteristics of each crude drug. Prolonged use of this drug will not produce the untoward effect. Probing into the application way of crude drugs is quite significant.

In actual clinical medicine, will the prolonged use cause any problems? Patients can be divided into two kinds of cases: one type of patients take considerable amount of drugs with no abnormalities. The curative effects appear slowly. Many patients have taken XZ-C_4 drugs for 3~5 years. They have high spirits and good appetites. Physical strength recovers better; body condition strengthens; state of an illness is stable; patient's condition is good. The daily clinical dosage is about 20g of coarse drugs, in which the basic remedy is anti-cancer drugs, accounting for about 10% (equal to 40g crude drugs). It is considerably different from the dosage of traditional Chinese medicine.

When will curative effects present after taking medicine? Usually 1~3 months reach peak. Therefore if patients can survive for more than six months, then about 90% patients' symptoms can be improved remarkably; 50% patients' cancer proliferation will stop; about 80% patients' survival time is lengthened.

The completely significant thing is that XZ-$C_{1\sim4}$ crude drugs preparations have favorable abirritation. Medium and advanced stages of liver cancer and cancer of pancreas both produce severe pain. Patients who have used this kind of crude drugs preparation for over one month hardly feel any pain. They even don't have to be injected with analgesic drugs. This is extremely amazing.

Extracts of single crude drugs and compounded crude drugs almost produce the same curative effect. But when decocted with traditional compound prescription, extracts of single crude drugs are less effective. Presumably this is caused by the existence of interaction among drugs. In terms of cancer treatment, the better choice is compounded medicinal preparations.

Please note that some crude drugs can also promote the reproduction of cancer cells but suppress normal cells' growth, especially mineral drugs and animal drugs. Such as pallas pit viper, hairy antler and others, even the microdosis can promote above reactions. The centipede can damage renal tubules.

Akihiko Sato says that cancer resistance of natural drugs can be divided into three categories. The first category is that ingredients of natural drugs have the effect on killing cancer cells, such as vinblastine. The second one is that polysaccharides of some drugs (e.g. purple ganoderma lucidum and evodia rutaecarpa), due to the action on enhancing immunologic function, is very popular as immunotherapy. While there is a limit that polysaccharides almost have no effect on progressive stage and advanced stage of cancer. But because of fewer untoward effects, they can be used as favorable adjuvanticity drugs. The third one is B-type anti-cancer drugs, whose active mechanism is not yet clear. When B-type drug is in high concentration, it can suppress the proliferation of cancer cells but not normal cells. Also it has fewer untoward effects and can be taken for a lone time. But it can neither kill cancer cells nor promote immunologic function. The B-type anti-cancer drug is considered as a kind of new drug.

In nearly a decade, with the intensive study, the writer has contacted with a large number of patients monthly, and collected much information that is not recorded in books and literature. And the writer has an intimate knowledge of many patients' epidemiology, clinical symptom, evolution of physical sign and analysis, evaluation and reflection on progress. Therefore the writer can carry out the following theoretic discussions.

II. Theoretic Discussion

1. Research on anti-cancer netustasis of traditional Chinese medicine from the level of modern molecular biology

In recent years, on the level of molecular immune pharmacology, domestic scholars have been carrying out a great deal of research on looking for traditional Chinese medicine and new drugs for anti-cancer, anti-metastasis and anti-relapse.

1. **From the perspective of increasing immunologic function to study traditional Chinese medicine with anti-metastasis** Tumor metastasis is a complex process, which is affected by many factors, such as wet ability and adhesiveness of cancer cells, hypercoagulable state of blood and low immunologic function, etc. Hypercoagulable state of blood plasma and low immunologic function play the major role in carcinomatous metastasis. While in microcirculatory system, detention of cancer cells is the key link in the formation of metastasis. Therefore, research is a must to exploit the traditional Chinese medicine, which can improve hypercoagulable state, low immunity and microcirculatory disturbance on the

molecular level. While XZ-C anti-cancer mixture can obviously suppress experimental lung metastasis in mice with Lewis lung cancer. The mechanism may be to enhance organism immunity, improve microcirculation and adjust immunologic function. Blood-activating and stasis-dissolving drugs, such as Elemene and others, can enhance immunologic function, reduce blood viscosity, eliminate microcirculatory disturbance and then decrease the formation and metastasis of cancer embolus.

2. **From the perspective of resisting platelet aggregation to study traditional Chinese medicine with anti-metastasis** Studies in recent years show that tumor metastasis is closely related to blood platelet. That cancer cells in blood circulation causing platelet aggregation of host is a critical step in the formation of metastasis. After cancer cells into blood circulation, they will activate platelet to produce cancer embolus. Some blood-activating and stasis-dissolving drugs have effects on resisting platelet aggregation, suppressing cancer cells and withstanding metastasis. Chen Jianmin has observed 440 cancer patients, in which 82.7% patients have high viscosity states in various degrees and are treated with stasis-dissolving prescription-xiong long decoction. Its curative effect is better. The effective rate is 65.2%. Some scholars combine red peony root and red sage root with small dose of chemotherapeutic drugs to obviously decrease metastases of cancer cells to lung. Cui Wei and other scholars use experimental studies to prove that leatherleaf milletia can obviously suppress platelet aggregation. Depolymerization rate is high. Observation under electron microscope shows that leatherleaf milletia can promote the increase of dispersive platelets. Clinically leatherleaf milletia is used to resist hematogenous metastasis of cancer embolus.
3. **From the perspective of anti-adhesion therapy to study traditional Chinese medicine with anti-metastasis** During the process of carcinomatous metastasis, cancer cells will adhere to various cells of host (e.g. endothelial cell, platelet and lymphocyte, etc.) and (or) extracellular matrix and basement membrane components. The above is also one of key factors for the occurrence of metastasis. Therefore, anti-adhesion therapy may be a new target for anti-metastasis. In recent years, studies discover that red sage root can suppress the adhesion of red blood cells in vitro with endothelial cells and platelet aggregation. It can also change tumor cell membrane to affect the affinity between tumor cells and host tissues. It has damaging effect on cancer cells. Results of animal experiments show that red sage root can decrease cancer cells into circulatory system, lessen the adhesion of cancer cells and vascular endothelial cells, reduce the capability of forming cancer embolus and lower the chance for cancer cells escaping from circulatory system.

   Pilose asiabell root and large headed atractylodes can obviously suppress metastases of cancer cells in tumor-bearing mice. Qiu Jiaxin and other scholars discover that large headed atractylodes can suppress Lweis tumor metastases to lung. This writer adopts BALB/C nude mice as models. 30d after inoculating with SGC-7901 human gastric cancer cells beneath the splenic envelope, nude mice are executed. Metastatic rate of control group is 83.33%. That of traditional Chinese medicine group is 16.67%. In clinical trials, the writer randomly classifies patients who have accepted radical operation for gastric carcinoma into two groups, involving group of taking traditional Chinese medicine that mainly invigorats the spleen and regulats the flow of qi and chemotherapy group. After one year, 35.87% patients of control group (chemotherapy) suffer from metastases of cancer cells. While metastatic rate of traditional Chinese medicine group is only 3.33%. Two years later, metastatic rate of traditional Chinese medicine group rises to 4.76% while metastatic rate of control group rises to 36.84%.

4. **From the angle of regulating signalling pathway of cancer cells to study traditional Chinese medicine with anti-cancer and anti-metastasis** Since 1980s, the study of signal system has always been the leading edge of cell biology. That is, various drug molecules in organism cannot directly enter into cells to take effect. They must combine with correlative receptors of cells. Then through signal transference, the correlative second signal system generates in cells. Finally information is transmitted to target location to take effect. In recent years, that through regulating and controlling cellular signal system to design and develop new anti-cancer and anti-metastasis drugs has caught redoubled attention from scientists.

Cuttlebones (white dragon tablets) have obvious effects on gastric carcer, lung cancer and bladder cancer, and also can obviously suppress the growth of animal solid tumor (liver cancer, lung cancer and cervical cancer). When cuttlebones are used in combination with chemotherapies, they also have effects on synergic action, toxin reduction and increase of immunologic function, etc. Liu Jun and other scholars have observed cuttlebones' regulating and controlling function to two sets of signal systems CAMP-PKA and DAG-PKC in human gastric cancer cells MGC80-3, cuttlebones' effect on suppressor gene of gastric cancer cells BGC80-3 in G_1 phase and their correlation with PKA signalling pathway. Scholars have found that cuttlebones have obvious inhibiting actions on proliferation of human gastric cancer cells. As seen from the signal system, 3h after cuttlebones' acting on MGC80-3 cells, they can increase cAMP level and PKA activity in cells, while decrease DAG content and PKC activity in cells. This indicates that cuttlebones' effects on MGC80-3 cells are realized by antagonistic regulation of two sets of signal systems.

2. Discussion on mechanism of action that effective elements of traditional Chinese medicine inhibit and kill cancer cells

1. **Traditional Chinese medicine that can inhibit and (or) kill cancer cells** Experimental studies prove that effective elements of some traditional Chinese medicines can inhibit or kill cancer cells. Such as curcumin has the cytotoxicity with concentration dependent to human gastric adenocarcinoma cells SGC-7901. It can obviously suppress the proliferation of SGC-7901 cells, and also have certain damaging effect. The electron microscope observation shows dissolution and necroses of cells.

    There are effective elements of other traditional Chinese medicines that can also suppress cancer cells, such as trichosanthin, elemene, glycyrrhizin, β-carotene and general ginsenoside, etc.

    Alcohol extractable matters of vietnamese sophora root have inhibiting effects on the proliferation of human liver cancer cells SMMC-7721 and mitochondrial metabolism.

    Elemene can obviously suppress the growth of leucemia HL-60 and K_{562} cells, prevent cancer cells to grow from S phase to G_2/M phase and finally induce apoptosis.

2. **Traditional Chinese medicine that can affect cells in proliferative stage of cell cycle** Most anti-cancer traditional Chinese medicines are cell cycle specific drugs, which mainly kill cells in the proliferative stage. Especially cells in S and M phases are most sensitive to traditional Chinese medicines. Tanshinone experiments in vitro show that it has obvious inhibiting effect on DNA syntheses of cancer cells. Tanshinone acts on S phase of cell

division cycle, suppresses DNA syntheses and has cytotoxic effect. Another example is American ginseng polysaccharides. They can effectively block DNA syntheses of cancer cells in S phase. Laiyang ginseng and fiveleaf gynostemma herb mainly act on G_2/M phase of SPC-A-1 cells and block cancer cells to proceed with mitoses. It can clearly be seen that those drugs affect proliferation and differentiation of cancer cells by changing cancer cell DNA and protein metabolism.

3. **Traditional Chinese medicine that can induce apoptosis of cancer cells** Along with the development of gene studies, it has been proved that the rapid growth, diffusion and metastasis of cancer cells are caused by too few dead cells and excessive cell proliferations. Disorder at this rate is due to the decline or loss of apoptosis ability. It is fully necessary to strengthen the research on apoptosis of cancer cells induced by drugs. Effective elements of some traditional Chinese medicines can induce apoptosis of cancer cells, such as trichosanthin has obvious inhibiting effect on melanoma cells of mice. It can cause the increase of tumor cells in G_0/G_1 phase and the decrease of cells in S phase, which show the obvious Blocking phenomenon for G_0/G_1 phase. That is, trichosanthin prevents the proliferation of cancer cells and induces apoptosis of cancer cells. Another example is the taxol. It is a kind of anti-cancer drug that is abstracted from the bark of natural drug—yew. Its cytotoxicity on cancer cells is relevant to its induction of apoptosis. Pharmacody and clinical experiments of elemene prove that it has exact curative effect on cancer. The flow cytometry proves that elemene can prevent cancer cells to grow from S phase to G_2/M phase and finally induce apoptosis.
4. **Traditional Chinese medicine that can affect genes of cancer cells and inhibit cancer gene expression** p53 gene is the cancer suppressor gene and can inhibit cell proliferation. Wei Xiaolong and other scholars have studied the effect of rehmannia root polysaccharide (LRPS) with low molecular weight on p53 gene expression. They have found that when optimal anti-cancer doses of LRPS are 20mg/kg and 40mg/kg, expression levels of p53 gene in Lewis lung cancer cells are respectively 1.52 and 1.48. While that of control group is 0.46, which explains that LRP can promote the obvious increase of p53 gene expressions in Lewis lung cancer cells. The conclusion is that the effect of LRPS on p53 anti-cancer gene expressions belongs to one of its anti-cancer mechanisms. Also icariin can decrease expression levels of bcl-2 and c-myc genes. Arsenic oxide in arsenic trioxide and arsenic disulfide can obviously lower bcl-2 gene and lead to the reduction of bcl-2/bax ratio.
5. **Traditional Chinese medicine that can induce the differentiation of cancer cells** Inducing differentiation therapy of tumor cells is a tumor research hotspot in the world. Its feature is not to kill tumor cells but induce cancer cells to differentiate into normal cells or cells that are similar to normal cells. In the past decade and more, domestic scholars have started the research on the differentiation of tumor cells induced by traditional Chinese medicine. Until now, they have found dozens of traditional Chinese medicine extracts show the effect on inducing the differentiation of tumor cells in experiments. Yi Yonglin and other scholars adopt general ginsenoside (GSL) to act on 58 cases of acute non-lymphocytic leukemia. The result shows that GSL has inducing differentiation effects with different degrees on various cells of this disease. Another example is notoginseng saponin R_1. It has the strong induction to make HL-60 cells (human promyelocytic leukemia cell strain) differentiate toward granulocyte series. The effective element—poriatin (F_{101}) extracted from poria cocos has effects on inhibiting the proliferation of tumor cells and activating macrophage in mouse' abdominal cavity. Many experiments have found that

there is a certain link between effective induction of leukemia cell differentiation and proliferation inhibition. Han Rui and other scholars have found that traditional Chinese medicines belonged to the sort of cassia have cassic acid and ramification. Cells of cloning high-metastasis giant cell carcinoma of lung ($PGCL_3$) are treated with cassic acid. Experimental results show that the form, proliferation rate, divisional index, agglomeration reaction and others of tumor cells totally convert to normal cells. At the same time, invasion and metastasis abilities of tumor cells are obviously weakened. Xu Jianguo and other scholars have found that water extracts of 22 kinds of traditional Chinese medicines have inducing differentiation effects with different degrees on HL-60 cells. For the emulsifying agent of effective elements of -elemenum emulsion radix curcumae, Qian Jun and other scholars inject 30μg/ml emulsifying agent into human lung cancer cells in vitro culture. Then they discover that the growth of lung cancer cells is inhibited. The flow cytometry analysis shows that 72h after injection, the proportion of lung cancer cells in G_0/G_1 phase increases. While proportion of lung cancer cells in S phase decreases. Observations under light microscope and electron microscope show that after the injection, the proliferation of cancer cells slows down, cells shrink and turn around, the number of microvilli decreases, nucleo-cytoplasmic ratio reduces and the number of heterochromatin increases. The above prompts that this medicine can reverse into lung cancer cell phenotype on the level of cytobiology and morphology. And finally these cells are induced to tend to differentiation.

Traditional Chinese medicines and their effective elements discovered in the above studies provide instructive train of thoughts and references for searching and preparing tumor differentiation inducer and studying the differentiation inducing mechanism in the future. And they also provide new idea, method and therapeutic evaluation standard for cancer treatment with traditional Chinese medicines. In the past, regulating dysfunction of organism with traditional Chinese medicines only means to regulate dysfunction of viscera. While inducing differentiation therapy with traditional Chinese medicines is on levels of cell, molecular organism and gene to regulate dysfunction of proliferation and apoptosis and dysfunction of proliferation and differentiation control. Cancer cell is the immature cell with incomplete differentiation. Differentiation inducer of traditional Chinese medicines promotes its further complete differentiation. Cancer cells grow to mature cells and lose malignant features. As seen from the level of cells, it can be called a kind of “strengthening vital qi” therapy. The therapeutic standards are the appearance of differentiation index, disappearance of tumor malignant features and survival time prolongation of tumor-bearing organism. The standard is not only the change of lump size. The appearance of differentiation index and prolongation of survival time are the most vital factors.

Tumor inducing differentiation therapy is the continuing discovery that develops the differentiation inducer with higher effective and lower toxic features. In this respect, traditional Chinese medicines have a big advantage. That is because that traditional Chinese medicines are rich in natural resources, traditional Chinese medicine and pharmacology have a long history. In several thousand years, abundant invaluable experience has been accumulated to provide extremely favorable conditions for developing and preparing Chinese materia medica preparation with higher effective and lower toxic features.

In studies, besides referring the above chemical structure of traditional Chinese medicine, effective elements and other factors, there are some other ideas for consideration, such as interferon (IFN). Especially IFN-γ can induce the differentiation of cancer cells. While many traditional Chinese medicines can induce IFN-γ in vivo. In conclusion, tumor inducing differentiation therapy is receiving more and more attention from foreign and domestic scholars. The research and application of traditional Chinese medicines in this field have an extensive future.

CHAPTER 27

Observation of Experimental and Clinic Curative Effect on Z-C Medicine Treating Malignancy

[Abstract] Objectives To find Traditional Chinese Medicines of Treating carcinoma which are good for curative effect and have no side effect. **Methods** We use liver cancer $H_{2,2}$ to inoculate 260 Kun Ming little white mice which are divided into group Z-C_1 and group Z-C_4, group of chemical treatment (CTX) and group of contrapose.

Results We observe that the repression rate of mice H_{22} in liver cancer to of group Z-C_1 for 2, 4, 6 weeks is 40%, 45% and 58%, and repression rate of mice H_{22} in liver cancer to of group Z-C_4 for 2, 4, 6 weeks is 55%,68% and 70%, while repression rate of group CTX for 2, 4 and 6 weeks is 45%, 45% and 49%. For ten years' clinic observation of 4277 middle and later period cancer patients, we find that Z-C medicine has good effect to prolong survival and has no side response for long time taking patients. **Conclusions** Through experimental research and clinic validation, it is proved that Z-C_1, Z-C_4 medicine can improve the survival quality and immunity of middle and later period patients, and control the increase of carcinoma cells to get a further curative effect.

[Key words] transplant of carcinoma cells; thymus atrophy; the repression rate of carcinoma

In order to look for the traditional herb medicine with actually curative effect and without toxication and adverse reaction, this surgical tumor research institute has screened 200 kinds of Chinese herbal medicines with so-called anticancer reaction recorded on Chinese herbal medicine books for tumor-inhibition reaction on the solid carcinoma in the tumor-bearing animal models one by one in the past 4 years. Through long-term in-vivo tumor-inhibiting animal experiments, we have screened 48 kinds of Chinese herbal medicines with relatively good tumor-inhibition rate that can prolong the survival time, protect the immune organ and obviously improve the immunologic function. According to the clinical conditions, the anticancer medicines screened are combined into 2 compounds including Z-C_1 and Z-C_4 with better anti-cancer reaction than each single medicine. In the original screening, we carried out the tumor-inhibiting animal experiment for each single medicine and now we further carry out the experimental study on these two groups of compounds for the tumor-inhibiting reaction in the solid tumor of the tumor-bearing rats.

I. Experimental Study on Animal

1. Materials and Method
   (1) Experimental animal: 260 Kunming clon white rats, half of male and female respectively, weight:21±2g, 8~10 weeks.
   (2) Cell strains and inoculation: hepatic carcinoma H_{22} cell strains, the fresh tumor bodies from the rats with tumor were prepared into the single cell suspended liquid, after

dyeing and counting of the cancer cells (1x 10^6/ml), 0.2ml normal saline of cancer cell was subject to subcutaneous vaccination at the front axilla at the right side of each rat.

(3) Drugs and experimental group: the traditional herb medicines Z-C_1 and Z-C_4 were entirely developed and prepared by Hubei Branch of China Anti-cancer Research Cooperation of Chinese Traditional Medicine and Western Medicine, the former was a compound and the latter was a medicinal powder. The chemotherapy control medicine used by the chemotherapy group was cyclophosphane (CTX).

Experimental group: the animals with H_{22} cancer cell transplanted were divided into four groups randomly: ① traditional herb medicine Z-C_1 group (90 rats). The rats were subject to gastriclavage once every day after 24h of transplantation of cancer cells, 0.8ml per rat every time, equivalent to 1.4mg of the dried medicinal herbs. ②Traditional herb medicine Z-C_4 group (90 rats), as to the dose and gastriclavage method, ditto. ③Chemotherapy group (50 rats), from the next day after transplantation of cancer cells, they were subject to gastriclavage with CTX50mg/kg weight every other day. ④Control group (30 rats), they were subject to gastriclavage with normal saline every day from the next day after transplantation of the cancer cells, 0.8ml/rat.

(4) Observation of indexes: measure the weight of the rats every 3d, measure the diameter of the tumor with vernier caliper, measure the immunologic function and blood picture. Half of each group as Group A, subject to tumor-bearing experiment, regular killing of the rats in batches, separation of tumor and weighing of the tumor and then calculation of tumor-inhabiting rate. The tumor was subject to the pathological section and a few of the specimens were subject to the observation of ultra-structural organization. The rest half of each group as Group B. The tumor-bearing experimental rats were drenched for a long time until they met with natural death. Then the tumor was separated and weighed, the long-term inhibition rate and life elongation rate of the tumor was calculated.

2. Experimental result

(1) The tumor-inhibition effect of Z-C Medicine on Rats bearing hepatic carcinoma H_{22}: in the second week after administration of Z-C_1, the tumor-inhibition rate was 40% and the one in the fourth week was 45% and 58% in the sixth week. The tumor-inhibition rate after administration of Z-C_4 was 55%, 68% in the fourth week and 70% in the sixth week. ($P<0.01$) the tumor-inhibiting rate after administration of CTX was 45% in the second week, 45% in the fourth week and 49% in the sixth week (See Fig. 27-1 and 27-2).

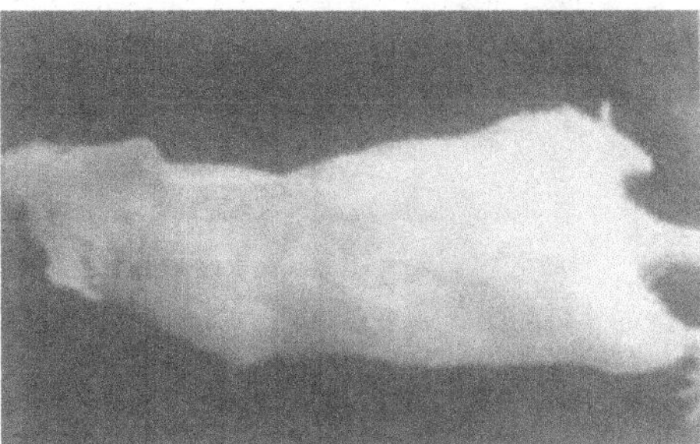

Fig. 27-1 Z-C_1 and Z-C_4 therapy group 30d after inoculation of hepatic carcinoma H_{22}

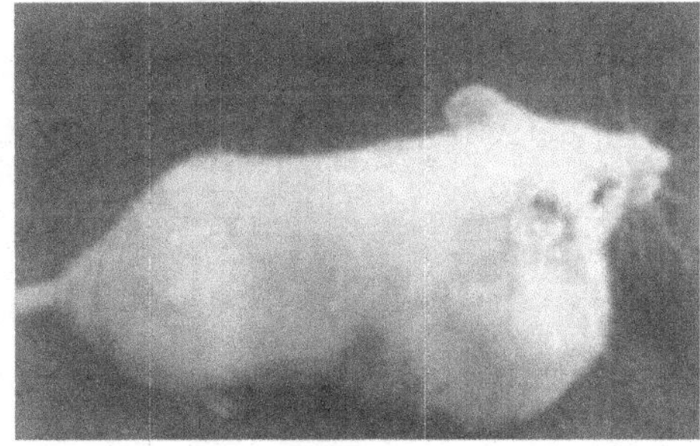

Fig. 27-2 Control group 30d after inoculation of hepatic carcinoma H_{22}

(2) The effect of Z-C medicine on the survival time of the rats bearing hepatic carcinoma H_{22}: the average survival time of Z-C_1, Z-C_4 and CTX was longer than the one of the normal saline control group ($P<0.01$); Z-C medicine played a role in obviously prolonging the survival time. Through comparison with the control group, the life elongation rate of Z-C_1 group was 85%, the one of Z-C_4 group was 200% and the one of CTX group was 9.8%. The rats in Z-C_1 and CTX in Group B met with death in 75d. 6 rats bearing carcinoma in Z-C_4 survived after seven months.

(3) Both Z-C_1 and Z-C_4 medicine improved the immunologic function and Z-C_4 obviously improved the immunologic function, increased the white blood cells and red blood cells, without any effect on the hepatic function and kidney function and without damage to the hepatic and kidney section. CTX decreased the white blood cells and reduced the immunologic function with the renal damage to the kidney section. The thymus in the control group was obviously atrophic (Fig. 1-4) while the one of Z-C_1 and Z-C_2 therapy group was not atrophic but a little hypertrophic (Fig.1-3).

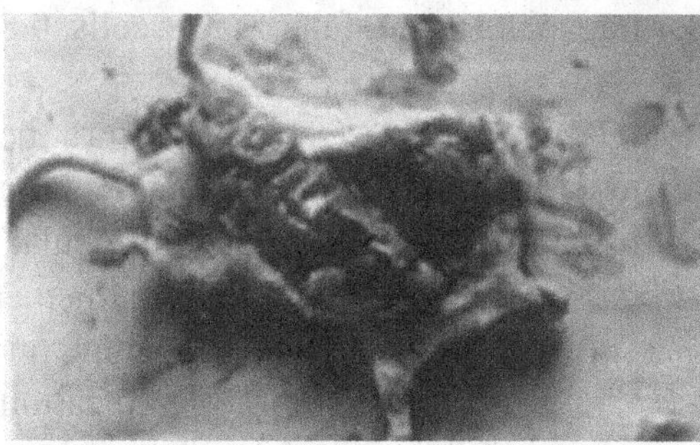

Fig. 27-3 Z-C_4 therapy group
The thymus was obviously hypertrophic in 30 days after inoculation of hepatic carcinoma H_{22}

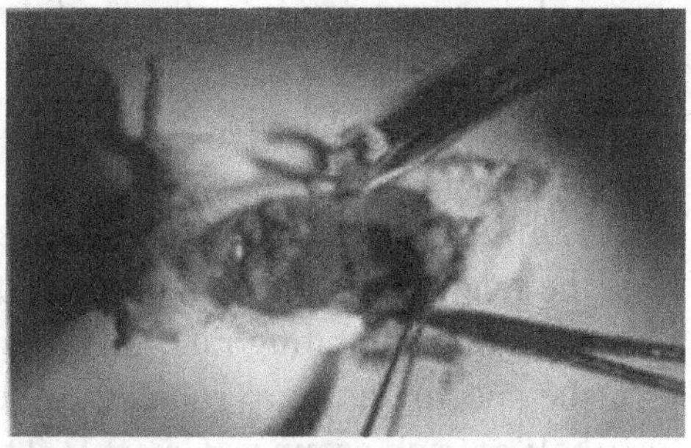

Fig. 27-4 Control group
The thymus was obviously atrophic in 30 days after inoculation of hepatic carcinoma H_{22}

Pathological section of thymus in the control group: the cortex of the thymus was atrophic, the cells were discrete and the blood vessel met with sludge (Fig. 1-5). The pathological section of the thymus in Z-C_4 therapy group displayed that the cortical area of the thymus built up, the lymphocyte was dense, the epithelium reticulocyte increased and the thymus corpuscles increased (Fig. 1-6).

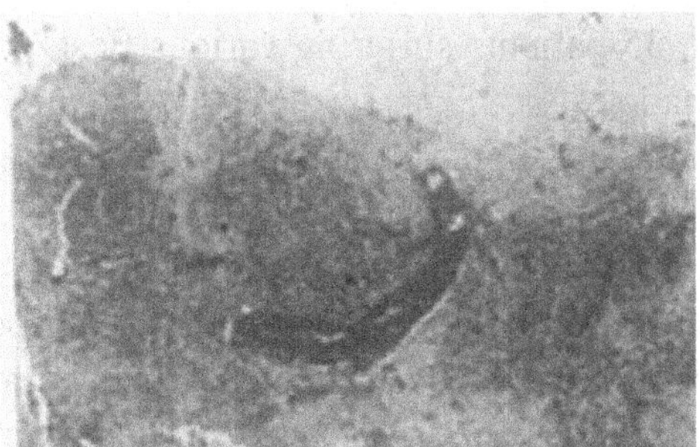

Fig. 27-5 Pathological section of the thymus in tumor-bearing control group HE x 100 cortex atrophia lymphocyte obviously decreased, cortical area formed an empty band of lymphocyte and the sludge appeared in the blood vessel.

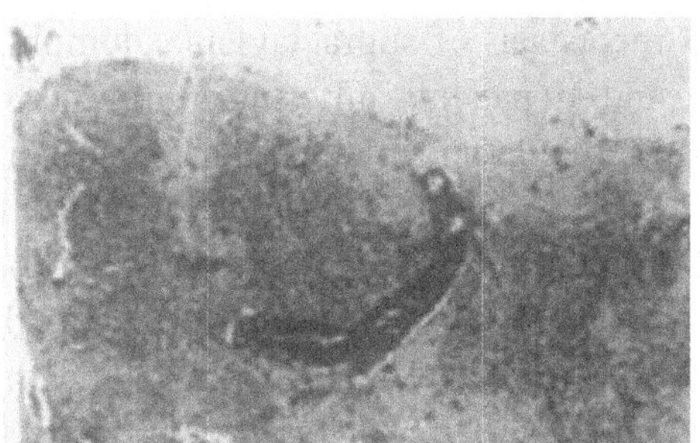

Fig. 27-6 Thymus of Z-C_4 control group HE x 100 the cortex and medulla of the thymus built up and the lymphocyte was highly dense

II. Observation on Clinic Application

1. Clinical information

(1) Hubei Branch of China Anti-cancer Research Cooperation of Chinese Traditional Medicine and Western Medicine, Anti Carcinoma Metastasis and Recurrence Research Office and Shuguang Tumor Specialized Outpatient Department had treated 4, 698 carcinoma patients in Stage III and IV or in metastasis and recurrence with Z-C medicine combined with western medicine from 1994 to Nov. 2002, among which there were 3, 051 men patients and 1,647 women patients. The youngest one was 11 years old and the oldest one was 86 years old, the high invasion age was 40~69 years. All groups of the patients were entirely subject to the diagnosis of pathological histology or definitive diagnosis with ultrasonic B, CT and MRI iconography. According to the staging standard of UICC, all the cases were entirely the patients in medium and advanced stage over Stage III. In this group, there were 1,021 hepatic carcinoma patients, among which there were 694 primary lesion hepatic carcinoma patients and 327 metastatic hepatic carcinoma patients; there were 752 patients suffering from carcinoma of lung, among which there were 699 patients suffering from the primary carcinoma of lung and 53 patients suffering from the metastatic carcinoma of lung; there were 668 gastric carcinoma patients, 624 patients suffering from esophagus cardia carcinoma, 328 patients suffering from rectum carcinoma of anal canal, 442 patients suffering from carcinoma of colon, 368 patients suffering from breast carcinoma, 74 patients suffering from adenocarcinoma of pancreas, 30 patients suffering from carcinoma of bile duct, 43 patients suffering from retroperitoneal tumor, 38 patients suffering from oophoroma, 9 patients suffering from cervical carcinoma, 11 patients suffering from cerebroma, 34 patients suffering from thyroid carcinoma, 38 patients suffering from nasopharyngeal carcinoma, 9 patients suffering from melanoma, 27 patients suffering from kidney carcinoma, 48 patients suffering from carcinoma of urinary bladder, 13 patients suffering from leukemia, 47 patients suffering from

metastasis of supraclavicular lymph nodes, 35 patients suffering various fleshy tumors and 39 patients suffering from other malignancies.

(2) Medicine and medication: the treatment aims to support healthy energy to eliminate evils, soften and resolve the hard mass and supplement qi and blood. Z-C_1 is the compound, 150ml to be taken on the daily basis, Z-C_4 is powder, 10g to be taken on the daily basis. According to the analysis and differentiation of the diseases, anti-cancer powder shall be taken orally and the anti-cancer apocatastasis paste shall be applied externally for the solid tumor or the metastatic tumor. In case of being in pain, anti-cancer aponic paste shall be applied externally. Icterus removal soup or dropsy removal soup shall be taken orally for the patients suffering from icterrus and the ascites.

(3) Therapeutic evaluation: it pays attention to the short-term curative effect and iconography indexes as well as the survival time of long-term curative effect, quality of life and immunologic indexes. Attention shall be paid to the changes in subjective signs in administration of drugs. It will be effective when the subjective signs are improved and last over one month; otherwise, it will be ineffective. As to the quality of life (Karnofsky Performance Status), it will be effective when it is improved and lasts over one month, otherwise, it will be ineffective. As to the evaluation standard of the curative effect of solid tumor, it can be divided into four levels according to the changes in size of tumor: Level I: disappearance of tumor; Level II: tumor reduces 1/2; Level III: softening of tumor; Level IV: no change or enlargement of level tumor.

2. Curative results

(1) The symptom was improved, the quality of life was improved, the survival time was prolonged: among the 4,277 carcinoma patients in medium and advanced stage who took Z-C medicine with the return visit over 3 months, the case history had the specific observation record of the curative effect, see Table 1-1. It improved the quality of life of the patients in an all-round way, see Table 1-2.

Table 1-1 General information about 4,277 patients suffering from recurrence and metastasis

		Hepatic carcinoma	Carcinoma of lung	Gastric carcinoma	Esophagus cardia carcinoma	Rectum carcinoma of anal canal	Carcinoma of colon	Breast carcinoma	adenocarcinoma of pancreas
No. of cases		1 021	752	668	624	328	442	368	74
Male: female		4:1	4.4:1	2.25:1	3.1:1	1:1	2.1:1	Female	3.2:1
Focus	Primary	694 (68.6%)	699 (93.9%)						
	Metastasis	327 (31.2%)	53 (6.1%)						

Usual metastasis part in this group		Metastatic lung (2) From the stomach (31.2%)	Metastasis of supraclavicular lymph nodes (11.6%)	Metastatic lever (23.8%) Lung metastasis (3%)	Upper metastasis of compact bone (13.1%)	Reoccurrence rate (14.8%)	Metastatic lever (16.0%)	Metastasis of supraclavicular lymph nodes (17.5%)	Metastatic lever (11.7%)
		From esophagus cardia (19.5%) From recta (31.2%)	Brain metastasis (3.1%) Bone metastasis (4.6%)	Metastasis of peritoneum (29.1%) Upper metastasis of compact bone (6.1%)	Metastatic lever (8.3%)	Metastatic lever (7.0%)	Metastasis of peritoneum (6.0%)	Metastasis of axillary lymph nodes (15.0%) Bone metastasis (5.0%)	Rear metastasis of peritoneum (39.1%)
Age	high invasion (year) %	30~39 (76.2)	50~69 (71.6)	40~49 (73.4)	40~69 (80.4)	40~49 (75.2)	30~69 (88.0)	40~59 (65.9)	40~59 (70.0)
	Oldest (year) %	11	20	17	30	27	27	29	34
	Youngest (year) %	86	80	77	77	78	76	80	68

Table 1-2 Observation of curative effect on 4 277 patients: fully improving the quality of life of the carcinoma patients in medium and advanced stage

Improvement	Vigor	Appetite	Reinforcement of physical force	Improvement in generalized case	Increase of body weight	Improvement of sleep	The restriction of improvement activity and capability released activity	self servicing normal walking	Resumption of work Engaged in light work
No. of cases (%)	4071	3986	2450	479	2938	1005	1038	3220	479
	95.2	93.2	57.3	11.2	68.7	23.5	24.3	75.3	11.2

In this group, all of them were the patients in medium and advanced stage. After taking the medicine, their symptoms were improved to different extents with the effective rate of 93.2%. With respect to the improvement of the quality of life (as per Karnofsky Performance Status), it rose to 80 scores on average after administration from 50 on average before administration; the patients in this group met with the different metastasis and dysfunction of the organs about Stage III. It was reported by the previous statistic information that the mesoposition survival time of this kind of patients was about 6 months. The longest time among this group of the cases reached up to 11 years; another patient suffering from hepatic carcinoma had taken Z-C medicine for ten years and a half; two patients suffering from hepatic carcinoma met with frequency encountered carcinomatous lesion in the left and right liver and it entirely subsided through secondary CT reexamination after the patient took Z-C medicine for half a year and the state of the disease had been stable over half a year. One patient suffering from double-kidney carcinoma met with the widespread metastasis of abdominal cavity after removal of one kidney, after taking Z-C medicine, he was entirely recovered and began to work again. 3 patients suffering from carcinoma of lung, with the lung not removed through explaraton, had taken Z-C medicine over three years and a half. 2 patients suffering from gastric remnant carcinoma had taken Z-C medicine for 8 years. 3 patients suffering from reoccurrence of rectal carcinoma had taken Z-C medicine for 3 years. 1 patient suffering from metastatic liver and rib of the mastocarcinoma had taken Z-C medicine for 8 years. 1 patient suffering from the recurrent bladder carcinoma after operation of renal carcinoma had not met with the carcinoma for 9 years and a half after taking Z-C medicine. All of these patients were the ones in the medium and advanced stage that could not be operated once more or treated with radiotherapy or chemotherapy. They only took Z-C medicine without other medicines for treatment. Up to today, they are reexamined and get the medicine at the out-patient department every month. Through taking the medicine for a long time, the state of the disease is controlled in the stable state to make the organism and the tumor in balanced state for a relatively long time and get a relatively good survival with tumor, in this way, the symptoms of the patients are improved, the quality of life is improved and the survival time is prolonged.

(3) As to 84 patients suffering from solid tumor and 56 patients suffering from enlargement of upper lymph node of metastatic compact bone, after taking Z-C series medicines orally and applying Z-C3 anti-cancer apocatastasis paste, they met with good curative effects, see table 1-3.

Table 1-3 Changes of 84 patients suffering from solid tumor and 56 patients suffering from metastatic mode after applying Z-C paste externally

	Solid tumor				Enlargement of upper lymph node of metastatic compact bone			
	Disappearance	Shrinkage 1/2	Softening	No change	Disappearance	Shrinkage 1/2	Softening	No change
No. of cases	12	28	32	12	12	22	14	8
(%)	14.2	33.3	38.0	14.2	21.4	39.2	25.0	14.2
Total effective rate (%)	85.7				85.7			

(3) 298 patients suffering from carcinoma pain obtained the obvious pain alleviation effects after taking Z-C medicine orally and applying Z-C anti-cancer apocatastasis paste externally, see Table 1-4.

Clinical menifetation	Pain			
	Light alleviation	Obvious alleviation	Disappearance	Avoidance
No of cases	52	139	93	14
(%)	17.3	46.8	31.2	4.7
Total effective rate (%)			95.3	

III. Discuss about Z-C Medicine Experiment and Clinic Curative Effect

1. Tumor-inhibition effect of $Z\text{-}C_{1\sim4}$ Medicine on hepatic carcinoma H_{22} rats bearing tumor

It was found that after the medicine was taken to H_{22} tumor-bearing rats for two weeks, four weeks and six weeks, the tumor inhibition rate increased with the prolongation of the administration time, the tumor inhibition rate of $Z\text{-}C_4$ in the 6th week reached up to 70%. Through two repeated experiments in succession, the results were stable, which indicated that the tumor-inhibition effect of Chinese herb medicine was slow and it would increase gradually, that is to say, the tumor-inhibition effect was of positive correlation to the accumulated dosage of Chinese herb medicine.

The effect on the survival time of hepatic carcinoma H_{22} tumor-bearing rats from $Z\text{-}C_1$ and $Z\text{-}C_4$ medicine: it was proven by the experimental results that $Z\text{-}C_1$ and $Z\text{-}C_4$ medicine could obviously prolong the survival time of the tumor-bearing rats, especially $Z\text{-}C_4$, it could prolong the survival time as long as 200%, more than that, $Z\text{-}C_4$ could remarkably improve the immunologic function of the organism, protect the immune organ and the bone marrow, alleviate the toxic action and side effect of the radiotherapy and chemotherapy medicines. Furthermore, no toxic action or side effect had been found in the past 12 months after the rats took the medicine. The above-mentioned experimental study offered the beneficial basis to the clinical application.

2. Clinical curative effect

Based on the experimental study, it had been applied to various clinical carcinomas, most of the patients were the ones over Stage III and IV, namely: the ones suffering from the cancer of late stage that could not be removed with exploratory operation; the ones with the exploratory operation without operation indication; the ones meeting with metastasis or reoccurrence in short term or long term after operation of the carcinoma; the ones suffering from hepatic metastasis, lung metastasis or brain metastasis in late stage or the ones accompanied with carcinoma hydrops and hydrops abdominis; the ones suffering from various carcinomas conservative removal operation with the exploratory operation only for the anastomosis of intestines and stomach or colostomy but not for removal and the ones not suitable for the operation, chemotherapy and radiotherapy and so on. Through over 10 years' clinical application and systematic observation, $Z\text{-}C_1$ and $Z\text{-}C_4$ medicine had obtained remarkable curative effect and no toxic action and side effect had been found after long-term administration. It had been proven by the clinical observation that $Z\text{-}C_1$

and Z-C_4 medicine could improve the survival quality of the carcinoma patients in medium and late stage in an all-round way, improve the whole immunity, control the hyperplasia of the cancer cells, consolidate and enhance the long-term curative effect. The oral-taken and external-applied Z-C medicine had good curative effect in softening and shrinking body surface metastatic tumor. With the assistance of intervention or treatment with cannula spray pump for medicine, it could protect liver, kidney and bone marrow hemopoietic system and the immune organ and improve the immunity.

3. Good pain alleviation effect of Z-C anti-cancer pain alleviation paste

   Pain is the relatively remarkable and painful symptom of the carcinoma patients in late stage, the common pain reliever had no remarkable effect on carcinoma pain, the stupefacient pain reliever had the addiction and dependence, Z-C anti-cancer pain alleviation paste had strong pain alleviation effect with a long maintenance time. It was proven through 298 cases of clinical verification that the effective rate was 78.0%, the total effective rate was 95.3%, after repeated application, there were no toxic action or side effect, without addiction. The paid alleviation effect was stable and it was an effective therapeutic method for the carcinoma patients to get rid of the pain and improve the quality of life.

IV. Z-C Medicine is a Modern Production of Traditional Herb Medicine

Z-C medicine was neither the experiential prescription nor the prescription made by the famous doctor of traditional Chinese medicine, but 48 kinds of traditional herb medicines screened from 200 kinds of common Chinese herbal medicines with so-called anticancer reaction after the animal screening test in batches and vitro screening and screening of tumor-inhibition rate in the tumor-bearing animal body one by one through over 4000 tumor-bearing animal models in the past 7 years with the modern medical method, experimental tumor study method and modern pharmacody and drug effect study method.

The substantial foundation of the traditional prescriptions that bring its unique curative effect into play in clinic was its chemical compositions. The changes in quality and quantity of the chemical compositions would directly affect the curative effect of the prescription in clinic. Therefore, it is necessary to study the changes in quality and quantity of the chemical compositions in the prescription and find out the main effective compositions in the prescription. Z-C medicine basically finds out its effect of medicine, action, molecular weight and constitutional formula and makes the study on the traditional prescription on a new step.

The prescription of Z-C medicine is the innovation and reform of the traditional herbal prescriptions, it is not the bonded solutions through mixing and boiling, but the granular concentration or powder of the medical compounds. The dried medicinal herbs in the medical compound still remain its original compositions without any change in pharmacological action, molecular weight and constitutional formula. It is made with modern scientific method but not through chemical combination, in this way, the original compositions and functions are remained for assessing and affirming the action and curative effect of the medical compounds.

References

1. Han Rui, editor-in-chief, Study and Experimental Technology of Anti-cancer Medicines. Beijing: Joint Press of Beijing Medical University and Peking Union Medical College, 1997
2. He Xinhuai, Xi Xiaoxian, editor-in-chief. Immunology of Traditional Herb Medicine. Beijing: People's Military Medical Press, 2002, 341-348
3. Zhou Jinhuang. Immunopharmacology of Traditional Herb Medicine. Beijing: People's Military Medical Press, 1994: 134-157
4. Xu Ze. New Concept and New Mode of Carcinoma Therapy. Wuhan: Hubei Science and Technology Press, 2001,171-173

CHAPTER 28

Study On Action Mechanism Of XZ-C Traditional Chinese Anti-Carcinoma Medicine For Immunologic Regulation And Control

With more and deeper researches on traditional Chinese medicine, it has been proved that many kinds of traditional Chinese medicine can regulate and control the production and biological activity of cytokine and other immune molecules, which is meaningful to explain the immunological mechanism of XZ-C traditional Chinese anti-carcinoma medicine for immunologic regulation and control from the level of molecule.

I. Protecting Immune Organs and Increasing the Weight of Thymus and Spleen

That XZ-C traditional Chinese medicine can protect immune organs resulting from the following active principles.

1. XZ-C-T (EBM):

   Using its 15g/kg and 30g/kg extracting solution (equivalent to 1g original medicine) along with 12.5mg/kg, 25mg/kg ferulic acid suspension to feed the mice for seven days in a raw can increase the weight of thymus and spleen obviously, especially the effects of the group with high dose are more apparent. Intraperitoneal injection of EBM polysaccharide can also alleviate thymus and spleen atrophy obviously caused by perdnisolone.

2. XZ-C-O (PMT)

   Extract PM-2, feed the mice with 6g/(kg·d) PMT decoction for successive seven days which can increase the weight of thymus and celiac lymph nodes and antagonize the reduction in the weight of immune organs caused by perdnisolone. Drenching the mouse of 15 months old with 6g/kg decoction (with the concentration of 0.5g/ml) for 14 days can increase the weight and volume of thymus, thicken the cortex and raise cellular density apparently. The combined use of PM and astragalus root can promote non-lymphocyte hyperplasia and benefit the micro environment of thymus.

3. XZ-C-W (SCB)

   SCB polysaccharide can gain weight of thymus and spleen of a normal mouse. Lavage with it enables cyclophosphane to control the gain in the weight of thymus and spleen.

4. XZ-C-M (LLA)

   Drench a mouse with LLA decoction for seven days resulting in increasing the weight of thymus and spleen.

5. XZ-C-L

For a 15-month old mouse, its thymus degenerates obviously. Astragalus injectio can enlarge the thymus significantly. The cortex under microscope is thickened and the cellular density increase obviously.

II. Effects on Proliferation, Differentiation and Hematopiesis of Marrow Cells

The following active principles of XZ-C traditional Chinese medicine have effects on hematopiesis of marrow cells.

1. XZ-C-Q (LBP) extracts (PM-2)

(1) Effects on the proliferation of hematopoietic stem cell (CFU-S) of a normal mouse: inject PM-2 with the dose of 500mg/(kg·d)×3d or 10mg/(kg·d)×3d LBP into the experimental mice respectively by venoclysis and kill them in the ninth day. It can be found that the number of spleen CFU-S in the group with administration increases obviously. The number of CFU-S in group PM-2 is 21% higher than that of the control group and it is 36% in the group with LBP.

(2) Effects on colony forming unit of granulocytes and macrophages (CFU-GM): the experimental results indicate that LBP with the dose of 5~30mg/(kg·d)×3d can increase the number of CFU-GM and PM-2 can also strengthen the effect of CFU-GM with the effective dose of 12.5~50mg/(kg·d)×3d. In the early stage of cultivation, most CFU-GMs are units of granulocytes and then units of macrophages increase gradually. In the anaphase units of macrophages take over the dominance.

From the above experiment, it can be found that PM-2 and LBP can promote hematopiesis of normal mice obviously. The experiment proves that during the process of restoring hematopiesis damaged by cyclophosphamide, PM-2 and LBP stimulate the proliferation of granulocytes at first, and then marrow karyocytes multiply; at last these two promote the restoration of peripheral granulocytes.

2. XZ-C-D (TSPG)

Ginsenoside, which is the active principle of ginseng to promote hematopiesis, can bring the recovery of erythrocyte in peripheral blood, haemoglobin and myeloid cell of thighbone in the mice of marrow-inhibited type, increase the index of myeloid cellular division and stimulate the proliferation of myeloid hematopoietic cell in vitro so as to make it into cell cycle with active proliferation ($S+G_2/M$ stage). TSPG can promote the proliferation and differentiation of polyenergetic hematopoietic cells and induce the formation of hemopoietic growth factor (HGF).

3. XZ-C-H (RCL)

Steamed Chinese Foxglove can promote the recovery of erythrocyte and haemoglobin for animals with blood deficiency and accelerate the proliferation and differentiation of myeloid hematopoietic cell (CFU-S) with the effect of predominance and hematosis significantly. Peritoneal injection of rehmannia polysaccharides for successive six days can promote the proliferation and differentiation of myeloid hematopoietic cells and progenitor cells as well as increasing the number of leucocytes in peripheral blood.

4. XZ-C-J (ASD)

   ASD polysaccharide has no effects on erythrocytes and leucocytes of normal mice, but for those damaged by radiation, injection of ASD polysaccharide can influence the proliferation and differentiation of both polyenergetic hematopoietic stem cells (CPU-S) and hemopoietic progenitor cells. But its decoction has no obvious effects.

5. XZ-C-E (PEW)

   Poria cocos (micromolecule chemical compound extracted from Tuckahoe polysaccharide) is the active principle that can strengthen the production of colony stimulating factor (CSF) and improve the level of leucocytes in peripheral blood inside the mouse's body. It can also prevent the decline in leucocytes caused by cyclophosphamide and accelerate the recovery with the effects better than sodium ferulic which is used to increase leucocytes.

6. XZ-C-Y (PAR)

   Its polysaccharide can obviously resist the decline in leucocytes caused by cyclophosphamide and increase the number of myeloid cells to promote the proliferation of myeloid induced by CSF as well as the recovery and reconstitution of hematopiesis for the mice irradiated by X ray. It can also increase the number of hematopoietic stem cells and myeloid cells along with leucocytes.

III. Enhancing Immunologic Function of T Cells

The active principles of XZ-C traditional Chinese medicine and their effects are following.

1. XZ-C-L (AMB)

   It can raise the percentage of lymphocytes in peripheral blood obviously. The LBP in small dose (5~10mg/kg) can cause the proliferation of lymphocytes, indicating that LBP can promote the proliferation of T cells apparently. 50mg/(kg·d)×7d is the best dose in that it will have no effects if lower than the level and it will bring the effects down if higher than the level. Oral administration of LBP can raise the conversion rate of lymphocytes for the sufferers who are weak and with fewer leucocytes.

2. XZ-C_4

   It can regulate immune system and active T cells of aggregated lymphatic follicles, as well as stimulate the secretion of hemopoietic growth factor in T cells. Among the crude drugs of XZ-C_4, the extract from the hot water of atractylodes lancea rhizome can obviously stimulate the cells of aggregated lymphatic follicles, which is regarded as the base of XZ-C_4 immunoloregulation.

IV. Activating and Enhancing NK Cell Activity

Natural killer cell, NK cell is another kind of killer cell in lymphocytes for human beings and mice, which needs neither antigenic stimulation, nor the participation of antibodies to kill some cells. It plays an important role in immunity, especially in the function of immune surveillance as NK cell is the first line of defense against tumors and has broad spectrum anti-tumor effects.

NK cell is broad-spectrum and able to kill sygeneous, homogenous and heterogenous tumor cells with special effects on lymjphoma and leucocytes.

NK cell is an important kind of cells for immunoloregulation, which can regulate T cells, B cells and stem cells, etc. It can also regulate immunity by releasing cytokines like IFN- α , IFN- γ , IL-2, TNF, etc.

The active principles in XZ-C traditional Chinese medicine and their effects are following.

1. XZ-C-X (SDS)

   Divaricate Saposhniovia Root can strengthen the activity of NK cells of experimental mice. When combined with IL-2, it can make the activity of NK cell higher, indicating that its polysaccharide can give a hand to IL-2 to activate NK cells and improve the activity.

   LBP can strengthen T cell mediated immune reaction and the activity of NK cells for normal mice and those dealt by cyclophosphamide. Peritoneal injection of LBP can improve the proliferation of spleen T lymphocytes and strengthen the lethality of CTL increasing the specific lethal rate from 33% to 67%.

2. XZ-C-G (GUF)

   Glycyrrhizin can induce the production of IFN in the blood of animals and human beings and strengthen NK cell activity at the same time. Clinical tests made by Abe show that after intravenous injection of 80mg GL, the raise of NK cell activity reaches 75% among 21 sufferers. Peritoneal injection of 0.5mg/kg GL on mice can strengthen the activity of NK cells in liver.

3. XZ-C-L (AMB)

   Its bath fluid can promote NK cell activity of mice both in vivo and in vitro, and can also induce IFN- γ to deal with effector cells under the certain concentration of 0.1mg/ml. Cordyceps sinensis extract can strengthen NK cells activity of the mouse both in vivo and in vitro. Fluids with the concentrations of 0.5g/kg, 1g/kg and 5g/kg can strengthen NK cell activity of mice.

V. Effects on LAK Cell Activity

Lymphokine activated killer cell, namely LAK cell can be induced by IL-2 cytokine. LAK cells can kill the solid tumors that are both sensitive and insensitive to NK cells with broad anti-tumor effects.

The active principles in XZ-C anti-carcinoma traditional Chinese medicine and their effects are following.

1. XZ-C-L (AMB)

   Its polysaccharide can strengthen LAK cell activity within a certain range of dose with 0.01mg/ml being the most effective, which is three times better than the damage effects of LAK cells. The concentrations of both higher and lower than this level can not achieve the effects.

2. XZ-C-U (PUF)

   It can significantly strengthen the spleen LAK cell activity of killing tumor cells and improve the activity of erythrocyte C3b liquid. PUF and IL-2 are synergistic that can be used as regulator for biological reaction in tumor biological therapy based on LAK/Ril-2.

3. XZ-C-V

   ABB polysaccharide can also raise LAK cell activity for the mouse and inhibit tumors remarkably. Its anti-tumorous mechanism relates to its strengthening immunity and changing cell membrane features.

VI. Effects on Iterleukin-2 (IL-2)

The active principles in XZ-C anti-carcinoma traditional Chinese medicine and their effects are following.

1. XZ-C-T

   EBM polysaccharide can enhance obviously the production of IL-2 for human beings when the concentration is 100ug/ml. At higher concentration (2500ug/ml and 5000ug/ml), it will lead to inhibition. Hypodermic injection of barrenwort polysaccharide for seven days in a row can significantly improve the ability of thymus and spleen of the mouse induced by ConA to produce IL-2.

2. XZ-C-Y

   PAR polysaccharide has strong immune activity and is able to promote the production of IL-2. For the mouse bearing S-180 tumor, it can raise the ability of spleen cells to produce IL-2 obviously

3. XZ-C-D

   Ginseng polysaccharide has great promotion on IL-2 induced by peripheral monocytes for both healthy people and sufferers with kidney troubles. The effects are relevant to the dose positively.

VII. Function of Inducing Interferon and Promoting Inducement of Interferon

IFN are broad-spectrum in resisting tumors and can regulate immunity. It can also inhibit the proliferation of tumor cells and activate NK cells and CTL to kill tumor cells. Meanwhile, IFN can cooperate with TNF, IL-1 and IL-2 to enforce anti-tumorous ability.

The active principles in XZ-C anti-carcinoma traditional Chinese medicine and their effects are following.

1. XZ-C-Z

   250mg/kg or 500mg/kg CVQ polysaccharide can improve significantly the level of IFN-γ produced by mouse spleen cells.

2. XZ-C-D

Ginsenoside (GS) and panaxitriol ginsenoside (PTGS) can induce whole blood cells and monocytes of human beings to produce IFN- α and IFN- γ . It can also recover the low level of IFN- γ and IL-2 to the normal.

The IFN potency of ASH polysaccharide on S-180 cell line of acute lymphoblastic leukemia and S_{7811} cell line of acute myelomonocytic leukemia produced after acanthopanax polysaccharide stimulation is 5~10 times more than that of normal control group.

3. XZ-C-E

Hydroxymethyl Poria cocos mushroom polysaccharide has many kinds of physical activity like immunoloregulation, promoting to induce IPN, resisting virus indirectly and alleviating adverse reaction resulting from radiation. Do IFN inducement dynamic experiment on S-180leukaemia cell line by using 50mg/ml Hydroxymethyl Poria cocos mushroom polysaccharide. The results indicate that its potency to induce interferon at all stages is better than that of normal inducement.

4. XZ-C-G (GL)

It can induce IFN activity. Make peritoneal injection of 330mg/kg GL on mice. IFN activity reaches the peak after 20 hours.

VIII. Function of Promoting and Increasing Colony Stimulating Factor

Colony stimulation factor, namely CSF is a kind of glucoprotein with low molecular weight that can stimulate the proliferation and differentiation of marrow hematopoietic stem cells as well as other mature blood cells. Cells that can produce CSF include mononuclear macrophages, T cells, endothelial cells and desmocytes. CSF not only take part in the proliferation and differentiation of hematopoietic stem cells and regulating mature cells, but also play an important role in anti-tumorous immunity of host cells.

The active principles in XZ-C anti-carcinoma traditional Chinese medicine and their effects are following.

1. XZ-C-Q

PAR polysaccharide is able to promote to produce CSF by spleen cells of experimental mice. 100~500ug/ml PAP-II can encourage spleen cells to produce CSF depending on the dose and time with the fittest dose of 100ug/ml and best time of 5d. Moreover, lentinan can also increase the amount of CSF.

2. XZ-C-Q

Injection of LBP can facilitate the secretion of CSF by mouse spleen T cells and improve the activity of CSF in serum.

3. XZ-C-T

EBM icariin can promote the proliferation of mouse spleen lymphocytes induced by ConA and bring CSF activity.

IX. Function of Promoting TNF

Tumor necrosis factor, namely TNF is a kind of cytokine that can kill tumor cells directly. Its main effect is to kill or inhibit tumor cells, which can kill some tumor cells or inhibit the proliferation both in vivo and in vitro.

The active principles in XZ-C anti-carcinoma traditional Chinese medicine and their effects are following.

1. XZ-C-Y (PEP)

   It can induce the production of TNF, so as PEP-1. Inject 80~160mg/kg PEP-1, once every four days. Collect peritoneal macrophages (PM), add 10ug LPS into culture medium to cultivate PM. Take the supernatant to determine TNF and IL-1. It can be found that PEP-1 can parallelly increase the auxiliary production of TNF and IL-1. The time of TNF inducement reaches the peak on the 8th day after the second intraperitoneal injection. Compared with the known startup potion BCG, the inducement of TNF has no difference.

2. XZ-C-E

   Carboxymethyl-pachymaran (CMP) is the principle essential component distilled from traditional Chinese medicine Tuckahoe. It can not only strengthen the ability of mouse spleen to create IL-2 and macrophages and promote the activity of T cells, B cells, NK cells and LAK cells; but also encourage the production of TNF. The experiment proves that CMP is an effective potion to promote and induce cytokines.]

3. XZ-C-V

   ABB polysaccharide can promote the production of TNF-b in mouse cells induced by ConA. It can also induce the synthesis of peritoneal macrophages and secrete 20ug/ml TNF-αachyranthes bidentata polysaccharides. The time of TNF-α to reach its peak is 2~6 hours after effects. Peritoneal injection of 100mg/kg achyranthes bidentata polysaccharides can accelerate the production of TNF-α, whose intensity of effects is comparable to that of BCG.

X. Effects on Cell Adhesion Molecule

Most adhesion molecules are glycoproteid and are distributed on cellular surface and extracellular matrix. Adhesion molecules take effect in the corresponding form of ligand-acceptor, resulting in the adhesion between cells, or between cell and stroma, or the adhesion of cell-stroma-cell. These molecules take part in a set of physical pathologic processes, like cellular conduction and activation of information, cellular stretch and movement, formation of thrombus as well as tumor metastasis, etc. Intercellular adhesion molecule-1, namely ICAM-1 is one kind of adhesion molecules in the super family of immune globulins.

The effect of corn stigma as an active principle in XZ-C traditional Chinese anti-carcinoma medicine: Hobtemariam has proved that alcohol extract from corn stigma has significant inhibition on the adhesion of endothelial cells to inhibit effectively the expression of ICAM-1 and the adhesive activity with TNF, LPS as agents.

CHAPTER 29

Bilogical response modification(BRM), traditional chinese anticancer medicine similar to BRM and tumor treatment

Biological reaction modification (BRM) explores the new field of the tumor biological therapy. Currently BRM as the fourth methods of the tumor treatment gets widely attention in the world.

1. The theory of biological reaction modification(BRM)

Oldham in 1982 built BRM theory. Based this in 1984 he advanced the fourth modality of cancer treatment—biological therapy again. According to this, in the normal condition, there is the dynamic equilibrium between the tumor and the body. The development of the tumors, and even invasion and metastasis, completely is caused by the loss of this equilibrium. If this unbland situation is adjusted to the normal level, the tumor growth can be controlled and will disappear. The anticancer mechanism of BRM in detail as the following:

a. Improve the host defence abilities or decrease the immune inhabitation of the tumors to the host to reach the immune response to the tumors.
b. Look for the biological active things in natural or gene combination to enhance the host defense abilities.
c. Reduce the host response induced by the tumor cells
d. Promote the tumors to division and mature to become the normal cells
e. Reduce the side effects of the chemotherapy and redio therapy and enhance

The host toleration.

The biological therapy is to adjust this biological reaction through from the outside of the body to add, induct or active the cell toxicities biological active factor or cells in. The biological theapy is different from the previous three therapy models such as surgery, radioactive and chemotherapy, to directly attack the target of the tumors. The biological reaction systems inside the host bodys. The therapy ranges of BRM is beyond the traditional immune therapy concepts, which the equilium between the body and the tumors is not limit to the immune reaction, but involved in all kinds of the regulation genes and cell factors related to the tumor proliferations.

The tumor biological therapy mainly includes :1). The injection of the immune active cells 2).The production /application of the cytokines and cell factors 3).Specific autoimmune including the application of the tumor cells groups xxxx, monoantibody and its crossing-thingsxxx.

The cytokines and liquid factors in the host immune system is in subtle control. If the balance of them was lost, the body response or the answer abilities will be affected significantly so that BRM can recover this unbalance condtion to the normal equilianume to reach the goal of treating the tumors.

BRM is a group of medicine which can adjust the host body immune function, recovering the immune function from the inhibition conditions, the function mechanism of which are active the immune function systems. Which are mainly from the microbiology agents and the plants, the former is the drugs as the immune strengthener and immune active agents and immune regulator, now the new name is the BRM.

Recurrently there are some BRM-similar medicine from the traditional Chinese medicine, which have excellent results.

2. The classifications of BMR

1). Cytokines: is the production from the immune effective cells and related cells, which are the cell-mediated proteins with the important biological activities. The types of their biological activities as the following: a. Interleukin 2, IL-2 is the molecules between the immune cells and active the T cells, Bcells proliferatin, and active the NK cells ect Killer cells b. IFN has three types of IFN-A, B, which are groups of glycoproteins. c. CSF is the factor which stimulated the blood stem cells growth an division into GM-CSF, M-CSF and G-CSF. d. TNF.

2). The immune active cells: so far there are four immune cells which are used to the tumor therapy: a. LAK b. TIL c. PWH-LAK and OKT3-LAK: The PBL or TIL from pwh, okt can stimulated LAK proliferation activity. d. CD8 CTL which can recognized the MHCI tumor groups has the strong activities which killed the tumor cells.

3). The vaccines of the tumor molecules: currently the main research on the tumor vaccination is the unique vaccine of antitumor monoantibodys, which can produce the anticancer response after imitating the antigen stimulation.

4). The natural medicine with BRM function: XZ-C have BRM function.

3. The function mechanism of BRM

BRM has the effects on the regulation of the host immmun response to the timor and killing the tumor s. The mechinsum are the following five aspects:

a. Directly regulating the growth and division of the tumors
b. Increasing the sensitivities of the tumors to the anticancer mechnisum in the body to benefit of killing the tumor cells.
c. Acting on the tumor vessels and affects the tumor's nutrition, blood supply so as to lead the death of the tumors and not damage the normal tissues
d. Stimulating the immune response to host antitumors
e. Stimulating the production of the blood to improve the inhibited bone marrow function to increase the tolerance of the the damage from the tumor therapy.

BRM can improve the body immune response and can strengthen the body immune surveillance to the tumors. The patients with the smallest size have good response to the BRM. BRM have very good effects on the early patients or the remaining tumor after surgery, or the tiny tumors and the xxxxx of the tumor cells.

BRM is one of the combination therapy methods to treat the malignant tumors, which some scientists said that immune therap just treat the 105 tumor cells such if the tumor cells formed clearly, the RRM functions will be limit the tumors to growth.

Even if the immune therapy have great development and attacted the whole world attentions, the mature degree of the tumor immune therapy is still in controevent., Currntly this is a worth research and there are some questions as the following:

1). It is difficult to have effects to the big tumors, only as the supply therapy to the therapy of the operation, chem. And radivation

2). Because the tumor antigen is specific, it is very difficult to produce the specific antibody.

Some researches showed that the antitumor therapy doesn't need absolute specificity, therefore, even if the tumors don't have the specific antigen, the immune therapy of the tumors is still acceptable. The concentration of the tumor relative antigens in the malignant tumor cells is higher than the normal cells, which this difference can make it possible for these antigens to become the effective attacked target. In addition, because the patients with cancer almost have the decreases of the immune function, and the increase of the immune inhibition factors, and the decrease of IL-2,TNF, and IFN ect, therefore, it is necessary to increase the immune function.

Because of the immune function decrease in the tumor patients, during the therap it should try to improve the immune function in the patients with the tumors. Because of the increaser of the immune inhibiting factors in the tumor patients, it should be treated to black ; because of the decrease of the IL-2, TNF and IFN etc, it should try to stimulate the production of these factors.

In order to improve the effects of the immune therapy, it is necessary to investigate how to get the best combinating forms of these therapies with the current therapy.

4. The research survey on the XZ-C traditional Chinese anticancer medicine for the immune regulation control similar to BRM

XZ-C immune regulation anticancer medicine have the functions and curative effects similar to BRM after four years experimental research and 16 years clinical research which are the drugs similar to BRM selected from traditional Chinese medicine.

XZ-C is the durgs that XU ZE in China professor selected from two hundreds of the anticancer herbs after the experiments. At first the culturing tumor were done. The in vitro was done One by one to select and abserve the direct damage to tumor cells in the culture setting and the control groups of the rate of the anticancer are the chemotherapyxxxx and the normal culture tube cells. The results are to select the a series of the medicine of the anti-cancer proliferation, then made the animal modes which 200 drugs were used on one by one. These experiments of the analysis and evaluation are steps by steps, scientific, practical and strict, etc. The results proved that48 of them have the excellent tumor inhibition effects, however the rest 152 of the tumors anticancer medicine are all common old anticancer medicine which proved no anticancer or less inhibition of the tumors in the animal models during these medicine selection experiments.

In the process of the experiments, the main work were conducted on the tumor animal models: one medicine was experienced on one group to observe them about three months and then selected 48 of the effective anticancer medicine, then combination of two or three medicine to do experiment on these animal models so that the single medicine has less effects than the multiple compound effects, which seems that the single medicine has the inhibition only on the tumor cell proliferation, however the multiple combination not inhibition to the tumor proliferation, but have the immune regulation control function of the body regulation, strengthen the energy, improvement of the immune system, promoting the production of the inhibiting cell factors, protecting the normal cells and promoting the anticancer factors etc.

Based on the author's experiments during four years of the single traditional medicine selection in the animal models, then the combination of the experiment, then set up again XZ-C 1-10 recepes of anticancer, antimetastasis and antireccurrency and last conducted the clinical verification. From 1992 the wide clinical tests were set up. After 16 years of the tumor specialty in outpatient centers there were 12000 cases of the tumor patients who were test and showed the excellent effects which their medical condition are stable, improved in there symptoms, the life quality improvement and the survival rates prolong. The medical condition in many metastasis patients were stable and didn't spread. Some of the patients with the number decrease of the white blood cells couldn't have chmetherapy and radicative therapy, however after taking these medicine, there were no metastasis and have excellent effects.

5. The function and curative effect of the XZ-C traditional Chinese anticancer medicine for the immune regulation control similar to BRM

BRM is in 1982 first was described by Oldham, which meaning is that the reaction to foreign attack or response ability is through the BRM.

The cell-mediated and antibody mediated immune response is in the subtle control situation. In the unbalance situation the host response or the response ability will be significantly affected. The application of the BRM regulator can recover the normal equilitiun from the loss of the equilitium to reach the goal of the disease prevention.

BRM explored the new field of the tumor biology therapy, which currently was used as the fourth medols and was great attentions from all over the world.

BRM have regulate the body's immune function, recovering the immune function which were inhibited. These medicine function mechanism are multiple, however no matter what mechanisum theirs, they are function through the activing the body immune systems.

BRM, mainly from the microorganism and plants, before called as immune strengthenor, immune stimulator, immune exciting factors or immune regulation, now called as BRM/

The medicine which the author selected on the tumor animal models and had excellent anticancer rat XZ-C can improve immune function, protection of the central immune organs such as thymus and, improving the cell-mediated immune functions, protecting the thymus function, protect the bone morrow function, increase the red blood cells and white blood cells number, active the immune factors, improve the immune surveilence in the blood ect. XZ-C the main anticancer pharmacology function si anticancer and increase of the immune function. After four years of the animal experiments of the selection of the medicine, 48 medicine were selected as the signle medicine for the high anticancer medicine., then after the immune and cell factors levele tests, got 26 medicine separately have phargocyte functions, immune cells function, or increase the antibody—liquid immune system, increased the thymus weight, and promote the bone marrow proliferatin, and improvement of the T cells, and increase the activities of the LAK cells, increasing the IFN activities levels, TNS activity level, strengthening the CSF factors, inhibition of the platelet anticoagulation to inhibiting the cancer thromobosis, antimetastasis, or clearing the free bases etc. The aboving XZ-C has the following function as :

1). activing the host immune system to promote the host immune function to reach the immune respond to the tumors.
2). Activing the host immune factors of the anticancer systems to strengthen the host immune function and improve the immunce surviellence of the host immune systems.
3). protecting the thymus and bone marrow, improve the immune system, and stimulate the bone marrow function to reduce the inhibition of the bone marrow and increase the white blood cell and red blood cells etc.
4). Reduction of the side effects of the chemotherapy and radioactive therapy to increase the tolerance of the hosts.
5). The development of the tumors is the imbalance between the biological characteristic of the tumor cells and the the inhibition of the host to tumor XZ-C is the improvement of the immune system and recover the balance of both them.
6). directly regulate the tumor cell growth and division to have the regulation function of the growth and division.
7). Increaseing thymus weight and stop the shrinkle of thymus because when the tumor develop thymus goes on shrinkles.
8). Stimulating the host immune response to the tumors and strengthening the host anticancer abilities and strengthening the sensitivities of the host anticancer mechanism so as to benefits of killing the tumor cells on the ways of the metastasis.

XZ-C can make the body to produce the strong immune reaction to the tumor cells so that it can treat the tumors, which can produce the following immune response: 1). Strengthen the regulation or recover the host immune response to the tumors;2).stimulate the host immune system to active the host immune defense system;3)recover the immune functions.

As the above statement, the basical mechanisu of XZ-C is similar to BRM and the clinical application is similar to those of the BRM.

6. The clinical application principle and the application range of the XZ-C anticancer immune regulation traditional medicine

1). The clinical application of XZ-C: BRM and XZ-C similar to BRM can increase the immune response and strengthen the host immune surveillance function. When the cells started the mutation or the tumors are small, the effects are good. After the surgery or radioactive therapy, the medicine therapy make the tumor shrinkle to the smallest size which therapy effects are the best.

For the patients who can not have the operation and are weak and cannot have the chemotherapy and radioactive therapy, the immune therapy has some effects and reduce the symptom and prolong the survival time.

After the removal of the tumor in order to reduce the mestastas and reccurency, the XZ-C can be used. After the operation removed the big tumors XZ-C can be use to get rid of the remaining tumr cells and the tumor which already spred further away.

IF the tumor is not removed, the chemotherapy or the radicaotive therapy can be used first, which kill the most of the tumor cells to reduce the number of the tumor cells, then XZ-C can be used to supply.

2). The clinical observation and application ranges of XZ-C

1). Antimestasticsid after the operation: recover and improve the immune response after the surgery to improve the life quality and kill the remaining tumor cells after the operatton to prevent the metastasis and inhibit the cell proliferation to prevent the recurrency an d strengthern the longterm curative effects.

The ranges of the application: a. all kind of the middle, and advanced tumor after the surgery. All kind of the tumor after the surgery c. the advanced tumor which can not be removel after the operation investigation d. only can have the intestine recombination or the opening of the colon during the operation. e. can not removal the advanced tumors and lost the indicaton for the surgery. f. the removed tumors plus the tube pump insections.

2). Improving the life quality, prolonging the survival rate, inhibiting the division of the tumors, control the tumor cell proliferation, improve the body immune response, mainly anti metastasis

Application ranges: a. all kinds of the tumors including the new, further metastasis after the operation; b. all of the cancer with the later metastasis such as the liver, lung, branin or chest cavity, abdominal cavity.

3). reduce the tumor pain: XZ-C can treat all kind of the pain from the advanced tumors and soft and reduce the tumor size.

4). Supply with the chemotherapy or the tube pump therapy to protect the liver, kidney and bone marrow and thymus etc immune organs to improve the immune response and change the whole body immune condition, to support and strengthen and increase the period and long time curative effects to prevent the metastasis and spreed and recovery and to improve thelife quality, prolong the life time after the liver cancer patient had the tubes and chemotherapy etc.

5). Combination with the chemotherapy and radiavivion therapy, can reduce the side effects and increase the curative effects to protect the liver, kindey and bone marrow and other immune organs fucnton to increase the white cell numbers/

6). the combination of the application of the XZ-C and the traditional xxx: such as the using with xxxx for the liver cancer and theascite or the matatstsis of the abdominal catiy ascite;used th the xxx for the treatment oft liver cancer and jaundice; wused with xxx for the liver tumor with HBSAG POSTIVE AND trf postitvie. Used with ccc for the white cell dectease casuse by the chemotherapy.

3). the application time of XZ-C:

The tumor patietnts mostly have the immune function decreases after the diagnosed, the treatment should be done soon, however the three therapy of the operation, chemotherapy and radicative therapy all can cause the immune function decrase and leasd the decraste the toleratance of the patatient to the surpery or chemotherapy radicative and decrase the immune surveilleance in the host immunce systym. Therefore, it is necessary to start theimmune therapy during the operation or eradicative herpy and chemoterrapy. XZ-C can take by oral as long the thepatiertnte can eart, this is can be taken by oral. After the 1-2 week of the operation, the patient can started to take them. Befre the chmotehrapy and radiative during the peroios beye the radicatcie and chemothery oand after the radicalctive and cheamotherpom the patoeint can comtinuce ot take ZX-C, SO THAT THESE WILL DECRASE OR CONTROL THE RECORURNENVT And metastasis. And decrase the side effect of the radiotherapy and terhotherpay; prevent theimmune system decrease by chemotherapy and imcrease the immn function; promote the bone marrow function, protect eh bone marrow functiinl active the immune cells systems and immune cytokines function to improve the immune surveillance and prevent the recurrenc and metastasis.

CHAPTER 30

The experimental research of the tumor inhibition and immunoenhancement of traditional chinese medicine for strengthening the body resistance and culturing foundation

1. The medicine of being applied in the advanced stage of carcinoma for enhancing the immune function

   a. The discovery from the tumor experimental research

      There are the decreases of the immune function in the advanced tumors in the mice and thymus shrinkled continuely.

      When the author made the tumor animal models, the animal models were made when the thymus were removed; the animal models were not made when thymus were not removed. These experimental results proved that the occurrence, development of the tumors have certain relationship to the host immune functions and thymus functions.

      The question is whether the immune function decrease first, then the cancer happen or the cancer occurs first, then the cancer will decrease the immune functions. The experimental result showed that the immune function will decrease first, then the cancer happen easily. If the immune function doesn't decrease, the inoculation is not easy to be successful. This research result showed that to improve and to maintain the good immune function and to protect the thymus functions are one of the important methods of preventing the occurrence of the tumors.

      When the author research the relation between the tumor metastasis and the immune functions, he set up the liver metastasis animal models, which are divided into A, B two groups. In group A the immune suppressor was used, however in group B the immune suppressor was not used. The results showed that the metastasis lesions in the livers in group A were more than those in group B. This research results showed that there are relations between the metastasis and the immune functions. The immune function decrease or the application of the suppressor of the immune function can promote the tumor metastasis.

      During the research of the effect of the tumors on the host immune functions, it was found that along with the tumor development, the processing cell proliferation in thymus was inhibited and the volume of the thymus significantly decreases. This research results showed that the tumors can inhibit thymus and causes the immune systems shrinkle.

      Above the research results showed that the tumor occurrence and development and metastasis have the significant relations with the decrease of the host immune functions. In the advanced stages of the tumors in the mice there were decreases of the immune functions and the shrinkles of the thymus. Therefore, in the therapy of the advanced stages of the tumors, the medication of enhancing the immune function should be used and the medication of decreasing or inhibiting the immune function should not be used.

b. The search for the medicine of improving the high immune function and inhibiting the tumors

In order to prevent the ongoing thymus shrinkls during the tumor development and to search for the methods of recovering thymus function and rebuilding the immune function, the author started to search for the anti-cancer medication of enhancing the immune function from the natural herbs. After long-term and in turn of selecting the efficient anti-cancer medication in the animal tumor models from 200 traditional herbs. The results showed that there are only 48 herbs which have the effective anticancer functions and at the same time have enhancing immune functions including 26 herbs which strengthen the phagocyte function or stimulate the increase of thymus weight in the animal immune organ thymus or increase the white cell counting ; promote the lymphocyte proliferation in the spleen to increase the transferring rate of the lymphocyte and strengthening the T cell function and NK cells activities and inducing IFN function and 152 herbs which don't have the results.

After combination of the components, we selected the effective combination and got rid of the unstable effective combination in the animal tumor models such as liver cancer, stomach cancer and S-180 etc so that further formed XZ-C immune regulation anti-cancer medication to protect the thymus function and protect the bone marrow and to improve the immune function. Based on the success of the animal selecting experiments, these were applied to the clinics. After 16 years of the huge clinical cases tests, XZ-C medication can improve the life survival qualities in the advanced cancer stages and increase the immune function and strengthen the ability of the body defense and improve the appetite and prolonged the survival time and the curative effects are significant.

2. The experimental research on effects of traditional Chinese medicine for strengthening the body resistance and chulturing foundation on tumor inhibition and immunoenhancement of mice bearing S-180

a. Objects

Through more than 50 years of the research and practice of our combination of the Chinese medicine and the western medicine, it was found that many of the Chinese medicine have certain effects on the tumor therapy, especially the research of culturing foundation on the tumor showed culturing foundation can strengthen the body, improving the human immune function, and improve the life quality and prolong the survival time. However in my therapy to the cancer, there are many clinical experience and we didn't do the experimental research. We conduct a series experimental research in order to investigate that the medicine which are the invigoration of the function of the spleen, help the circulation of the bloodxxxx and increasing the function of the kidney can inhibit the tumor growth and do a series of the experimental research.

b. Methods:

1). The experimental animals: Qiuming mice 160, 5-6weeks old, body weight:27+2.0g, no gender differences

2). The tumor animal models: S-180 ascite tumor cells group, inoculating 1x107/ml 0.2ml/per mice in the right front armtip under the skin
3). The experimental groups:

The animals were divided into the following groups:
A group: enrich the function of the vital energy(n=20)
B group: enrich the blood tonic and vital energy.(n=20)
C group: enrich the negative (n=20)
D group: enrich the positive (n=20)
E group:ATCA combination therapy group(n=20)
F group: xxxx group
G group: combination of the capsule group(n=20)
H group: The tumor control group(n=20).

Each group will start to use the traditional medicine 0.4ml/per mice by the ngt in the second days after the injection, the tumor control group is the normal control saline group.

4). The preparation of each medicine: the medicine concentration is 200% according to the exchange method from the original recepes amonts into the modern ways. All of the amounts which were given to the mice as the exchange from the normal adults amounts into the mice amounts.

In this experiment the tradition medicine were used to treat S-180 mice with culturing foundation of enriching the vital energy, enriching the blood, the kidney of the positive and the negative and enrich the ATCA combination, xxxx and combination of the capsule etc.

5). the items of the observation:systematically observing the tumor occurring time, existing time, to measure their serium proteins, T cell number counting in the peripheral blood and the weithg of the immune organ.

c. Results: The culturing foundation and ATCA combination which are mainly function as the culturing foundation can significantly prolong the occurring time after inoculation of the tumor cells, inhibited the tumor growth(A, B, C, D, E groups the inhibiting rates are the 40%, 45%,44.5%,31% and 36%), prolong the tumor mice survival time(A, B, C, D, Egroup survival times are the 27.5%m45%,38.5% 25% and 26.5%). The xxx, combination capsule of the get rid of the wrong things can not inhibit the tumor growth and prolong the survival rates(compared with group e, $P>0.05$). A, B, C, D, E groups the serium proteins amount are increase, A/G the ratio were improved, the counting numbers of the T cells in the periphery blood(compared to G group $P<0.05$, B, C group $P<0.01$). Thymus shrinkle significantly.

d. Conclusion:This research showed that the culturing foundation or mainly culturing foundation medicine can inhibit the tumor growth and increase the immune function which can improve the T cells liver in the peripheral blood some degrees, which are more effective than the medicine of get rid of the wrong thins.

e. Discussion

1). Culturing foundation on the tumor and prolonging the survival function

Many of the tumor patients can present the "weak" symptom such as the deficiency of vital energy, deficiency of blood, deficiency of yin(insufficiency of body fluid) and deficiency of yang etc. In the treatment the medicine of the culturing foundation are used. This experiment investigated the culturing foundation and the inhibition of the tumor with offensive and supplement. The results showed that the culturing foundation medicine which enhanced the vital of the energy, both blood and vital energy, enhancing the yin and warming the yang ect and the medicine of mainly effects on the culturing foundation which ATCA combination all can prolong the occurring time after the inoculation in the mice, inhibiting the tumor growth, and prolong the survival time in the tumor mice. From each group of the inhibiting rates, the inhibiting rates in enhancing both blood and vital of the energy is 45%, is 44.5% in enhancing the yin kidney group, is 40% in enhancing the vital of the energy, which the effects are very good, is 36%in enhancing ATCA group, is 31% in the warming yang kidney groups which the curative effects are weak. In inhibiting the tumor, it is better to use the enhance of the vital of the energy and enrich the yin. From the prolong the survival rates, the enhancing both blood and vital of the energy is 45%, the longest group; next is 38,5% in the enriching the yin group, with the better results. About the enhance of the vital of the energy, warming the positive kidney function and ATCA combination group can prolong the survival time, however less than the former two. The xxx and the compound capsules which mainly get rid of the wrong thing can not clearly inhibit the tumors, can not prolong the survival rates, it s effects are weak. Therefore, in the prolong the survival time the enhancing both blood and vital energy, and the yin thereapy are the first, next is to enhance the vital of the energy and warming the yang and enhance the attack. From both the inhibition of the tumor and prolonged the survival rate, the best way is to enhance the both blood and vital energy, the second is the enrich of the yin, then is the enhance of the vital energy and ATCA compound, the effects of the enrich of the yang is not significant. There is no effect on the xxxx and compound capsules which got rid of the wrong things.

In summary, Culturing foundation and the medicine mainly based on the cuturing function have differenct degree of the inhibition timor growth and prolonged the survival time, however the therapy of getting rid of the wrongthings have no clearly function of inhibition of the tumors an d prolong the survival time.

Our experiment showed that Culturing and the medicine mainly cultring have excellent inhibition to the small size of the tumors, and prolong the survival rates a nd improve the life qualities so that in the clinics it was used as the supplement therapy of the operation and the radioactive and chemotherapy. Many literature reported that Culturing foundation therapy treat the malignant tumor very good. The results from our experiments showed that the therapy of both enhancing the blood and the vital energy, the yin, and vital energy etc can inhibit the tumors and prolong the survival time and provide the experimental basis of the combination of the western and Chinese medicine in the clinical therapy.

2). Culturing foundation on strengthening the immune functions: this experiments showed that culturing function and the medicine mainly functioned in the culturing function can improve the T cell level in the peripheral blood, such as in the fourth week the level of the T cells is 41.5% in the groups of enriching of the vital energy, 44.8% in the groups of enriching blood and vital energy, 38.6% in the groups of strengthening the yin kidney and 37.5% in the groups of enriching the yang kidney and 35.6% in ATCA combination groups; inhibiting the thymus shrinkle, such as in 2nd week, Index of thymus in the group of enhancing the vital energy, both the blood and vital energy, enhancing the yin and yang kidney and ATCA combination is significantly different from the control group of the tumors. These suggest that the inhibition of the tumor in culturing foundation is related to strengthening the body immune function. Some researchers suggest that many plants include the effective elements of the immunoregulators, called as anticancer multiglycerals, which can not kill the tumor cells directly, however it can active the immune systems to release the anticancer cell factors or increase the LAK cells to kill the tumor cells. Culturing foundation included the rich plant multiglyceral, such as XXX reported that the extra xxx multiple sugars, molecular amount 200000-250000, which have clearly promote the PBMC to secret the TNF in the blood. XXX etc reported that the traditional medicine can promote the activities of natural killer cells in S-180 mice and IL-2 and promote the activities fo T cells and improving the phagocyte function and increase the spleen and thymus weight. In summary, culturing foundation can prolong the occurring time of the tumor after inoculation and inhibit the tumor growth and prolong the tumor survival time, and strengthening the immune function against the diseases, improve the life qualities so that the anticancer research of the clinical traditional medicine provide the experimental basis.

3. The immunological function of traditional Chinese herbs on cancer patients in Advanced stage

The patients in advanced tumor stage often present the deficiency of vital energy and lowering o f body resistance and have the decreases of their immune functions. Strengthening the host immune system can increase the body immune function and is the important meaning for preventing the decreases of the host immune system.

1). The strengthen of the non-specific immune function

a. The increase of the weight of the animal immune organs thymus and spleen:

Ren sheng soup can increase the mice thymus weight, 2.2 time than the contral groups

b. The increase of the phagocyte function: such as the Rensheng, xxx, xxx, xxx and xxx ect can improve the hagocyte function so that it increased the vital energy distanctly.

c. The increase of the white blood cells in the peripheral blood: Such as xxx, xxx, xxx, xxx, and xxx etc can increase the number of the white blood cells

2). The increase of thc cell-mediated immune functions:

a. Improvement of the proliferation of the lymphocyte of the spleen: such as rensheng can increase the amount of the lymphocytes, xx and xxx can improve the Tcell in the peripheral blood.

b. Improvement of the transformation rate of the lymphocyte: the medicine such as RENSHENG, xxx, xxx and xxx etc, which enrich the weak, can improve the transformation of the lymphocyte.

c. Strengthen red blood cells immune function: such as xxx and xxx can improve the RBC-C3B ring rates and RBC-IC rings formation rates.

3). Increasing the antibody immune function:

a. Promoting the antibody production: such as xxx, xx, xxx, xxx, xxx, xxx and xxxx etc can promote the production of the antibody and increase the level of the serum IgG, IgA, IgM etc.

b. Increasing the cells numbers of forming the antibody in the spleen: XXXX can increase the antibody production one time in mice spleen cells comparing to the control groups. XXX can increase the cells numbers which can produce the xxxxxx in the spleen. However some of enhancing the weak medicine have two-way functions both enhancing and inhibiting.

CHAPTER 31

New Cognition of Treatment of Carcinoma Immunity

[Abstract]

Objectives: Probe into the theoretical basis of immunological therapy of carcinoma, its important role in anti-metastasis and the approach to evaluate the curative effect of immunological therapy.

Methods: experimental findings through the in-tumor animal model by means of animal experiment.

Results: it is shown by the results of experimental study that the occurrence and development of the carcinoma is obviously related to the thymus of immune organ of the host and its functions, the inferior immunologic function may easily cause carcinoma. Suggestion: improvement and maintenance of the good immunologic function is one of the important measures to prevent the occurrence and development of carcinoma. It is shown by another experiment that the metastasis is related to the immune, the inferior immunologic function or application of immunologic inhibitor may promote the metastasis of tumor.

Conclusions: it is found from the experimental study that the occurrence, development, metastasis and reoccurrence of carcinoma are closely related to immunologic atrophia and inferior immunologic function of the host. The immunological therapy for improving the immune is one important measure for anti-cancer and anti-metastasis, especially the anti-metastasis is very important to eliminate the cancer cells in routing of metastasis. The immunological therapy is of great advantage for in-tumor host to improve the survival quality and obviously prolong the life period.

[Keywords]: Thymus; In-tumor animal model; immunologic therapy

I. General to the Headway of Treatment of Carcinoma Immunity

Since 19th century, the field of immunity treatment has gone through success and failure, the scientists have always been making efforts to probe into it. With the further search on immunology and the rich clinical experience, the immunity treatment has played a more and more important role in treatment of tumor.

Since the early of 1980s, with the rapid development of cell biology, molecular biology, molecular immunology, gene engineering and biotechnology, the new favorable turn and expectation have come up to the treatment of carcinoma immunity. In 1982, Biological Response Modifier (BRM) Theory was put forward, which made people cognize the theory and practice of traditional immunity treatment again and established the 4th treatment method besides operation, radiotherapy and chemotherapy, namely the biological therapy of tumor. The establishment of BRM Theory enables the biological treatment of tumor to own the theoretical basis while the development and utilization of biotechnology makes it possible to put the clinical application of the biological treatment of carcinoma into operation. The gene engineering technology can produce a large quantity of interleukin, interferon, tumor necrosin, immunoglobulin factor and over 10 kinds of cytokines of BRM including colony stimulating factors [1, 2].

The progress of the above-mentioned biotechnology and the further understanding of the cellular immunity, molecule immunity and molecule biology provide the development opportunity of treatment of carcinoma immunity.

In the recent years, some herbs with the roles of BRM samples have been found from the traditional Chinese herbal resources and the delightful effects have been realized from the experimental study and clinical application. These natural traditional Chinese botanicals with the roles of BRM samples realize the anti-carcinoma-metastasis through enhancing the immunologic functions of the organism and activating the activity of the immune factors, undoubtedly, it is a promising research field.

Z-C immune regulation and cancer inhibition medicine studied by us is the 48 kinds of traditional Chinese herbs with good curative effects screened from 200 kinds of traditional Chinese herbs with role of so-called cancer inhibition through tumor-inhibiting experiment in the tumor-bearing animal model body and screening via animal experiment for 3 years, with 152 kinds of traditional Chinese herbs eliminated. Based on the successful animal experiment, it has been applied to the clinical experiment and remarkable curative effects have been obtained through the clinical verification on over 12000 clinical cases over 11 years. Z-C immune regulation and cancer inhibition medicine is the natural botanical with the similar role of BRM and delightful effects have been obtained in experimental study and clinical application. Z-C_4 can promote the hyperplasia of the thymus and improve the immunity; Z-C_8 can protect the bone marrow and realize the hematopiesis and protect the function of the hematopiesis of the bone marrow. Z-C immune regulation medicine can improve the subsistence quality of the cancer patients in middle and late stage, enhance the immunity, enhance the anti-carcinoma ability of the body, improve the body condition, improve the appetite and obviously prolong the survival time [3].

II. Findings from Experimental Tumor Study by this Lab

① When this lab made the tumor-bearing animal model, we removed the thymus of the mouse to make the animal model. In addition, the injection of immune inhibition medicine can be of help to establish the tumor-bearing animal model. It was proven by the study conclusions that the occurrence and development is obviously related to the thymus of the immune organ of the host and its functions. ② As regards whether the inferior immune results in the carcinoma or the carcinoma results in the inferior immunity, the experimental findings were as follows: firstly the immunity was inferior, and then the carcinoma occurred and developed; if without the inferior immunologic function, it was not easy to realize the successful inoculation. It was clewed by the experimental findings: it was one of the important measures to improve and keep the good immunological function so as to prevent the occurrence of the carcinoma. ③ When studying the relationship between carcinoma metastasis and immunity, we established the animal models of metastatic carcinoma of the liver and divided them into two groups, namely Group A and Group B, Group A adopted the immunity inhibition medicine and Group B did not adopt it. Results: the metastatic lesions in the livers of Group A were obviously more than the ones in Group B. It was clewed by the experimental findings that metastasis was related to the immunity, the inferior immunological function or the application of the immunity inhibition medicine may promote the metastasis of tumor. ④ In the experiment to probe into the influences on the immunological organ of the body from the tumor, it was found by us that with the development of the carcinoma, the thymus was in progressive atrophia, the thymus of the host would be in progressive atrophia after inoculating cancer cells, the cell increment was suffocated and the volume was obviously shrunk. It was clewed by the experimental findings that the tumor cells may inhibit the thymus, resulting in the shrinkage of the immunological organ. ⑤ it was found through the experiment that if some experimental mice failed to be successfully inoculated or the tumor is too small, the thymus would not be obviously shrunk. In order to understand the relationship between the tumor and the shrinkage of the thymus, we removed the inoculated solid tumor of a group of the experimental mice after it grew up as big as a thumb. After one month, it was found through anatomy that the thymus did not meet with the progressive atrophia any more. As a result, we hereby presumed that the solid tumor may produce a kind of unknown factor to inhibit the thymus, which should be further studied through experiment. ⑥ It was proven by the above-mentioned experimental findings that the progress of the tumor may make the thymus in progressive atrophia; in this way, could we take any measures to prevent the shrinkage of the thymus of the host? Therefore, we tried to find the method or medicine to prevent the shrinkage of the thymus of the tumor-bearing mice through the animal experiment study. And then, we adopted the cellular transplantation of immunological organ to recover the functions of the immunological organ. We were probing into the shrinkage of the thymus of the immunological organ while preventing the progress of the tumor, finding the method to recover the functions of the thymus and reestablish the immune and carrying out the experimental study to reestablish its immunological function through adopting the immune via cellular transplantation of fetus liver, fetus spleen and fetus thymus of the mice. It was shown by the results: after joint cellular transplantation of Group S, T and L, the entire extinction rate of the tumor in the near term was 40%, and the one in the long term was 46.67%; the one with the entirely extinct tumor would survive for a long time.

III. Immunity of Carcinoma Patient Descends slowly

The inferior immunologic functions of carcinoma patients, especially the abnormal local immunologic micro-environment of the tumor, resulting in ineffective immune defence reaction of the body, is the important factor for the carcinoma to meet with immunologic escape and metastasis and reoccurrence easily. How to effectively regulate the immunologic functions of the host, how to improve the local micro-environment of the tumor so as to be good to bring the anti-carcinoma effect of the host into play and how to improve the micro-environment obstacle to reduce the implantation of the metastatic lesion of the cancer cells are the important and effective measures to prevent the reoccurrence and metastasis of carcinoma after operation, eliminate the metastatic lesion due to the implantation of the remained cancer cells in the chest cavity and abdominal cavity after operation.

IV. How to Evaluate Immunity Measure, BRM Treatment and Curative Effect and Value of Chinese Traditional Medicines Similar to BRM

As to the evaluation standard of the curative effect, there are two different understandings.

The traditional curative measure holds that the evaluation standard of the curative effect is: the traditional therapeutics concept of the carcinoma holds that the cancerous protuberance is caused by the crazy cleavage and proliferation of the cells, so the cancer cells are the arch criminal. Therefore, the target of tackling the key problem is to kill off the cancer cells and the therapeutic methods include operation, radiotherapy and chemotherapy and the objective or target of the treatment is the primary lesion or (and) metastatic lesion. The evaluation standard of the curative effects of the three largest traditional treatment measures is to relieve the primary carcinoma block or the shrinkage or disappear of the metastatic lesion, in other words, it takes the tumor as the evaluation standard.

XU ZE New Concept holds: the goal of tackling the key problem is the metastasis. It is necessary to pay attention to the treatment of the primary lesion and metastatic lesion as well as the treatment of the cancer cells in routing of metastasis. These cancer cells or cancer cell groups or micro-thrombus in the routing of metastasis cannot be seen or touched at present or be displayed through iconography such as B ultrasonic, CT and MRI and so on, therefore, it cannot evaluate it through the size of the carcinoma lesion. Generally, the evaluation standard for the curative effect of the chemotherapy is relief and shrinkage. However, relief and shrinkage are not the goal of treatment of the carcinoma patient, "being effective" that it means only refers to the shrinkage of the cancerous protuberance and it does not obviously prolong the life of the carcinoma patient and improve the survival quality of the patient. The basis to evaluate the shrinkage is generally the size of the occupation of the iconography such as B ultrasonic, CT and X-ray, which is very scientific, correct and reasonable. Shrinkage is better than non-shrinkage. However, it is not so absolute. Some cancerous protuberances shrink, but they meet with metastasis rapidly; some do not meet with shrinkage or metastasis. Maybe the occupation is small, but inside it are the cancer cells; or the occupation lesion may be large, there are not only the cancer cells but also the liquefacient organization with cellular necrosis inside it. In the recent 10 years, we have seen from so many metastatic and recurrent patients from time to time in Shuguang Tumor Clinic that the tumor is obviously shrunk after radiotherapy and chemotherapy, however, the patients meet with reoccurrence and metastasis after a long time or several months; after radiotherapy, there is a little metastasis; after chemotherapy, it is easy to meet with metastasis. In this tumor clinic, after assistant chemotherapy, it was found by us that some patients met with fewer metastasis when they were subject to chemotherapy not exceeding 4 times after operation compared to the ones subject to over 4 chemotherapies. The more the chemotherapy times, the easier the remote metastasis, chemotherapy while metastasis, more chemotherapy, more metastasis. Maybe the radiotherapy is the local treatment and the chemotherapy acts on the whole body, killing off the cancer cells in the whole body as well as the immunological cells and stem cells in the whole body, making the whole immunologic function inferior, making the immunological survelillance of the body of the host weakened, in this way, the remote metastasis may easily appear, it even promotes the metastasis. With respect to the evaluation of its curative effect and value, the more important is to whether it prevents the occurrence of the metastatic lesion and controls the metastasis. Since one of the goal of carcinoma treatment is to improve the immunity of the patient and improve the inhibition ability of the host to the carcinoma. Anti metastasis is to control the cancer cells in routing of metastasis and improve the immunological surveillance of the blood circulation system. The immunity treatmemt or BRM treatmemt or Z-C immune regulation medicine similar to BRM that can kill off 10^5~10^6 cancer cells, cannot make the primary lesion or metastatic lesion shrink or disappear, however, the new metastatic lesions obviously reduces or no new metastatic lesions appear any more, controlling the metastasis. Therefore, if the immunity treatment is evaluated with the shrinkage of the carcinoma lesion, its curative effect is just so so. If it improves the survival quality and prolongs the survival period through improve the immunological surveillance of the body of the host and kill off or inhibit the cancer cells in routing of metastasis, its effect is very remarkable. Immunity measure and the therapy with Z-C immune regulation and anti-tumor medicine can obviously improve the survival quality of the patients, improve the symptom, enhance the body condition, improve the spirit and appetite for food, obviously prolong the survival period and improve the long-term curative effect.

References

1. Zhou Xiong, Zhang Lining. Molecular Immunology and Clinic. Jinan, Shandong Science and Technology Press, 2003, 283~290.
2. [Germany] Gernot Stuhler, Peter Walden. Cancer Immune Therapy. Beijing: Chemical Industry Press, 2004, 85~89.
3. Xu Ze. New Concepts and New Methods of Treatment of Carcinomatous Metastasis. Beijing: People's Military Medical Press, 2006, 155~162.
4. He Xinhuai, Xi Xiaoxian. Immunology of Traditional Chinese Medicine. Beijing: People's Military Medical Press, 2002: 341~348.

CHAPTER 32

Typical cases of treatment for malignant tumor by XZ-C traditional Chinese anticancer medicine through immunological regulation and control

Typical cases of treatment of liver cancinoma

Case 1. Mr. Mao, male, 48 year-old(yo), Taimen, officer. Medical record numbers: 100014

Diagnosis: primary liver cancinoma

Disease course and treatment:

On August 1, 1994 becasue the patient felt fatigure and tired, he had Ultrasound in the local hospital and found a 4.1cm x4.5cm nodule in the left lobe of the liver. On August 26, 1994 the left lobe of the liver was removed in the Xian Ha hospital. Pathological slides showed: liver cell carcinoma without any treatment. After operation, the patient was treated with anticancer immunological traditional medicine **XZ-C1+XZ-C4+XZ-C5 in** our outpatient center. After taking these medicine, the patient's appetite increased and energy level increased and was happy. He takes medicine regularly and comes to our office every month for following up and refilling the medicine. He feels very well and goes back his work. On December 14 1996 there was another 1.3cmx1.8cm nodule which was found by B ultrasound in the edge of the left liver. On December 30 1996 he had that nodule removed again. After the operation, he continued to take the medicine. After that, this patient takes his medicine persistently and regularly. In May 2010 when he came to follow-up, his general condition is good and his face was glowing in the health, his body was strong as a healthy person and came back to labor work for more than 11 years. His appetite is great and his emotion is very good. He eats 600g food per day and his Ultrasound is normal.

Commons: on August 26 1994 this patient had a 4.1cmX4.5cm nodule removal of left liver. After the operation, the patient take XZ-C to treat. On December 30 1996 another 1.3cmx1.8cm nodule was found and removed again. After that, this patient continues to take XZ-C. While he came back to follow-up for 16 years, his health condition is good and can do labor work for many years. This patient is still alive very well while we wrote this book.

Implication: After the removal of the liver carcinoma the patient took XZ-C1-XZ-C4+XZ-C5 persistently, these medicine can improve the thymus function and protect bone morrow function of the producing blood cells, protect the liver function and improve the whole body immunology function against the diseases. The operation and the medicine XZ-C can increase the long-term treatment of the cancer patients.

Case 1 primary liver cancer

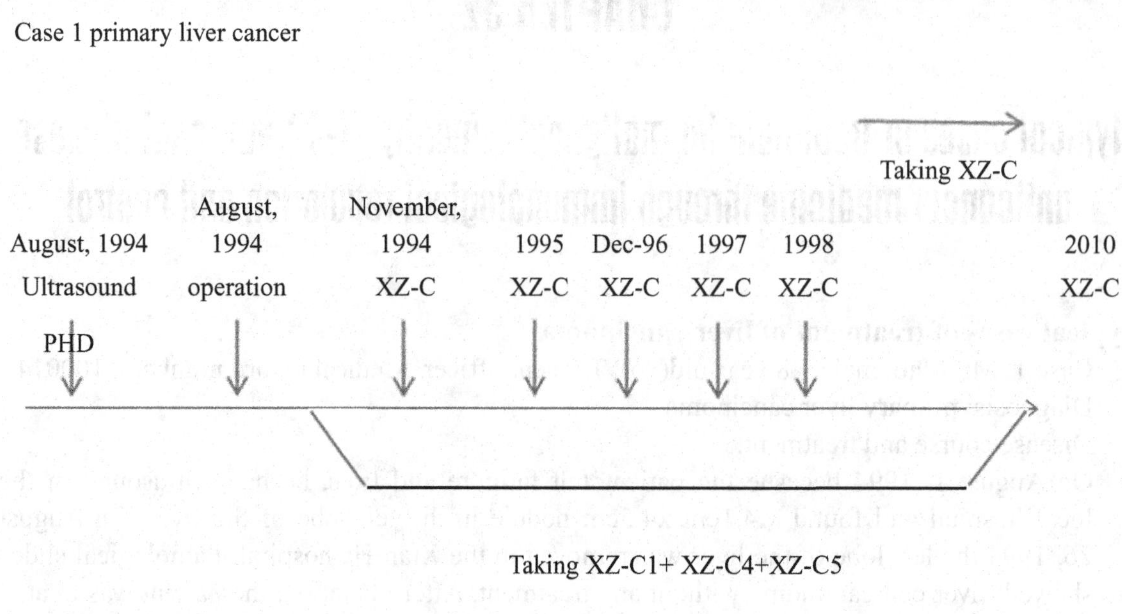

Case 2. Ms. Liu, female, 65yo, Jianxian in Hubei, officer, Medical record number:110201

Diagnosis: primary huge liver carcinoma

Disease course and treatment: Because of the uncomfortable in upper abdomen, the patient had CT in xxx hospital which found that a 6.7cmx7.1cmx9cm nodule in right liver, then diagnosed as primary liver carcinoma. He refused to take operation and chemotherapy. In July 11 1995 he started to take the XZ-C1+XZ-C5. After 2 months, his emotion and appetites get better and his weight increased. In September 20 1995 while follow-up ultrasound, the nodule was reduced. In November 1995 she had a xxx(gen shai therapy) and didn't have any other therapy. She continues to take the XZ-C for more than 6 years and continues to follow-up more 10 years. This patient's condition is good. In May 2005, this patient is healthy as the normal person.

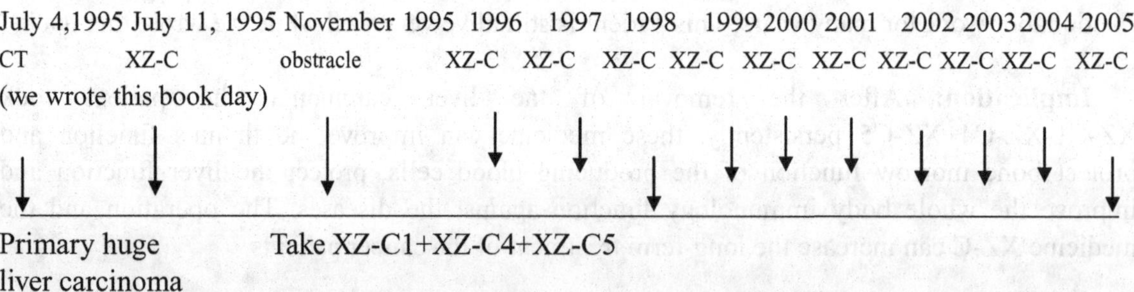

Commons: In July 4 1995 this patient was diagnosed as primary liver carcinoma by CT and then took XZ-C after 1 week. After 2 month, the CT scan showed that the nodule become smaller. In November 21 the obstruo procedure was conducted, then she continues to take XZ-C regularly and persistently for 10 years. Now this patient is healthy as the normal individual.

Implication: The obstractin+XZ-C have good results on liver carcinoma treatment. The obstracle can stop the blook supply for the cancer nodulae and chemotherapy can kill the parts of cancer cells. There are living cancer cells inside and under the tumor nodule membrane after obstraution, the tumor cells didn't die completely and then grow fast after its circulation built up. XZ-C can protect thymus and improve the immune ability, protect the bone morrow function and to improve the body immune function. In addition, 85% hepatic cancer occurred in the cirrhosis patients so that sophagipy throught the tube artery obstract will damage the liver function. XZ-C will protect the liver. The combination of obstract+XZ-C will inhibit the tumor and protect the host to improve the long-term treatment. This is called take out the bad and keep the good in Chinese.

Case 3 Mr. Kei, male, 54 yo, Yanxi in Hubei, officer. Medical record: 6301244.

Diagnosis: primary liver canceromal

Disease course and treatment: The patient had pain on the upper right abdomen for half of month and his appetites decreased. CT in Yanxia showed the nodules in the right front and back lobe and left lobe. Diagnosis: primary liver carcinoma. On Auguat 20 1998 the patient had opening surgery which the main tumors were in the entrance of common duct and there were the metastasis in both of left and right liver, which could not be removed so that a tube for the chemotherapy was placed through the hepatic artery. After the operation, the chemotherapy of xxxxxxx was used once. In Octocber 1998 the second chemotherapy of xxxxx was used. Because the tube was blocked, the patient stopped using the tube. On September 8 1998 he started taking XZ-C1+XZ-C4+XZ-C5. After taking this medicine one month, the patient emotion and appetite were good and her body weight increased and her face was glowing in the health. On her physical exam her abdomen was soft and flat and the spleen and liver could not be felt, Her general condition was good. She could support herself very well and picked her medication by her own. On June 4 2002 when she came back for her following up, her healthy condition was good, her face was glowing of the health. Her walking, acting and smiling liked the normal healthy persons. On the physical exam there was no abnormal found.

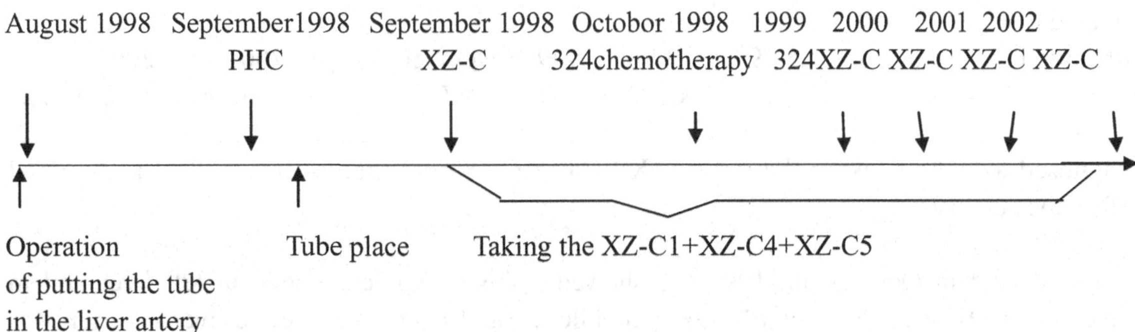

Commons: On August 20 1998 the liver cancinoma was found in the right and left liver and could not be removed and put a chemotherapy tube through which the twice chemotherapy was given after CT scan showed many occupation disease changes in the left lobe, right front and right back lobe. On September 8 the patient started to take XZ-C1+XZ-C4+XZ-C5 until 2002 this patient condition was good and didn't have metastasis.

Implication: When liver cancer could not be removed, the liver artery tube could be placed, then XZ-C1+XZ-C4+XZ-C5 was used to protect Thymus, bone morrow, liver to improve the host immune system function and induces the host to produce more anticancer factors to control the tumors and to control the development of the cancers.

Case 4 Mr. Pu, male, 51 year-old, YinZheng, officer, medical record: 500989

Diagnosis: primary liver caner

Disease course and treatment: there is a 4.6cm X3.6cm nodule in left liver and a 1.6cmX 1.6cm nodule in right liver after the patient had CT on October 30 in 1997. Diagnosis was liver carcinoma. There is a 5.9cimX4.0cmX5.4cm nodule in the left liver lobe and a 2.1cmX1.8cm lesion in the right liver lobe when the patient had Ultrasound in the XieHei hospital. Liver angiography showed that the patient had liver cancer. HbsAg(+), AFP(-). Because this patient's liver function was poor, he couldn't stand the operation and put on the tube for chemotherapy. This patient is alcohol drinker for 40 years(250ml/per meal average). In 1996 he had Hapetitis B. In 1966 he had blood fluke. On November 25 the patient starts to take XZ-C1+XZ-C4+XZ-C5. In 1998 and 1999 the patient continued to take the medicine. The patient condition is good, and his face is red and smiles. On November 2 1999 he came to follow-up and the ultrasound showed the lesion got small. He can do light work and feels very well. For more than 2 years, he continues to take XZ-C1+XZ-C4+XZ-C5. After these medicine the patient's energy lever is improving and appetite is improving. In June 2002 he went to Beijing for treatment (befpre he went to Beijing, he is good and walking as the normal person). During the operation there is a 5cmx6cm nodule in the liver which is the same as 5 years ago and there are cancer cells in the common duct and now metastasis and no fluid in the abdominal cavity. There is no metastasis in liver, however because the nodule is close to the sophagi entrance, it is very difficult to remove the cancer nodule and then put the Ttube to drainage. After surgery, this patients didn't have urine and had acute renal failure. He passed away during the 6th days.

October 30, 1997
CT diagnose
ultrasound November 25,1997 1998 1999 November 1999 2002 June 2002
XZ-C1+XZ-C4+XZ-C5 XZ-C XZ-C XZ-C XZ-C pass away after operation

---

Diagnosed as cancer taking the XZ-C1+XZ-C4+XZ-C5 only the patient condition was good before the surgery

Commons: In October 30, 1997 CT showed a 4.6cm X3.6cm nodue in left liver and in November 1997 there is a 1.6cmX 1.6cm nodule in right liver. Because the liver function was poor, the patient didn't have operation and tube placement and other treatment. On November 25 he started to take XZ-C1+XZ-C4+XZ-C5 and continued for 5 years. His healthy condition was fine.

The experience: XZ-C can improve the host immune system ability(including the cell and antibody immune function) to protect the central and peripheral immune organ and to protect the liver, kidney, and to produce anticancer factors and sophagi the cancer cells and prevent the cancer cells to metastase and spread. XZ-C is no side effect medicine and help the patient in fight with bad and help the right. In addition the patient had very good emotional condition which was sophag to overcome the diseases and to get recovery so that therapy effect was very good. This patient took XZ-C for 5 years and his condition is stable and the liver cancer lesion was not increasing and no metastasis. His general condition was good and no uncomfortable and walked as the normal person. He went to Beijing for surgery and diagnosed as liver cells carcinoma which was in the entrance of the liver and couldn't remove because of the cancer cells in the common duct and placed the T-tube to drainage. After the operation, this sophag didn't have urine and died of acute renal failure. If he didn't have operation which destroyed the liver and kidney function, he might survive by now.

Case 5 Huang, 53 year-old, Wuhan, medical record: 11202225

Diagnosis: primary huge liver cancer, liver cirrhosis after hepatitis, the later stage of Japanese blood fluke, Portal hypertension.

Disease course and treatment: In September 2000 CT showed there is 13.6cmx11.8cm in the right liver because the patient's appetite deceased and he felt uncomfortable in his sophag. In September 7 2000, MRI showed a huge 13.1cmx11.4cmx12.5cm lesion in right lobe, diagnosed as huge liver cancer in right lobe. The patient had hepatic arterial chemoembolization (HACE) and embolization (HAE) and the chemoembolization medicine were xxxx 25mg+xxx1000g: xxxx10ml+xxxx10mg. Currently his general condition is good. The change of his liver lesions are the following which are stable and getting small:

CT showed a 11.1cmx11.8cm lesion in the right liver lobe on October 12, 2000, a 10.8cmx9.8cm lesion in the right liver lobe on December 14 2000, a 10.5cmx9.5cm lesion on Feb 2001 and a 9.8cmx8.9cm lesion on September 3 2001 in the right liver lobe. This patient started to take XZ-C1+XZ-C4+XZ-C5 on January 9, 2002 and his general condition is good such as his emotion, appetite and sleep are very good. He comes back for check-up every month and takes his medicine regularly. On October 21 2002 during his follow-up, his general condition is good, emotion is stable, and appetite is good and bowel movement is good and his routine is regular and exercise regularly. He never got any cold during the last four years. He lived as the normal healthy person.

September 2000 October 19,2000 Jan 2 2001 March 30,2001 November, 12 2001 Jan.9 2002, 2003, 2004, 2005

CT, embolization embolization embolization embolization embolization XZ-C XZ-C XZ-C XZ-C

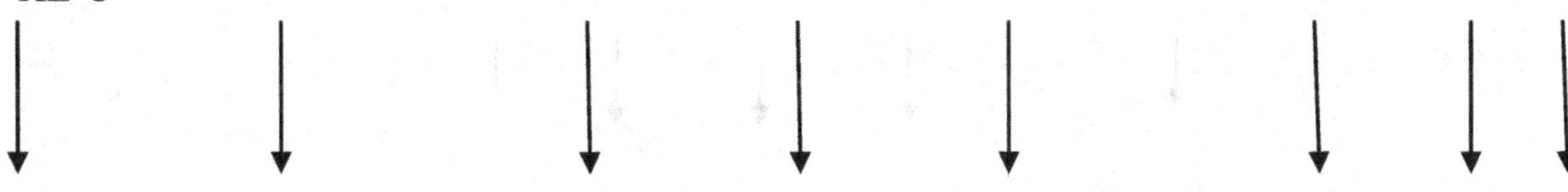

Lesion in the right liver embolization

13.6cmx11.8cm

Commons:this case is primary huge liver carcinoma which had five times emboliztion and the lesion was getting smaller and had very good response. Last embolization is on November 12, 2001 and the lesion is 9.8cmx8.9cm. He started to take XZ-C1+XZ-C4+XZ-C5 on Jan 9, 2002. The XZ-C1 can kill the cancer cells and not kill the normal cells;XZ-C4 protect thymus and inhibit thymus shrink; XZ-C5 protect the liver function and continues to take this medicine for more than 3 years, however when he came back for follow-up in the fourth year, his health condition is general, disease is stable and there is no metastasis and no further development. His emotion is stable, his appetite is good and walks as the normal healthy person. The experience from this case is for primary huge liver cancer, first embolization treatment are given to make this lesion smaller and stable, later use XZ-C to support the long-term therapy and to protect the liver function and to improve the immune system and to contral the metastasis.

Case 6 Mr. Lee, male, 53 yo, Wuhan, parents medical record: 9901979

Diagnosis: primary huge liver carcinoma, late stage Japanese blood fluke hepatic cirrhosis.

Disease course and treatment:In January 22 2001 the patient felt painful in the right back. In Feb 26 2001 Ultrasound showed a nodule in liver. In January 31 2001 CT showed a 14cmx1cm lesion in the right liver lobe diagnosed as primary huge liver cancer in the right liver. On March 1 2001 the open abdomen surgery was done in Tongjin Hospital and the pump implanation in the portal vein because the lesion was huge and couldn't be removed. After the surgery the patient had once pump with xxxxx and xxxxx. This sophag had 30 years Japanes blood fluke. On March 9, 2001 this sophag started to take XZ-C medicine. He used XZ-C1+XZ-C4+XZ-C5, LMS, MDZ, and XZ-C3 placed on the fist-size lump in the right rib edge area. After one month of taking this medicine, the patient's condition is getting better, his emotion is stable and happy. His appetite is increasing. The lump in the right rib edge area is getting smaller and softer than before. After he continued to take this medicine for three months, his general condition is good and his appetite and sleep are good. His energy level is recovering and walking as the normal person. On October 22 2001 Ultrasound showed a 6cmx7.8cm lesion in the right lobe liver and he continues taking XZ-C1+XZ-C4+XZ-C5 and using XZ-C3 on the lump. On November 19 2003 during his follow-up, ultrasound showed this lesion size the same as before, Kidney function is normal and CXR didn't show abnormal, there is no positive lymph node adn the lump on the right rib edge is soft and getting smaller and the bound is clear and no painful. This patient continued to use XZ-C1+XZ-C4+XZ-C5 .

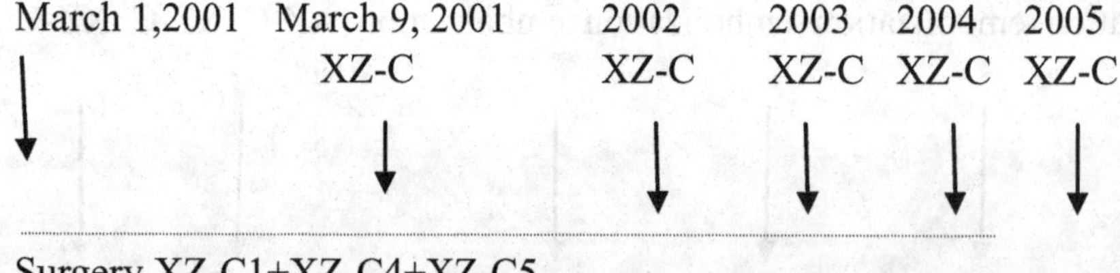

Surgery XZ-C1+XZ-C4+XZ-C5

Commons: this case is diagnosed as primary huge liver cancer and the lesion can not be removed so that the portal vien pump was placed for chemotherapy once. In March 2001, he started to use the XZ-C1+XZ-C4+XZ-C5 and topical XZ-C3 for 4 years. His general condition is stable and didn't develop further and didn't metastase.

Case 7 Mr. Wang, male, 40 yo, Shangdou, teacher, medical record: 900164

Diagnosis: primary liver cancer

Disease course and treatment: the tumor was removed in the mediastinum on June 28 1989, the pathology showed the thymoma with lymphocyte type and high malignant tumor and without treatment. In Feb 1995 Ultrasound showed a lesion in liver. On Feb 23,1995 CT showed a 8.2cm x8.7cm lesion in right posterior lobe and many nodes mixed together. On June 5, 1995 the hepatic artery graph embolization was done. The chemotherapy was injected in the lesion and on November 10, 1995 this right liver lesion was removed and the pathology showed that liver cell cancer. On December 21, 1995 Ultrasound showed a 3.8cmx3.2cm lesion in the right liver lobe which was the recurrent lesion after the surgery and there was fluid in the right cheat cavity and the right low lung is not distend and CXR showed the right low lung metastasis. On December 23, 1995 this patient took the XZ-C1+XZ-C4+XZ-C5 for more than two years and follow-up more than five years. His general condition is good and continued to teach and work normally without other treatment.

June, 1989 Feb 1995 June 1995 November1995 December1995 December1995 1996 1997 1998 1999
Thymus

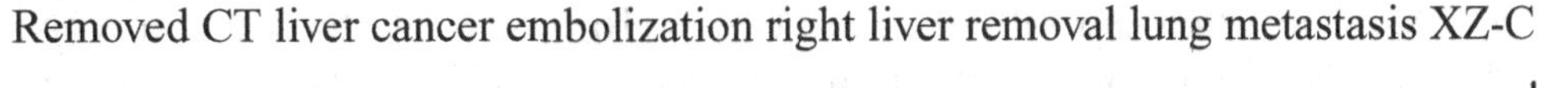

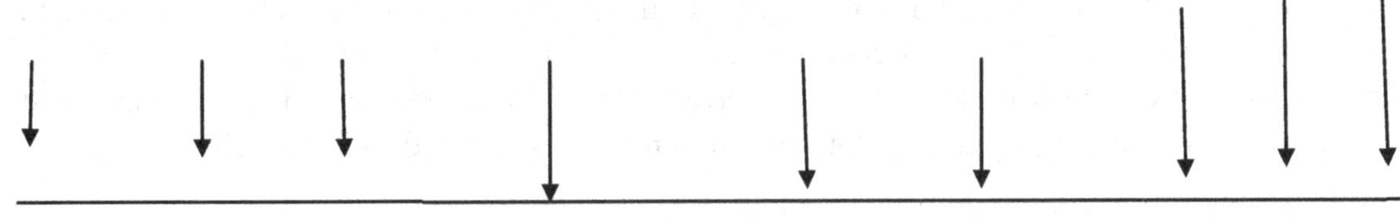

taking XZ-C1+XZ-C4+XZ-C5

Commons: In May 1995 CT showed a 7.1cmx6.6cm lesion in the right liver lobe. In 1995 the embolizatin was done once. On November 10, 1995 this right liver lesion was removed and diagnosed as liver cancer. On December 21, 1995 Ultrasound showed a 3.8cmx3.2cm lesion in the right liver lobe which was the recurrent lesion. On December 23, 1995 this patient took the XZ-C1+XZ-C4+XZ-C5 and his condition is good for more than four years.

Implicatin: there is very good result for liver cancer while using the combination of embolization +operation removal+XZ-C immune anticancer medicine

Case 8 Mr. Zhao, 34 yo, JinZhou, anounting, medical record: 380742

Diagnosis:primary huge liver cancer

Disease course and treatment: On Feb 26, 1997 there was a 13cmx10.4cm lesion between the liver quadrate lobe and left lobe because the patient feel uncomfortable about her stomach and had ultrasound test, then MRI showed a 7.9cmx11.2 cmx11.0cm lesion and portal vein had the cancer emboliz. On March 1, the patient had fever as 39C. On March 2, the patient was transferred to the XieHE hospital because of high fever and there is a 5cmx6cm hard lump under sternum. On March 10 the embolization was performed and the patient had great reaction to this. This patient had embolization on April 30, on July 9, on September 18. Then lump decrease significantly. On March 4 the patient started to take XZ-C1+XZ-C4+XZ-C5 to stable the lesion and to control the spread and to provent the metastasis. After taking the medicine, the patient's emotion and appetite are getting better and the general condition is getting better and life quality is getting better. The lump under the sternum couldn't be palpated.

Feb 26 March 3, 1997 March 10,1997 April 30,1997 July 9, 1997 Sept 18, 1997, 1998 1999 2000
,1997 XZ-C Embolization Embolization Embolization Embolization XZ-C XZ-C XZ-C
CT |
MRK |

Taking the XZ-C1+XZ-C4+XZ-C5

Commons: for this primary huge liver carcinoma, four times embolizations were performed and the patient took XZ-C persistently so that the combination of embolization and XZ-C had good treatment result and life quality increased. The lump under sternum went away. In the past three years the patient's general condition is good.

Implication: The combination of embolization and XZ-C had good results and support the long-term results and embolization can kill the parts of cancer cells and lump decreased, however there are alive cancer cells and continues growth so that after embolization he took the XZ-C1+XZ-C4+XZ-C5, which can kill 105 cancer cells. To take XZ-C for long-term can control tumor and stable the lesions and to prevent metastasis. Embolization chemotherapy had a big problem because cancer cells continues divisions and chemotherapy just is used peroidly. The cancer cells can grow back during the interrept period. The embolization can damage most of the cancer cells and XZ-C can support our immune ability to kill the cancer cells.

Case 9 Mr. Zheng, male, 48 yo, Enshi, officer, medical record 500987

Diagnosis: primary liver carcinoma

Disease course and treatment: In January 1996 a thumus-size lesion was found in the right liver lobe and was treated with protection of liver treatment. In Octocber 1997 a 5.7cmx5.7cm lesion was found by Ultrasound. In October 1997 the patient had open abdominal surgery and the lesion couldn't be removed so that a hepetic tube was placed for pump chemotherapy. Pathological diagnosis is Liver cells carcinoma.

In December 23, 1997 the second time chemotherapy was given, however the reaction is great so that the patient didn't have chemotherapy again. In December 25 1997 the patient started to take the XZ-C. Until he come to follow-up, his condition is stable and healthy and is happy. His appetite is good and energy lever is up and walk and other activities as the normal individual. In Nevomber 1998 the patient come back to regular work as teacher and his energy lever is great.

Jan Oct Dec Dec 25 April May July Aug 1998 Oct 1998 Dec 1998 Jun1999
1996 1997 1997 1997 1998 1998 1998

CT CT lesion operation,
Increase XZ-C ....
....

Taking XZ-C1+XZ-C4+XZ-C5

Commons: In January 1996 a lesion was found in the right liver and In Nevomber 7,1997 the chemotherapy pump was placed during the surgery which chemotherapy was used twice. After the second time in Dec 23, 1997, the patient only received XZ-C1+XZ-C4+XZ-C5 for more three years. His condition is good.

Implication: The hepatic arterial chemoembolization and XZ-C1+XZ-C4+XZ-C5 had good result because the chemotherapy can kill most of cancer cells and XZ-C1+XZ-C4+XZ-C5 can kill cancer cells and protect hosts as well to improve the host immune function and to get rid of the rests of cancer cells.

Case 10 Mr. Wei, female, 36 yo, Chibi in Hubei, medical record:15603095

Diagnosis: Liver cell cancer

Disease course and treatment:The patient had pain in upper abdomen and his appetite decreased and he was tired for more than half month so that he had CT which showed a lesion in left liver and AFP is more than 400ug/L. On June 6,2004 the left half liver was removed and a portal vien chemotherapy pump was placed in Chibi hospital. During the operation, a lesion was found in most of the left liver so that the pump was placed after the removal of the left liver lobe(the end into hepatic portal vien). After operation, the chemotherapy was used twice throught the pump and Ultrasound showed a 1.7cmx1.8cm lesion in right liver. Pathology show:XXX liver cells cancer. On Sept 27 2004 the patient started to take XZ-C1+XZ-C4+XZ-C5, LMS and MDZ and follow-up every month to fill up the medicine. On April 2008 Ultrasound showed no lesion in the liver and AFP is normal. The patient general condition is good. His emotion is stable and his appetite is good. His body weight is increased and her energy lever is good and works in other city. She continued taking medicine for more than 7 years and she is healthy.

Jun 6 2004	Sept 2004	Sep 27 2004	2005	2006	2007	2008	2009	2010
Left liver Removal Placed pump	Ultrasound	XZ-C						

a 1.7cmx1.8cm taking XZ-C1+XZ-C4+XZ-C5, LMS and MDZ
in right liver

Commons: After left liver removal and pump chemotherapy which was used twice with right liverlesion, the patient still continued to take XZ-C to protect thymus and bone morrow for more than seven years and her health condition is good. Recently she works in another city and filled up her medicine every month.

Case11 Mr. Huang, male, 38 yo, Hubei, worker, medical record : 13402661

Diagnosis: primary liver carcinoma

Disease course and treatment: In Feb 16, 2003 during physical exam, the ultrasound found that liver tumor and CT showed a 9.8cmx5.8cm lesion in positive right lobe which boundary line is not separate clear diagnosed as liver cell carcinoma. AFP is 91.875 ug/l. In March 8 2003 the right half liver was removed which Pathology diagnosis is liver cell carcinoma. The patient only takes XZ-C after operation. He takes XZ-C regularly and persistenly for more than 8 years which he follow-ups every 2 month. His general condition is good. He come back to work for more than four years and energy level is great. In December 10 2009 he come back to follow-up and filled his medicine and his general medical control was great and appetite is good and no other complains. This year he works in another city and he is healthy.

This is the case which after operation the patient survives more than eight years through only taking XZ-C medicine.

March 8,2003	April 2003	2004	2005	2006	2007	2008	2009	2010
Right half liver removal	XZ-C	XZ-C	XZ-C	XZ-C	XZ-C	XZ-C	XZ-C	XZ-C
Liver cell cancers	taking XZ-C1+XZ-C4+XZ-C5							

Commons: This is the case which after right half liver removal, the patient only taking XZ-C medicine to improve thymus function to improve the immune function and survives more than eight years. He comes to work four years now.

Implication:XZ-C medicine can work as an assistant therapy for the surgery to improve the host immune function and to prevent recurrence and metastasis.

Case 12 Mr. Lee, male, 60yo, Wuhan, officer, medical record:270003392

Diagnosis: liver cells cancer

Disease course and treatment: in November 2005 during the physical exam B showed a 5.4cmx4.0cm lesion in right liver lobe. In the same month the patient had right half liver removal. Pathology diagnosed as liver cell carcinoma. After the operation, on November 28 2005 he started to take XZ-C1+XZ-C4+XZ-C5, LMS and MDZ to protect thymus and bone morrow. He takes the medicine regularly for more than five years and his general condition is good and his appetite is great and he is healthy.

November 2005	November 28 2005	2006	2007	2008	2009	2010
Right half liver removal	XZ-C	XZ-C	XZ-C	XZ-C	XZ-C	XZ-C
Liver cell cancer	taking XZ-C1+XZ-C4+XZ-C5, LMS and MDZ					

Commons: The patient had a lesion in the right liver, which had right half liver removed. After operation, the patient only takes XZ-C1+XZ-C4+XZ-C5, LMS and MDZ for more than five years and his health condition is good.

2. Typical cases of assistant treatment after operation in pancreatic canrcinoma

Case13 Mr. Yao, female, 73 yo, Wuhan, medical record:240469

Diagnosis: gallbladder adenocarcinoma

Disease course and treatment: the patient felt pain in right upper quadrant in Dec 1995 getting worse, then admitted to hospital in Feb 1996. On March 26 1996 the patient was diagnosed as gallbladder cancer during operation, then removed of the gallbladder and put T-tube placement to have bile draigage. Pathological diagnosis is papillary adenocarcinoma involved in muscle layers with gallbladder stones. On April 26 1996 the tube was removed and started to take XZ-C1+XZ-C4. On Jan 23 1997 the patient had severe pain and was diagnosed as common duct blockage and jaundice by Ultrasound. Common duct dilated into 1.5cm. After taking the medicine for 2 months, the jaundice went away, appetite increased, energy level increased. He took the medicine regularly for 15 months. In July 1997 the patient recovered completely, walked normally, activites as the normal individual. She did the chores every day. On December 4 1999 her son come to office for follow-up:after taking this tradition medicine for one and half years, the patient did ifne, happy, energy level recovery and does chores, play cards and toto shop, her activities are the same as the other women.

March 26, 1996	April 26,1996	Jan, 1997	Sept 1997	Dec 1999
Gallbladder removal	XZ-C	XZ-C, JAUDICE	XZ-C,	FOLLOW UP

TAKING take XZ-C1+XZ-C4 ______________________________HEALTHY

Commons: On March 26, 1996 the patient was diagnosed as gallbladder cancer and removed it. The patient didn't' take any other treatment becaseu of ther age and weekness. On April 26,1996 he start to take XZ-C1+XZ-C4. On Jun 1997 the jaundice came after obstacle of common duct. He continues to take XZ-C for 2 month and the jaundice went away. She took XZ-C regularly and persistently. Follow-up the pateient for four years, she is fine.

Sugguestion: taking XZ-C1+XZ-C4 for long term treatment can improve life qualities and prevent mestatasis and improve the patient's survival rate.

Case 14 Mr. Zhou, male, 53 yo XiaoGan, officer, medical record: 950004284

Diagnosis: Pancreatic adenocarcinoma

Disease courses and treatment:In August 15 2007 the patient was diagnosed as hepatitis and had CT which showed tumor on the pancreas and obstacle of the common duct. Then had operation of the removal of the pancreas and dueducal. The pathology showed that malignant pancreas adenocarcinoma and metastasis of the common duct and dueduan wall and the membrance of the pancreas. There are no lymph node metastasis around the pancreas. After four weeks chemotherapy, the wbc and plaletet and other side effects were significant. On June 16 2008 the patient started to take XZ-C1+XZ-C4+XZ-C5+LMS+MDZ. This patient's general medication is fine and his appetite is great. He takes his medication regularly and fills his medication regularly for more than four years. In Sept 2010 when he came back to follow up, his medical condition is good and there was no lymph node enlargement and his abdomen is soft and there is no lump palpation. Now the patient went back to work for one year and he is healthy.

August 21, 2007 June 2008 2009 2010

Removal of pancreas and duedual chemoth chemoth chemo chemo XZ-C

Pancreas cancer Taking the XZ-C1+XZ-C4+XZ-C5

Commons: this patient had the removal of the pancreas and duedual and after four times chemotherapy, the side effects were significant and then started to take XZ-C for more than four years and now goes back work.

Suggestion: After the pancreas adenocarcinom operation, the XZ-C can protect thymus and to protect the bone marrow to control the metastasis and to improve the survival rates.

Case 15 Mr. Fong, male, 50 yo, Hubei Lou Tang, peasant, medical record: 330651

Diagnosis: Pancreas cancer

Disease course and treatment: Because of uncomfort in upper abdomen for more than three months, he had jaundice and had opening abdomen surgery showing : no stones in the bile system and the enlargement of the pancreas and couldn't be removed and Pathology showed that pancreatic cancer. CT showed that the enlargement of pancreas head and dilation of the bile duct in liver. After the operation the jaundice extended persistently. On December 11 1996 he started to take the XZ-C and after one month his medical condition got better and his appetites increased, however he still had little juandic and weekness and sweeting. After taking XZ-Cand soups two months the jaundice and pain reduced and got better. After four months, the jaundice was gone away completely and his appetites and energy lievel are good. His pain in abdomen was mild. In July 1998 he came backto work and did mild labor work and his face looks red. He continues to take his medicinefor many years. On April 6 2004 his family introduced a new patient to us and told us that this patient was fine and his activities as the normal and does his chores very well.

November, 1996	December, 1996	1997	1998	1999	2000	2001
	XZ-C	XZ-C				

Operation

Showed pancreas head cancer taking the XZ-C1+XZ-C4

Commons:this patient has pancreas head cancer and jaundice. On November 28 1996 during the operation, this tumor can not removed and Pathology: pancreas cancer with the dilation of the bile duct system in the livers. On December 11 1996 this patient took ZX-C and soup. After seven months his jaundice reduce and he continues to take medicine to improve his immune system. Until July 1998 his condition is completely normal. He continues to take his medicine for more than four years and later changed into periodly taking the medicine to support his healthy condition. Now this patient follow us for more than nine years and his condition is very well.

3. Typical cases of assistant treatment after operation in stomach carcinoma:

Case 16 Mr. Chan, male, 65 yo, Wuhan, retired officer, medical record:280555

Diagnosis: adenocarcinoma in the pyloric area of the stomach and recurrence after the surgery in the remain stomach.

Disease course and treatment:This patient had pain in the upper abdomen for more than one year and in June 1993 he was diagnosed as stomach cancer and had the removal of the great curvature in the stomach. After the operation, he had FM chemotherapy once to cause the anemia ane weekness and WBC counting is 1900. After operation 8 months, the patient had abdomen pain with vomiting and had left upper abdominal pain for half years. On March 25

1994 the Barium showed: there was no filled on the upper area of the stomach and part damage of the membrance and the narrow change in the cutting parts. A barium swallow showed that recurrence of the stomach cancer. On May 3 1996 Ultrasound showed that there is no lesion inside the liver. Because this patient couldn't eat rice and just eat the noodle and fuild food so that he had fatigue and no energy and and didn't want to have operation. In June 1996 he started to take XZ-C. After that he is fine and appetites increase and he takes this medicine regularly for more than four years. On May 6 2000 when he came back to follow-up, his general condition is great and his face looks red and healthy. Walking and activities are normal as the others and he eats rice soup and bannon often as his meal.

June 1993 March 1994 June 1996 June 1997 June 1998 June 1999 Dec 1999 May 2000
Stomach operation

---

taking XZ-C

Commons: In June 1993 the patient had the stomach removal. In March 1994 the cancer recurred and the junction part turned narrow. After taking XZ-C+XZ-C4 only, for more than six years his health condition is great.

Sugguestion: For the recurrence of the stomach cancers, the junction of the surgery was not closed completely and still could eat the food. After taking the medicines to improve thymus function to control the tumor growth and prevent the tumor growth and metastasis. The patient's medical condition is stable and is still alive.

Case 17 Mr. Liu, 65 yo, Wuhan, economist, medical record: 2200421

Diagnosis: fundus and cardia stomach cancinoma

Disease course and treatment: In Jan 1995 the patient had the stomach pain for six months and had the endoscopy which showed stomach pyloric adenocarcinoma and had surgery which had the primary stomach removal and connect the esophagus with stomach body. After the operation the patient is week and thin so that he didn't have chemotherapy. On March 16 1996 he started to take the XZ-C1+XZ-C4 only formore than five years persistently, then change into periodly taking the medicine.

Jan 1995 March 1996 1997 1998 1999 2000 2001 2002 2003
Operation XZ-C XZ-C

Taking the XZ-C1+XZ-C4

Commons: In Jan 1995 this patient had the removal of the cardia and fundus of the stomach which connected the esophagus with the stomach body. Because of his weekness, he didn't take chemotherapy and takes the XZ-C1+XZ-C4 only for more than ten years and his medical condition is fine.

Sugguest: After the operation, the medicine XZ-C can control the cancer to recure and to metastasis and has very good curevature results.

Case 18 Mr. Cheng, male, 65yo, worker, medical record:260518

Diagnosis: the recurrence and metastasis of the stomach cancer

Disease course and treatment: On June 1 1994 the endoscope showed that 3cmx3cm ulcer in the stomach pyloric area and Pathology: the adenocarcinoma in the pyloric. In June 1994 the patient had the surgery to remove the cancer. Pathology showed: the cancer cell into the muscular layer and not the lesser curvature and mucous adenocarcinoma. In May 1996 the patient felt painful in the upper abdominal area and appetites decrase and fatigue. On May 14 1996 he was admitted into the hospital and had fever, pain in the abdomen, low protein and ascite and fuild in the chest. There were many cancer cells in the ascite. Because of the heavy ascite the patient came to our office and started to take our medicine. After taking this medicine the patient general medication condition is very well and appetites was great and his ascite is reduced and his energy level is increased. He came back to follow-up regularly. After the surgery six years and recurrence for four years the patient condition is great and appetites are great and activities are as the normal persons.

June 1994
Surgery

Commons: This patient had surgery in June 1994. After that he didn't have any treatment. In May 1996 he had fulid in his chest and his abdomen cavity. Becaue the ascite is heavy, he started to take the XZ-C and his general medical condition is good and follow-up with us for more than four years.

Suggestion: After one year surgery this patient had fuild and cancer cells in his chest and abdominal cavity. He takes the medicine persistenly and his medical condition was controlled and his life qualities are improved and survives very well with his cancer.

Case 19 Mr. Wang, male, 53yo, Xinzhou, peasant, medical record:800157

Diagnosis: the recurrence in the stomach carcinoma.

Disease courses and treatment: In February 1994 the patient felt uncomfortable and the Endoscopy show the stomach carcinoma. In June 1994 he had the stomach removal and followed with chemotherapy for two course of treatment with xxxx+xxxx. On May 30 1995 the barrumm scan showed that the damage of the conjuction sides and had narrow area for more than five cm and partially obstructed and there is a 5 cm diameter masses in the junction area. On June 2 1995 he started to take XZ-C1+XZ-C4. After taking his medicine his general medical condition is great and appetite is increased and can eat the rice and bannes. He comes back to follow up regularly for more than two and half years. His healthy condition is great.

June, 1994	July, 1994	August, 1994	May 30, 1995	June 2,1996	1996	1997
Operation	336soph.	Chem.	GI recurrence	XZ-C	XZ-C	XZ-C

Taking the medicine

Commons: the patient had the recurrence of the stomach cancer after the conjuction of the stomach partial removal. In June 1995 he started to take the xz-c and follow up with us for more than two and half years. His condition is great.

Sugguests: XZ-C can stable the recurrence of the cancinoma and improve the patient's condition well and had very good results.

Case 20 Ms. Zhang, female, 39 yo, Wuhan, account, medical record:1700321

Diagnosis: the stomach cancer from the stomach ulcer, low differential adenocarcinoma

Disease courses and treatment: in March 1994 because of the uncomfortable in the upper abdomen for one month and getting worse for one week so that the endoscopy showed the stomach ulceration. On April 20 1994 the major stomach was removed and had chemotherapy for six courses of the treatment after the operation with xxxxx+xxxxx to protect the livers. Pathology showed the low differential stomach canciroma and had lymph nodes metastasis. On November 22 1995 he started to take XZ-C1+XZ-C4+XZ-C8 only to protect the bone marrow and follow up with us for more than ten years. He doesn't have metastasis and recurrence and his condition is great.

April 20,1994	Chem 6 times	November 22,1995	1996	1997	1998	1999	2000	2005
Operation		XZ-C		XZ-C	XZ-C			

Taking XZ-C1+XZ-C4+XZ-C8

Commons: this patient had low degree adenocarcinoma in the stomach and lymph node metastasis. On April 20 1994 he had the removal of his major stomach, then he had six courses of the chemotherapy. On November 22 1995 he took the medicine only and followed up with us for more than ten years. His medical condition is great.

Suggustions: After the operation the combination of the chemotherapy and XZ-C medicine can improve the long-term treatment. XZ-C can prevent the cancer recurrence and metastasis.

Case 21 MR. Zhou, male, 57 yo, officer, medical record:1900368

Diagnosis: pyloric and greater curvature of the stomach carcinoma from the ulceration

Disease courses and treatment: In September 1995 after the removal of the stomach caner, he had two courses of the chemotherapy and the side effects were significant and his hair lost. Pathology:medium differential adenocarcinoma without the lymph nodes metastasis. On January 5 1996 he started to take the medicine and his medical condition is getting better and his appetite is good. He persistenly takes his medicine for more than four years and his medical condition is stable.

September 1995	1995	1995	Jan 5 1996	1997	1998	1999
The removal of His stomach	Chem(1)	337soph.(2)	XZ-C	XZ-C	XZ-C	XZ-C

Commons: the patient had the cancinoma from the stomach ulceration, with medium differential. On September 25 he had the operation and took two period of the chemotherapy after the operation, however the reaction was strong so that he took the XZ-C only since then to prevent the recurrence and metastasis of the cancinoma. He took this medicince for more than four year and his medical condition is great.

Sugguest: After his opearation his immune system function is decreasing so that the chemotherapy was used for short-term and XZ-C1+XZ-C4 for long-term to protect thymus and to prevent the recurrence and metastasis.

Case 22 MR. Yi, male, 58yo, Shanxing, medical record:8801750

Diagnosis: stomach carcinoma

Disease courses and treatment: after the pain in the stomach two years, on April 27,2000 he had the endoscope which showed the stomach cancer which low-grade adenocarcinoma in the body of the stomach so that he had radical removel. After five days of his surgery, he had a chemotherapy. On June 19 2000 he started to use XZ-C1+XZ-C4 to protect his thymus and the patients took the medication persistently. So far he takes this medication for more than eleven years and continues to follow up with us. On Jan eight 2010 when he came back to follow up, his general medical condition was very well.

April 27 2000
Operation Chemotherapy once June 19 2000 2001 2002 2003 2004 2005 2006 2010

Commons:after the radical operation, there is once chemotherapy. Because of the reaction, he kept using the XZ-C to protect his thymus and bone marrow to prevent the immune system and protect the metastasis and recurrence. He kept using the small amount medication to get good health.

Case23 Ms. Zheng, female, 54 yo, worker medical record:12602507

Diagnosis: the stomach adenocarcinoma

Disease courses and treatment: in September 2002 the endoscope showed that stomach cancer. On Octocber 14 2002 he had radical operation. Pathology showed I-II stages and in the deep muscular layer and 2/3 lymph nodes metastasis and once chemotherapy after the operation. WBC decreases and then stop. On Octocber 25 2002 he started to take XZ-C1+XZ-C4. After that he is llively and his appetite is good and his physical strengthen gradually increase and have continues to take this medicine for more than eight yo. On September 4 2010 when he follow up to us, his healthy condition was great.

Octocber 14, 2002 chemotherapy Octocber, 25 2002 2003 2005 2006, 2007 2008 2009 2010
Radical once XZ-C

Commons: after this patient had operation and once chemotherapy, his reaction is strong so that he started to take XZ-C to protect his thymus and to prevent his bone marrow to inhibit the recurrence and metastasis. For eight years he takes this medication persistently and his medical condition is healthy.

Case 24 Mr. Liao, male, 60 you, Wuhanjiongxia, medical record:7101403

Diagnosis: the pyloric carcinoma

Disease course and treatment: Because he had pain in the upper back and under stern for more than four months, he had endoscopy and bisopy done which showed the low grade pyloric adenocarcinoma. In December 1998 he had the radical removal of the total stomach the xian hei which the Pathology showed the same results as before and had the metastasis of the lymph nodes in the lesser and greater curvative. He had once chemotherapy and on Jan 31 1999 he started to take XZ-C1+XZ-C4 and he is spirited and his appetite is good and his physical lever is great. He followed up with us for more than twelve years and his general medical condition is great.

December 1998
Stomach removal Jan 31 1999
XZ-C

Commons: this patient had the stomach removal and chemotherapy. After one month later he started to take the XZ-C to protect the thymus and bone marrow. For 12 years his healthy condition is good.

4. Typical cases of assistant treatment after operation in lung carcinoma:

Case 25 Mr. Liu, male, 68yo, Changzhou, officer, medical record:8701735

Diagnosis: the central lung cancer on the right upper of the lung with the metastasis

Disease courses and treatment: in Octocber 1998 he coughed two weeks with the pain in the right shoulder and was treated with inflammation. In Jan 1999 his cough is getting worse and this appetite is decreased and fatigure and getting weak. On CT there is mass on the right upper lung showing the central lung. He had endoscope and biopsy which showed that lung adenocarcinoma in the xxxxxx. He and his family member don't want to have operation. In Feb 1999 after chemotherapy for one course, his reaction to the chemotherapy was strong and stopped to use it. This patient had metastasis in the left lung which showed there are two lesions and he coughed with mucous and blood sputdu and difficult walking. On April 23 2000 he started to take the XZ-C1+XZ-C4+XZ-C7, LMS+MDZ for three months and his general condition is good and he is lively and his appetite is great. In December 2000 his medical condition is stable, and he is lively. His appetite is good and his breath is smooth and his face is red. He walked as the normal person and sometimes he coughs. He persistently takes this medication for more than four years and when he comes back to follow up during the five years, his general condition is great and he walked as the normal healthy person.

1999
CT

Commons: this patient has the central lung cancer in the right upper lung. In April 2000 he started to use XZ-C1+XZ-C4+XZ-C7. XZ-C1 is used to kill the cancer cells only without kill the normal cells; XC-C4 protect the thymus and increase the thymus weight and to protect the bone marrow, XZ-C7 inhibit the lung cancer cells and protect the lung and solve the suptid. After short-term chemotherapy he started to take the XZ-C to strengthen his long-term therapy. XZ-C improve the whole body immune system and he is lively and his appetite is good and his spleen is great and help the patients against the diseases and help the patient's organ functions and the nutrition condition and metabliztion recover so that the patients' healthy condition is recovery.

This patient didn't have the operation. In Feb 1999 he had chemeotherapy, however there is left lung metastasis after chemotherapy. Afterh that, he only took the XZ-C to control the metastasis. He persistently took the medicine for more than four years and his medical condition is great without any complaints. He followed up with us for more than seven years. In May 2005 when he came back to follow up, his general medical condition is great and his appepital is good without other symptoms. His walking and activities and he talks cheerfully and humorously.

Case26 Mr. Zhou, male, 49yo, Wuhan, officer, medical records: 410804

Diagnosis: lung cancer in the right low labor

Disease courses and treatment: In 1996 the patient started to have cough and chest tightness and low fever and difficult breath and was treated as the Cold. In April 1997 he suddenly started to cough blood and X-ray and CT showed the right lung cancer in low lobe. And at the same month he had right low lobe lung removal and Pathology showed that lung low grade adenocarcinoma. After the operation, his condition is stable and didn't have chemotherapy and radioactive therapy. On May 15 1997 he started to take XZ-C:1,4,7,vitamin C, B6 E, A. After he took these medicine his energy level is increase and appetite was great and his face is red and there were no recuurence and metastasis and no complaints. In June 2004, the patient came back to follow up with us he continues to take these medicine more than three years. Everything is stable. So far his condition is stable as the normal healthy person after he took his medication more than eight years.

Commons: this patient has right low lobe low grade adenocarcinoma. After the operation, he didn't have radioactive and chemotherapy treatment and he only takes the XZ-C medication XZ-C1+C4+C7. After taking these medicine more than eight years, his energy level is high and appetite is good and his healthy condition is great.

Case 27 Mr. Zheng, male, 52 yo, Wuhan, driver, medical record:11302254

Diagnosis: right lung low grade adenocarcinoma with lymph node metastasis

Disease courses and treatment: because of bloody cough he had the CTscan which showed that right low lung tumor and the bronchoscopy didn't show abnormal. On December 12 2001 he had the removal of the right middle and lower lobe and one lymph node between lobe and two lymph node in the entrance were found. Pathology showed that low grade adenocarcinoma with lymph node mestastasis. After the operation he has once chemotherapy. In 2002 he started to take XZ-C to prevent the tumor recurrence and metastasis. He continues to take the XZ-C1+C4+C7+LMS+MDZ for more than three year and his condition is stable and he is energetic and his appetite is great.

Commons: this patient has the right low lobe adenocarcinoma with lymph node metastasis. After the chemotherapy once, then using the XZ-C1+C4+C7 as the supplement treatment. XZ-C1 kills the cancer cells without killing the normal cells. XZ-C4 protects the thymus and bone marrow; XZ-C7 to protect the lung function. He continues to take his medication for more than three years and there was not metatastasis. When he came back to follow up for his fourth year treatment, his condition is stable and his appetite is great and walked as the normal healthy person.

Case 28 Mr. Long, male, 60 yo, Huangguang, officer, medical record; 521028

Diagnosis: Right lung middle and low lobe adenocarcinoma with diaphragm lymph node metastasis

Disease courses and treatment: In January 1997 he started to cough and fever and was treated as pneumonia. In December 1997 CT showed right lung cancer. The bronchoscopy showed that right side central low grade adenocarcinoma with diaphragm lymph node metastasis and then he was treated as xxxx and XZ-C treatment. He had his first chemotherapy through the brochial artery on Dec 31 1997 and the second chem. On Jan 20 1998, The third chemotherapy in March 1998. On July 8 1998 he received the 35th radioactive therapy. In September 1998 after the radioactive therapy, the twice chemotherapy were given(one months). From February 14 1998 to March 14 1998, May 9 1998 to June 9 1998, July 1 1998 to August 1 1998 the patients took ZX-C1 +XZ-C4+XZ-C7 by oral. After that the cough decreased an general conditions well, the vital energy and appetites are good, the energy level come back, he walked and acted as the normal person, dry cough. On Auguest 9 1998 because of the radioactive esophagitis which cause the swellon, congestion and difficulty swallowing, horse voice, then XXXX the XZ-C2 and inhaling the Chinese herbs, continue to take XZ-C medicine, his vital viguour and appetites are very well and can take the food.

Common: This patient have the right low lobe lung cancer with diaphragm lymph nodes mestatasits which was treated with XXX+XZ-C, after the long-term usage of the XZ-C regulation and control medicine, his general medical condition is good and appetite is good. Follow-up with us more two years and eight month, the condition is stable.

Suggestion: Left lung cancer with diagraph lymph node metastasis cannot be operated so that he was treated with XXX+Radiavtive+Chinese medicine, first radi+chem to kill the tumor cells, then continue to use the XZ-C immune medicine to protect thymus and improve th whole body immune level, so that to strength the curative therapy and protect the recurrence which has the effective effects.

Case 29 Mr. Xie, male, 55 yo, Xiang Fen, medical record:340663

Diagnosis: Right upper lung adenocarcinoma

The disease courses and treatment: The activities of the right shoulder and right hands decreased about half of years and two months cough and little XXX without blood. On November 26, 1996 Chest X-ray showed that there is round lump on the right upper lung, which was confirmed by CT. On December 16 1996 he had the removal of the right upper lung and the pathology showed that right upper lung adenocarcinoma. On December 23 1996 he started to take XZ-C to prevent the recurrence, metastasis and he didn't take any other therapy. After taking XZ-C for a long-term, the patient is stable and his appetite is good and the vigour is very well and the energy level recovered and didn't have any other symptoms. His face glow with health so far it has been three and half years and everything is good as the normal healthy persons. He had many times of Chest X-ray which showed the normal. Ultrosound is normal.

Commens: this patient took XZ-C1+XZ-C4+CX-C7 for three years after the operation, so far he still used the XZ-C without other therapy. He is healthy as the normal persons.

Suggestions: After the lung operation, to take XZ-C for a long term can prevent the reccurence and metastasis for longterm. Because XZ-C protect thymus and bone marrow and can improve the immune function, the immune function of the patients can keep the high level without using radioactive and chemotherapy. Only treated by XZ-C for more than three years, he is well and as healthy as the normal persons.

Case 30 Mr. Huang, male, 54year olds, Xiaogan, the officer, medical record: 4600907

Diagnosis: Lung cancer

Diseases courses and treatment conditions: In September 1996 cough blood and recovered with the antiinfection. In Aprle 1997 coughed again the symptoms can not be treated in the local hospital. On August 15 1997 the bronchoscopy and biopsy showed that lung squamous carcinoma. On August 31 1997 he have the left low lung removal and the pathology showed that left low lung squamous carcinoma with the lymph nodes of the lung entrance metastasis(1/3). Since September 1997 he took XZ-C to prevent the recurrence and matastasis. After taking the medicine, he is vagorous and his appetite is good. Every month he came back to get the medicine. In April 1999 when he came back to follow-up, he is healthy and his face is glowing with health, walking and acting and talk cheerfully and humorously, the superclavica, xxx, xxxxl lymph nodes and liver and spleens have no lesions, his body weight is 63kg. Chest X-ray and CT have changed sincere the surgery. After the surgery he started to take the medicince XZ-C1+XZ-C4+XZ-C7 for more than two and half years without other therapy. He is healthy.

Comments: This patient had the removal of the left low lung on Auguest 31 1997 and the pathology showed that left lung squamous carcinoma with the lymph nodes in the lung entrance metastasis(1/3). On September 19 1997 he started to XZ-C1+XZ-C4+XZ-C7 without other therapy for more than three years and he is healthy.

Suggestions: after the lung removal, to take XZ-C can improve the immune function and strengthen the body and maintain the curative therapy which can form the environment of no benefits for the tumor growth to prevent the tumor recurrence.

Case 31 Mr. Wang, male, 61yo, Machen, officer.

Diagnosis: the central left lung cancer.

Disease courses and the treatment condition: On July 29 2006 the left lung cancer was found during the physical examinatoion. On August 21 2006 the total lungs in Tongjin hospital and cleaned the lymph nodes and part of the heart capsule+left part of artrium+ the xxx nerve removal. After seven days the left chest cavity had pneumothorax and induced by the tube. After the operation the patient was weak without the chemotherapy and radioactive. On October 10 2006 he started to take XZ-C and he is energetic and his appetite is good. He persistently took his medicince for more than five years. On Octocboer 8 2010 he came back to followup and his health condition is good.

Comments:this patient has the left central lung carcinoma which the surgery is very difficult and have the removal of the total parts of the lung in the heart cavity+ lymph nodes in the digraph+parts of the heart capsule+parts of the left antrium+ xxx nervous. After the operation, the tube was used to induce the fluid. Because of the age he didn't receive any therapy. On November 11 2006 he started to take XZ-C and he took them regularly and he is vagour and his appetite is good formore than five years.

Suggestions: Left central lung cancer, the surgery removal is a difficult procedure. After the operation, the immune function decreases and the patient was weak. After taking XZ-C to protect the thymus and bone marrow, the therapy is excellent. This patient medical condition is stable.

Case 32 Mr. Guang, male, 64 yo, Fushan in Guangdou, business man, medical record:220003302

Diagnosis: right lung adenocarcinoma

Disease course and treatment:in May 2005 CT in the southern hospital showed tha the right lung cancer in the peripheral. On May 16 2005 he had the removal of the right upper lobe lung and Pathology showed that peripheral lung adenocarcinoma in the right lung with XXXXX and no lymph node metastasis. After the surgery once chemotherapy. On July 13 2005 he came to our office for XZ-C1+XZ-C4+XZ-C7+LMS+MDZ, and continued to take them for more than five years without other therapy. His condition is stable

Comments: this patient had the right upper lobe lung cancer with the removal. After the chemotherapy, he had great reaction so that he stoped. In July 2005 he started to take XZ-C which he refilled every three months. He persistently took his medicine for more than five years and his medical condition is good.

Case 33 Mrs Ling, female, 64yo, Danan, medical record:670003868

Diagnosis: after the removal of the right lung cancer, with both of the sizes metastasis and bone metastasis

Disease course and treatment condition: in March 2006 the patient coughed without the reasons. In May 2006 CT showed the right upper lung cancer and In June he had the removal of the right upper lobe + lymph node in the secondary hospital in the Daniang. The pathology showed that small cell lung cancer. In July 2006 after chemotherapy, CE xxx for two weeks the bone marrow were inhibited for the three degree. In September after the operation CT showed that both lung had metastasis nodules. Because of read my book<< the new ways and new concepts of the cancer treatment>>, he started to take XZ-C1+XZ-C4+XZ-C7+LMS+Vit. He took the medicine persistently for more than four years. His healthy condition is fine and he is energetic and his appetite is good and walking as the normal healthy persons.

Comments: this patient had right upper lobe small cancinoma. After the operation, he had twice chemotherapy and the bone marrow were inhibited to three degree so that he started to use XZ-C medicine to protect his thymus and bone marrow as the supplemental therapy to prevent the recurrence and metastasis.

Suggestions: XZ-C can be used as the assistant therapy after the surgery to improve the immunce function and to prevent the recurrence and metastasis.

5. Typical cases of assistant treatment after operation in esophagus carcinoma

Case34 Mr. Ding, male, 63yo, Wuhan, officer, medical records: 600106

Diagnosis: the middle esophagus cancinoma

Disease course and treatment:in January 1994 the patient had the xxx difficulty of the swallow and after the barium swallow tests the diagnosis was confirmed. On Feb 3, he had the removal of the cancer with the reconixxxxx of the esophague and stomach. After one month of the radioavitvotherapy, because of the heart problems, he didn't use the chemotherapy, On April 5 1995 he started to take XZ-C and then he is energetic and appetite is good. From 1996 to 1999, he refilled his medicine every month and take the medicine persistently. In July 2005 his hair was gray. Recently one year his hair started to turn black and currently his black hair is full of his head and his facial skin is mor tenderer than before, his face is glowing of the health. He is the same as the normal persons. So far he has taken the medicine more than 16years and will continue to take his medicine.

Comments: The patient had the removal of the esophageus on Feb 3 1994. After 40 days of the operation he had radioactive and immune therapy and continued to take the medicine more than 16 years and his healthy condition is good.

The experience of this treatment: During the fourty days after the surgery, he received the radioactive and immune therapy. After that he took the immune therapy persistently to protect his bone marrow and thymus. XZ-C1 can inhibit the cancer mutation and XZ-C4 can improve the immune functions and induced the anticancer factors to protect the immune organs and stop the rest cells into the proliferation stages. If persistently using, the body will be the high immune function level and to prevent the recurrence and the health will recover.

Case 35 Mrs. Huang, femal, 66 yo, Wuhan han yan, medical record:10102008

Diagnosis: the squamous carcinoma of the low esophagus

Disease courses and treatment: in December 2000 the patients started to vomit and to have progressively swallow difficultly and only swallow the half of xxxx food. EGD showed that there was narrow in the low esophagus, congestion, ulcer and xxx. Pathology showed squamous carcinoma in the lower esophagus. According to his medical condition he should be treated for a surgery, however because he could afford to the medical cost, he started to take XZ-C. After one month, he is energetic and his appetite is getting better and can eat the soft food, noodle and rice soup. After she continued to take these medicine for six months, he is vagour and his appetite is good and can eat the soft food and noodle and rice soup. Until June 2003 she took the medicine more than two and half years and his health condition is good and can eat the regular rice and felt fine as the normal healthy persons. However she stopped to taking the medicine for more than four and half months. Until Octocber 16 2003 he suddenly had the difficulties to swallow the food and vomit the brown food. She could not eat for more than three days. After adding her some fluids and continued to take XZ-C until Octocber 31 2003 she can eat the food again. After that, she never stopped taking the medicine again. Now she is 70 year-old and healthy the same as the normal persons. She is energetic and her appetite is good and can eat regular food. She lived in the seventh floor and everyday she will come down the first floor and sometimes she help others to fill the bicycle wheels.

Comments: This patient had the low grade squamous carcinoma in the low esophagaus which was diagnosed by EGC and pathology. At that time he could only eat the liquid food and half ofXXXX food. She makes her living by filling the bicycle wheels and didn't have money for her surgery so that she started to take XZ-C medicine. After taking the medicine half of year her symptoms turned good. Aftertaking the medicine two andhalf years she recovered as the normal person and didn't have any complain. Because of her incoming condition, she didn't get any other tests and treatment. When she came back to followup, she had taken the medicine more than five years and her condition is good.

To take XZ-C for longterm can improve the patients immune function and the pateitns energy level will increase and the appetites will increase and the sleep will be good. XZ-C4 can protect the bone marrow and thymus to improve the nutrition and the metabolism will turn good and will get rid of the free bases to control and to repair the diseases.

Case 36Mrs Hang, female, 65yo, Huangpi in Hubei, medical record:10402074

Diagnosis: the middle esophogus carcinoma

Disease courses and treatment condition: In April 2001 the patient had difficulty swallowing and chest and back pain and gradually increased. Until June only can eat the liquid food and vomit the mucous staffs. On June 6 2001 the barium swallow tests in the xxx showed under the aorta branch xxxx 2cm there is a 10cm lenghth narrow and 6cm xxxxxlump in the left wall and the muscous stop. Because of the cost, she didn't have the operation, radioactive and chemotherapy. On June 25 she started to take XZ-C. After three months, her general condition is better and her appetite is getting better and the difficultying swallowing is getting better and can eat the rice soup, noodle. She continued taking the medicine until March 2002 then can take the rice and regular food. In July 2003 she just took XZ-C4+XZ-C2. In April 2005 when she followed up with us, she is energetic and her appetites was great at that time she had been taking XZ-C for more than five year. He condition is stable and can eat the regular food and can do light house work.

Comments: This patient had esophageal cancer which she only took XZ-C to control her condition without the operation, radiactiv therapy and chemotherapy. For more than four years, there was no metastasis and her condition had been controlled and can eat the regular food and rice. She is as healthy as other old persons and can do some choresevery day.

She kept taking her medicine regularly.

Case 37 Mr. Huang male, 66yo, Huanpi, officer, medical record:300584

Diagnosis: the middle and low esophagous carcinoma

Disease courses and treatment:in March, he had the difficulty to swallow and the barium swallow test showed that the middle and low esophagum cancer. In May 1996 he had the removal of his cancer without other therapy. On June 19 1996 he started to use the XZ-C as the supplemental therapy to prevent the reccurrence and metastasis. He only takes XZ-C to protect his thymus and bone marrow for more than three years, then he changed into periodly taking the medicine. He is energetic and his appetite is good and walking and other activities are the same as the normal persons. In April 2005 when he came back to follow up with us, his condition is stable.

Comments: after the operation of his esophague, this patient only took XZ-C to assisting his therapymore than nine years, his condition is stable.

6. Typical cases of assistant treatment after operation in breast carcinoma

Case 38 Mr. Zhen, female, 44 yo, Wuhan, medical records: 700121

Diagnosis: Breast adenocarcinoma

Disease courses and treatment: right breast lump was found for three months which the needle biopsy showed breast cancer. On February 20 1995 she had the removal of the breast cancer and once radioactive therapy after the operation. Because of the weakness, she couldn't tolerate it. On May 11 1995 she started to take XZ-C1+XZ-C4 and continued to take them for more than three years. After she took the medicine, her energy level was improving and her appetite was increasing and her weight is increasing. Following up with us every month and her medical condition is stable.

Comments: this patient had the removal of the breast on Feb 20 1995 and once radioactive therapy after the operation. Because of the weakness the radiative therapy was stopped. In May 1995 she started to take the XZ-C1+XZ-C4. After three years her condition is stable. When she came back for her five year follow-up, she is healthy.

Case 39 Mrs Pan, female, 68yo, Shengyang

Diagnosis: multiple bone metastasis after the removal of the breast cancer.

Disease courses and treatment: in 1984 the patient had the removal of the right breast cancer I stage, the pathology showed that simple breast cancer without lymph node metastasis. After the xxx +xxxx chemotherapy for two years, she started to use some immune enhancing drug. In January 2001 she felt the right shoulder pain and ECT showed that multiple bone metastasis and the supericlavical lymph nodes enlargement. Since March 27 she had 25 times radicacto therapy on the sites of the right superoclaviceal lymph nodes and the whole blood counts decreases and the white cell counts decrease into 2.9x109/L. After the radiactherapy, her condition stable.

On June 15 2001 he started to take XZ-C such XZ-C1+XZ-C2+XZ-C4+LMS+MDZ+VS for two months and her symptom significantly increased. After six months ECT was normal and she is stable. On September 2 2002 on the phone she told us that she is stable and takes her medicine regularly for more than four years. In April 2005 She called us that she is energetic and her appetites is great and walking as the normal healthy persons. On her physical examination, Ultrasound of her liver and gallbladder, Chest X-ray, ECT etc she is normal.

Comments:this patient had right breast cancer after the operation for more than 17 years with bone metastasis and right shoulder pain. After the radiactiv therapy her medical condition is getting better. After taking XZ-C for a long period to protect thymus and bone marrow function, her metastasis was controlled well.

Case 40 Ms. Liu, female, 49yo, Wuhan, account, medical record: 4500884

Diagnosis: Left breast ductal adenocarcinoma

Disease courses and treatment: on May 19 1997 left breast had a lump 3cmx3cm. after the removal, the Pathology showed that left ductal infiltrated cancinoma. On June 3 1997 the second operation of the radiactie left breast cancer was done, which showed that there is no lymph node metastasis. Twice chemotherapy by taking XXXX were used after the operation. Because of the strong reaction to the chemotherapy, she started to take the XZ-C on August 24 1997. After that she is energetic and her appetite is increasing. After three months, she can go back to her work. After four months, the 3cmz3cm of the two lumps were found and the adjecxxxx is not clear, which the biopsy is breast proliferatin. After using the XZ-C1+XZ-C4 the lumps went away. For three years, she only takes the XZ-C medicine and her medical condition is stable and worked as the normal persons.

Comments: this patient had the removal of the breast cancer with twice chemotherapy. On August 24 1997 she only takes XZ-C to protect her thymus and bone marrow. For more than eight years, she is stable.

Suggestions: after the surgery she used twice chemotherapy for short time which the reaction is great so that she only used xz-c to induce the production of the anticancer factors to improve the immune function and to protect the host immune functions.

Case 41 Ms. Lee, female, 33 yo, Changda in Hunan, worker, medical record:3400667

Diagnosis: Left simple breast cancer.

Disease courses and treatment: On November 29 1996 she had the removal of the breast cancer in Changda which showed the right armpit lymph node metastasis(3/5). After one month, CMF was done which she used once/week, for more than four weeks.

On December 25 1996 she started to use XZ-C to protect her bone marrow. After taking the medicine, her whole blood went back to the normal level. From April 2 1997 to May 14 1997 she had radioactive 15 times in right breast inner line, 15 times under the armpit right and 25 times in the right breast outside lines. XZ-C were taken as the supplement therapy without the side effects. The patients is stable and reaction small and even no side effects when she took XZ-C with radiactherapy and chemotherapy. In June 2004 she only took XZ-C. Every three months she came to Wuhan to refill her medicines. Her condition is stable. In Dec 2004 when she came back to follow up with us, she is energetic and appetite is good and her face is glowing of the health. Acting is as the normal healthy persons. She came to refill her medicine from XXXX to WuHAN.

Comments: the curative experience of the treatment:1). During the radiacti and chemotherapy the XZ-C4 can reduce the reaction, during the interval time between the radiac and chemotherapy and after them XZ-C can strengthen longterm curative effects to protect the recurrency.2)after the surgery about six months the radia+chemotherapy +XZ-C can kill the remaining tumor cells or the small tumor lesions, meanwhile to protect the host immune organs. After taking the medicine for six months, the patient's general condition is good so that XZ-C can get rid of the wrong and strengthen the long-time curative effects. After 9 years of the operation, XZ-C can strengthen the long-term therapy.

Case 42 Ms Zhang, female, 65yo, officer, medical record:13502682

Diagnosis: Breast ductal adenocarcinoma

Disease courses and treatment conditions:in 2002 on PE, a small lump was found in the breast, which is considered as breast cancer. In 2003 she had breast radiacal removal in Wuhan center hospital, which the Pathology showed that breast ductal adenocarcinoma without metastasis. She has the Diatebite and chronic renal inflammation. On April 2003 she started to take XZ-C1+XZ-C4 and has been taking the medicine for more than eight years. Every month she come back to refill the medicine and her healthy condition is well.

Comments: This case is the removal of the breast cancer, after the operation due to the chronic renal inflammation so that she started to take XZ-C and XXX soup to protect the thymus and bone marrow for more than eight years to prevent the reccurrency and metastasis. In addition, her kidney inflammation was getteing better and never recurrent. She come back to refill her medicine every two weeks. She is healthy and stable.

Case 43 Ms Liu, female, 49 yo, Changsha in Hunan, teacher, medical record:260003372

Diangosis: breast infiltrating ductal cancer.

Disease courses and treatment condition: in February 2005 a left breast lump was found which is 2cmx1.5cm, biopsy showed that high degree mutation. On March 8 2005 she had CAF. On May 30 2005 the breast cancer was removed partially, pathology showed the breast cancer so that the breast cancer radiact removal was performed Pathologyshowed that left breast cancer infiltrated ductal cancer. LN0/20 with the C-erB2(++), P53(+), PR(-),ER(-),nm23(+). After the surgery the chemotherapy was used for six cycles. On Octocber 22 2005 she started to take XZ-C to strengthen the curative effects and to prevent the recurrence and metastasis.

Comments:in this case before the operation the lymph nodes under armpit were palpatited. Chemotherapy for six cycle was used before the operation and after the operations to strengthen the long time curative effect. She persistently takes these medicine more than six years and her healthy condition is stable.

7. Typical cases of assistant treatment after operation in colon and rectal carcinoma

Case 44 Mr. Yan, female, 71 yo, Wuhan, teacher, medical records:100188

Diagnosis: ascending colon carcinoma

Disease courses and treatment: Because of abdomen pain and bloody stool, the patient was diagnosed as colon cancer by colonoscopy with biopsy. On December 19 1994 he had half of the right colon removal. Pathology showed the medium grade of colon adenocarcinoma involved in serosa. After the operation, he didn't accept other therapy. On July 4 1995 he started to take XZ-C1+XZ-C4 as assistant therapy to prevent the recurrence and metastasis. He only takes XZ-C more than ten years and his healthy condition is very good. In April 2005 when he was 81 years old and came back to follow up with us, he was healthy and played the card every day in the afternoon.

Commons: this case is that after the removal of the ascending colon, the patient just takes XZ-C medicine as the assistant therapy to protect recurrence more than 10 years and his condition is stable.

Case 45 Mr. Yin, female, 60 yr, Huangpu, medical record:8301655

Diagnosis: sigmoid colon cancer and the removal of half of the left colon.

Disease courses and treatment: In August 1998 the patient had bloody stool and was treated as hemorrhoid. In Octocber 1999 when he had the colonoscopy in Xiehu hospital which there is narrow in the 32cm from the anus. On December 3 1999 he had the removal of half of the left-colon. Pathology showed:sigmoid xxxx adenocarcinoma involved in the whole layers of the colon and the metastasis of the nearby lymph nodules(6/8). On Jan 12 2000 he started to take XZ-C: XZ-C1+XZ-C4+LMS+MDA+VT to protect recurrence and metastasis. After he continues to take the XZ-C more than three years and eight months, his son came to refill the medicine on August 4 2003 and told us that his medical condition was good and did the chores every day and planted a lot of different kinds of flowers and vegatables watering them with ten buckles of water. The patient has been in the good condition and happy and has good energy. After his operation, he continues to take the XZ-C medicines only everyday without other chemotherapy. When he followed up with us, he already took the medicine more than five and half years.

Commons: the case is that sigmoid colon carcinoma with metastasis of the nearby lymph nodes. After the removal of the operation the patient didn't have chemotherapy because of the decrease of the white blood cells so that he took the XZ-C as the assistant therapy to protect the bone morrow and thymus to improve the body immune system to protect the reccurrence and the metastasis. After five and half years, his condition was good.

Case 46 Ms. Yun, female, 63yo, Jiling, officer, medical record:8601705

Diagnosis: the rectal adenocarcinoma

Disease courses and treatment: in Octocbor 1999 the patient has the bloody stool and the the rectaoscopy showed there is a flower-like tumor in the 10cm distance from the ana and Pathology showed the rectal cancer. On November 22 1999 the rectal radioactive surgery was done in the affliatite hospital with Dixon ways. After the operation the patient's condition is stable. On December 2 the chemotherapy was done(urine xxxx 1.0g/day, for five days, xxx 100mg/day for three days). On December 9 the white blood cell counts decrease into 0.09x109/L, on December 10 the white blood cells decrease into 0.06x109/L, injection of the medicine of increasing the white blood cells for five days, the white blood cells into1.1x109/l and had the pneumonia and fever with 40C. On January 2 xxxx after treatment with xxxx+xxxx, the patient still has fever and had the throat infection with three bacteria and can not eat and drink anything. After using XXX for five days, the temperature dropped into 38C. Because this patient had hypertension, diabetes and lung diseases, her medical condition is weak and severe and had twice warrancy from the hospitals. After two months of the treatment, she is stable. On March 20 2000 she started to take XZ-C for half of the years and her medical condition is stable and can do a little chores and can support her daily life by her own. On September 2000 she recurred very well and can shop in the nearby market and do little chores. She has been taken the medicine for more than five years consistently. In May 2005 her daughter come to refill the medicine and told us that she is totally fine and still do some house chores as healthy as other normal healthy individuals.

Comments: this case is the radial rectal cancer removal and the chemotherapy. After these her immune function and bone morrow function were inhibited so that she had throat and both the lung infections, which later are two fungus infections. After the treatment her condition started to get better and started to take the XZ-C which XZ-C1 only inhibited the tumor cells without affecting the normal cells and improve the immune fucntions, XZ-C4 to protect thymus and bone marrow to improve the immune function. The chemotherapy can inhibit the bone marrow so as to lead the bone marrow inhibition to some degrees which can affect the patients for more than 2 to 3 years so that XZ-C which have protect thymus and bone marrow function need to be taken for several years to benefit the bone marrow and immune functions

Case 47. Mr. Qian, male, 66yo, Wuhan, accounting, medical record:5401066

Diangosis:rectal carcinoma

Disease courses and treatment conditions:occasionally diarria and constipation with bloody stool for two years. The rectal examination showed that there was a 3cmx3cm lump at the 6 clock point in the xxxx position. On January 20 1998 the colonoscopy showed the polypoid mutation of the rectal colon. On January 24 1998 Dixon which the 40cm of the colon were cut off was done in the xiehae hospital, Pathology showed that rectal cancer with middle division and invade into the muscular layer without lymph nodes metastasis and the margin clear. After thesurgery, on March 3 1998 he started to use the XZ-C and took this medicine persistenly for more than eight years and he come back to work for more than five years He is stable and still continued to use these medicine.

Comments: this case is rectal adenocarcinoma. In January 1998 Dixon was done and Pathology showed that rectal adenocarcinoma, middle-degree. After the operation he only took the XZ-C1+XZ-C4 for more tha eight years. His medical condition is stable.

Suggestions: After the rectal Dixon without the chemotherapy, he only took the immune regulation medicine XZ-C to protect his thymus and bone marrow to improve his immune functions to improve the life quality and prevent the recurrence and metasatasis. He was stable.

Case 48. Ms Yong, female, 32yo, Zhaoyang, accounting, medical record:500993

Diagnosis: rectal villious adenocarcinoma

Disease courses and treatment condition: the patient had bleedy stool. In September 1997 the Colonoscopy and biopsy showed the rectal cancer. On September 17 1997 she had the rectal radial operation which showed that the lump was 1.0cmx1.0cm on the bases and was 4cm distance from the ana. Pathology reported the rectal villious adenocarcinoma and invaded into the all of the wall of the intestines with the menstema lymph node metastasis. After the operation she had chemotherapy once. Because of the decrease of the white blood cells she stop chemotherapy and started to use XZ-C1+XZ-C4. Her medical condition is well and stable. She continued to take the medicine for more than eight years only without chemotherapy and other therapy. She did her chores as the normal persons.

Comments:this case is the rectal radial removal on September 17 1997, during the operation, the metastasis were found in the mestaen membrane lymph nodes and invades the whole wall of the intestines. After the operation she had the chemotherapy once which had been stopped because the side effects were severe. Since December 3 1997 she started to take XZ-C only for more than eight years to prevent the reccurrence and metastasis after the surgery. Her medical condition is well.

Case 49. Ms. Cheng, female, 68yo, physician, medical record: 15403059

Diagnosis: Colon cancer

Disease coursed and treatment condition: Because the treatment for the obstracle didn't improve, the operation was done in XinHua hospital on April 30 2004 and found the colon cancer, then the right half of the colon was removed. Pathology showed : the colon capillary adenocarcinoma and the obstracle. After the operation, she received once chemotherapy which she can not tolerate. She started to take XZ-C. After that she is energetic and her appetite is good. She took the medicine persistently for more than six years and she is healthy.

Comments: this patient have obstracle from the Colon cancer and had surgery to remove the right half of the colon. After once chemotherapy she couldn't tolerate and then she started to take the XZ-C for more than six year. Her medical condition is well and she is healthy.

Case 50. Ms Zhang, female, 38yo, Hanchuan, medical record:400003595

Diangosis: colon cancer

Disease courses and treatment conditions: the patients had occasionally abdominal pain for more than five months and the Colonoscopy showed the colon lump in the descending colon. On Octocber 4 2005 the left half of the colon and right overian were removed and Pathology showed that the low grade adenocarcinoma and the metastasis to mesentery and right overain. After the operation six cycle of the chemotherapy were done. On August 18 2006 she started to take the XZ-C medicine such as XZ-C1+XZ-C4+LMS+MDZ persistently for more than five years. She is healthy and refilled the medicine every month.

Comments:this case is left half of the colon and right overian removal. After the operation, the six cycle of the chemotherapy was used, then take XZ-C to strengthen his immune systems. She is healthy after she takes the medicine persistently for more than five years.

Case 51 Mr. Luong, male, 60yo, Shichuang, professor medical record:8801759

Diagnosis: rectal carcinoma

Disease courses and treatment: in November 1999 there was blood in the stool and he was treated as hemorriod. In Febrary 2000 he was diagnosed as rectal cancer by the colonoscopy with biopsy. On March 2 2000 he had radical rectal cancer removal in Tongjing University, which is Mile models, Pathology: medium grade rectal adenocarcinoma. After the surgery, he had 12 radiactive therapy and once chemotherapy. On May 30 2000 he began to take XZ-C1+XZ-C4+LMS+MDZ. After he took this medicine, his appetite is good and persistently takes small amount medicine to protect thymus and to protect the bone morrow and follow-up with us monthly for more than ten years and his healthy condition is good and every test is normal.

Comments: this patient had the Mile surgery. After theoperation, he had 13 radiactive and one chemeotherapy, then only take the XZ-C to protect thymus and bone marrow. He persistently takes his medicine and every month he refilled his medicine. So far he has been taking his medicine more than ten years and his medical condition is stable.

8. Typical cases of assistant treatment after operation in galdbladder carcinoma

Case 52 Mr. Shong, male, 51 yo, Tianmen, officer, medical record:14302843

Diagnosis: adenocarcinoma in the distant common ducts

Disease courses and treatment: After one week painless jaundice, the CT showed the tumor of ampulla of vater. On September 7 2003 he had pancreas and duodenum removal in Zhanjiang xxxx central hospital and the operation was done very well and the size of the tumor is the same as the thumb. Pathology: high-grade adenocarcinoma involved in the whole lumon layer and the head of the pancreas. After twice chemotherapy he came to our outpatient center to take XZ-C :XZ-C1+XZ-C4+XZ-C5+LMS+MDZ+Vit. He continued to finish Chemotherapy so that he had chemotherapy and immune regulation medicine. After finished six periods and continued to take XZ-C4+XZ-C5 to protect thymus and to protect his bone morrow. After taking the medicine, his general medical condition is good and his appetite is increasing. So far he had taken XZ-C for 7 years and his general medical is good and his healthy condition is good and healthy condition is good. He comes back to work more than three years and he is physical strength and he look a regular heathy person.

Case 53 Ms. Dai, female, 59yo, Wuhan, medical record:790003988

Diagnosis: Gallbladder adenocarcinoma

Disease courses and treatment condition: because of the gallbladder stone found in PE, the gallbladder was removed on March 22 2007 in Zhengshun Hospital. After the operation the sample was grossed as 1.8cm in the base of the gallbladder ranges from 2.5cmx3cm. Pathology showed that high division of the adenocarcinoma and IHC showed CK(++), CEA(+). EGD showed that the chronic ulcerative gastritis with bile gastritis. H.pyloric (+), after the operation she took the xxxx. She started to take XZ-C such as XZ-C1+XZ-C4+XZ-C5+ LMS+MDZ and treatment of H. Pyloric bacteria. After one month of the XZ-C he is stable and his appetite is good. She have been taken the XZ-C for more than four years and her medical condition is stable.

Comments: This case is gallbladder cancer. Before the operation the diagnosis is gallbladder stone. After the gallbladder removal through laparoscopy, the Pathology showed that high division of the adenocarcinoma. He took XXX for two cycles of the chemotherapy and took XZ-C to assisting the therapy. For more than four years he has been taken XZ-C and his appetite is good and his energy level is good.

Case 54 Mr. Guong, male, 57yo, Wuhan, medical record:260003376

Diagnosis: middle degree of adenocarcinoma in the gallbladder.

Disease courses and the treatment condition: Because of the abdominal pain in September 2005, the test was done and showed polyp in the gallbladder. The gallbladder was removed with laparoscopy on October 18 2009 in Wuhan first hospital. Pathology showed that middle degree gallbladder cancer without the liver metastasis. After the operation, he didn't have the chemotherapy and radioactive therapy. On Octocber 31 2005 he came to our outpatient center and started to take XZ-C1+XZ-C4+XZ-C5+LMS+MDZ to assisting his therapy. After he took his medicine for more than five years, his medical condition is stable.

Comments: this case is gallbladder carcinoma was diagnosed as the polyp of the gallbladder and the removal of the gallbladder through the laparoscopy. Pathology showed that gallbladder carcinoma. Because of the early stage of the carcinomam, he didn't receive other therapy. He only takes XZ-C to assisting his surgery for more than five years. He is healthy as the normal persons.

9. Typical cases of assistant treatment after operation in kidney and bladder carcinoma

Case 55: Mr. Cheng, male, 62yo, Wuhan, engineer, medical records: 210412

Diagnosis: Renal pelvis carcinoma in the right kidney and the recurrence after the bladder carcinoma operation.

Diseases courses and treatment: the patient had cytoscopy which showed the bladder carcinoma in November 4 1995 afterthe bloody urine for two years. On November 21 1995 CT showed that rght renal pelvis tumor. On December 6 1995 the right kidney and urother were removed and his bladder was removed by the xxx and after the operation the local xxxx chemotherapy was used for seven times. On March 8 1996 the cystoscopy showed there was the hard lump in the left wall of the bladder in order to prevent the reccurrence of the tumor, he started to take XZ-C1+XZ-C4+XZ-C6. After taking this medicine he is well and his appetite is getting better. On June 24 1996 the cytoscopy showed that the bladder walls are smooth and the surface is smooth and the new things were gone. He continued to take XZ-C medicine to prevent the recerence and metastasis. Until June 11 1997 the cystoscopy showed the bladder is normal. On December 28 1998 the cystoscopy is normal. On June 26 1999 when he came back to follow up, his condition is stable and he continues to take the XZ-C1+XZ-C4+XZ-C6 for more than ten years to prevent the recurrence and metastasis. On May 6 2005 when he follow-up, he is stable and his condition is good and is the same as the normal individuals.

Comments: this case is the recurrence of the bladder cancinoma after the operation. After taking this medicine more than ten years to prevent the recurrence and metastasis, his medical condition is good and after many cystoscopy, the bladder is normal.

Suggestion: XZ-C can improve the patients immune function and prevent the tumor recurrence and metastasis and control the primary lesions. He is healthy and is in the good condition.

Case 56. Mr. Lin, male, 68yo, Wuhan, Professor, medical record: 7701534

Diagnosis: the recurrence of the bladder cancer operation.

Disease courses and treatment conditions: After the removal of the bladder cancer was done in April 1994 in the hospital, Pathology showed: transitional cell carcinoma. After the operation the bladder was poured with chemotherapy. Because of the decrease of the white blood cells the chemotherapy stopped. In 1996 he came back to check up and found the cancer recurrence so that the second operation was done by the removal of eight tumors. After the surgery the patient's bladder was poured with XXX+XXXX twice every month for three months. After three months, repeat these medicine for another three months. Twice per month until 1997. In May 1998 the cystoscopy in the XXX hospital showed the xxx in the bladder. In December the ultrasound showed the bladder infection. In April 1999 because of the bloody urine, the cystoscopy showed that there were a four cm2 of the tumor and CT biopsy showed that bladder cancer. In May 1999 the arterial chemotherapy was poured. In June the second time of the poured the XXXX+XXXX+XXX was done. After that the white blood cells decreased into 2x109/l. In September the third time of the poured medicine with xxx+xxxx+xxx, the white blood cells decreased into 1.2x109/L, then inject the XXX to increase the white blood cells. His medical history: stroke in 1992, Hypertension(160/90mmHg), Diabete. In 1984 he had hepatitis and in 1998 had cirrhosis. Family history : two brothers had hepatitis B and then liver cancer, another brother had rectal cancer.

In July 1999 because of the white blood cells decrease after the chemotherapy, he started to take xxxx to protect the bone marrow and take XZ-C1+XZ-C4+XZ-C6. After taking them more than six months, the whole blood count come back again. His energy level is increased and his appetite is getting better and continue taking the medicine. In July 2000 the cystoscopy showed that the bladder was filled well and a 1.3cmx0.6cm xxxxx in the xxxx ranges, considering as the recurrence of the tumors and continued to take the medicine until June 2001, because of the prostate enlargement which caused the frequency and urgency of the urine. CT showed that this lesion was getting bigger than before(in February in 1999), then had arterialy poured once. He continued to take XZ-C1+XZ-C4+XZ-C6 untill July 2002 CT showed that the lesion in CT shrinkled. After taking the medicine, his general medical condition is better and his appetites is good without the bloody urine. He kept coming back to followup and take his medicine for more than six years. His lesion in his bladder is stable without metastasis and enlargement.

Comments: This case is transitional cell carcinoma. After the removal of the cancer, the long-time chemotherapy didn't stop the recurrence. Because of many years of the poured bladder and many times of the cystoscopy with the enlargement of the prostate and the narrowness of the urother, the cystescopy is difficult to be done. After taking XZ-C such as XZ-C1+XZ-C4+XZ-C6, the neoplasm in the bladder didn't develop and didn't metastes. Since he had this disease, it has been 11 years. His general medical condition is well and his appetite is getting better. When he walked more, sometimes the bloody urine occurred.

Case 57. Mr. He, male, 76yo, Henan, officer, medical record;9201839

Diagnosis: left renal clear cell cancer.

Disease courses and treatment condition:in 1996 there is a kidney cyst, in 2000 on PE there is a 7.5cmx6.5cm cysts in the left renal. CT and MRI showed that left kidney tumor. On August 31 2000 the removal of the left kidney was done in Tongjing hospital. Pathology showed that middle degree of kidney clear cells carcinoma. After the surgery he started to take the xxxx without chemotherapy and radiactvie therapy. On September 28 2000 she started to take XZ-C1+XZ-C4+XZ-C6 to protect thymus ad bone marrow. After taking the medicine one month, he is vigour and his appetite is still low and contine taking the medicine for three months, his general condition is good and his energy level is high and his sleeping is good. After taking the medicine for one year, Ultrasound of the abdomen, Chest X-ray, and others regular tests are normal and he continues to take XZ-C1+XZ-C4+XZ-C6 to prevent the metastasis and recurrence. After five years of taking these medicine, his healthy condition is stable. On April 10 2005 when he follow-up with us, he is healthy and his face is glowing of the health and his voice is xxxx, and he is energetic and had the hear decrease due to his age. His medical condition is100 by CCCCCC.

Comments: this case is left kidney clear cells. He was 76 year-old when he had his surgery. Because of his age, he didn't have the chemotherapy and radioactive therapy and only take the XZ-C immune therapy as the supplement therapy to protect his thymus and bone marrow to improve the immune functions and protect the recurrence and metastasits. He has been taking the medicine for more than five years and when he came back to followup he was 80 years old. His general medical condition is good and his appetite is good and his face is glowing of the health and his energy level is high and his voice is xxx as the normal healthy person.

Case 58 Mr. Yu, Male, 69yo, Heilunjing, officer, medical record:6001181.

Diangosis: the bladder transitional cell cancer

Diseases courses and treatment condition: The bloody urine on Februay 27 in 1998. On March 2 the cystoscopy and ultrasound showed that there was the round lump in the front wall, which is 1.6cmx1.4cm and growed toward to the cavity of the bladder and is the neoplasum of the front wall of the bladder. On March 10 in 1998 the surgery removed the tumor tissues in the bladder and Pathology showed that the bladder transitional cell tumors. He was told that this tumor is the recurrence of the tumors. After the surgery, he had once chemotherapy(on May 26 1998). His reaction to chemotherapy is severe such as the vomiting, nausea, and the whole body is uncomfortable. The left testicule enlarges so that he stop chemotherapy. On June 18 1998 he started to take the XZ-C. He follow up with us very month and his condition is good and his urine is normal and he doesn't have any other symptoms. He follow up with us for more than six years and he is healthy.

Comments: in this case on March 10 1998 the surgery removed three tumors in the bladder and Pathology showed that bladder transitional cell carcinoma. After the operation once chemotherapy was done which the patient had severe reaction to this chemotherapy. On June 18 1998 he started to take the medicine XZ-C1+XZ-C4+XZ-C6. He continued to take this medicine for more than seven years and his healthy condition is good without other therapy and without the recurrence and metasatasis.

Case 59. Mr. Zhong, male, 66 yo, Wuxiu, officer, medical record: 11602315

Diagnosis: right kidney clear cell tumors with the bone marrow metastasis and superclavaical lymph node metastasis.

Disease courses and treatment condition: Because of the pain in the right should, the diagnosis was "the inflamtion of the sourround shoulder", which there was a lump as big as XXX behind the right clavical and stern bone, the biopsy showed adenocarcinoma. After CT of abdomen and chest Ultrasound, there was no lesion found. On March 2002 he started to take the XZ-C such as taking XZ-C1+XZ-C4 and plastic XZ-C3. After the plastic gels, the lump was getting soft and shrinkle into small. On March 24 2002 Ultrasound showed a lump of 3.1cmx4.3cm in the right kidney. CT showed : L2,L4 had bone damage and still took the XZ-C and GEM+XXX chemotherapy once. On May 16 2002 the right renal was removed which there was a lump of the size of table tennis. Pathology showed clear cells. Because he was on the immune function medicine, his medical condition was stable and his appetite is good. Although he had the metastasis of his whole body, he still walked as the normal persons. In 2002,2003 and 2004 he came back every month to refill his medicine and his medical condition is stable. Until July 2004 he suddenly lost the ability of speech and headache. CT showed that the bleeding of the brain. After three weeks of the hospitalization, his medical condition was stable and CT showed that the brain bleeding was absorbed and he continues to take XZ-C1+XZ-C2+XZ-C6+LMS+XXX+XXX+xxxx etc. His medical condition is good and he is vigour and his appetite is good.

Comments: this case is the right metastasis lump of the clavic bone with L2 and L4 bone metastasis, the biopsy showed the metastasis adenocarcinoma. After the whole examination the right kidney tumor was found. On May 16 2002 he was diagnosed as right kidney clear cell cancer and the kidney was removed. On March 16 2002 he started to use the XZ-C by taking and plastic. After three years his medical condition is stable and his appetite is good and he is vigour.

Case 60. Mr. Shi, female, 61yo, Hunan, medical record:790003989

Diagnosis: left kidney clear cell tumors

Disease courses and treatment condition:on Octocbr 27 2006 on PE the Ultrasound showed the left kidney lump. On November 8 2006 the left kidney was removed and Pathology showed that clear cell tumors with 0/2 lymph node. After the operation, the treatment of INF and IL-2 for three months without the radiactiv and chemotherapy. On May 10 2007 she started to take ZX-Csuch as XZ-C1+C4+C6+LMS+MDZ etc. She came back to refill up her medication every month for more than four years now. Her medical condition is ok and she is healthy now.

Comments: this case is left kidney clear cells tumor. After the operation, she took XZ-C only and persistently for more than four years. Her medical condition is good and after many tests she is healthy.

Sugguestion: XZ-C immune function medication can improve the immune function and to prevent the recurrence and metatastasis.

Case 61. Ms. Shi, female, 61 yo, Hubei, Medical Record:790003989

Diagnosis: the kidney cell tumor

Disease courses and treatment condition: in October 2006 PE showe the right kidney lump and no other syptom. On October 2006 the right kidney lump was removed(partial) and Pathology showed the renal cell tumor. After theoperation, the chemotherapy was used. In September 2007 she started to take XZ-C such as XZ-C1+XZ-C4+XZ-C6+LMS+Vit and then every three month she came back to fill her medicine for more than four years now. She is healthy.

Comments:this case is the removal of the partial right kidney and Pathology showed that kidney cell tumors. Since September 2007 she started to take XZ-C1+XZ-C4+XZ-C6+LMS for more than four years. Her medical condition is stable.

10. Typical cases of assistant treatment after operation in Thyroid cancer and peritoneum carcinoma

Case 62 Ms Pen, female, 39 yo, Shichuang Luchang, officer, medical record:7801545

Diagnosis: Thyroid cancer

Disease course and treatment: On April 27 1999 after the removal of the right neck lump, diagnosed as lymphocyte thyroid cancer. On May 6 1999 he had the radical total removal of the thyroid, then he had hourse voice and didn't have chemotherapy. On July 24 he started to take XZ-C:XZ-C1+XZ-C4, LMS, VS and follow-up with us every month and continue to use more than half years. Until Jan 2000 his voice gets better and after continue to take XZ-C another three months his voice come back to the normal. His general conditions get better and his emotion is stable and appetite is good and his energy level came back and he can go back his work. He persistently takes XZ-C1+XZ-C4 to improve his immune function and followed with us more six years and in May 2005 when he came back to us, his general condition is very good.

1999,5	1999,7	2000	2001	2002	2003	2004	2005
Thyroid operation	XZ-C						Follow-up

Commons: this patient has capillary thyroid cancer. After operation his voice was housral and didn't have radiology and chemoactive therapy. He only took the XZ-C to improve his immune function and to prevent recurrence and metastasis.

Case 63 Mr. Cheng, male, 64 yo Hubei Xin Zhou, officer, medical record:7301454

Diagnosis: the tumor of the mesentaic membranexxxx.

Disease courses and treatment condition:On January 6 1999 the patient suddenly had the uncomfortable in chest and pain and vomit. The emergency diagnosis was "actual GI infection", the surgeons thought of that he had the pancreatitis. On March 3 EGD showed the obstractle of the duodenum. On March 6 1999 during the survey of the abdomen, the tumor which was behind the abdominal membrance including big vessals which during the operation a 6cmx9cm lump in the roots of the small intestine membreance xxxx of hard, stable, fixed and unsmooth on the surface, connected to aorta and the xxxx arterial and pressed the duodenum which it was difficult to remove so that the connection of the duodenus and colon was done because the tumor can not be removed and the patients was told to be treated by the combination of the western and Chinese therapy. On April 1999 she started to take XZ-C1Z+C4. From May 15 1999 to February 2002 she continued to take the medicine and refill her medicine. She is stable and her medical condition is good.

Comments: On March 6 1999 the tumor from the abdomen membrane was found by the survey of the operation. Because it is connected to the small intestine membrance including the

Case 64. Mrs. Pu, female, 67yo, Shiyiazhoung, worker, medical record:7601511.

Diagnosis: The recurrence after the surgery of the abdominal cavity serous tumors

Disease courses and treatment conditions:because of the belly was getting bigger and ascites, in May 1999 he was hosptilizated in Tongjing and ascite(++) and his belly was like to frog and the tumor can be touched. On April 9 the surgery found that there were very many different sizes of the tumor, which were gel-like lump full of the abdominal cavity. One by one were removed, the total weight are 2.5g. During the operations, the chemotherapy tube was put with XXX 500mg. After the operation of four days xxx500MG once/per day and continued to use five days and xxx 100mg once/per day and continuing three days. On June 16 1999 he started to take XZ-C1+XZ-C4 andd after two months she is vigour and her appetite is good and her weight increases. PE: there were no lymph nodes in the superclavial, the abdomen is soft and flat, the ascite(-) and continue to take the XZ-C and refilled her medicine every month until November 26 2000, PE: there was a lump of the fit=size, hard, many nodual on the surface and deep and the clear edges which showed the tumor recurrence. The patient refused to the operation again and to chemotherapy, however he continued to take the XZ-C medicine: XZ-C1+XZ-C4+LMS+MDZ and the anticancer gel on the skin patched. Until Febrauay 24 2002 PE: there was on abnormal and her abdomen was soft and there was a lump which was hard, deep and clear edge and the size is smaller than before and her medical condition is stable. Until December 15 2004 her medical condition is good and her appetite is good and her abdomen is little enlarge and her ascite(++) and there is a fit-size lump with unsmooth surface and many nodule and deep and fix without the metastasis further. After her operation until now she has been following up with us more than six years and her medical condition is stable and the tumor is not metasatasis further.

Comments: This case is the serous tumor in the abdominal cavity. After the removal, the tumor recurrence. After the chemotherapy one week, the reaction is great so that in June 1999 she started to take XZ-C1+XZ-C3+XZ-C4 and she continued to take this medicine for more than six years and her medical condition is stable without the far metastasis and the tumors didn't grow big. She lives well with the tumors.

11. Typical cases of assistant treatment of non-Hodgkin lymphoma

Case 65 Ms. Liu, female, 34 yo, Xinzhou, medical record:7701538

Diagnosis: Non-Hodgkin lymphoma in stomach and liver metastasis

Dieasce course and treatment: in Feb 1999 the patient has little difficulty swallowing and didn't pay attention to. In April he have significantly difficulty swallowing and have difficulty to swallow the water and other fluid foods. In May the endoscopy showed that stomach body and stomach pyloric cancer. And had total stomach removal in June 1999. Pathology showed: Stomach non-hodgkin lymphoma and liver metastasis and lymph node metastasis in the spleen and the stomach lesser and greater curvature. Because her condition is week, she didn't have any chemotherapy after her surgery. On August 18 1999 she started to take XZ-X1+XX-C4. After 2 months, her general condition get better and emotion is stable and her appetites get better. After taking this medicine for more than 3 years, there is not abnormal during her Ultrasond. In November 2002 he feel find and appetites get better so that he takes the medicine peroidly. On Jan 18 2004 When he came back to follow up, her general condition is good and appetites are great. On her PE, her abdomen is soft and there is no lump. Sometimes she felt weak on her right hand, however her left arm can work very well and do all of the chores. In April 2005 during her following-up, her general condition is well and everything is find, however she takes the medicince periodly to support her longt-term therapy.

June 29,1999	August 18 1999	2000	2001	2002	2003	2004	2005
Operation	XZ-	XZ-C	XZ-C	XZ-C	XZ-C	XZ-C	XZ-C

Taking the XZ-C medicine

Case 66 Ms Mei, female, 42 yo, Wuhan, worker, medical record:400003599

Diagnosis: Non-hodgkin lymphoma

Disease course and treatment: in November 2005 the patient has pain in both of shoulder, fatigue and there is a thumb-size lump in low jaw. Then there are some egg-size lymph in both of inguinal areas. The lumps were not painful and the patient didn't have fever, however she felt fatigue. Pathology showed that non-hodgkin lymphoma, B cell large cells types which the immunohistochemistry showed:CD30(+), ALD(++), EMA(+), CD20(+),CD79(+),CD3(+),CD 43(+),CD15(-). On Auguest 16 2006 the patient didn't have radiative and chemotherapy. On August 22 2006 She came to our office and started to XZ-C4+XZ-C2+LMS+MDZ=XX after PE which showed that the patient's general condition is fine and had a cutting scar in low jaw and there were xxx-size lymph nodes in the back of the neck and there were many lump in both of inguinal area. After 3 months she felt good and appetites increased and continued for three months to take XZ-C2+XZ-C4+XXS+DIANSHEN, the patient's energy level improved and continued to take XZ-C2+xz-c4+xx+dianshen+ganchao for three months, her medical condition turn better. She continues to take the medicine regularly and fills her medicine every month for more than 5 years, which she only takes. On September 26 2010 when she came back to follow up, she is fine and working and acting as the normal individual and her emotion is stable and her appetites are fine and is happy and playing card with her friends.

November 2005	August 2006	2007	2008	2009	2010
Lump biopsy	XZ-C	XZ-C	XZ-C	XZ-C	XZ-C

Non-Hodgkin Lymphoma — taking the medicine

Commons: The patient had egg-sized lumps in both of inguinal area. Biopsy showed that non-hodgkin lymphoma with B large types. She didn't take chemotherapy and radioactive therapy. On August 22 2006 she started to takeXZ-C2+XZ-C4+LMS+Dianshen+qindai for more than five years which she fills up her medicine every month. Her medical condition is fine.

Suggestion: Non-hodgkins diseases can be treated by takeXZ-C2+XZ-C4+LMS. The patient continues to take her medicine only for more than 5 years and her medical condition is fine.

Case 67 Mr. Gao, female, 38 yo, worker, medical record:550003745

Diagnosis: Non-hodgkin lymphoma, marginal zone lymphoma, recurrence after spleen removal and chemotherapy

Disease course and treatment: in June 2000 the 2cmx3cm lymph nodes on the right neck was biopsied and pathology showed that follicule lymphoma. The chemotherapy was given from June 29 2000 to July 10 2000, from September 2000 to March 2002, from June 2002 to May 2004 because of lung metastasis. In 2005 the spleen enlarged and was removed. Pathology showed: xx lymphoma, small cells types. CT showed that the lymph node in left lung and in both armpits and in diaphragm. After chemotherapy for three weeks, the lymph node disappeared. In November 2005 the lymph node in the back of right ears enlarged and chemotherapy was given for two weeks. In April 2006 the lymph nodes were enlarged in the back of right ear and the left neck. Biopsy showed: marginal Zone lymphoma. Ct showed that LN enlarged in the sizes and increased in the numbers in the entrance of the lungs and central veins.

After the spleen removal and many times chemotherapy this disease came back again. On Jan 7 2007 the patient started to take XZ-C4+XZ-C2+LMS+MDZ+XX+XXX+Vit. After the patient took this medicine, her general medical condition is getting better and stable, her appetite is good and now she has been only using these medicine for more than four years regularly.

June 2000 Jun 29 2000 Sept 2000 June 2002

Common: This case is non-hodgkin lymphoma which was treated by chemotherapy. Since Jan 7 2007 She only took these medicine for more than four years. Her medical condition is stable and appetite is improved. She filled up her medicine regularly once per three month.

12. Typical cases of treatment of acute leukemia through chemotherapy +XZ-C

Case 68 Mr. Zhao, female, 34 yo, Wuhan, officer, medical record: 9801953

Diagnosis: Acute leukemia

Disease course and treatment: On Novermber 29 the patient was diagnosed as acute leukemia in Beijing hospital and was treated by chemotherapy for seven months. In August 2000 he was treated by bone morrow transplantation, however the results were not good after that because WBC, RBC and platelets are low. Such as wbc0.5x109/l, platelets were 5x100/l, HB46g/l. He depended on the blood transfusion, which were performed once per 8-9 days for 250ml. During his inpatient in Beijing, He had 10 times blood transfusion and 14 times platelets (once per 10 days).In Feb 2001 he came to Wuhan and on Feb 2, 2001 he started to use XZ-C1+XZ-C2+XZ-C8 to protect his thymus and his bone morrow. In April 2001 his WBC and RBC and Pletelets increase and stop to get transfusion. He takes XZ-C1+XZ-C2+XZ-C4 for more than one year and seven months and feel fine and he looked good and healthy and appetites increases and walking and runnig as the normal individual. In September 4 2003 he traveled to America and took his medicine XZ-C1+XZ-C2+XZ-C4 with him and he takes his medicine persistently.

In 2004 he immigrate into Canada and took his medicine XZ-C1+XZ-C2+XZ-C8 regularly and increase blood soups which will be filled once per 3 months. In April 2005 He called me and told us that he was healthy and his medical condition was controlled very well and appetite and sleep very well and started to work on business and energy level is perfectly well.

November 29, 1999 2000 August, 2000 Feb 2,2001 2002 2003 2004 2005

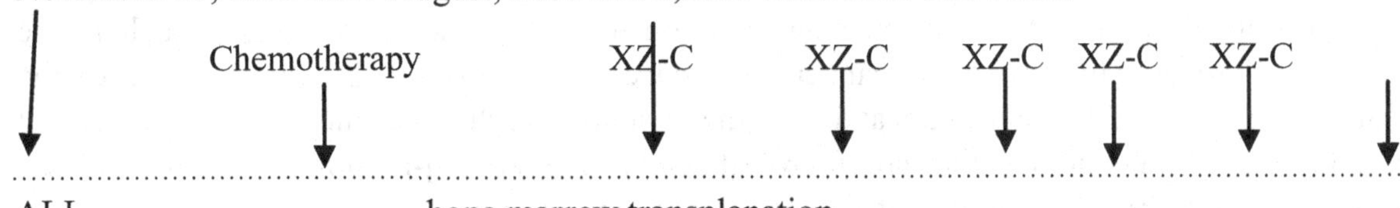

ALL bone marrow transplanation

Commons: This patient has ALL and after seven months chemotherapy in August 2000, he had bono marrow transplantation. However the treatment results were not good because his blood counts were still low which he depended on the blood transfusion. On Feb 2 2001 he started to take XZ-C1+XZ-C2+XZ-C4. And increase blood soups etc. and after four months his blood counting went back the normal. After one year and seven months his blood counting keeps normal and he is healthy and has taken these medicine for more than 4 years and work in the business field and energy level is normal.

Suggustion: All can be treated satisfiedly by chemotherapy and XZ-C to protect the bone marrow and improve the immune system function. Now he has been followed up more than seven years and his healthy condition is very well.

Case 69 Ms. Hu, female, 64 yo, Xisui, account, medical record: 850004087

Diagnosis: Hypothyroidism +multiple bone marrow tumor with toung amyloid change

Disease courses and treatment: In December 2005 the patient's low jaw was sollowed and snored heavily and on Physical exam his tongue was big and after radiative treatment the enlargement tongue got better, howevery after stop treatment, the large tongue came back again. In December 2007 the soft tissue biopsy in the low jow was done and found that amyloid change of the low jaw amyloid change. Bone marrow biopsy showed that multiple bone marrow tumor. After six weeks chemotherapy, he came to our office. PE: his general condition is find and emotion is stable. His tongue was enlargement and couldn't speak clearly and his low jaw was firm and bougle. He was in chemotherapy and start to take XZ-C on Octocber 10 2007. This patient had multiple bone marrow tumor and was treated by chemotherapy and had tongue amyloid change and his microcirculation need to improve and his blood need to be active and his swellen need to be treated. After taking XZ-C4+XZ-C2+XZ-C3 +XXX+XXX+XXX+XXX for three months, his medical condition is stable and after six months his medical condition is significantly improved and his appetites is good and general condition is fine. He fills up his medicine every two months for more than four years.

Feb 2007 March, 2007-June, 2007 Oct, 2007 2008 2009 2010
Low jaws biopsy Chem1 chem2 chem3 chem4 chem5 chem6 XZ-C XZ-C XZ-C XZ-C

Multiple bone marrow XZ-C4+XZ-C2+XZ-
XXX+XXX+XXX
Tumor

Commons: This patient has the enlargement of low jaw and tongue enlargement. The biopsy showed that multiple bone marrow tumor and amyloid change in the low jaw muscle. On OCtocber 10 2007 he started to take XZ-C to control his immune function and active his blood circulation to improve his circulation. He takes these medicine for more than four years and his medical condition is stable and general condition is good.

Suggestion:1. After surgery XZ-C can be used as assistant therapy to improve thymus function and to protect the bone marrow function to protect the central organs to help the patients to recover to protect the cancer recurrence and metastasis. 2. Above the cases the patients take the XZ-C many years and after the patients take the medicine the patiens' general condition get better and appetites are improved and have good long-term results. XZ-C is safte, effective, and there is not significant side effects for long-term use.

How can we evaluate the curative effects after the surgery? It should be evaluated by survival quality and survival time, but the tumor size. From the above cases, after surger the patients who take the XZ-C to assist the treatment survive more than five or ten years and the medical condition were controlled well.

CHAPTER 33

Future Development Of Newtraditional Chinese Medicine For Prevention Of Cancer And Anti-Cancer

Now, there are extensive researches on prevention and treatment of malignant tumors all over the world. Almost in every country, a large amount of experts and scholars with the ability of experimental researches and experience of clinical practice are researching on it and trying to overcome cancer. Hence, it is necessary for China to exert her advantages and catch up with the international advanced level.

In the field of researching into cancer, traditional Chinese medicine is the advantage of China. So it can be used in the filed field of researching into cancer to find out and develop traditional Chinese medicine to prevent and cure cancer. It should have strategic vision with international meaning to exert this advantage.

I. Reason and Background

1. Currently, except synthetic drugs, many herbal medicine and indigenous remedies have been studied in every country all over the world as scientists came back to nature to look for new anti-cancer drugs. American researchers are studying a kind of local natural herbs called taxol; in UK, a kind of African dwarf willow are studied; in Osaka, Japan they are studying bamboo leaves and ginseng. For Taiwan, China, it is a kind of tea to be researched; in Austria, they are studying a kind of natural herb that can activate macrophages to kill cancer cells and in Germany, they have distilled active principle of anti-cancer from urine. At the same time, scientists are also researching into the immunological therapy of biological reaction regulator, such as lymphokine activated killed cells, LAK and Interleukin-2 found by Britain and America as well as OK-432 in Japan, which are all T cellular, B cellular or lymphocyte immunity from the perspective of principle.

   In China, there are many natural herbs (proved recipe, local and folk recipe) like rue polysaccharides K, lentinan, Ganoderma Lucidum Polysaccharide, Hericium erinaceus polysaccharide, etc. Many natural herbs contain all kinds of histone, polysaccharides, etc. that have good effects as biological reaction regulator and can be used as anti-carcinoma medicine for immunological therapy. Many folk and proved recipes contain this sort of medicine and most of them are from folk and tried in clinic without correct research and verification. They need to be strictly and objectively studied further and developed by experts with modern scientific techniques in the laboratory for experimental tumor research. This is the unique precious natural wealth that may be a gold mine to overcome cancer. As Chinese researchers, the foreign also pay attention to the studies on folk remedies and herbs. In China, there are abundant sources of natural herbs and traditional medicine for thousand years, which is the advantage to research and overcome cancer for China. It is necessary to do experiment to research and develop new anti-carcinoma preparation of Chinese herbs through revising and concluding with modern scientific techniques and methods.

2. Many of traditional Chinese herbs are immunopotentiator, regulator for biological reaction or the herbs for nourishing that can reinforce immunity and anti-carcinoma capacity. Currently, cancer and acquired immune deficiency syndrome are the two worldwide diseases threatening human beings. The former results from weak immunity, but the latter is from immunological deficiency. Now, scientists around the world have consistent thought that the formation of tumor includes three processes: first, carinogenic factors act on bodies and disturb cellular metabolism; second, they destroy the genetic information in caryon, resulting in cancerization; third, cancer cells escape from immune system of precaution. Immune defense is the internal cause, through which external causes can act. Cancer cells must escape from the monitor of body's alarm system and break the immune defense, so as to grow into tumors. Therefore, improving immunity is the key to prevent and resist cancer. As to the question how to improve immunity, traditional Chinese herb is very important to this question, for the preparations of many traditional Chinese herbs (like ginseng, astragalus root, aweto, etc.) have abundant sources of medicine herbs and can improve immunity, which should be used as important sources of prevent and resist cancer as well as AIDS to be studied and developed.

3. in the later of 1980s, the new reorganization, new theory of "teeterboard" put forward the fourth generation of therapy, that was biological immunological treatment (surgical operation, radiotherapy and chemotherapy are the three previous ways). As mentioned above, traditional Chinese herbs belong to the fourth therapy. Therefore, in 21st century, using traditional Chinese medicine to prevent and resist cancer plays an important role, which is the advanced science and need to be studied and developed urgently.

   On the road of conquering cancer for human beings, it must be promising to study, to find out and develop effective and repeatable new-typed preparation of traditional Chinese herbs to prevent and resist cancer. However, it is necessary to do strict and objective researches through repeated verification with modern scientific methods of experimental surgery. All experimental researches must pass rigid clinical verification, that is to say the medicine must be proved to be effective on a large amount of sufferers evaluated by the standard of improving life quality and prolonging lifetime.

II. Study and Prospect

In the past years, many scientists spared efforts to study and develop anti-tumor vegetable drugs. Many kinds of traditional Chinese and western medicines have been developed with favorable and precise curative effects as well as low toxicity, which bring the treatment of malignant tumors from horrible situation of "chronic death" to the present achievement that generally more than one third can recover. There is no doubt that this is due to the development of modern medicine. However, the new researches into drugs with the ability to resist the activity of tumors play an important role in the new development, especially those natural active constituents with precise curative effects and little toxicity, which is the hot spot of current researches of human beings.

Making a general survey of the researches and development of anti-tumor drugs in the past decades, people can definitely feel the profound changes. Especially after 1980s, thanks to the development of medicine, people have made further studies on the cause, physical and pathological changes of malignant tumors. The new studies have brought new thoughts to the researches and development of anti-tumor drugs like computer aided drug design, the combination of combinatorial chemistry and screening technique of drugs, which made the abstraction, screen, reorganization and synthesis more reasonable with new dose types and drugs published. At the same time, researches into the system of administration, structure of acceptors and functional regulatory mechanism have become the popular contents. Looking back to the changes in these years and looking forward the prospect, many experts anticipate that research and development of anti-tumor drugs, especially the natural ones will step much further in the 21st century.

China is possessed with a large amount of herbs with long history of developing and utilizing natural herbs and glory achievements. Especially in recent decades, researches into traditional Chinese herbs have become more extensive and profound by using modern technology and instruments for analysis and test, which enable many applications of traditional medicine more scientific and reasonable and provide them with theoretical bases.

Natural medicaments can inhibit the activity of tumors, and have many irreplaceable advantages compared with chemosynthetic ones. Except the advantage of little untoward reaction to human bodies, they can also reduce environmental pollution by pharmaceutical industry. Although these natural medicaments have strong anti-tumor activity, their contents in plants are very micro, so that their applications are limited in some degree. Although it has been proved that taxol, vinblastine, caamptothecine, etc. have broad-spectrum effects to resist tumors with contents being a few hundredths of a percentage point, the costs of abstraction and preparation are expensive, which constraint the clinical application. As to another kind of active constituent with strong activity of resisting tumors, the content is not very small, but its toxicity and side effects are strong which also limit its clinical application. In order to overcome these shortages, scientists worldwide make use of modern industrial means like microbe metabolism and tissue culture, etc. to produce these kinds of medicine on one hand; on the other hand they reform the structure of active constituents that have untoward reactions and are limited in clinical applications, so as to reduce the untoward reactions and enlarge the clinical applications. In the author's opinion, studies of this aspect will be the major coverage of anti-tumor medicaments in a long period.

Today, as human beings pay increasingly attention to the living environment, researches on the medical speciality has extended into the field of biological genetic engineering. If combined with researches on natural medical sources, they will combine medical high-tech in 21st century and the exploration and utilization of natural sources perfectly.

CHAPTER 34

Study On Reform And Development Of Caronima Therapy

I. How to Summarize, Sort and Express the Clinical Scientific Research Data

It is useful to expound scientific research data or articles by forms. This way is not only concise and clear, but also comprehensive and detailed, which can be understood easily. A large amount of scientific research material and experimental data that was gained from hard and delicate clinical research in several decades can be summarized, sorted and collected by forms concisely, clearly and orderly so that readers can understand the core contents within about ten minutes.

China is a large country with populations of 1.3 billion, so it is a great source of tumor cases. In China, there are a large amount of cancer cases that can be used in clinical observation and analysis. If a clinician observes and analyzes the state of diseases, and positively researches on it, he can find out some new and step further continuously through the accumulation of practical medical experience in long period. As medical research is to improve clinical diagnosis and treatment, as well as medical quality and level, clinical scientific research is an important part of clinic medical work.

1. Preserve clinic case history to keep the information of diagnosis, treatment, recovery and follow-up survey. So it is necessary to fill in form-typed clinic case history in detail completely to gain complete material of clinical verification, which is easy to analyze and do statistics. Without preservation of clinic case history, scientific research on the analysis, statistics and follow-up survey of curative effects can not be developed. Preserving case history is to observe the curative effects. Moreover, restoration and preservation of material are in favor of scientific research on clinic and improving medical quality.
2. Build a schedule to display the treatment of cancer for outpatients, which should be complete and in detail. Those who have return visit after more than three months should fill in the schedule. Filling the schedule with registration in long term is easy to classify, to collect, to sort and count a large amount of material.
3. How to summarize, sorting, analyze and express the clinical scientific research data and experimental scientific research data.

This book is the production of author's practical experience of clinical treatment over fifty years combined with the collection, sorting and classification of research data and experimental data of cancer research in laboratory over thirty years. All the clinical and experimental data come from real work. Actually, it is the collection of articles or material of serial scientific payoffs.

Through experimental research and practical clinic experience combined and many cases of clinical verification over the past fifty years, the author reviews and analyzes the traditional treatment in clinic cases, evaluates and reflects them. He also concludes his own experience of clinical practice from both positive and negative aspects and puts forward new findings, new concept and methods of treatment.

The summarization, sorting, classification and conclusion of such clinical and experimental research data, scientific articles and theoretic creation and development can be explained with the forms as following.

II. Study on New Concept and Way of Treatment of Carcinoma (1)

The pattern of medical research is clinic-centered and focuses on sufferers, finding out and raising problems

↓

Do follow-up surveys in clinical practice and discover problems from them, which means after operations relapse and metastasis are the key.

↓

Basic research on the problems proposed. Without breakthrough on basic research, it will be difficult to improve clinical curative effects.

↓

Looking back to the history of development of surgery in 20th century, every achievement and step are related to experimental research closely.

↓

When surgeons find out problems in clinical work, he should study them by means of experiments and apply the study to solve clinical problems

↓

Through animal experiment with more than 6000 cancer bearing animal models to do a series of basic clinical research; explore basic problems one by one to gain large number of research and experimental data.

↓

Professor Xu Ze is the first one to discover and propose the following four items of creative theoretical creation.

↓

- Advocating new pattern of comprehensive treatment covering several subjects Principle axis: surgery + biological immunological therapy Auxiliary axis: radiation, chemotherapy in short term
- Putting forward that the cause and pathogenesis may result from low thymus atrophy and weak immunity
- Putting forward theoretical and experimental basis for the treatment of XZ-C Immunological regulation—protection thymus and improving immunity, protecting marrow and hematopiesis
- Advocating that treatment of cancer should target on tumors and host cells simultaneously; build comprehensive view on treatment and change partial view of killing cancer cells purely.

III. Study on New Concept and Way of Treatment of Carcinoma (2)

Through looking back, reflecting and concluding successful experience and failed cases, problems and disadvantages that exist in systemic venous chemotherapy for solid tumor are recognized gradually

↓

Analyze and research on the problem why chemotherapy does not prevent relapse and metastasis; reflect and come up with queries

↓

It needs to be discussed that whether the administrative approach of systemic venous chemotherapy and the dose are reasonable or not

↓

As the above problems have been existed, further studies are needed. Improve traditional therapy according to traditional trail of thoughts on one hand, on the other hand it is more important to create and change opinions to move forward.

↓

Creations must challenge traditional ideas and overcome their shortages to make it improved. So reforms and creations are needed.

↓

Advocate to change systemic venous chemotherapy into chemotherapy inside blood vessels of target organs

↓

In order to bring chemotherapy inside blood vessels of target organs, it is necessary to make clear where is the target organs; as chemotherapy means using cell toxicant to kill cancer cells, it is essential to definite the location of cancer cells so as to be clear about target and control the treatment

↓

Professor Xu Ze put forward the following five items of proposals on reform and development

↓

- Queries on systemic venous chemotherapy: ①query on the approach of administrative ② query on the calculation of dose ③ query on the standard of curative effects
- Propose basic pattern and particular Rx of anti-carcinoma metastasis; carry out the therapeutic schedule and solution to metastasis
- Propose new concept and pattern for the treatment of cancer, so as to strengthen immunological treatment and eliminate untoward reaction; change therapy with damages into that without damages; put forward the idea of immunity plus chemotherapy
- Advocate changing systemic venous chemotherapy into chemotherapy inside blood vessels of target organs; propose the detailed approach and methods; point out the problem and abuse: ①abuse of approach;②abuse of dose; ③abuse of standard; ④abuse of untoward reaction
- Advocate reforming and develop postoperative auxiliary chemotherapy; in intraperitoneal surgery, it should try to insert pump into the gastroepiploic vein catheter and take cancer tissue sample to cultivate cancer cells and test the drug susceptibility

IV. Study on New Concept and Way of Treatment of Carcinoma (3)

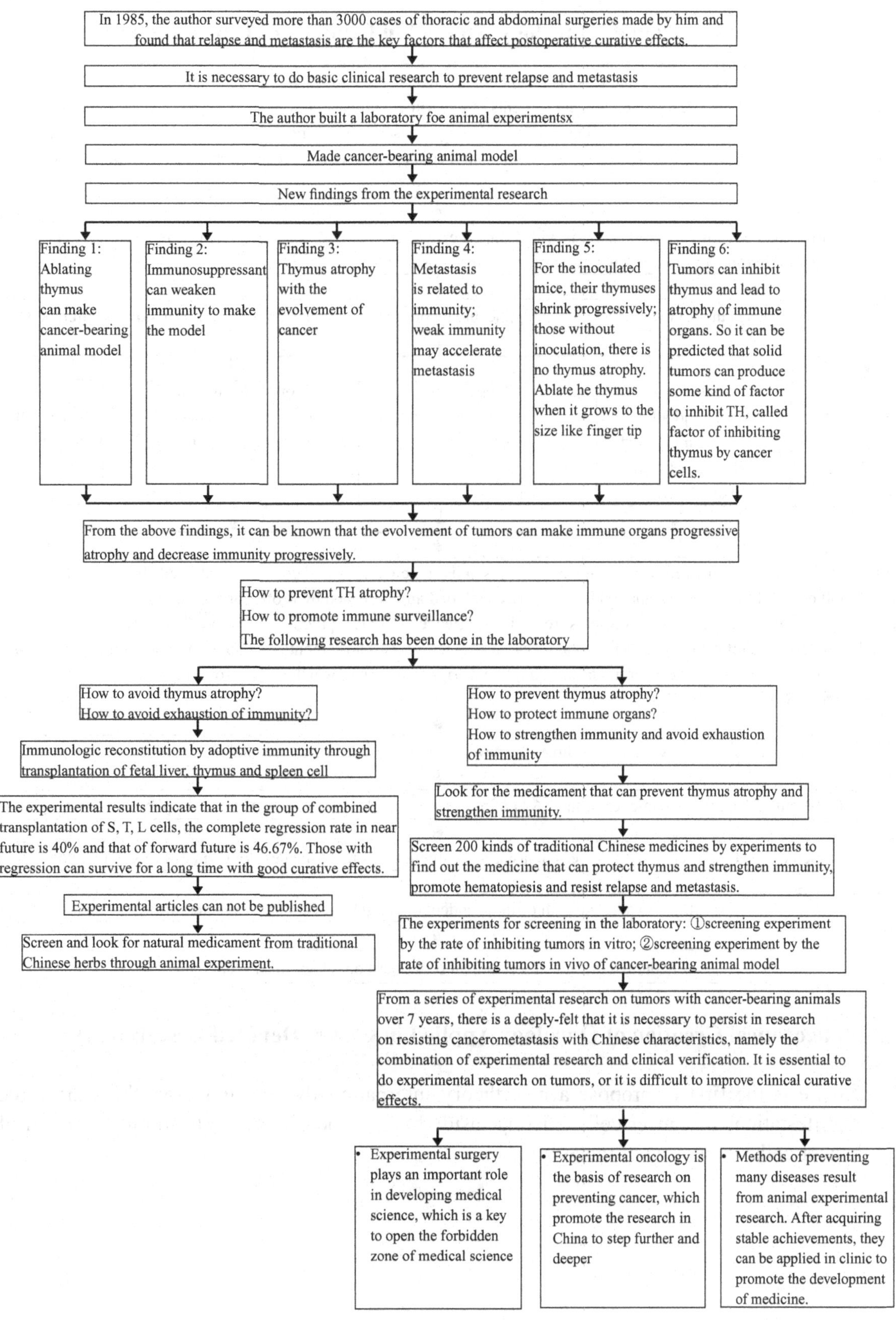

In 1985, the author surveyed more than 3000 cases of thoracic and abdominal surgeries made by him and found that relapse and metastasis are the key factors that affect postoperative curative effects.
It is necessary to do basic clinical research to prevent relapse and metastasis
The author built a laboratory foe animal experimentsx
Made cancer-bearing animal model
New findings from the experimental research
Finding 1: Ablating thymus can make cancer-bearing animal model
Finding 2: Immunosuppressant can weaken immunity to make the model
Finding 3: Thymus atrophy with the evolvement of cancer
Finding 4: Metastasis is related to immunity; weak immunity may accelerate metastasis
Finding 5: For the inoculated mice, their thymuses shrink progressively; those without inoculation, there is no thymus atrophy. Ablate he thymus when it grows to the size like finger tip
Finding 6: Tumors can inhibit thymus and lead to atrophy of immune organs. So it can be predicted that solid tumors can produce some kind of factor to inhibit TH, called factor of inhibiting thymus by cancer cells.
From the above findings, it can be known that the evolvement of tumors can make immune organs progressive atrophy and decrease immunity progressively.
How to prevent TH atrophy?
How to promote immune surveillance?
The following research has been done in the laboratory
How to avoid thymus atrophy?
How to avoid exhaustion of immunity?
Immunologic reconstitution by adoptive immunity through transplantation of fetal liver, thymus and spleen cell
The experimental results indicate that in the group of combined transplantation of S, T, L cells, the complete regression rate in near future is 40% and that of forward future is 46.67%. Those with regression can survive for a long time with good curative effects.
Experimental articles can not be published
Screen and look for natural medicament from traditional Chinese herbs through animal experiment.
How to prevent thymus atrophy?
How to protect immune organs?
How to strengthen immunity and avoid exhaustion of immunity
Look for the medicament that can prevent thymus atrophy and strengthen immunity.
Screen 200 kinds of traditional Chinese medicines by experiments to find out the medicine that can protect thymus and strengthen immunity, promote hematopiesis and resist relapse and metastasis.
The experiments for screening in the laboratory: ①screening experiment by the rate of inhibiting tumors in vitro; ②screening experiment by the rate of inhibiting tumors in vivo of cancer-bearing animal model
From a series of experimental research on tumors with cancer-bearing animals over 7 years, there is a deeply-felt that it is necessary to persist in research on resisting cancerometastasis with Chinese characteristics, namely the combination of experimental research and clinical verification. It is essential to do experimental research on tumors, or it is difficult to improve clinical curative effects.
• Experimental surgery plays an important role in developing medical science, which is a key to open the forbidden zone of medical science
• Experimental oncology is the basis of research on preventing cancer, which promote the research in China to step further and deeper
• Methods of preventing many diseases result from animal experimental research. After acquiring stable achievements, they can be applied in clinic to promote the development of medicine.

V. Study on New Concept and Way of Treatment of Carcinoma (4)

1. Theoretical Creation of Oncology Applied in Clinic (Brief Introduction)

The author combines his experience and lessons from both positive and negative experience of clinical practical cases in surgical oncology over fifty years with the achievements of experimental research over more than ten years to do analysis and conclusion. He got several new understanding as followed and proposes new theoretical concept, advocated carrying out new therapeutic strategy, which formed the new understanding and concept of cancerometastasis and new techniques and methods of treatment.

↓

Take a creative road of anti- cancerometastasis with Chinese characteristics with transition from clinic to experiment and adverse transition in order to pioneer a new way to overcome cancer.

↓

Xu Ze proposed the following five clinical applicable theoretical creations firstly in an international conference.

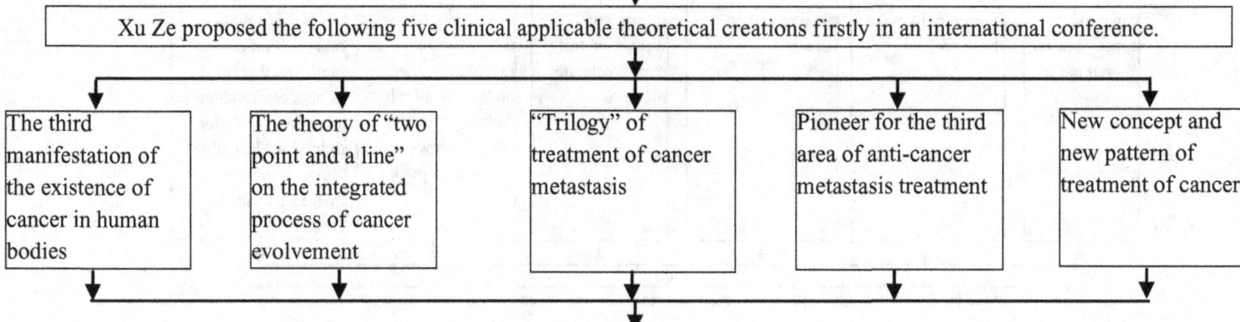

↓

So far, there has been no any reference on the new understanding, new theory and concept mentioned above in both literature and schoolbook. All these clinical applied theories are concluded and proposed by Professor Xu Ze in an international conference firstly which are the achievements from his experience of clinical practice over more than fifty years combined with the analysis and reflection of experimental research over ten years. Those mentioned above are the unique theoretical system of new concept of anti- cancerometastasis treatment applied in clinic, which are all from independent creation and possess intellectual property rights.

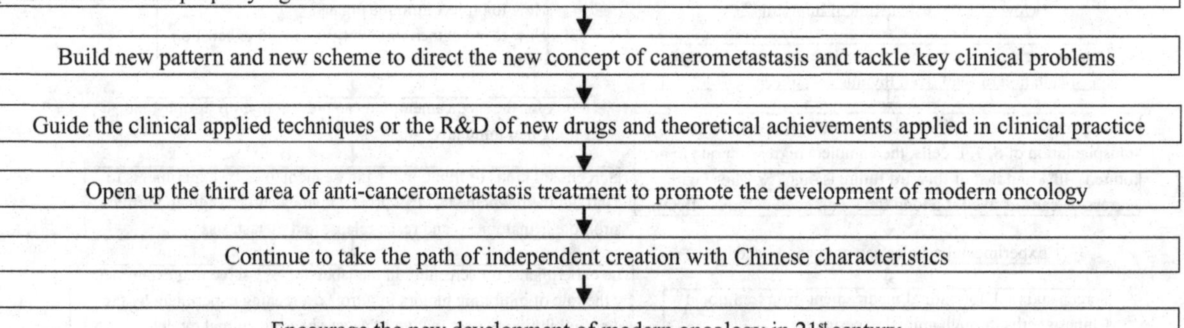

Build new pattern and new scheme to direct the new concept of canerometastasis and tackle key clinical problems
Guide the clinical applied techniques or the R&D of new drugs and theoretical achievements applied in clinical practice
Open up the third area of anti-cancerometastasis treatment to promote the development of modern oncology
Continue to take the path of independent creation with Chinese characteristics
Encourage the new development of modern oncology in 21st century

2. Theoretical Creation of Oncology Applied in Clinic (Detailed Description)

1. Xu Ze is the first to propose a new theory internationally, that is to say, there are three manifestations of cancer cells existing inside human bodies and the third one is crowd of cancer cells on the way of metastasis.

It is necessary to update thoughts and change concepts to overcome cancer that therapeutics of cancer should have comprehensive therapeutic concept

(1)Two manifestations in traditional therapeutics of cancer:
1st manifestation—primary lesion
2ndmanifestatio—metastatic lesion

Traditional therapeutics is targeted on these two manifestations:
One is to the 1st manifestation—primary lesion
The other is to the 2ndmanifestatio—metastatic lesion

The traditional therapeutics has been used for more than 100 years, which separates the above two targets and ignore the dynamic connection, causal relation and subordination between them. If there is no prevention of cancer cells that are on the way of metastasis, cancerometastasis can not be controlled. Thus, traditional therapeutics holds that there are only two manifestations, which is partial and defective.

(2) Three manifestations of cancer existing in human bodies in Xu Ze's theory:
1st manifestation—primary lesion
2nd manifestation—metastatic lesion
3rd manifestation—cancer cells, crowd of cancer cells on the way of metastasis and micro cancer embolus

The new concept holds that the aims or the "targets" of treatment should point to these three manifestations:
1. to the 1st manifestation—primary lesion
2. to the 2ndmanifestatio—metastatic lesion
3. to cancer cells, crowd of cancer cells on the way of metastasis and micro cancer embolus

Once the new theory or the new understanding was proved effective and recognized by public, it will cause a series of reforms and renovations of oncotherapy (especially for the cancer cells that are on the way of metastasis) as chain reaction.

The new concept holds that cancer cells exist in human bodies in three manifestations, which is more complete and comprehensive. It illustrates the dynamic connection, causal relation and subordination among the three manifestations, so it is a complete therapeutics of cancer that explains the whole process of cancer evolvement and gives answer to the question how to control the whole process of canerometastasis in all its aspects. This new theory sheds a great deal of light on the solution to cancer.

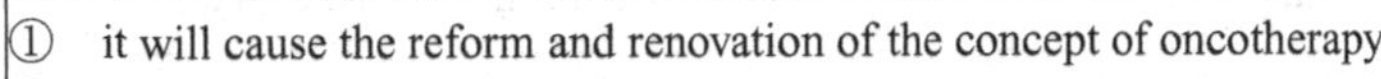

① it will cause the reform and renovation of the concept of oncotherapy.
② it will bring into the significant reforms and renovations of diagnostic methods
③ it will lead to important reforms and renovation of research and development of anti-cancer and anti-metastasis drugs.
④ it will result in reforms updates of the pattern and methods of oncotherapy.
⑤ it will cause the reform and renovation that guide the research on metastasis and relapse from oncology of cellular pathomorphology on cellular level to molecular organism and genetic expression on molecular level.

Why it is necessary to come up with that the third manifestation is the crowd of cancer cells on the way of metastasis?

Because this problem has been neither recognized by people, nor attached with adequate attention without any reference in literature and schoolbooks.

Actually, the new concept that aims at preventing cancer cells on the way of metastasis and the new therapeutic pattern that cut off metastatic approach are the key.

2. Xu Ze has proposed another new theory firstly on the international conference that is the "two points and one line" theory of the whole process of cancer evolvement. So far, scholars in home and abroad have only realized the "two points" but ignored the "one line"

about oncotherapy. However, treatment of cancer should not only emphasize "two points", but also the "one line". Cutting off the "one line" is the key of anti-metastasis.

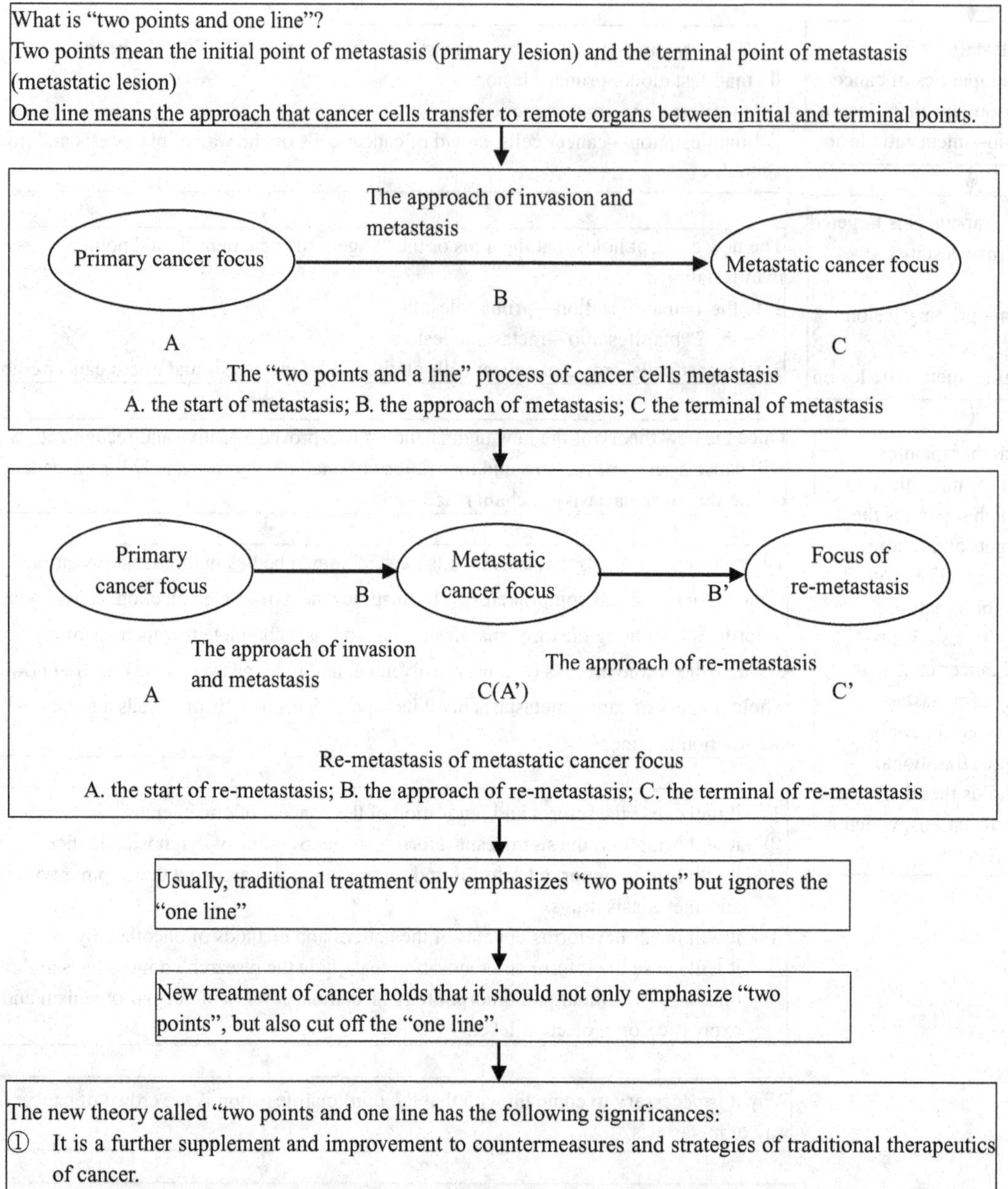

What is "two points and one line"?
Two points mean the initial point of metastasis (primary lesion) and the terminal point of metastasis (metastatic lesion)
One line means the approach that cancer cells transfer to remote organs between initial and terminal points.
The approach of invasion and metastasis
Primary cancer focus
Metastatic cancer focus
B
A
C
The "two points and a line" process of cancer cells metastasis
A. the start of metastasis; B. the approach of metastasis; C the terminal of metastasis
Primary cancer focus
Metastatic cancer focus
Focus of re-metastasis
B
B'
The approach of invasion and metastasis
The approach of re-metastasis
A
C(A')
C'
Re-metastasis of metastatic cancer focus
A. the start of re-metastasis; B. the approach of re-metastasis; C. the terminal of re-metastasis
Usually, traditional treatment only emphasizes "two points" but ignores the "one line"
New treatment of cancer holds that it should not only emphasize "two points", but also cut off the "one line".
The new theory called "two points and one line has the following significances:
① It is a further supplement and improvement to countermeasures and strategies of traditional therapeutics of cancer.
② It emphasizes not only "two points", but it is necessary to pay more attention to that "one line". Only preventing cancer cells on the way of metastasis can resist cancerometastasis and improve curative effects.
③ If people have a clearer concept of cancerometastasis and a particular outline, the proposal of this new theoretical basis will benefit clinicians to design and apply all kinds of the existed treatment means reasonably and seek for new therapeutic methods.
④ It craves out a new area of basic experimental research and clinical practical research on cancer.

3. Xu Ze has been the first to come up with the "Trilogy" of treatment of cancer metastasis internationally.

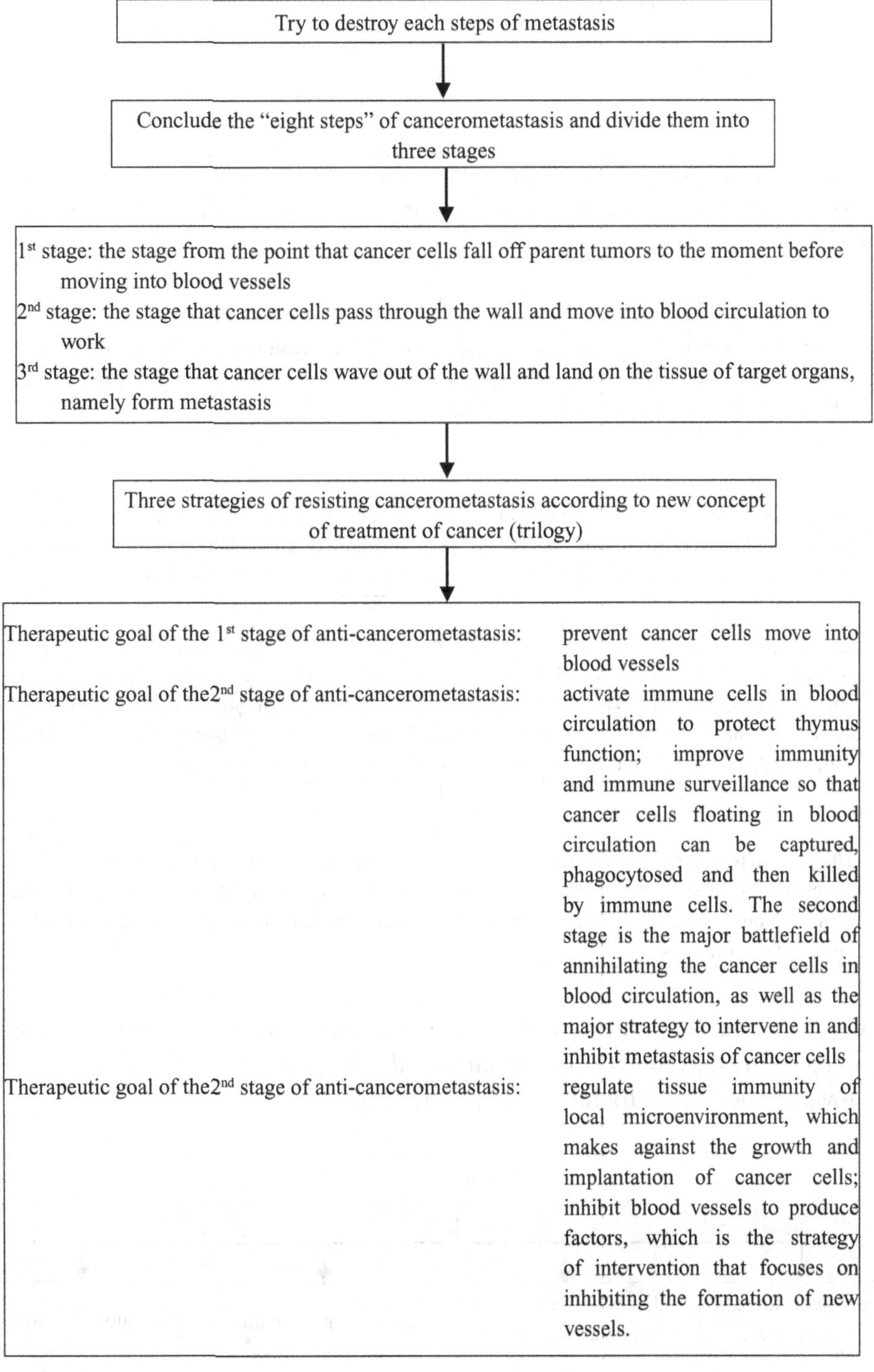

4. Xu Ze is the first to put forward the third area of anti-cancerometastasis treatment internationally.

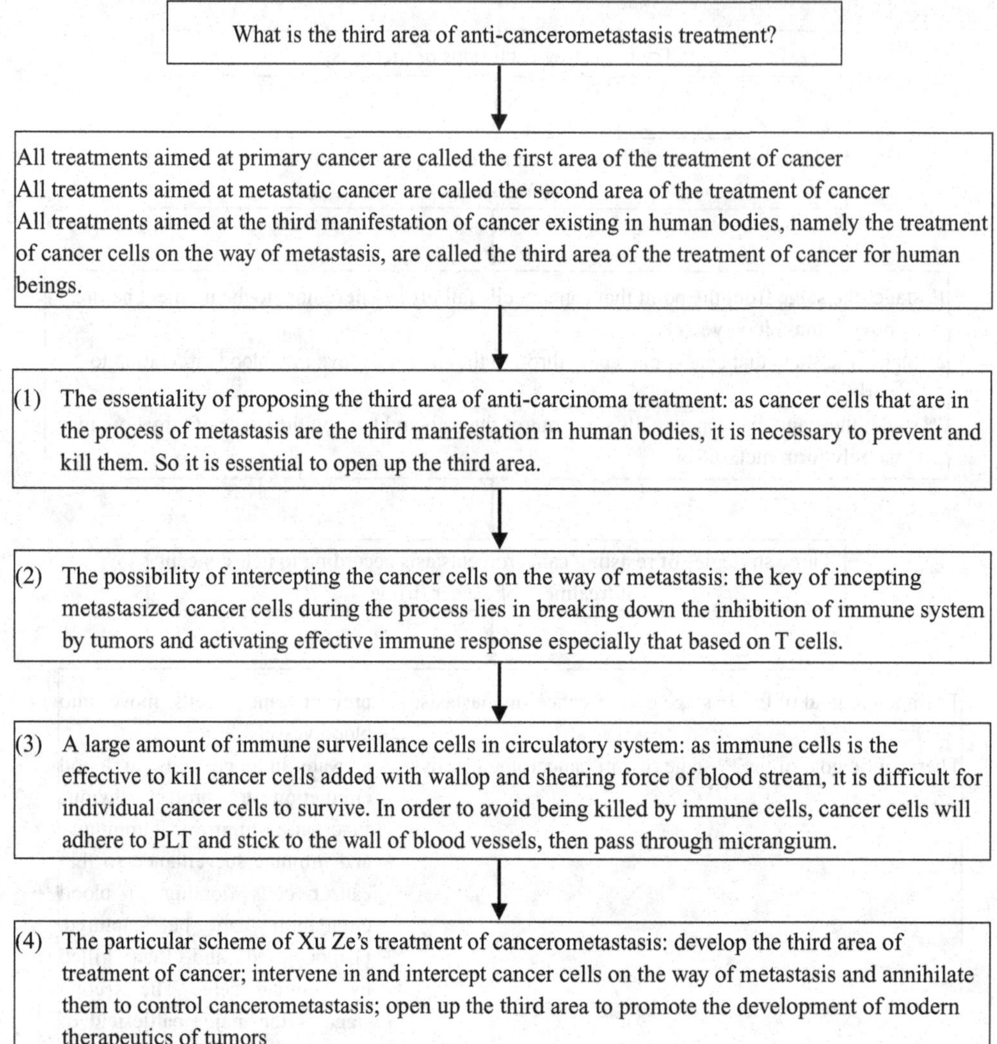

What is the third area of anti-cancerometastasis treatment?
All treatments aimed at primary cancer are called the first area of the treatment of cancer
All treatments aimed at metastatic cancer are called the second area of the treatment of cancer
All treatments aimed at the third manifestation of cancer existing in human bodies, namely the treatment of cancer cells on the way of metastasis, are called the third area of the treatment of cancer for human beings.
(1) The essentiality of proposing the third area of anti-carcinoma treatment: as cancer cells that are in the process of metastasis are the third manifestation in human bodies, it is necessary to prevent and kill them. So it is essential to open up the third area.
(2) The possibility of intercepting the cancer cells on the way of metastasis: the key of incepting metastasized cancer cells during the process lies in breaking down the inhibition of immune system by tumors and activating effective immune response especially that based on T cells.
(3) A large amount of immune surveillance cells in circulatory system: as immune cells is the effective to kill cancer cells added with wallop and shearing force of blood stream, it is difficult for individual cancer cells to survive. In order to avoid being killed by immune cells, cancer cells will adhere to PLT and stick to the wall of blood vessels, then pass through micrangium.
(4) The particular scheme of Xu Ze's treatment of cancerometastasis: develop the third area of treatment of cancer; intervene in and intercept cancer cells on the way of metastasis and annihilate them to control cancerometastasis; open up the third area to promote the development of modern therapeutics of tumors

5. Xu Ze's new concept and pattern of the treatment of cancer, namely strengthening immunological therapy and ameliorate untoward reactions.
   (1) Untoward reactions of traditional chemotherapy

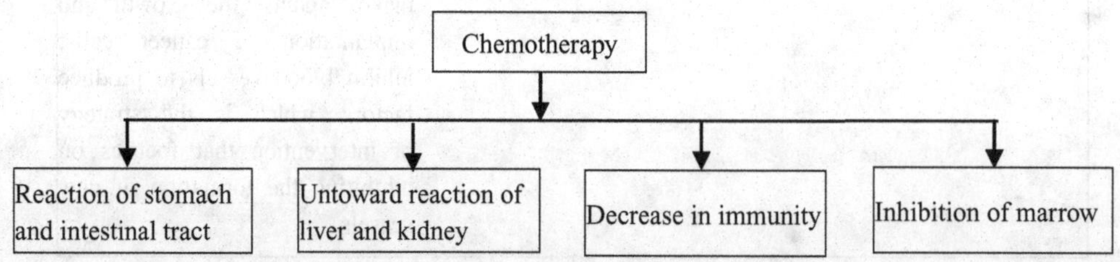

   (2) methods in the treatment of cancer with new concept, which is to take effective actions to protect host cells.
   (4) Changing intermittent treatment into success ional treatment

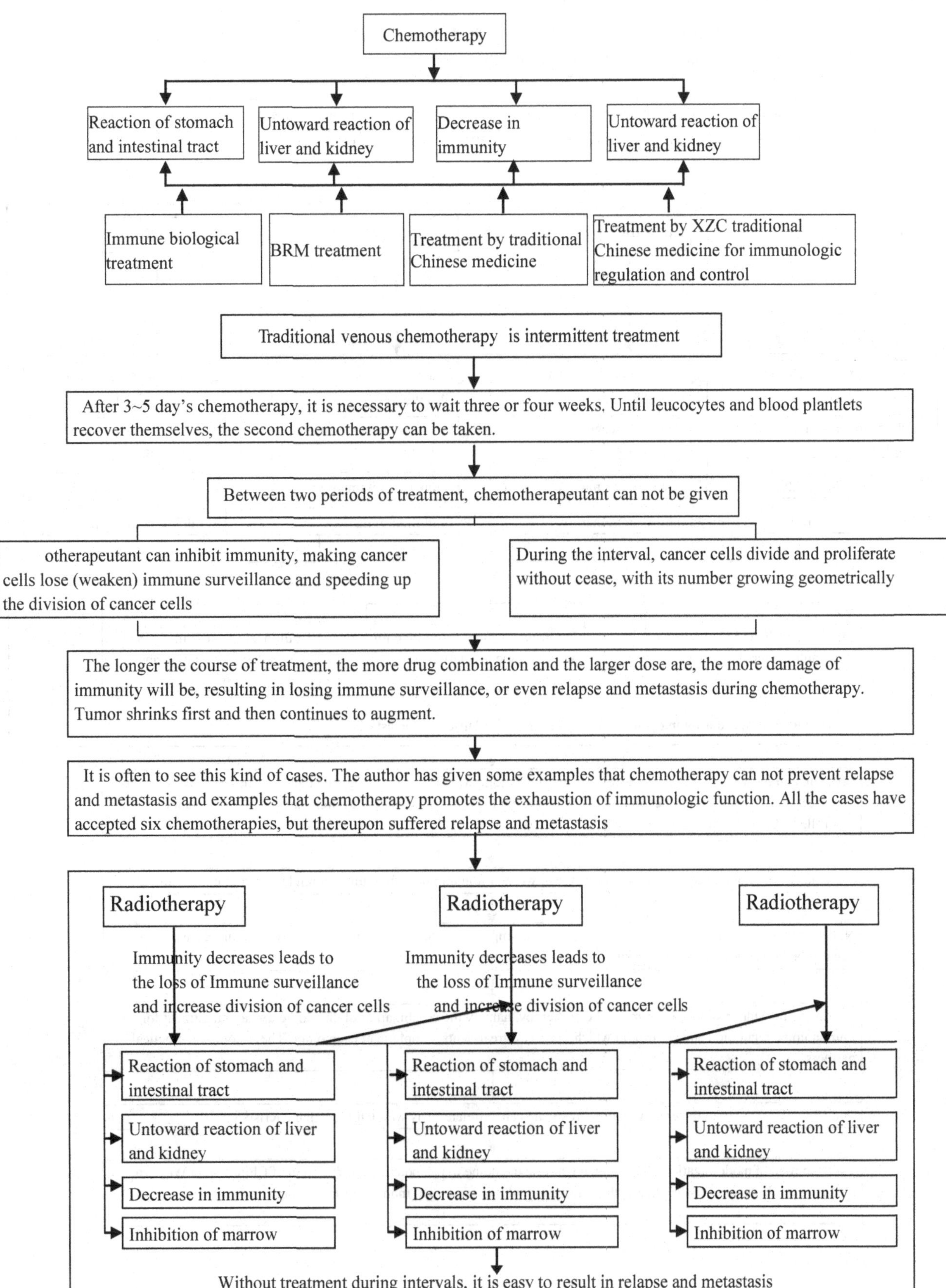
Chemotherapy
Reaction of stomach and intestinal tract
Untoward reaction of liver and kidney
Decrease in immunity
Untoward reaction of liver and kidney
Immune biological treatment
BRM treatment
Treatment by traditional Chinese medicine
Treatment by XZC traditional Chinese medicine for immunologic regulation and control
Traditional venous chemotherapy is intermittent treatment
After 3~5 day's chemotherapy, it is necessary to wait three or four weeks. Until leucocytes and blood plantlets recover themselves, the second chemotherapy can be taken.
Between two periods of treatment, chemotherapeutant can not be given
otherapeutant can inhibit immunity, making cancer cells lose (weaken) immune surveillance and speeding up the division of cancer cells
During the interval, cancer cells divide and proliferate without cease, with its number growing geometrically
The longer the course of treatment, the more drug combination and the larger dose are, the more damage of immunity will be, resulting in losing immune surveillance, or even relapse and metastasis during chemotherapy. Tumor shrinks first and then continues to augment.
It is often to see this kind of cases. The author has given some examples that chemotherapy can not prevent relapse and metastasis and examples that chemotherapy promotes the exhaustion of immunologic function. All the cases have accepted six chemotherapies, but thereupon suffered relapse and metastasis
Radiotherapy
Radiotherapy
Radiotherapy
Immunity decreases leads to the loss of Immune surveillance and increase division of cancer cells
Immunity decreases leads to the loss of Immune surveillance and increase division of cancer cells
Reaction of stomach and intestinal tract
Untoward reaction of liver and kidney
Decrease in immunity
Inhibition of marrow
Reaction of stomach and intestinal tract
Untoward reaction of liver and kidney
Decrease in immunity
Inhibition of marrow
Reaction of stomach and intestinal tract
Untoward reaction of liver and kidney
Decrease in immunity
Inhibition of marrow
Without treatment during intervals, it is easy to result in relapse and metastasis

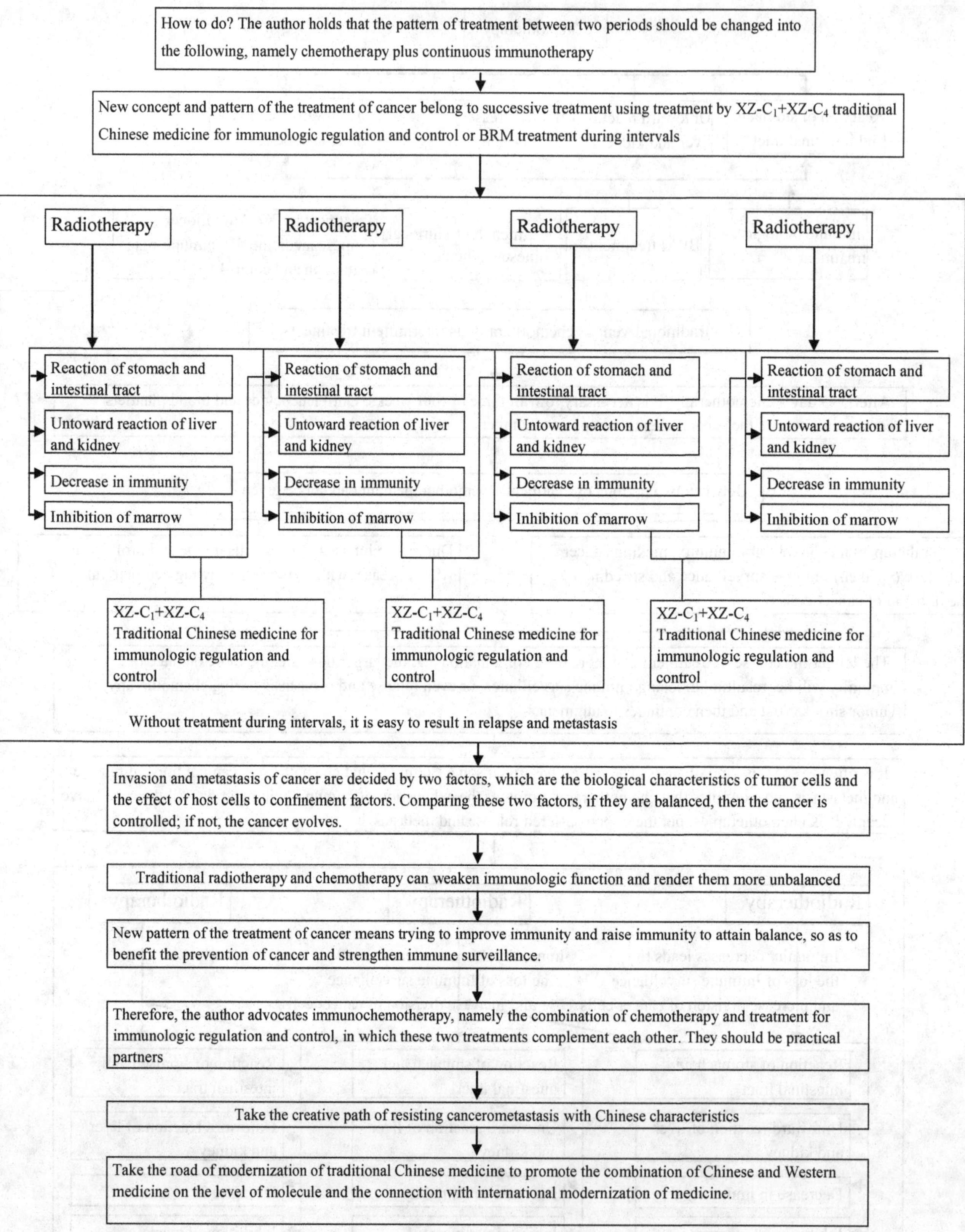

How to do? The author holds that the pattern of treatment between two periods should be changed into the following, namely chemotherapy plus continuous immunotherapy
New concept and pattern of the treatment of cancer belong to successive treatment using treatment by XZ-C1+XZ-C4 traditional Chinese medicine for immunologic regulation and control or BRM treatment during intervals
Radiotherapy
Radiotherapy
Radiotherapy
Radiotherapy
Reaction of stomach and intestinal tract
Untoward reaction of liver and kidney
Decrease in immunity
Inhibition of marrow
Reaction of stomach and intestinal tract
Untoward reaction of liver and kidney
Decrease in immunity
Inhibition of marrow
Reaction of stomach and intestinal tract
Untoward reaction of liver and kidney
Decrease in immunity
Inhibition of marrow
Reaction of stomach and intestinal tract
Untoward reaction of liver and kidney
Decrease in immunity
Inhibition of marrow
XZ-C1+XZ-C4 Traditional Chinese medicine for immunologic regulation and control
XZ-C1+XZ-C4 Traditional Chinese medicine for immunologic regulation and control
XZ-C1+XZ-C4 Traditional Chinese medicine for immunologic regulation and control
Without treatment during intervals, it is easy to result in relapse and metastasis
Invasion and metastasis of cancer are decided by two factors, which are the biological characteristics of tumor cells and the effect of host cells to confinement factors. Comparing these two factors, if they are balanced, then the cancer is controlled; if not, the cancer evolves.
Traditional radiotherapy and chemotherapy can weaken immunologic function and render them more unbalanced
New pattern of the treatment of cancer means trying to improve immunity and raise immunity to attain balance, so as to benefit the prevention of cancer and strengthen immune surveillance.
Therefore, the author advocates immunochemotherapy, namely the combination of chemotherapy and treatment for immunologic regulation and control, in which these two treatments complement each other. They should be practical partners
Take the creative path of resisting cancerometastasis with Chinese characteristics
Take the road of modernization of traditional Chinese medicine to promote the combination of Chinese and Western medicine on the level of molecule and the connection with international modernization of medicine.

VI. Study on New Concept and Way of Treatment of Carcinoma (5)

Professor Xu Ze is the only one to research on and develop the particular experimental program of XZ-C traditional Chinese medicine for immunologic regulation and control of anti-cancer and anti-metastasis.

Goal: to find out and pick up the traditional Chinese herbs for anti-cancer and anti-metastasis.

Purpose: to pick out the "intelligent anticancer drugs" that can be taken orally during a long period with high selectivity but without drug resistance and untoward reactions

Approach: from experimental research to clinical research, applying the successful animal experiments to clinical practice.

Methods: the author has done the screening test on 200 kinds of traditional Chinese herbs that were thought to have anti-cancer effects by traditional Chinese medicine with the expectation to find out new anti-cancer and anti-metastasis drugs.

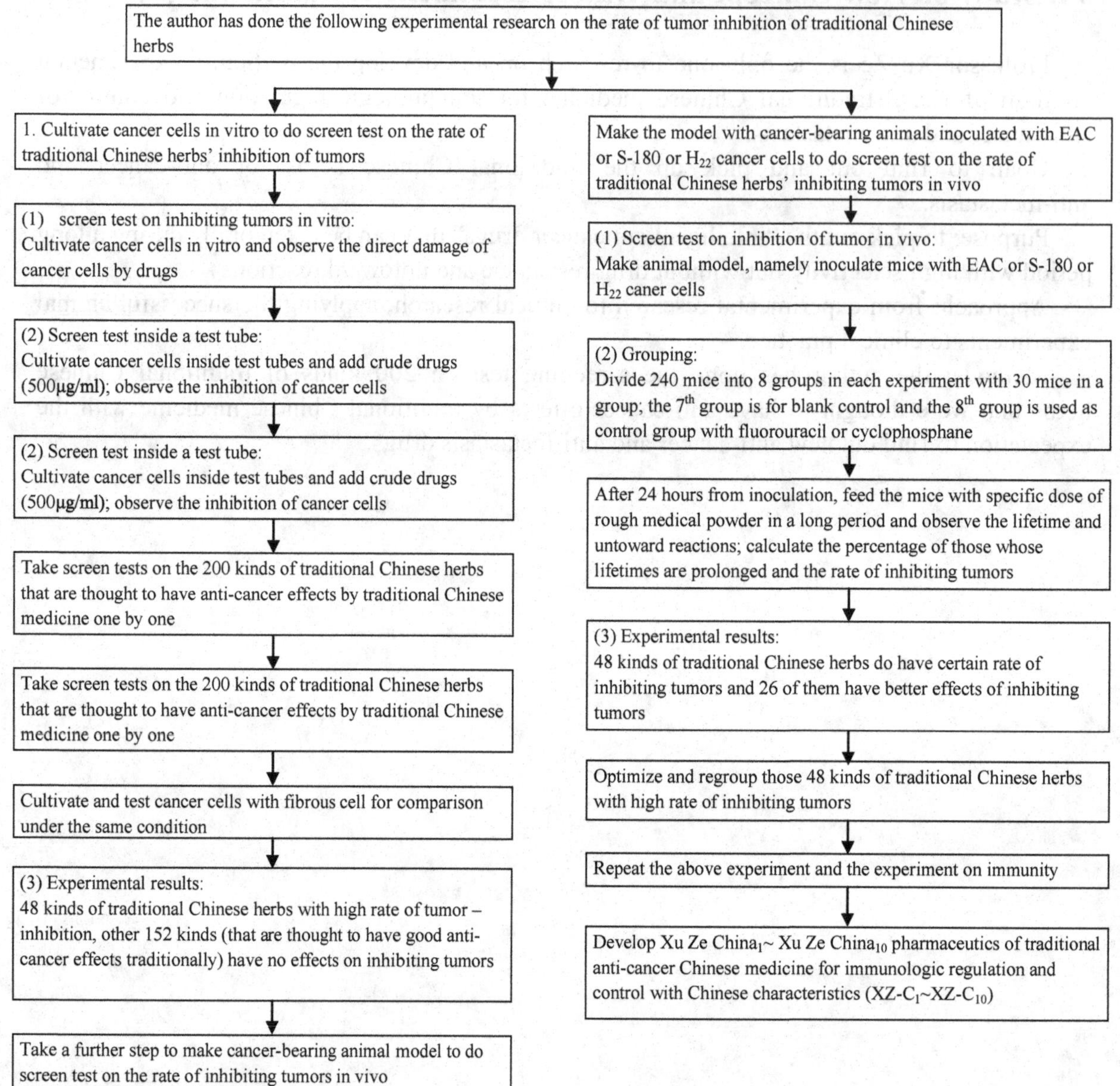

The author has done the following experimental research on the rate of tumor inhibition of traditional Chinese herbs
1. Cultivate cancer cells in vitro to do screen test on the rate of traditional Chinese herbs' inhibition of tumors
(1) screen test on inhibiting tumors in vitro: Cultivate cancer cells in vitro and observe the direct damage of cancer cells by drugs
(2) Screen test inside a test tube: Cultivate cancer cells inside test tubes and add crude drugs (500μg/ml); observe the inhibition of cancer cells
(2) Screen test inside a test tube: Cultivate cancer cells inside test tubes and add crude drugs (500μg/ml); observe the inhibition of cancer cells
Take screen tests on the 200 kinds of traditional Chinese herbs that are thought to have anti-cancer effects by traditional Chinese medicine one by one
Take screen tests on the 200 kinds of traditional Chinese herbs that are thought to have anti-cancer effects by traditional Chinese medicine one by one
Cultivate and test cancer cells with fibrous cell for comparison under the same condition
(3) Experimental results: 48 kinds of traditional Chinese herbs with high rate of tumor – inhibition, other 152 kinds (that are thought to have good anti-cancer effects traditionally) have no effects on inhibiting tumors
Take a further step to make cancer-bearing animal model to do screen test on the rate of inhibiting tumors in vivo
Make the model with cancer-bearing animals inoculated with EAC or S-180 or H_{22} cancer cells to do screen test on the rate of traditional Chinese herbs' inhibiting tumors in vivo
(1) Screen test on inhibition of tumor in vivo: Make animal model, namely inoculate mice with EAC or S-180 or H_{22} caner cells
(2) Grouping: Divide 240 mice into 8 groups in each experiment with 30 mice in a group; the 7th group is for blank control and the 8th group is used as control group with fluorouracil or cyclophosphane
After 24 hours from inoculation, feed the mice with specific dose of rough medical powder in a long period and observe the lifetime and untoward reactions; calculate the percentage of those whose lifetimes are prolonged and the rate of inhibiting tumors
(3) Experimental results: 48 kinds of traditional Chinese herbs do have certain rate of inhibiting tumors and 26 of them have better effects of inhibiting tumors
Optimize and regroup those 48 kinds of traditional Chinese herbs with high rate of inhibiting tumors
Repeat the above experiment and the experiment on immunity
Develop Xu Ze China$_1$~ Xu Ze China$_{10}$ pharmaceutics of traditional anti-cancer Chinese medicine for immunologic regulation and control with Chinese characteristics (XZ-C_1~XZ-C_{10})

The particular experimental program on the immunologic function of XZ-C traditional Chinese anti-carcinoma herbs for immunologic regulation and control on the level of molecule:

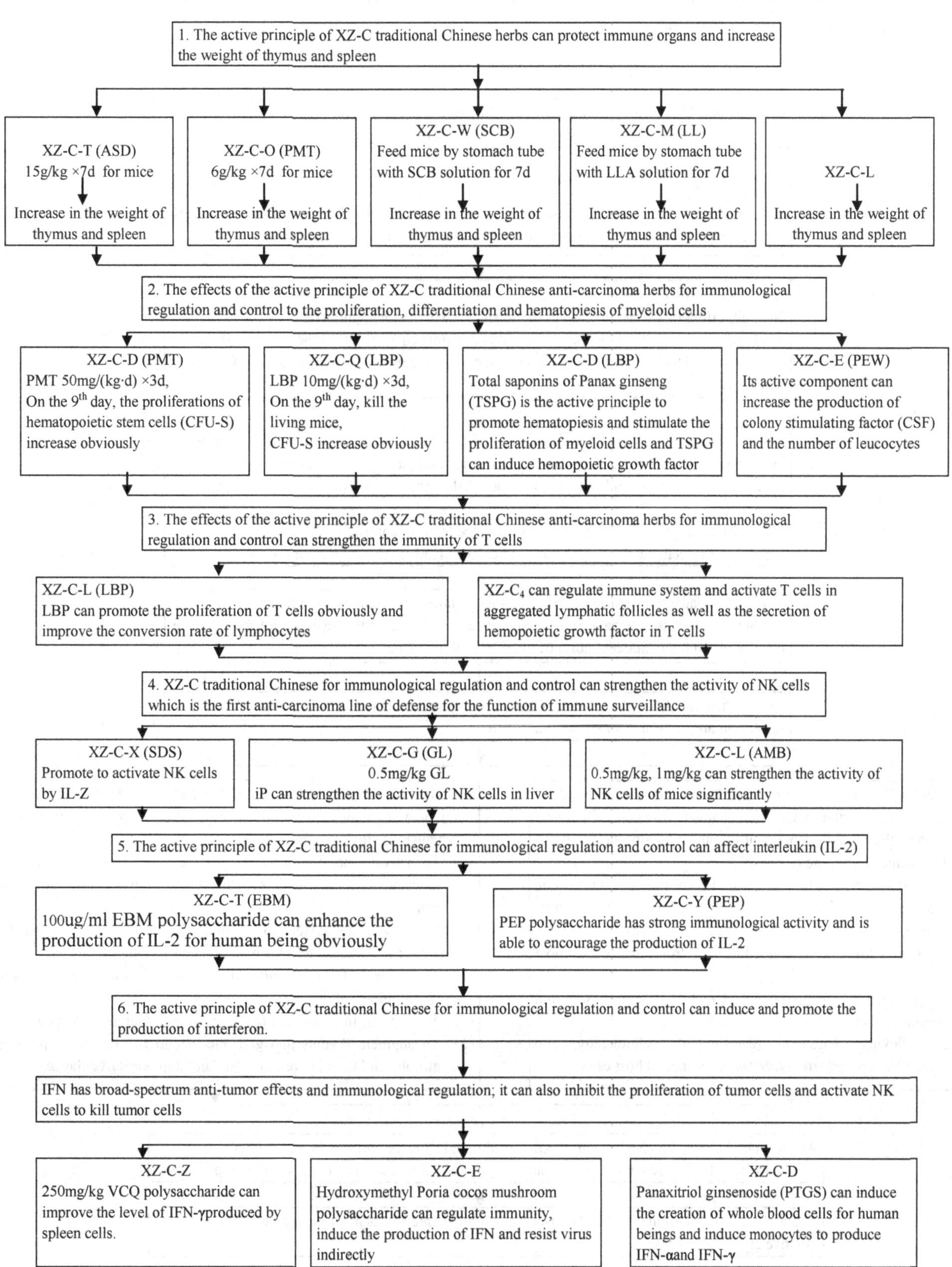
1. The active principle of XZ-C traditional Chinese herbs can protect immune organs and increase the weight of thymus and spleen
XZ-C-T (ASD)
15g/kg ×7d for mice
Increase in the weight of thymus and spleen
XZ-C-O (PMT)
6g/kg ×7d for mice
Increase in the weight of thymus and spleen
XZ-C-W (SCB)
Feed mice by stomach tube with SCB solution for 7d
Increase in the weight of thymus and spleen
XZ-C-M (LL)
Feed mice by stomach tube with LLA solution for 7d
Increase in the weight of thymus and spleen
XZ-C-L
Increase in the weight of thymus and spleen
2. The effects of the active principle of XZ-C traditional Chinese anti-carcinoma herbs for immunological regulation and control to the proliferation, differentiation and hematopiesis of myeloid cells
XZ-C-D (PMT)
PMT 50mg/(kg·d) ×3d,
On the 9th day, the proliferations of hematopoietic stem cells (CFU-S) increase obviously
XZ-C-Q (LBP)
LBP 10mg/(kg·d) ×3d,
On the 9th day, kill the living mice,
CFU-S increase obviously
XZ-C-D (LBP)
Total saponins of Panax ginseng (TSPG) is the active principle to promote hematopiesis and stimulate the proliferation of myeloid cells and TSPG can induce hemopoietic growth factor
XZ-C-E (PEW)
Its active component can increase the production of colony stimulating factor (CSF) and the number of leucocytes
3. The effects of the active principle of XZ-C traditional Chinese anti-carcinoma herbs for immunological regulation and control can strengthen the immunity of T cells
XZ-C-L (LBP)
LBP can promote the proliferation of T cells obviously and improve the conversion rate of lymphocytes
XZ-C4 can regulate immune system and activate T cells in aggregated lymphatic follicles as well as the secretion of hemopoietic growth factor in T cells
4. XZ-C traditional Chinese for immunological regulation and control can strengthen the activity of NK cells which is the first anti-carcinoma line of defense for the function of immune surveillance
XZ-C-X (SDS)
Promote to activate NK cells by IL-Z
XZ-C-G (GL)
0.5mg/kg GL
iP can strengthen the activity of NK cells in liver
XZ-C-L (AMB)
0.5mg/kg, 1mg/kg can strengthen the activity of NK cells of mice significantly
5. The active principle of XZ-C traditional Chinese for immunological regulation and control can affect interleukin (IL-2)
XZ-C-T (EBM)
100ug/ml EBM polysaccharide can enhance the production of IL-2 for human being obviously
XZ-C-Y (PEP)
PEP polysaccharide has strong immunological activity and is able to encourage the production of IL-2
6. The active principle of XZ-C traditional Chinese for immunological regulation and control can induce and promote the production of interferon.
IFN has broad-spectrum anti-tumor effects and immunological regulation; it can also inhibit the proliferation of tumor cells and activate NK cells to kill tumor cells
XZ-C-Z
250mg/kg VCQ polysaccharide can improve the level of IFN-γproduced by spleen cells.
XZ-C-E
Hydroxymethyl Poria cocos mushroom polysaccharide can regulate immunity, induce the production of IFN and resist virus indirectly
XZ-C-D
Panaxitriol ginsenoside (PTGS) can induce the creation of whole blood cells for human beings and induce monocytes to produce IFN-αand IFN-γ

Treatment of tumors by biological response modifier (BRM) and analogous BRM traditional Chinese medicine

BRM opens up the new area of biological treatment of tumors. Currently, it has been regarded as the fourth modality of treatment of tumors which is widely appreciated in medical field.

↓

What is BRM?
Oldham founded biological response modifier, namely theory of BRM in 1982 and proposed the fourth modality of cancer treatment, namely biological treatment later on this basis.

↓

According to BRM theory:
Normally, tumors and the defense of organism are in dynamic equilibrium. The occurrence and even metastasis of tumors result from this dynamic equilibrium. If the disordered state can be adjusted to the normal, it is possible to control the growth of tumors and make them fade away.

↓

According to the research on the mechanism of XZ-C traditional Chinese anti-carcinoma medicine for immunological regulation and control exclusively studied and developed by the author, cancer invasion and metastasis are decided by the comparison of two factors, which is:
Biological characteristics of cancer cells — balance leads to control
Effects of host cells by the constraints — unbalance leads to the evolvement of cancer

↓

Taking the road of modernization of traditional Chinese medicine is good for the combination with traditional Chinese and Western medicine on the level of molecule and the connection with the modernization of international medicine.

↓

The mechanism of XZ-C traditional Chinese anti-carcinoma medicine for immunological regulation and control is similar to that of BRM

↓

The effects of biological response modifier include the following:
(1) To strengthen the defense mechanism of host cells or to weaken the immunodepression of cancer-bearing host cells so as to achieve immune response
(2) To add natural or biological active substance with genetic recombination to strengthen the defense mechanism of host cells
(3) To modify tumor cells and induce the strong response of host cells
(4) To promote the proliferation and mature of tumor cells and normalize them
(5) To alleviate untoward reaction of radiotherapy and chemotherapy and strengthen the resistance of host cells

The main pharmacological action of XZ-C traditional Chinese anti-carcinoma medicine is to resist cancer and strengthen immunity, whose mechanism is similar to that of BRM
(1) To activate the system of immune cells and strengthen the defense mechanism of host cells to achieve the immune response to cancer cells
(2) To activate the system of immune cytokine of the organismal anti-cancer mechanism to improve immune surveillance
(3) To protect thymus and strengthen immunity and to protect hematopiesis of marrow
(4) To alleviate the untoward reactions of radiotherapy and chemotherapy
(5) To augment thymus and gain the weight to prevent its progressive atrophy and to improve immunity and immune surveillance

↓

As mentioned above, the mechanism of XZ-C traditional Chinese anti-carcinoma medicine is similar to that of BRM generally, which can also get analogous curative effects in clinical practice

↓

Therefore, XZ-C traditional Chinese anti-carcinoma medicine has as analogous function and curative effects as BRM

↓

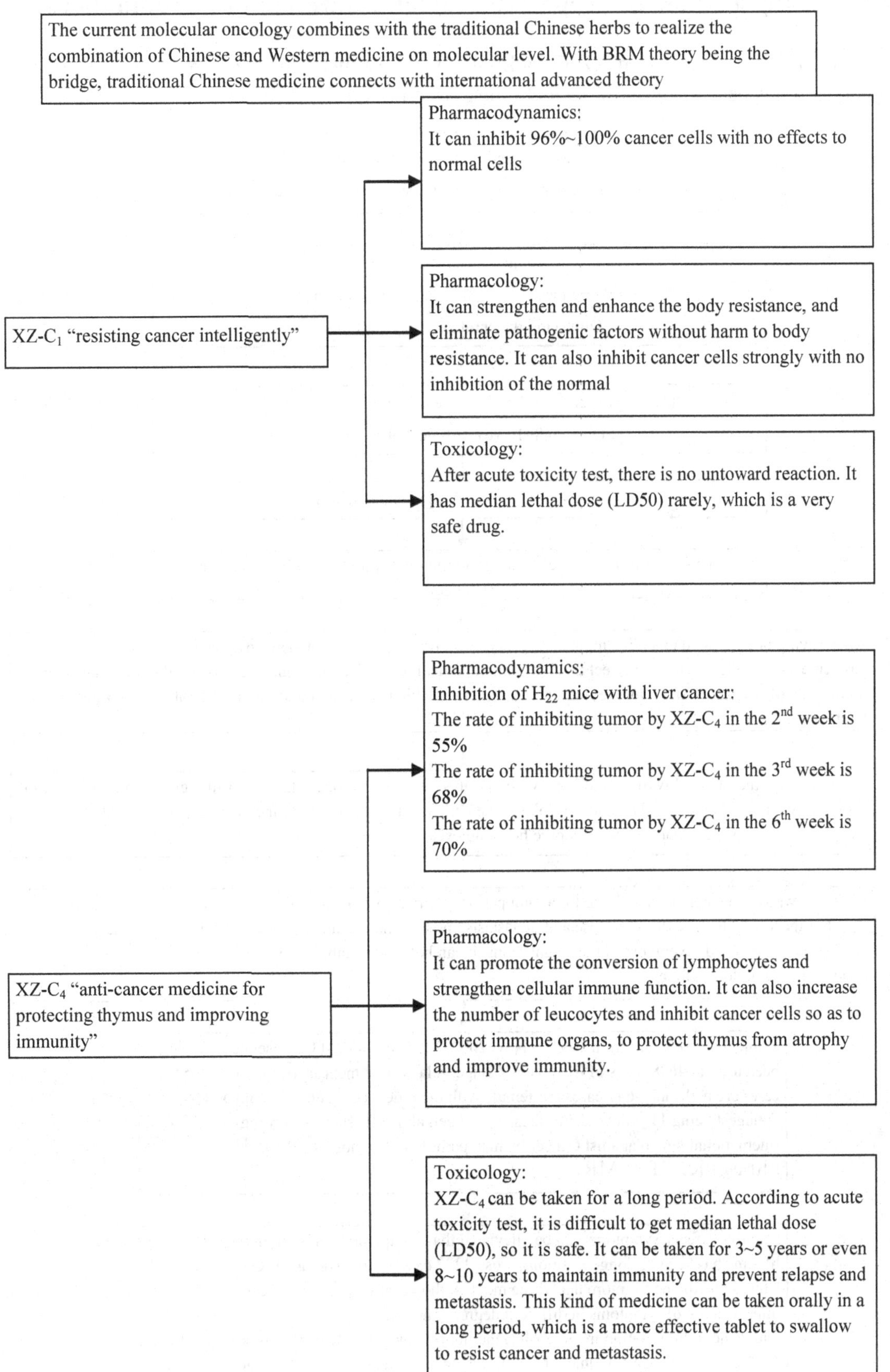
The current molecular oncology combines with the traditional Chinese herbs to realize the combination of Chinese and Western medicine on molecular level. With BRM theory being the bridge, traditional Chinese medicine connects with international advanced theory
XZ-C_1 "resisting cancer intelligently"
Pharmacodynamics:
It can inhibit 96%~100% cancer cells with no effects to normal cells
Pharmacology:
It can strengthen and enhance the body resistance, and eliminate pathogenic factors without harm to body resistance. It can also inhibit cancer cells strongly with no inhibition of the normal
Toxicology:
After acute toxicity test, there is no untoward reaction. It has median lethal dose (LD50) rarely, which is a very safe drug.
XZ-C_4 "anti-cancer medicine for protecting thymus and improving immunity"
Pharmacodynamics:
Inhibition of H_{22} mice with liver cancer:
The rate of inhibiting tumor by XZ-C_4 in the 2nd week is 55%
The rate of inhibiting tumor by XZ-C_4 in the 3rd week is 68%
The rate of inhibiting tumor by XZ-C_4 in the 6th week is 70%
Pharmacology:
It can promote the conversion of lymphocytes and strengthen cellular immune function. It can also increase the number of leucocytes and inhibit cancer cells so as to protect immune organs, to protect thymus from atrophy and improve immunity.
Toxicology:
XZ-C_4 can be taken for a long period. According to acute toxicity test, it is difficult to get median lethal dose (LD50), so it is safe. It can be taken for 3~5 years or even 8~10 years to maintain immunity and prevent relapse and metastasis. This kind of medicine can be taken orally in a long period, which is a more effective tablet to swallow to resist cancer and metastasis.

VII. Study on New Concept and Way of Treatment of Carcinoma (6)

The animal experiment of XZ-C traditional Chinese medicine for immunological regulation and control has been successful, so it can be applied to clinic to verify its curative effects.

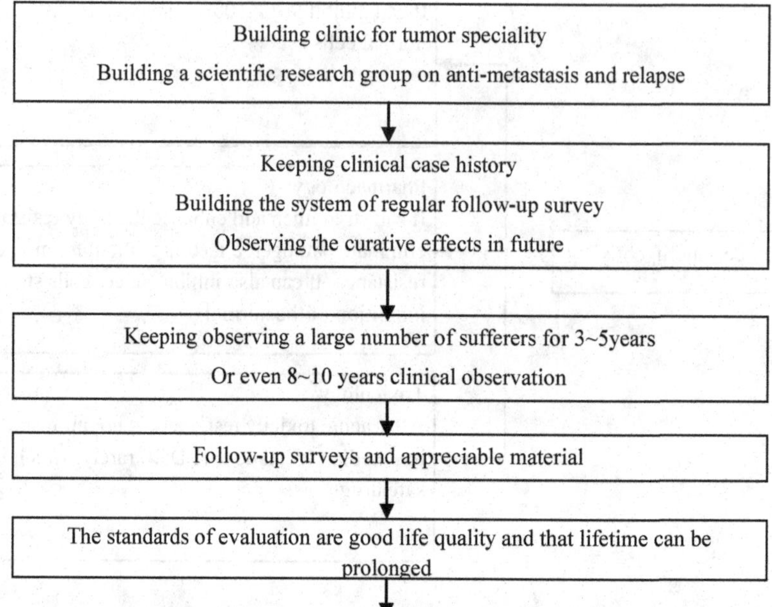

After having been applied to a large number of cancer sufferers of intermediate and advanced stages for 12 years, it has achieved significant curative effects. XZ-C immunological regulation and control can be used to kill cancer cells on the way of metastasis and improve immune surveillance, which opens up the third area of anti-cancerometastasis treatment

It can improve the life quality of the sufferers with intermediate and advanced stages and strengthen immunity. It can also improve the ability to regulate and control and the ability to resist cancer. By increasing appetite and physical strengthen, it can protect marrow and reinforce hematopiesis.

For those who have taken this medicine for a long period, the rates of postoperative relapse and metastasis is very low. For those who have suffered relapse and metastasis, most of them can keep stable with no further metastasis. For those who experienced several organ transplantations, it can help them stabilize the state of an illness, control metastasis and prolong lifetime.

Clinical information: from 1994 to Nov. 2002, XZ-C traditional Chinese medicine has been used in 4698 cases of III stage, IV stage, relapse and metastasis, in which 3051 cases are male and 1647 cases are female with the oldest being 86 years old and the youngest being 11 years old. All these have been above III stage according to TNM of International Union against Cancer by histopathology diagnosis or type-B ultrasonic, CT or MRI.

Curative effects: symptoms can be alleviated that life quality has been improved and lifetime has been prolonged. Among those 4277 cases who have taken XZ-C traditional Chinese medicine for more than three months, those with advanced cancer have had improvement of symptoms in different degree. The effective rate has researched 93.2% with general information in table 34-1, the improvement of life quality is seen in table 34-2, and the changes in tumors have been showed in table 34-3 and analgesia in table 34-4

Table 34-1 general information about 4277 cases of relapse and metastasis

		Liver cancer	Lung cancer	Gastric cancer	Cardia Cancer	Rectal and anal cancer	Colon cancer	Breast cancer	Cancer of pancreas
Cases		1021	752	668	624	328	442	368	74
Male: Female		4:1	4.4:1	2.25:1	3.1:1	1:1	2.1:1	All female	3.2:1
Focus	primary	694(68.8%)	699(93.9%)	-	-	-	-	-	-
	metastatic	327(31.2%)	53(6.1%)	-	-	-	-	-	-
General parts of metastasis		from lung (2%) from gorge (27.2%)	lymph nodes metastasis in clavicle (11.6%)	from liver (23.8%) from lung (3%)	from clavicle (13.1%)	rate of relapse (14.8%)	from liver (16.0%)	lymph nodes metastasis in clavicle (17.5%)	from liver (11.7%)
		from cardia (19.5%) from recta (31.2%)	from brain (3.1%) from marrow (4.6%)	from peritoneum(29.1%) from clavicle (6.1%)	from liver (8.3%)	from liver (7.0%)	from peritoneum (6.0%)	lymph nodes metastasis in armpit (15.0%) from bone (5.0%)	behind peritoneum (39.1%)
Age (year)	popular (%)	30-39 (76.2)	50-69 (71.6)	40-49 (73.4)	40-69 (80.4)	40-49 (75.2)	30-69 (88.0)	40-59 (65.9)	40-59 (70.0)
	youngest	11	20	17	30	27	27	29	34
	oldest	86	80	77	77	78	76	80	68

Table 34-2 the life qualities of the sufferers with advanced cancer among the 4277 cases with comprehensive improvement in observation of curative effects

	Spirit	Appetite	Physical strengthen	Improvement of general situation	Gain in weight	Improvement of sleep	Improvement of mobility and alleviation of movement restriction	Living by oneself and ambulating normally	Recovery of the ability to do light muscular work
Cases with improvement	4071	3986	2450	479	2938	1005	1038	3220	479
Percentage (%)	95.2	93.2	57.3	11.2	68.7	23.5	24.3	75.3	11.2

Table 34-3 the changes in metastatic nodes after the external application of XZ-C medicine among 56 cases

	The enlargement of lymph nodes in cervical clavicle			
	Disappear	Shrink by 1/2	Become to be soft	No changes
Cases	12	22	14	8
Percentage (%)	21.4	39.2	25.0	14.2
Total effective rate			85.7	

Table 34-4 the situation of analgesia after oral administration and external application of XZ-C medicine among 298 cases

Clinical performance	Analgesia			
	Alleviated lightly	Alleviated obviously	Disappear	No effects
Cases	12	22	14	8
Percentage (%)	21.4	39.2	25.0	14.2
Total effective rate			85.7	

On the aspect of improving life quality (according to KPS)
The average score is 50 before administration; it increases to 80, even 90 or 100 after 3 months

Analysis of lifetime: it is difficult to compare clinical sufferers as their stadiums and degrees are different. In this group, all sufferers are above third stage with different organ transplantations and dysfunctions. According to former statistics in this sort, the medium lifetime is about six months. In this group, the longest case is 14-years with the average lifetime of other cases being more than 1 year.

↓

The sufferer in one case who experienced relapse and re-ablation after surgery of liver cancer has been taking XZ-C medicine for 14 years; that in another one case of liver cancer has been taking XZ-C medicine for ten and a half years; the sufferers in three cases that the lung cancer can not be cut off have been taking this medicine for three and a half years; two cases of cancer of gastric remnant taking XZ-C medicine for 8 years; three cases of rectal cancer with postoperative relapse have been taking XZ-C for 3 years; one case of mastocarcinoma with metastasis from liver and rib has been taking it for 8 years and another one case of renal carcinoma with postoperative relapse has been taking it for 9 and a half years. These sufferers have rechecked in clinic, got the medicine and taken them so as to keep the state of illness stable with lifetime being prolonged obviously.

↓

Analysis of prolonging lifetime:
without surgeries, radiotherapies and chemotherapies, cases that have been taking XZ-C traditional Chinese medicine for immunological regulation and control solely for 5 years are: ① Di, central type carcinoma of lung in left top lung accompanied by metastasis in left lung, has been taking $XZ\text{-}C_1+XZ\text{-}C_4+XZ\text{-}C_7$ for 5 years; ② Huang, with esophageal carcinoma has been taking this medicine for 5 years; ③ Huang with cancer in the middle place of oesophagus has been taking this medicine for 5 years; ④ Huang, with primary massive type cancer has been taking this medicine for 5 years; ⑤ Qi, primary liver cancer, has been taking this medicine for 5 years.
Typical cases whose cancer can not be cut off by exploratory surgeries and can not use radiotherapies and chemotherapies to treat, have been taking XZ-C traditional Chinese medicine for immunological regulation and control for 4 years: ① Cheng, with tumors after abdominal distention which can not be cut off by exploratory surgery, has been taking this medicine for 4 years; ② Fang, with cancer of pancreas which can not be cut off by exploratory surgery, has been taking XZ-C medicine for 7 years; ③ Li, with primary massive type liver cancer that can not be cut off by exploratory surgery in Tongji Hospital, has been taking XZ-C medicine for 4 years; ④ Ke, with primary liver cancer that can not be cut off by exploratory surgery in the PLA general hospital, has been taking XZ-C medicine for 5 years.

CHAPTER 35

The form process of the new concept and new way of the tumor therapy

1. From the follow-up to build the surgical experimental laboratory

   Since 1985 the author follow up the 3000 cases of the chest-abdominal cancer patients after the surgery. The result showed that most of them recurred or metastased around 2 or 3 years, even several months, one year, then died.

   These patients often went to oncology department or oncology hospital to have chemotherapy and radiotherapy, not went back to surgery.

   1. After many following-up, the author found an important thing which the recurrence and metastasis after the surgery is the key to affect the long-term curative effects.
   2. Therefore, we realized that to research the prevention and therapy of the recurrence and metastasis after the surgery is the way to the key to improve the long-term curative effects after the surgery and the key to improve the survival time after the surgery.
   3. Therefore, the clinician must conduct the clinical basic research to prevent the recurrence and metastasis of the cancer. If there is the basic research, it is difficult to improve the clinical curative effects.

      According to the following-up results, set up the following research goals: a. it must conduct the clinical basic research to prevent the recurrence and metastasis after the surgery to improve the long-term curative effects. b. it must build the tumor animal models to do the experimental research to research the prevention of the tumor recurrence and metastasis.

      Therefore, we set up the experimental surgical lab to conduct the tumor research to do tumor cells transplantation to build up the animal models.

      a. Search the mechanism and rules of the tumor recurrence and metastasis to find the relation between the tumors and the immune system and immune organs, and the immune organs and the tumors.
      b. Search the methods to inhibit the immune organscontinuing shrinkles and rebuild the immune system during the tumor growth.
      c. Search the effective methods of the regulating the tumor invasions and recurrence and metastasis.
      d. Do the tumor animal experiments to select the antitumor medications from 200 anticancer Chinese herbs which were considered as the anticancer herbs in the literally.
      e. The experimental research of searching the anticancer and antimetastasis and antirecurrence from the natural herbs to use the modern science technology to research and to discover the anticancer Chinese herbs.
      f. Conducting the strict, scientific, and repeating animal models selecting research of the traditional anticancer Chinese medicine. To get ride of the unstable medication to select 48 kinds of the good effective XZ-C medication.

g. On the base of the successful animal experiment, applying them into the clinical practice. After 12 years of the huge clinical tests, the curative effects will be significant.

2. The new discovery
   a. The results after the following-up:
      1. The key of affecting the long term therapy is about the recurrence and metastasis after the surgery, therefore an important question which was posted : the physicians must pay attention to and research the prevention methods for the tumor recurrence and metastasis to improve the longterm curative effects.
      2. It must conduct the basic and clinical research about the recurrence and metastasis. If there is no basic research, it is very difficult to have the clinical improvement.

   b. The discovery from the experimental tumor research
      1. The tumor animal models can be set up after the removal of thymus and injection of the immune suppressors. The research showed that the tumor occurrence, development have the close relations to the immune organ functions.
      2. Which will be the immune function decrease first, then to get the cancer or the tumor occur first, then the immune function decrease: the research showed that the first is the immune function decrease, then the tumor happened. If there is no immune fucnction decrease, the inoculation of the tumor will not be successful.

         The experimental results showed that to improve and maintain the good immune function and to keep the good immune organ thymus is one of the important ways to prevent the tumor occurrence.

      3. During the research of the relation between the tumor metastasis and immune function, to set up the liver metastasis animal models, separating into A, B groups, A group is the immune suppressor, B group is control without the immune suppressor. The results are the lesion numbers in A group are significant more than B group.

         The results showed that the metastasis and immune function have the relations such as the decrease of the immune function or the application of the immune suppressor can promote the tumor metastasis.

      4. When conducting the experiments of the tumor effects on the immune organs: along with the development of the tumors, thymus continued shrinkled and the host thymus immediately shrinkled and the cells were inhibited and the volumes decreases.

         These results showed that the tumors can inhibit thymus and cause the shrinkles of the immune organs.

      5. The experiments showed that thymus will not significantly decrease if the inoculation of the tumor cells was not successful or the tumors grew very small.

In order to investigate the relationship between the tumors and thymus function, to remove thymus when the tumors grew into the thumb-sized. After one month to get thymus, it was found that thymus didn't shrinkle.

Therefore, the tumors maybe can produce some unknown factors which can inhibit thymus, called "tumor inhibiting factors", which need to further investigate.

6. From the above experiments, it showed that the tumor development can make thymus shrinkle, however can thymus shrinkle be inhibited ?Therefore, we did the experimental researches to recover the immune organs function by thymus transplants. During the experiments of inhibiting thymus shrinkle the ways of recovering thymus function and rebuilding the immune function were searched such as transplanting the embroyee liver and spleen and thymus to the mice.

   The results showed that S, T, L can be combined to transplant. The recent tumor disappearing rates are 40%, the long time tumor disappearing rate are 46.67%. The mice can survive for a long time when the tumor completely disappeared.

7. When investigating the tumors affect the immune organ functions, the results showed that the spleen can inhibit the tumor growth in the early stages. In the tumor later stages, the spleen started to shrinkle.

   The experiment results showed that spleen had the two-way effects on the tumor growth: in the early stage the tumor has some inhibition function, later stages the spleen can not inhibit the tumor growth.

8. The key to the tumor therapy is to control the metastasis. Currently it was known that the tumor cells metastasis had many steps. In order to stop a step to inhibit the tumor metastasis, in 1986 the author conducted the microvascular research lab which observed the microvascular formation and its circulation information in the transplanting tumor nodules under the microscopy.
9. To look for the medication which could inhibit the microvessel formations from the natural herbs. Using the Olympus microscopy to observe the new vessels formations and count the blood flow ad blood amount in the micro-arterial and micro-vein. TG was found from the Chinese herbs to inhibit the vessel formation. The results showed that after inoculation of the tumor 24hours, there was no new vessel formation, on the second day the microvessel grew and TG could decrease the new entering and outing microvessel densities.
10. It was found that some tumors grew bigger in the inoculation skin and the cells in the centers of the tumors and the peripheral areas of the tumors had the difference such as the centers were necrosis or dead tissues, the peripheral areas are the activating tumor cells. Therefore, the sterile-death therapy methods can be used in the clinics.

    The goals of the research and therapy are : a. protect thymus shrinkle and increase thymus weight and increae the immune function, such as protect thymus and the bone marrow. B. On the basis of the above experiments the new concepts and ways of the cancer therapy were found which are to protect thymus and to increase thymus functions and to protect the bone marrow function and to increase the immune organs functions. C. Set up the new ways and new concepts of the cancer therapy and the experimental rules and theory: XZ-C regulation and control medication therapy or Biology immune therapy.

How to protect thymus shrinkles and to protect thymus?

After three years of the basic animal experiments, it was found that thymus got shrinkle in the tumor animals; the tumor models can be made after the removal of thymus and the immune function decrease is related to the tumor occurrence and development and metastasis. Based on the experiments, the therapy goals are set up as protecting thymus and bone function and increase thymus weight to increase the immune function to anticancer and to antimetastasis.

How can thymus be protected from shrinkles and to protect the thymus function? The author found that after the transplantation of the same specied embryo liver, thymus and spleen the tumors would disappear into 46.7%, however these experiment results were not used to the clinical patients because the human embryo tissues were not used now. Therefore to start to seek the anticancer medications from the natural herbs to protect thymus shrinkle and to protect the thymus.

3. The experimental research of searching the anticancer and antimetatasis new medications from the natural herbs

The experimental ways of search for the new anticancer and antimetastasis from the natural herbs:

1. The experimental selection in vitro: with the tumor cells culture to observe the direct damage of the tumor from the medication and measure the inhibition rate of the cell proliferation from the toxicities.
2. The experiments of the inhibition rate in the tumor animals: Each experiment had 240 Qui Ming Mice, divided into 8 group. In each group there are 30 mice, which from group 1 to group 6 those are experimental groups for selecting one herb, Group 7 is the control group for no medication, Group8 is the control group for Fluenceor xxxx. All of the mices injected EAC or S-180 or H22 tumor cells under the skin of the front armpit. After 24 hours of the inoculation, the mices were fed as the mice raw powder by the oral, 1000mg/kg, 1/d for four weeks to observe the survival rate, side effects, the survival time and count the inhibiting rates.

   48 herbs which had the excellent inhibition rates were selected from the 200 raw herbs, which the inhibition rates to the tumor cells are up to 70% or 90% or above, the rests of the Chinese medication had no inhibition to the tumors.

   After the tumor animal experiments, XZ-C1 to XZ-C10 were made up of as the immune function regulation and control. XZ-C1 can inhibit the tumor growth, however it doesn't affect the normal cells, XZ-C4 can protect the thymus function and improve the immune function, XZ-C8 can protect the bone marrow to improve the life qualities and to increase the appetites and strengthen the host body to prolong the survival time.

4. Clinical tests a. After seven years of the experimental scientific experiment. The author made XZ-C immune regulation and control anticancer and antimetastasis Chinese medication from natural herbs to protect thymus and bone marrow and to activate the blood circulation which all of these were done on the tumor animal models and on the clinical aspects. b. Since 1985 while we did the experiment on the small animal, we conducted the clinical tests of the curative effects. However the patient cases are not enough and are without the medical records because the medical records were given to the patients so that there were no good ways to gather all of the information. Now we have to get support from different places to completely finish these projects.

 3. Set up the anticancer association and collaborate with different oncology clinical and build XX oncology outpatient center.
 4. Starting to keep the medical records in the outpatient center and filled the full medical records in the outpatient center so as to get the full information and easily to analyze and statasis the data and help the outpatient clinical research and improve the medical care qualities.
 5. Keep the outpatient medical records and follow up the patients periodly and briefly summarized the experience and lesions from the clinical therapy so as to observe the patients for long-term.
 6. The medical records for oncology are the table forms including all of diagnosing and treatment information and epidemiology information so that they can be used as analyzing the etiology factors.
 7. After one year of following up in the outpatient centers, the case summary will be written for every case and put it together with the big tables. Every item in the big form includes the contents in the outpatient medical records briefly and completely. xxx oncology outpatient center has tested these medications for more than 14 years and in the big tables there are more 10,000 cases in this outpatient center for these research.
 8. From the experiment to the clinics and from the clinics to the experiments. The associate has the experimental base and the clinical base. The former is in the university lab, the later is in the xxxx outpatient center. From the lab to the clinics is that after the success in the experiment then use them into the clinics and find the new questions during the clinics and went to do further the base experimental research, then applied the new results into the clinics. For instance, in the outpatient centers some patients have liver cancers and the tumor thrombosis in the portal veins, the kidney cancer with the tumor thrombosis in the xxx vein. Some are reported by CT and some are reported by pathology slides after the surgery removals. In fact, the tumor thrombosis is the tumor cells during the metastasis ways, the third forms of the tumors I the human body. In order to discover the tumors thrombosis, we conducted the experimental research of the tumor thrombosis to search for the new ways against the tumor thrombosis and to solve the tumor thrombosis. The results is

that we found the four kinds of the Chinese medications to help solve the tumor thrombosis and found their effective elements.

Such as the experiment to the clinics to the experiments again to the clinics, the continue recycles again. After 12 years of the clinical practices, we summarized the practices and analyzed and think of them again and evaluation them again then up to the theory to post the new concepts and new therapy ways.

9. After 12 years of analysis and evaluation and rethinking there are some clinical questions which were found and need to be further researched and perfected.
10. From lots of the outpatient clinical medical records we realized that the chemotherapy can not stop the recurrence after the surgery, even promote the immune function worse so that the chemotherapy need to do further research again.
11. From lots of the outpatient medical records we found that after the surgery many patients had the recurrence and metastasis. The "radical therapy" need to be further researched and completed. How to keep the free-tumor skills during the surgery and to prevent and to deal with the tumor cells in the chest cavities or abdominal cavities or the laid-off and plants of the tumor cells is the important ways to prevent the recurrence and metastasis after the surgery.
12. The following experiences were gotten from therapy practice in the lots of the cases through the associate: a. in many cases the chemotherapy can not stop the tumor recurrence and metastasis after the surgery. b. The key to anticancer is to stop the recurrence and metasatasis, which is the key to improve the long term curative therapy after the surgery. c. The anticancer keys are three early. d. Antirecurrence must be done from the operation. From the information in the outpatient patients, some basical hospital operation didn't follow the rules so that the recurrence happened early and metastasis widely in the abdominal cavity. It is very important to strength education and study of the surgery rules and the standards. e. After some radial operation the patients were weak and the chemotherapy for four months or six months further decreased the immune function. Why will it need to have four cycles or six cycles of the chemotherapy? Where are these experimental data or the therapy bases? From the literatures in China there are the therapy bases of the four or six cycles of the chemotherapy.
13. Through 14 years of the practices in the outpatient centers we found that the tumor diagnosis mainly depended on Pathology slides, however Pathology samples only can be gotten during the operation, after the operation or biopsy under the endoscopy or needle biopsy, which the patients are the advanced stages so that the tumor new marker and the new ways of the early diagnosis should be searched.
14. If the patients in the outpatient centers had the positive signs on CT and MRi and Ultrasound, etc, they were in the advanced stages, sometimes they lost the operation opportunities, therefore it is necessary to look for the new knowledge and new skills and new tumor marker to diagnose them.

15. The observation of the clinical curative effects: on the basis of the experimental research, since 1994 these research results were applied into the clinical on the different tumors, mostly III stages, IV stages, all of them the later stage of the cancer patients which had lost the surgery opportunities; the recurrent patients after the surgery;the late stages of the liver metastasis tumors and lung metastasis tumors and brain metastasis, bone metastasis or with the tumors in the chest cavities, abdominal cavities; all of the polpy removals surgery, the unable removal of the tumors after the surgery survey; the patients unable to have surgery, chemotherapy and the radiotherapy etc. XZ-C have been used in the clinics more than 14 years and observed carefully and systematically and have very excellent effects. There are not side effects for the long term to take. The clinical experiments showed that XZ-C can improve the life qualities in the advanced cancerpatients and improve the body immune function and control the tumor cell proliferation and strengthen and increased the longterm effects after the surgery or after the chemotherapy or radiotherapy.

16. These medications have good effects on softening the tumors and shrinkling the sizes of the tumors in taking by oral or by skin and support the chemeotherapy by the tubes or the medication pump and can protect the liver, kidney and bone marrow function and the immune organs to improve the immune functions.

    In XXXXX outpatient center from 1994 to 2005 4698 cases of the patients in the III, IV stages or the metastasis were followed up.

17. The life qualities evaluation for the advanced cancer patients who are taking XZ-C medication: in this group all of the patients are in the advanced stage after taking the medication the effective rate of changing the symptoms is 93.2%;95.2% of the improvement in the emotion; 93% of improvement on the appitite; 57.3% of strengthening the body. These medication completely change the patients' life qualities in the advanced patients. In the 42th ASCO posted that one of the main goals of the therapy is to increase the patients' life qualities. In 2006 in the ASCO meeting articles there are 223 which are related to the patient's lifer qualities, occupied 5.8% of the total articles. The lifer qualities have been an important factor which the patients were used as selecting the ways of the therapy and lots of research have started to use the life qualities as the main idex.
18. XZ-C function of stopping the pain: pain is the significant symptom. For example, the pain medication doesn't have effects, theanesthesia can lead the adduation and stopped the pain, XZ-C have the strong pain inhibition function and last longer function. In 298 of the clinical cases theresults showed the effective rates are 78%, the total rate is 95.3%. After the medications were used many times there were not side effects and noaddiction and the function of stopping the pain is stable which is the effective method of reducing the pain and improving the life qualities.
19. The curative effects: we should pay attention to not only the recent therapy effects and the index of the imagines, but also the long term survival period, life qualities and the index of the immune system. The goals are to keep the

patients to live longer and good life qualities. If the patients can watch their symptoms, which if the improvement can be seen to last more than one month it was considered as it had the clinical effect. Otherwise it was considered as no effects; Pay attention to the improvement of the patients' energy level, the appetite, the life qualities(xxx score) lasting one month, otherwise it was considered as no effects. The standard of the tumor curative effects according to the tumor sizes are the following: four grades : first lump disappeared, II lump decrease into half of the size, III lump turned soft, IV grade lump no changes or increases.

5. The research background and experiences a. The process of the research coming background and of the research completion

In April 1991 the author applied for the "85" critical research and technology projects from China scientific department, which this project was named as "further develop the preventing the cancer and anticancer Chinese herbs which can treat the stomach cancer an liver cancer and the precancer of the stomach with the combination of the Chinese medicine and western medicine in the basic and the clinical research". In June the xxx in Hubei organized three persons who is responsible for these projects to report to Hygience and health department in Beijing. After two months the providence xxx with these three persons went to Beijing to further report these projects and accepted these important projects. After two months, these projects were approved as << 85 Chin national important scientific and technology projects>>, however the author suddenly had the heart attack which he had acute myocardiac infarct in the anterior walls and lateral walls. After the therapy of hospitalization half years, he was discharged and his health was recovered gradually. However this critical project was stopped since then.

In 1993 the author started to conduct these projects again after his healthy condition was getting better so that he followed up his patient who had the cancer surgery done. The results showed that the recurrence and metastasis after the surgery is the key toaffect the treat the long-term treatment and must be researched to prevent the recurrence and metastasis for the basic and clinical concept and the effective method. He set up his mind to do good research on these topics and started to raise money for this research. In 1993 his wife was retired and opened her own private practice, which she used these income to help with these research projects. He also applied the support from the university such as sharing the small animals and other instruments for these projects. In brief, these projects started soon after the author got small amount funding, later he built the animal experimental laboratory which is a building with two floors and six rooms. In 1996 the author was already 63 year old and retired from the university, however he continued to do the research and clinical research under the low income. After 10 years of the hard work, he almost finished these national projects and gathered all of the experimental and clinical research material and data together and summarize them, consistencely published two books which are : 1. << the new concepts and ways of treatment of the cancer>>, Xu Ze, Jan, 2001, published in book press by Hubei Science and technology company. 2. << the new concepts and ways of treatment of the cancer>>, Xu Ze, published by People's military medical press. b. Some experiences:

In the past the author did research work in the hospital and under the help of the supervisors and co-workers, the experimental conditions are good and finished two research projects: a. the advanced level in China. B. the international advanced level, which received the second award in Hubei Provence scientific and technology research and the first award in Hubei Provence hygience scientific and technology.

However currently it is different. Under this condition such as in a private clinics or outpatient center, there is no condition or no instrument, how to finish this national research projects? The author have the following experience:

a. Indepedence and Raise the money : the research fee from the payment of our outpatient clinics
b. Keep the medical record in the outpatient center and follow them up
c. Build the specialty research groups and follow the research plans and support each other between groups.
d. Build up the detail medical records including the epidemiology information
e. Sharing the instruments and material and the research awards. Don't buy the big instrument and colaboratory with the university.
f. Build up my own research projects and did not apply for the research project through the government. However we report my research project to the officer in Provence, city and Department.
g. The elder Professors can do and complete the research projects when we share the scientific instruments and sharing the plans and the good condition in the hospital with my many years of the experiences.

CHAPTER 36

Scientific study route and research method of the new concept and new way of carcinoma therapy

Science is no ending. Our scientific research continuously obey the scientific development and is based on the known science knowledge and face the future medicine. After 16 years of hard work, we practice the concept of the scientific development, face the edge of the science and try to innovate and move on. To overcome the tumors must be guided by the concept of the scientific development; must move from the clinics to the experiment research, then go back the clinics to solve the patients' problems; must be practical and realistic and provide the data and the facts; must continuously overstep self and move on independently; in the scientific research we must open the minds, break the traditional concepts and be based on the independent and original creativities; the scientific routes f in our decade years are to discover the questions provide the questions research the questions

solve the questions or explain the questions. The routes were made up by walking hard one step by one step hard. Under the concepts of the scientific development we hope to create an innovating anticancer way which has Chinese characters and have the independent knowledge property rights.

Our oncology medical models are : the patients are centers, to discover and post the questions from the clinics, then to do the animal experiments, then applied these basic research results into the clinics to improve the medical care level and finally help the patients.

Why are these theories need to innovate? Because all of the clinical therapy and medication and diagnosis must have the reasonable theories and the clinical guides. After more than half of century surgery practices, recalling and thinking, I felt the current oncology is the most backward subject in all of the specialties. Why? Because the etiology and mechanism and pathophysiology are unclear. The researches on oncology are very new and there are many basic and clinical researches and the combination of the basic and clinical research needs to be further done.

Since 1985 the author followed up 3000 of the cancer patients who had surgery for their cancers. The result found that most of them had the recurrence or metasatasis after two or three years, even some had the recurrence or metastasis within several months or one year after Surgery, even died. After lots of following-up a very important question was found that the keys of affecting the long-term surgery effects are the recurrence and metastasis, then the author built up the experimental surgery research lab and did the tumor research: spent four years on doing the research about the anticancer mechanisms and rules to look for the effective ways to overcome the tumors. The results are that 48 of the Chinese herbs were selected as the anticancer medication XZ-C, then applied these basic researches in the clinical more than 16 years in the advanced cancer patients and had excellent effects. Based on the clinical practice and combination with half century of the clinical experience and recalled, up to the theory and posted the new concepts and ways and new theory so as to put all of the experimental research and clinical tests and data and material into the book collection. In this book the new concepts and ways and theories were posted and have our own authorization rights. The new theories and new concepts have important scientific meaning and values which will have important impacts on the oncology medical science and help with millions of the cancer patients and created the new ways to overcome the tumors. How to create the new ways to antimetastasis and where can we start? Chinese medications are our country characters which we can use to develop our advantages and to compete with the advanced international level. XZ-C medications after three years of the selection experiments on the animal models and 16 years of the clinical practice, which was introduced by this book, not only helped millions of the patients, but also will make the huge economical benefits for our country.

This book is my own innovation or the original creativity and created a new China character anticancer and antimetastasis way on the molecular oncology level combining with the Chinese and western medicines from the clinics to the experiments, then from the experiments to the clinics.

1. Scientific study route

The clinical work in our oncology outpatient center was following the rules:

a. Discover the questions to post the questions to research the questions to solve the questions

   Through following up most of the patients, it was found that the keys of effects on the longterm curative effects are the reccurence and metastasis after the surgery.

   Suggest that research and solve the recurrence and metasatasis problems can improve the long term curative effects which set up the targets or aims of how to antimetasatasis.

   Set up the research center and do some research to investigate the mechanism of the metastasis and antirecurrence reasons and to look for the new drugs such as 48 chinese herbs of 200 chinese herbs were selected as anticancer and antimetastasis medications.

   Conduct the clinical research to investigate the rules of the tumor metastasis and to find the new anticancer therapy models and upto the automatic new theory and new anticancer therapy models.

b. This research is from the clinical to the experiments to the clinics to the experiments to the clinic again, to solve the clinical problems

c. Combined the theory and the practice : these research started from the clinics, searched the questions and the clinical breakthrough. After experimental research and clinical research, then applied into the clinics again to solve the clinical practical questions.

   This research took the combination of the Chinese medicine and the western medicine to macroscopic combination to molecular level combination, and use the new theory of the modern tumor molecular transferring mechanism and eight steps, three stages to search and to select the new anticancers from 200 oldest herbs to protect the immune organs and activate the cell factors and immune factors and make the old medication into the modern medicine and to merge them into the international levels and combined the modern medicine with the older Chinese herbs in the molecular level and BRM level.

d. Obey the medicine rules and keep the truth and scientific facts. To prove the facts by the evident and get the experimental research and the clinical verified.
e. The curative therapy evulation standard and the long term curative effects: living longer and observed in the clinics 3-5 years, even 8-10 years so as to evaluate the longterm curative therapy.

2. Research methods

Antirecurrence and antimetasatasis laboratory and XXX outpatient center were built and obeyed the all the research ways:

1. Raise money by our own and independent work: the incomes from the private outpatient service were used as a research fee.
2. Build the outpatient medical records and kept them and follow the patients up: many years of the following up and called them to aske the questions and educated the diet habits and other important things to pay attention to be healthy. Kept the following tables and chemotherapy tables and the medication tables.
3. Build up the associate of the research group and the projects associate and do the research according to the research plans such as the research tables.
4. Build the detail medical records such as the patients' epidemiology and deeply analyze the successful experience and failure of the experience and specific medical condition for each cases such as analysis of the medical records.
5. Write the summary of analyzing the cases after following up more six months to one year. After three year of the follow-up the cases have the written summary of the analysis of the curative experience and lessons such as the medical summary.
6. Build the big tables and statistic one by one such as on the wall put the big tables includeing all of the epidemiology information, the tumor metastasis rules and information and the curative therapy experience and lessons.
7. Sharing the instruments and the materials and sharing the research awards and we didn't buy the big instruments which we used them in the university.
8. Didn't apply for money from the Province, however we reported our research results and scientific evaluation to Province and the city.

3. Academic values and position

Science is the front edge without the ending. Our research work are always following the scientific development and based on the known medicine and faced the future medicine. After 12 years of hard work and practice the scientific development and face the front edge of the science to create the new things and move on.

1. Modern molecular tumor transferring mechanism The old Chinese herbs selection

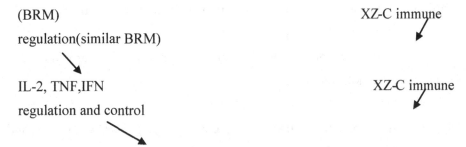

Merge the old chinese herbs into the international level in the molecular transferring mechanism to select the new drugs.

2. Modern molecular tumor immune cell factors XZ-C immune regular products,

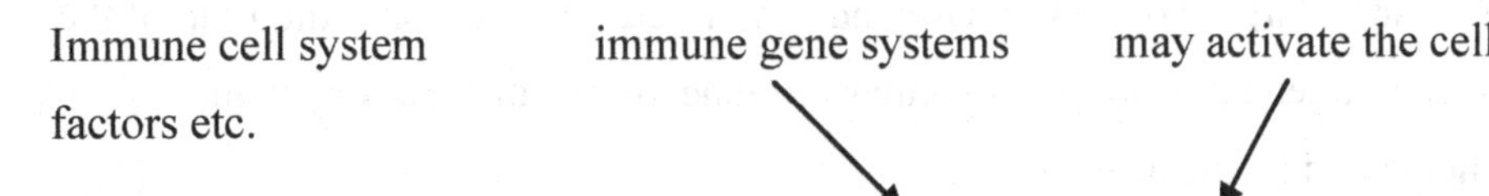

XZ-C is the combination of the Chinese and western medicine in the molecular levels

3. The new concept of the tumor therapy:

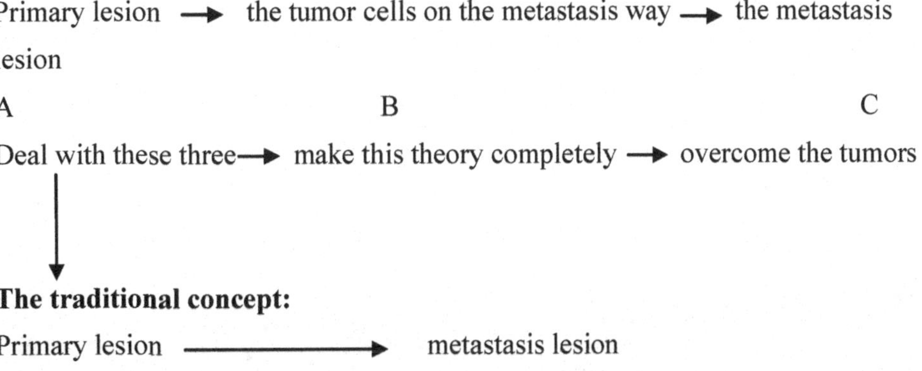

The isolated two points ⟶ the theory is not complete and can not overcome the tumors

4. Found the direction of the tumor development, research and breakthrough initially and recalled, thinking and summary so as to see the future:

The success and failure in the past

↓

Search for the existing questions

↓

Realized that the tumor diagnosis and therapy in 20 century is in the cell levels

↓

Found the future direction and post the tumor diagnosis and therapy in the 21 century is in the molecular level.

From the cells become the maligance to the imaging diagnosis by CT, MRI and Ultraosound , there is a big gap between them. Currently there is no effective method. Next step is to search the effective measurement method to check the tumors so as to diagnose the tumor early

↓

21 century " target" is the premaligance and micro metastasis, in the field of the molecular , gene diagnosis, molecular immune , molecular biology, Chinese medicine and medication, gene therapy.

↓

Create the new way to antimetastasis with China characters and independent knowledge property right.

4. Scientific research spirits of Shuguang tumor research institute

Hard work and strive---------ten years of work

↓

Recalling and thinking----------follow up and summary of the successful experience and recall the failure lessons

↓

Create and innovate-----select 48 chinese herbs which have the good inhibition rate from the 200 chinese herbs through the animal experiments, XZ-C immune regulation and control medication products, 11 years of clinical tests and understand them very well and up to the theory and the new concepts and new models.

Face the future medicine------realize the shortage and questions in the 20 century of the tradition therapy and realize the future direction in the 21 century.

↓

See the future direction

CHAPTER 37

Task, Mission, Opportunity and Challenge of Study on Anti-cancerometastasis

[Abstract] Why the study on anti-cancerometastasis shall be made? Because cancerometastasis is the core of anti-cancer and the bottle neck of anti-cancer at present.

What to do? Make the fundamental study on cancerometastasis (including experimental study on animal and clinical study).

How to do it? From the clinic, and to the clinic; from the clinic to the experiment and then from the experiment to the clinic; combination of Chinese medicine and Western medicine at the molecular level.

Study route: disclosing the problem→ putting forward the problem→ studying the problem →resolving or explaining the problem.

[Keywords] Cancerometastasis and reoccurrence; fundamental study; clinical study; molecular level;

I. Why the study on anti-cancerometastasis shall be made? Because it is the active demand of the present situation.

(I) We must make clear which problem exists at present and how to resolve the problem

1. The fundamental problem is that the death rate of the cancer patients receiving the three therapies still takes the first place over 100 years? How to do it? We should analyze, reflect and study it.
2. The recurrence after operation is still serious, the patients and their family numbers are afraid of the reoccurrence after operation, some patients are in fear and trembling all day long after operation and in a state of anxiety and desperateness. How to prevent the reoccurrence and the metastasis after operation by the surgeons? How to do it? We should study it.
3. Metastasis is the core of the cancer and the key of the survival time. Everyone is afraid of cancerometastasis. How to effectively prevent the cancerometastasis? How to control the metastasis of cancer cells? How to do it? We should make the fundamental and clinical study.

(II) We must make clear which problem exists in the current therapeutics and how to resolve it

1. The chemotherapy shall be further studied and perfected. Whether the assistant chemotherapy after operation prevents the reoccurrence and the metastasis or not? How to prevent the reoccurrence and metastasis after operation? It shall be studied.

We should make clear how to further study and perfect it based on our own data and experience.

2. The radiotherapy shall be further studied and perfect. The radiotherapy is for local treatment and the metastasis exists in the whole body. How to play its role in anti-metastasis treatment and how to further study and perfect it?
3. The design of radical operation shall be further studied and perfected to reduce the reoccurrence and metastasis after operation. In respect that it is radical operation, why it cannot realize the objective of radical treatment? In respect that the lymph clearing is made, why the metastasis exists? All of these issues shall be further studied. How to stress on the tumor-free technology in operation? How to reduce and prevent the ablation of the cancer cells in operation? How to reduce the metastasis of cancer cells in operation? How to reduce the spread in the vein? (The operation shall be gentle, stable and accurate). The fundamental experimental study shall be made on all of these issues and the experimental observation and study on the tumor-bearing animal model in operation shall be made. The operation is to prevent the metastasis.

II. Why we make the study on anti-cancerometastasis? It is the need of the present situation of the oncology.

We must make clear which problem exists in the present situation of the oncology by all means and how to deal with it

1. Oncology is the most behindhand subject among the medicine subjects at present? Why? Because we have been not making clear the pathogenic factor, pathogenesis, pathophysiology of the oncology, which is a scientific virgin soil for the scientific research and shall be further fundamentally studied.
2. Although lots of expenses have been invested in treatment of the cancer patients at home and abroad, although these three traditional therapeutics have been used for the clinical application over 100 years, the death rate of the cancer has been taking the first place among the causes of death of the urban and rural residents in China? Why? Mainly because:
   (1) The pathogenic factors of cancer have been not entirely making clear; Pathogenesis and metastasis mechanism of cancer cells have been not making clear sufficiently;
   (2) The complicated biological behaviors of cancer have been not making clear sufficiently;
   (3) Rx is of rather blindness;
   (4) The means of diagnosis are behindhand, once the cancer is found, it is in metaphase and advanced stage, the curative effects are bad;
   (5) Many large-sized hospitals have not established the labs, in this way, they cannot carry out the fundamental study on cancer, anti-cancerometastasis and anti-metastasis. It is necessary to make the fundamental study on cancer-bearing animal model and establish the cancerometastasis animal model with nude mice to study the rules and mechanism of the metastasis of cancer cells (this lab have made the experiments on cancer-bearing animal model with pure-blood Kunming mice over 10000 times). Therefore, without the breakthrough of fundamental study, it is difficult to improve the clinical curative effects.

III. Our scientific research must face the scientific cutting edge and walk up to the way of anti-cancerometastasis with Chinese characteristics with the guide of scientific development concept

The academic study on anti-cancerometastasis shall stress on studying the unknown knowledge and the researchers shall go ahead and face the future science. Science is the endless cutting edge and the scientific research must pass beyond the previous old knowledge with the foresight of development for uninterrupted updating, surpassing, development and advance.

The clinical medical workers, especially the professors, the associate professors, the chief physicians and the associate chief physician, undertake double task, one is to treat the patients and another is to develop the medicine. Why do we publish the papers? Just to develop the medicine and work together to build the medical palace.

1. The core of study is to base ourselves upon the study, develop the medicine, face the future medicine and study the prevention and treatment of cancerometastasis with the foresight of development and innovation. The oncology in 20th century was at cellular level and the one in 21st century shall be at molecular level. The study on oncology must uninterruptedly surpass the knowledge of the predecessors, and the latercomers shall surpass the formers in learning. The medical experts of the older generation are willing to act as the human ladder to enable the latercomers to surpass the formers in learning, technology and achievements.
2. The study shall be based on the patients and the new fruits and methods helpful to the patients, improve the medical quality, abate the paints of the patients and prolong the survival time. What is the medical quality? The quality refers to the curative effect. What is the curative effect of the cancer patient? It is long survival time, good survival quality and little pain.

IV. What to do? How to do?

1. What to do? Make the fundamental study on molecular biology and genetic engineering biology. Make the fundamental clinical study and clinical follow-up retrospective analysis and study. Carry out the evidence-based medicine and make the experimental study for evaluation and the evaluation study on the long-term curative effects with the clinical verification data. Probe into the cancerometastasis and recurrence mechanism and strive for the effective measures for regulation and control. The animal experimental surgery is extremely important in developing the medicine and it is a key to open the forbidden zone of medicine and promote the development of medical career. So many new drugs and new technologies are applied to the clinic based on the successful animal experiment.
2. How to do? Our scientific study route: ① disclosing the problem→ putting forward the problem→ studying the problem→ resolving or explaining the problem. ② Theory shall be closely integrated with practice. The topics in the study are selected from the clinic and they shall be studied to find the focus of the problems in the clinic and the clinical breakthrough and then they will be applied to the clinic to resolve the actual problems through experimental study and clinical verification.③ Walk up to the way of combination of Chinese medicine with Western medicine→ macroscopic combination→ experimental study→ combination at molecular level. ④ The combination of

tumor foundation and clinic will play a leading role in conquering the cancer. ⑤ We exert our existing advantages in the existing fields with advantages to surpass the international advanced level. In the field of cancer study, traditional Chinese medicine and combination of Chinese medicine and Western medicine are our advantages. It is internationally strategically significant to exert the roles of these advantages in cancer study.

3. The anti-cancer study needs a batch of scientific researchers to undertaken the scientific study topics and make study on the micro-metastasis. All of them have rich clinical experience and they will be the engine of the development of oncology. The anti-cancerometastasis study shall base ourselves upon the scientific study, development and transformation of achievements and walk up to the way of the trinity enterprises, campuses and institutes. We should hold the flag of scientific development concept and stand at the cutting edge of scientific study (this research institute are right standing in the cutting edge of the oncology), walk up to the road of study and development so as to make great achievements of conquering the cancer.
4. All of the attendants are the outstanding scientific researchers, some even the leading persons in this field. It is necessary for us to make scientific achievements and walk up to the anti-carcerometastasis innovation way with Chinese characteristics and make great achievements in the scientific study on cancerometastasis. Let's advance hand in hand on the way of scientific study and strive for the papers on Science without a stop. We should face the science, face the future and dare to develop and innovate it.

CHAPTER 38

Strategic Thoughts And Suggestions For Overcoming Carcinoma

Nowadays, cancer has become the main serious disease threatening human health. Its number of cases steadily increases at an average annual rate of 3%~5%. The morbidity and mortality respectively rise by 24.7% and 19.2% compared with those of ten years before. Three traditional therapies have a history of nearly one hundred years. But the mortality of cancer patients is still the number one. What is to be done? How to continue the road of researches? Those deserve our analysis, reflection and study.

Where is the way to overcome cancer? The writer holds that the right way is to carry out scientific researches. That is to say, overcoming cancer needs the scientific researches on cancer prevention and cure, the fundamental experimental researches on exploring cancer's cause, pathogenesis and pathophysiology, the scientific researches on studying the whole process of cancer generation and development, the reform and development of traditional therapies, multidisciplinary researches, cancer researches on prevention and cure of metastasis and relapse, and researches on "early detection, early diagnosis and early treatment".

Through the scientific researches on cancer prevention and cure, humans will certainly conquer cancer and finally overcome cancer.

My thoughts on how to overcome cancer: the first part—the road of scientific researches lies in the fundamental experimental researches on exploring the cause, pathogenesis and pathophysiology of cancer

1. The writer holds that conducting scientific researches on cancers is a desperate need for the current situation of tumor subject. Researchers must recognize that what the problems are in the current situation of tumor subject? What is to be done?

   Cancer therapy has developed for over a century and now it has stepped into the second decade of the 21st century, but "oncology" is still the most backward branch among all the current medical subjects. Why? That's because the cause, pathogenesis and pathophysiology of "oncology" are not clear or definite. Oncology is a piece of scientific virgin soil for scientific research, and needs numerous basic scientific researches and clinical basic researches.

   Although three traditional therapies (surgical operation, radiotherapy and chemotherapy) have been applied for nearly one hundred years and thousands upon thousands of cancer patients have undergone radiotherapies and chemotherapies, what the consequence is? So far cancer mortality still occupies the number one in causes of death of China's urban and rural residents. How to open up the road demands an intensive reflection, analysis and study.

   Why it should have been so can be mainly divided into the following points.

   (1) The cause, pathogenesis and pathophysiology of cancer are not clear. Enormous basic theoretical questions are not definite yet.

(2) There isn't an adequate understanding of biological characteristics and behaviors of cancer cells.
(3) There is insufficient appreciation of the molecular mechanism of metastatic cancer cells.
(4) There isn't an adequate understanding of cancer's complicated biological behaviors of generation, growth, clone, proliferation, invasion, metastasis and implantation, which await scientific researches by units that meet the necessary conditions.

The current cancer therapeutic schedules still have the considerable blindness. Means of diagnosis are unprogressive; as soon as the cancer comes to light, it has reached the middle or advanced stage; therapeutic effects are poor. The above are due to the insufficient understanding of cancer's cause, pathogenesis and pathophysiology as well as inadequate fundamental experimental studies. Therefore, the current understanding of oncology seems not clear enough and shows a fuzzy or twilight state. The tumor knowledge is still in a very backward stage.

Many large-scale tumor hospitals or affiliated hospitals of university have not yet established a cancer laboratory to carry out fundamental researches of cancer. There is also no laboratory of cancer animals to conduct experimental researches of cancer-bearing animal models. Anti-cancer metastasis and relapse must carry out fundamental researches of cancer-bearing animal models. Researchers should use nude mice to build cancer-metastasis animal models for studying the law and mechanism of cancer cell metastases. Why should we pay attention to the fundamental research in laboratory? That's because if there is no breakthrough in the fundamental research, clinical efficacy will be hard to increase.

2. Experimental surgery is the key to open up the forbidden zone of medical science.

Experimental surgery plays a very important role in developing medical science, which is the key to open up the forbidden zone of medical science. The pathogenesis and control methods of many diseases have been achieved after countless animal experimental researches. The research results with stability can only be applied to the clinic, which promotes the progress of medicine, improves medical quality and develops new control methods.

The laboratory of experimental surgery in our college was set up in May 1980. Under the charge of Professor Xu Ze, researchers have carried out experimental researches of surgical therapy of refractory ascites caused by hepatic cirrhosis and the pathogenesis; have adopted the method of experimental surgery to explore the cause, pathogenesis and pathophysiology of pathological change of schistosomiasis japanica on lung; have studied the pathogenesis of hepatic portal vein hypertension caused by the hepatic cirrhosis of schistosomiasis japanica; have transplanted hepatic cells in the spleen to produce the second liver for treating hepatic failure. The above national-level and provincial-level scientific research items have laid a good foundation for experimental research.

In early 1987, this laboratory began to turn to the experimental tumor research. Researchers have carried out the transplantation of cancer cells, built experimental tumor animal models, explored the pathogenesis and pathophysiology of tumor, and investigated the law and mechanism of cancer cell metastases in cancer-bearing animal models and changes of the host's immune function. And then researchers have discussed Chinese herbal medicines with good anti-cancer effects, made a strict and scientific screening study of Chinese herbal medicines with anti-cancer and cancer inhibited effect in vivo of cancer-bearing animal models. In order to develop the career of cancer prevention and treatment, researchers commit themselves to the experimental researches of exploring the cause, pathogenesis and pathophysiology of cancer and further extracting Chinese herbal medicines with the effect of cancer prevention and cure.

With the practical requirement in our college's medical science situation, Institute of Experimental Surgery of Hubei College of Traditional Chinese Medicine was set up in March 1991 on the basis of experimental surgical laboratory. Professor Xu Ze serves as director of the institute and Academician Qiu Fazu is invited as the mentor. Their research target and task are: Institute of Experimental Surgery is mainly to tackle key problems of cancer. The emphasis is to adopt the method of experimental surgery to carry out fundamental researches of experimental tumors and control researches of clinical patients. This research laboratory of experimental tumor adopts biological engineering technology and genetic engineering technology of cancer cells, exploits the fundamental research and clinical practice of tumor biological therapy and immunization therapy, develops and promotes the career of cancer prevention and treatment.

3. Our laboratory has found the following understandings from the experimental tumor research.
   (1) Our laboratory has found that removal of mouse's thymus will not affect the buildup of cancer-bearing animal model and injecting immunosuppressant can also contribute to the buildup of cancer-bearing animal model. The research results indicate that there is an obvious link between the generation and growth of cancer and the host's immune organ—thymus and its function.
   (2) The experiment, which explores tumor's effect on the host's immune organ, shows that with the gradual growth of cancer, thymus presents progressive atrophy. That is to say, the host's thymus presents acute progressive atrophy after inoculation of cancer cells.
   (3) This experiment has also found that some experimental mice, which are inoculated unsuccessfully or have a very small tumor, do not have an obvious atrophic thymus. In order to know the relationship between tumor and atrophy of thymus, researchers resect the transplanted solid tumors in a set of experimental mice when the size of tumors equals to the size of thumb. The anatomy after one month shows that their thymus does not have a further progressive atrophy. Therefore, it can be speculated that the solid tumor may produce a kind of unknown factor to inhibit thymus. But accurate results still need the further experimental researches.
   (4) The above experimental results prove that the growth of tumor can lead to the progressive atrophy of thymus. Then can we adopt some methods to prevent the host's thymus atrophy? Therefore, the writer starts to carry out animal studies to look for a way or drug to prevent the thymus atrophy of tumor-bearing mouse. He adopts cellular transplantation of immune organs to restore the function of immune organs, which is to explore a way to inhibit thymus atrophy of immune organs as the tumor grows and look for a method to restore the thymus function and reconstruct immunity. Then the writer conducts transplantations of fetal liver cells, fetal splenic cells and fetal thymocytes on mice, which is to reconstruct mice's immunologic function through adoptive immunity. The result indicates that after combined transplantation of three groups of cells (S, T and L), the completely regressive rate of short-term tumor is 40% and the rate of

long-term tumor is 46.67%. The patient whose tumor has completely regressed can get the chance for long term survival.

4. The experimental study result reveals that one of cancer causes and pathogeneses may be the atrophy of thymus and the hypo-function of immune organs.

   A series of animal experimental studies have been done for exploring the cause, pathogenesis and pathophysiology of cancer. The analysis and think of experimental results produce new discovery, new thinking and new revelation. That is, one of cancer causes may be the atrophy of thymus, the damage of thymus function and the hypo-function of immune organs. Therefore, Professor Xu Ze first proposes the idea in the world that one of cancer causes and pathogeneses may be the atrophy of thymus, the function damage of central immune organs, the hypo-function of immune organs, the reduction of immune surveillance function and immunologic escape. But what leads to the host's thymus atrophy? The writer ruminates over this question and speculates that the solid tumor might produce a kind of factor that can suppress thymus; nevertheless, the speculation needs further experimental researches. This kind of factor is temporarily called "thymus suppressor cancer-factor".

5. Subsequently, the writer raises the theoretical and experimental basis of "thymus protection for enhancing immunity; pulp protection for hemogenesis" in XZ-C immunologic mediation and control therapy.

   Based on the inspiration from the above experimental results about the cause and pathogenesis of cancer, the new theory and new method of XZ-C immunologic mediation and control targeted therapy that first proposed by Professor Xu Ze have their theoretical and experimental basis. Our presented therapeutic principle and theory of "thymus protection for enhancing immunity; pulp protection for hemogenesis" are reasonable and scientific. Through sixteen years' clinical observation of over 12,000 patients with intermediate- or advanced-stage cancer in Twilight Specialist Out-patient Department, it can clearly show that this therapeutic principle with sixteen years' clinical application is correct and reasonable. The therapeutic effectiveness is satisfactory and trusted by patients.

   As an old saying goes, "Once the headrope of fishing net is pulled up, all its meshes open." As long as the thymus atrophy might be one of cancer causes and pathogeneses, then theoretical basis of therapy must emerge at its proper moment.

6. Review the research history of cancer causes over the past one hundred years.

   In the history of medicine, more than 2500 years ago, the scholar of ancient Greek-Hippocrates used a word "Cancer" to describe tumor. From then on people started the study and understanding of malignant tumor.

Until 1775, British doctor found that boys who sweep air flue for a long time are easy to suffer from carcinoma of scrotum. Then this doctor proposed the theory that the production of tumor is closely related to environmental factor.

In the late 19th, German doctor discovered that workers who touch dye have an impressively high proportion of suffering from bladder carcinoma. Afterwards some chemical substances successfully induce tumor in animals; tobacco components exert an influence on lung cancer; Aspergillus flavus has a definite relation with liver cancer. All these have provided direct evidences for the theory of cancer caused by chemical substances.

In 1908, Danish pathologist Ellerman and Bang found that chicken's leukemia can pass to healthy chickens through the filtered solution without cells. Two years later, American pathologist Rous proved that a kind of sarcoma in chicken is caused by virus, which establishes the theory of oncogenic virus.

The relation between human tumor and virus was established after EB virus was found in Burkitt lymphoma in 1964. The following researches show that EB virus and nasopharyngeal carcinoma, hepatitis b virus and primary carcinoma of liver, human papilloma virus and cervical carcinoma have an intimate relation. Those all lay a solid foundation for the theory of oncogenic virus.

People's knowledge of tumor causes continues to expand. Finding that sailors who often expose to the sun have a high risk of contracting skin carcinoma, people start to consider physical factors which may cause cancer. Until discovering that rate tumor can be induced after a large dosage of X-irradiation, people begin to confirm the theory of cancer caused by physical factors. In 1940s, after the explosion of atomic bombs in Japanese cities of Hiroshima and Nagasaki, various tumors and leukemias in survivors occur in high incidence. In the process of clinical cancer therapy, iatrogenic leukemia appears after the primary lesion is controlled. The two facts provide evidences for the theory of cancer caused by physical factors.

Although having had a preliminary knowledge of the tumor etiology, people still feel indefinite about the pathogenesis and pathophysiology of malignant tumor, and also lack effective preventive and therapeutic measures. Therefore, it is urgently necessary to have an extensive, in-depth and detailed study of tumor's pathogenesis and pathophysiology as well as prophylactic-therapeutic measures.

Reviewing the above research history of cancer over the past one hundred years, we can find that researches about cancer's cause, pathogeny, pathogenesis and pathophysiology are still quite rare. Until now whether or not cancer is a kind of disease can hardly be explained. That's because according to the definition, a disease must have the pathogeny, cause, pathogenesis, pathophysiology and pathology. But for one hundred years, people have always applied themselves to clinical and clinical fundamental researches of surgical operation, radiotherapy and chemotherapy. But in aspects of regular laboratory fundamental and clinical fundamental researches of cancer cell mutation, clone, proliferation, invasion, metastasis and implantation, people have done a little, such as invasion, metastasis, cancer embolus, immunization, endocrine and virus, etc. Exploring cancer's cause, pathogenesis, pathophysiology, metastasis and relapse must depend on the fundamental research of cancer-bearing animal models. All sorts of cancer animal models should be built with nude mice, in order to study the law and mechanism of cancer cells' invasions and metastases.

My thoughts on how to overcome cancer: the second part—the road of scientific researches lies in the study of the whole process of cancer's production and growth as well as the scientific study of prevention and treatment

1. The thought, strategy and program against cancer are shown in the following schematic drawing.

How to overcome cancer?

↓

Where is the way?

↓

Our thought, strategy and experience should be divided into three parts

↓

Before the formation of cancer——prevention part——anti- mutation

↓

Precancerous lesion with possible tendency of malignant change——intervention part

↓

The therapeutic part of primary cancer with the formation of focus and anti-metastasis

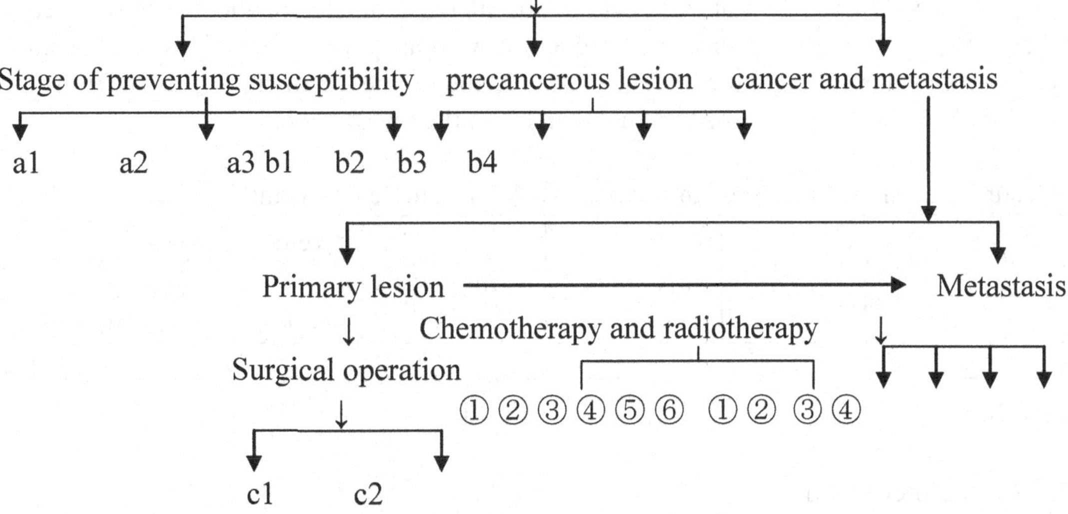

a1. "Two-oriented society" contains essences and measures
a2. "Lift scientific research" makes plans and measures of cancer control
a3. Propaganda, education and study of popular science

b1. General investigation of physical examination
b2. Selective examination of high risk group
b3. Outpatient service of "early detection, early diagnosis and early treatment"
b4. Induced differentiation

c1. Improve free-tumor technique
c2. Prevent intraoperative implantation of cast-off cells

① with indication
② individuation
③ scientization
④ drug sensitive test
⑤ try to reduce untoward reaction
⑥ "intelligent resistance to cancer" of target administration

① targeted therapy
② anti-metastasis and anti-relapse therapies
③ BRM biological therapy
④ immunoregulation therapy

2. Cancer treatment lies in "early detection, early diagnosis and early treatment"; anti-cancer method lies in prevention.

   Cancer's production and growth will go through stage of susceptibility, precancerous lesion and invasive stage. All the present tumor hospitals or tumor departments mainly focus on the cancer treatment in middle or advanced stage. The Therapeutic effects are poor. If patients in middle or advanced stage can accept surgical operation, then they will be treated surgically. But if not, they will only receive palliative treatment. Therefore, cancer treatment lies in "early detection, early diagnosis and early treatment". Generally, patients in the early stage will get a better therapeutic effect. The increase of therapeutic effect will certainly reduce the fatality rate of cancer. Consequently, we must put much emphasis on the study of early-stage diagnostic and therapeutic methods, and on the treatment of precancerous lesion for lessening medium-term or terminal patients in the invasive stage.

   Occupying lesion can be seen through CT or MRI, middle or advanced stage

stage of susceptibility	precancerous lesion	early stage	no metastasis	have metastasized	
				local position	amphi position
①	②	③	④	⑤	⑥

① Cancer prevention
② Outpatient service of "three kinds of earliness"
③ Surgical operation
④ Place surgical operation first, radiotherapy, chemotherapy and biological TCM second
⑤ Possible to undergo surgical operation
⑥ To give treatment as carcinomatous metastasis

If patients have been treated well in the stage of precancerous lesion or early stage, then the number of patients in middle or advanced stage of invasion and metastasis will fall off. Thus, the cancer incidence rate will also decline. Therefore, we hold that the present tumor hospitals in various places mainly focus on the cancer treatment in middle or advanced stage. Even though the therapeutic result is effective, it can only bring the reduction of cancer mortality rate. But if ignoring the stage of susceptibility, precancerous lesion or early stage, it will be impossible to reduce the cancer incidence rate. Therefore, we must put much emphasis on the whole process of cancer production and growth. After all this is the real global change of strategic importance.

The writer has engaged in surgical oncology for over fifty years. More and more patients suffer from cancer, and the cancer incidence rate also rises. The writer deeply feels that people should emphasize not only therapy but also prevention. Only in this way could the cancer be killed in the source. Cancer treatment lies in "three kinds of earliness" (early detection, early diagnosis and early treatment); anti-cancer method lies in prevention.

As stated above, the strategic center of gravity of tumor treatment and prevention moves forward. There are two aspects in its meaning. One is to prevent cancer by changing life style and improving environmental pollution; the other is to cure precancerous lesion for inhibiting cancer's development to the invasion stage, middle stage or advanced stage.

In 1990, our institute's specialist out-patient department of tumor surgery once opened the outpatient service of "three kinds of earliness" to carry out various endoscopies and biopsies, through which have found many atypical hyperplasia of stomach, intestinal metaplasia, atrophic gastritis and hyperplasia of mammary glands, etc. These "precancerous lesions" are difficult to treat. Then how to handle these precancerous lesions or precancerous conditions so as to prevent their cancerations urgently needs clinical researches to look for better treatment methods.

3. Put emphasis on fundamental and clinical researches of precancerous lesions with diagnosis and treatment techniques.

"Three kinds of earliness" is the key to cancer treatment. While how to handle precancerous lesion is the key stage for cancer prevention and treatment.

The present cancer diagnosis mainly depends on image examinations of type-B ultrasonic, CT and MRI. But as soon as the cancer comes to light, it has reached the middle or advanced stage. Many patients have lost the chance of radical excision. Although the complex treatment has been done, the therapeutic effects are still poor. If the cancer is in the early stage or belongs to the carcinoma in situ, then the curative effect of operation will be better and the cancer can be cured. Therefore, the cancer treatment should strive for "three kinds of earliness", which refers to early detection, early diagnosis and early treatment.

Because cancer's pathogenic factors are not very clear, the primary prevention is still quite difficult.

Studies in recent years indicate that malignant tumor rarely has a direct carcinomatous change in normal tissues. Before the occurrence of tumor in clinical diagnosis, cancer often goes through quite a long evolution stage, which is the stage of precancerous lesion. Early identification and control of these precancerous lesions will bring positive significances for the secondary prevention of cancer.

What is precancerous lesion? The precancerous lesion is a histopathology concept, which refers to a kind of tissues with the dysplasia of cells. Precancerous lesion has the potential to become cancerous. If there is no cure in a long period, precancerous lesion will evolve into cancer. In other words, precancerous lesion just has the possibility of changing into cancer. But not all the precancerous lesions will eventually become cancer. Through proper treatments, precancerous lesions may return to their normal states or have a spontaneous regression.

Canceration is a developing process with several stages. There is a stage of precancerous lesion between normal cells and cancer. It is a slow process from precancerous lesion evolving into cancer, which needs many years or even more than ten years. The length of canceration course is closely related to the strength of carcinogenic factors, individual susceptibility and immunologic function. Therefore, the study of precancerous lesion is of great importance to cancer's prevention and control.

4. More than one third of cancers can be prevented.

The tumor formation is a long process with several factors and stages. Precancerous lesion is of reversibility, so cancer is preventable.

The several factors, steps and stages of tumor formation have the following features.

The generation and growth of tumor can be roughly divided into several stages of initiation, promotion, metastasis and others. Cellular canceration induced by chemical carcinogen is a multistage process. The chemical carcinogenesis process of Experimental animals and the generating process of human tumors (such as colon cancer) have a series of changes, which are hyperplasia → pathological changes → benign tumor → malignant tumor → tumor metastasis, etc. The whole change process is complicated with multiple stages of initiation, promotion and evolution, etc. It often takes a long cytometaplasia time to change from normal cells to the tumor that can be detected clinically, which is a long cumulative process.

(1) Two-stage theory of tumor formation: In 1942, Beremblum carried out the experimental study of mouse's skin canceration induction, in which he used benzoapyrene to treat mice's skins for about one year, and only three out of one hundred and two mice suffered from skin tumors. If mice's skins were treated with benzoapyrene for several months and then treated with the tumor promoter-croton oil, thirty-six out of eighty-three mice suffered from skin cancers, whose incidence rate was ten times higher than that of using benzoapyrene alone. If mice's skins were first treated with croton oil for several months and then treated with a carcinogenic substance, there would be no induced tumor. If mice's skins were only treated with croton oil for a long time, whose incidence rate of tumor would be lower than that of using benzoapyrene alone (1/106).

On the basis of this study results, Beremblum and Subik have proposed that cancerous process contains two different but intimate stages. One is a specific provocation stage. Small dosages of carcinogenic substance induce normal cells to become potential cancer cells. The other is nonspecific promoting stage. Potential cancer cells are further promoted to suffer from mutation and evolve into tumor under the action of tumor promoters, such as croton oil and others.

People hold that provocation process refers to the process that normal cells change into potential cancer cells under the action of carcinogenic substances. The time of promoting process is fairly short and generally irreversible. While promoting process is the process that potential cancer cells change into cancer cells under the action of tumor promoters. The early promoting stage is reversible but the late stage is irreversible.

Carcinogenic substance is a kind of mutagen, which plays a decisive role in canceration process. While cancer promoters do not have the mutagenicity, which can only promote potential cancer cells to have a further proliferation change and gradually evolve into cancer cells. During these two processes of provocation and promoting stages, induced cells grow out of control, escape from the host's immune surveillance, gradually form tumor cells with malignant phenotype and then evolve into tumor cells with infiltration and metastasis. This theory recognizes that tumor generation is quite a long process (months, years and even more than ten years) and will be impossible through a single factor or stage, which is very important to cancer prevention and control. It prompts that people have enough time to build up cancer-fighting ability, strengthen immunity, change life style and improve environmental pollution to prevent cancer. Intervention measures should be emphasized to tackle the reversible stage of cancer promoting.

(2) Multi-factor and multi-stage model of tumor formation: Vogelstein proposed the multi-stage model of genetics of colon cancer and histological change, which makes people get a better idea of the formation of human colon tumor and molecular events happening in the process of development. It proves that the synergic action between cancer gene and cancer suppressor gene is the key factor for cellular canceration. The study conclusion is that canceration process of colon is a process with multiple involving genes and developing stages (Fig. 38-1).

5. Anti-cancer method lies in prevention.

For almost half a century, human spectrum of disease has undergone a drastic change. Most communicable diseases have been effectively controlled. Chronic diseases, such as cardiovascular diseases and malignant tumors have been the most serious diseases threatening human health.

Carcinogenic action
Genetic change Variance of cancer suppressor gene
Genetic change Oncogene abnormality
Genetic change Oncogene abnormality Abnormality of cancer suppressor gene
Cloning expansion
Genetic change Oncogene abnormality Abnormality of cancer suppressor gene
Normal cells transformed cells precancerous lesion malignant cells clinical diagnosis of tumor metastatic tumor
Initiation stage promoting stage evolutional stage metastatic stage

Fig. 38-1 Multi-factor and multi-stage model of tumor formation
(Quote from *Molecular Oncology*, written by Zhan Qimin)

Cancer has become the most serious public health problem in the world. Compared with other chronic diseases, cancer's prevention and control face a greater challenge.

Over the last thirty years, the fatality rate of cancer in China is on an obvious rise, which has occupied the number one in causes of death of urban and rural residents. On average, one out of every four deceased persons dies from cancer.

Cancer not only seriously threatens human health but also causes the rapid rise of hospitalization costs. The direct costs of cancer treatment in China are about one hundred billion RMB every year, which makes patients and the whole society bear a huge economic burden.

Although each country inputs a large number of funds to treat cancer patients, the five-year survival rate of some common cancers has no obvious improvement in the recent twenty years. For instance, during the years from 1974 to 1990 in USA, the five-year survival rate of esophagus cancer only rose from 7% to 9%, stomach cancer from 16% to 19%, liver cancer from 3% to 6%, lung cancer from 12% to 15% and that of pancreatic cancer remained the same as 3%.

What's to be done? Anti-cancer method lies in prevention. Prevention and intervention is the most important thing in the field of public health.

As for the malignant cancer, prevention outweighs therapy. Worldwide tumor researchers have reached a consensus of adjusting public health resources and policies, shifting strategic focus from therapy to prevention, and carrying out positive and effective studies of pre-warning, early diagnosis and intervention to lower tumor incidence rate and raise curative rate.

The evidence in *Cancer Report* provided by World Health Organization proves that up to one thirds of cancers can be prevented. As long as every national government, medical workers and the common people actively take actions and shift the research emphasis of tumor prevention and treatment to tumor prevention, they can prevent above one thirds or even about half of the cancers.

My thoughts on how to overcome cancer: the third part—the road of scientific researches lies in carrying out multidisciplinary researches, organizing relevant professional research team and deeply specializing in fundamental and clinical discipline researches

1. Oncology study is the most complicated and difficult subject in the study of medical science. It ranges over multi-disciplinary knowledge and theories, which involves pathology, cytology, immunology, virology, molecular biology, medical genetics, immunopharmacology and molecular oncology. On the level of molecule, studying tumor pathogenesis and learning diseases causes can provide intervening and therapeutic measures for effective tumor prevention and treatment.

   The present surgical operation is still the most important, frequently used, definite and effective therapeutic methods to treat malignant tumor. But relapse or metastasis often appears in the short or long term after surgical operation. Follow-up results of more than 3,000 patients who have accepted cancer surgeries of chest and abdomen discover that postoperative relapse and metastasis are key factors for long-term therapeutic effectiveness of surgical operation. Therefore, an issue is raised that the method and measure of preventing and treating postoperative relapse and metastasis are important for improving long-term therapeutic effectiveness. There is a must to carry out fundamental and clinical interdisciplinary study on resisting relapse and metastasis.

   Since 1970s, in view of extremely high recurrence and metastatic rate after cancer operation, in order to prevent postoperative recurrence and metastasis, patients accept a series of adjuvant chemotherapies. Some patients have even started to accept preoperative chemotherapies, but the results are not fully up to expectations. Postoperative relapse and metastasis still come out in a short time. How to prevent recurrence and resist metastasis to get a good long-term effect is the matter that really deserves clinicians' serious and objective analysis, reflection, consider and study.

   Now in the early 21st century, cancer recurrence and metastasis have become the "bottleneck" in cancer treatment. The main problem of cancer treatment still focuses on how to fight against metastasis. If not solving the metastasis after radical operation of cancer, cancer treatment cannot have a further improvement. We hold that tackling key cancer problem mainly depends on the resistance to metastasis. The key problem of cancer treatment is to tackle metastasis and recurrence.

2. Organize multi-disciplinary joint researches with large-scale cooperation among hospitals.

   It is a must to carry out fundamental and clinical studies on resisting relapse and metastasis as well as multi-disciplinary joint researches with large-scale cooperation among hospitals. Organize professors, experts, scholars, doctors, master, and physicians in universities and colleges as well as their affiliated hospitals, independent hospitals and special hospitals on the level of Hubei province or Wuhan city and anti-cancer persons with lofty ideals to carry out research cooperation and walk the way of joint researches with large-scale cooperation. Advocate large-scale research cooperation, pay attention to organize scientific and technical force of each side and raise anti-cancer force on resisting cancer, metastasis and relapse.

   Anti-cancer study needs to cover a wide range of subjects, which involve not only clinical medicine but also many borderline subjects, interdisciplinary subjects and basic subjects. The study of cancer metastasis and recurrence ranges over internal medicine, surgery, radiation, endocrine, drugs, immunity, molecular organism, virus, biological information, genetic engineering, life science, molecular chemistry, enzyme chemistry, environmental protection, traditional Chinese medicine and laboratory, etc. Wuhan city has talented persons in all of the above fields. Therefore, our city has a certain foundation to organize scientific and technical force of each side, pool the wisdom and efforts of everyone, walk the way of joint researches with large-scale cooperation, and raise the anti-metastasis and anti-relapse level together to benefit ten million of cancer patients.

   Anti-cancer study, which is to overcome cancer, must involve fundamental and clinical studies on resisting relapse and metastasis, multi-disciplinary joint researches with large-scale cooperation among hospitals and the establishment of Wuhan anti-cancer institute.

   With the energetic support of academician Qiu Fazu, through the declaration and preparation of Xu Ze, Li Huiqiao and other professors, upon the local tax authorities' approval, they finally set up Wuhan anti-cancer institute on June 21, 2009. Then they establish a special committee for treating cancer metastasis and relapse, also organize academic and research team of tackling cancer metastasis to carry out academic research, academic discuss and academic propaganda, and open academic workshop or seminar. Thu they have trained many batches of senior talented young and middle-aged people on the study and treatment of resisting cancer metastasis for our province and city.

   The goal in anti-cancer study relies on "research". Under the guidance of scientific outlook on development, take the view angle of development and innovative spirit, focus on the front sight and look into the future to develop medical science, research into the cancer prevention and control, the generation and growth of cancer, the pathogenesis of cancer metastasis relapse as well as the prevention and treatment of cancer. The research line is to discover, raise, study, solve or explain the problem.

3. Assemble the following professional research groups which are closely related to cancer; deeply specialize in fundamental and clinical discipline researches.

   In view of oncology study ranging over multi-disciplinary knowledge and theories, the related personnel must assemble relevant professional research groups to further specialize in and reply on the known knowledge and medical science in this subject, study and explore the unknown knowledge and future medical science in this subject, borderline subjects and interdisciplinary subjects to help conquer cancer. The following professional research groups should be set up. In the future, new subjects, interdisciplinary subjects or new industries may come out.

(1) Immunity and cancer research group: in the modern history of tumor treatment, surgical operation, chemotherapy and radiotherapy are basic treatment methods. They have made some progress, but the whole curative effects are still not fully up to expectations. Cancer still occupies the number one in human causes of death.

The modern immunological therapy of malignant tumor began in the early 1970s. Through decades of unremitting efforts, with the development of technology, different treatment methods and drugs, such as interferon, interleukin and LAK cells appear in succession and have also got certain curative effects. But the successful application of anti-CD20 monoclonal antibody (rituximab) in lymphoid tumor just truly realizes immunization therapy and also opens up a new tumor therapeutic area—immune targeted therapy.

The earlier chapters in this book have already made some introductions. After four-year experimental research history of exploring pathogenic factors, pathogenesis and pathophysiology with cancer-bearing animal models, our laboratory have found that removal of mouse's thymus will not affect the buildup of cancer-bearing animal model; injecting immunosuppressant can also contribute to the buildup of cancer-bearing animal model and with the gradual growth of cancer, thymus presents progressive atrophy. Therefore, Professor Xu Ze first proposes the idea in the world that one of cancer causes and pathogeneses may be the atrophy of thymus, the function damage of thymus and the reduction of immune function. He also raises theoretical basis and experimental evidence of new theory and method—XZ-C targeted therapy of immune regulation.

The latest clinical research task of immunity and cancer research group should be: ① to assess the condition of immunologic function in cancer patients; ② to monitor the curative effect of immune regulation therapy in cancer patients; ③to quantitatively measure the condition of immunologic function in radiotherapy and chemotherapy patients.

(2) Virus and cancer research group should consider the relevant treatment measures to cure some cancers closely related to virus.

① The pathogenesis of some cancers is virus: As early as 1908 and 1911, people have found in succession that leukemia cells of chicken and filtering medium of chicken sarcoma can induce leukemia and sarcoma. In 1951, leukemia virus is found in mice. In the recent ten years, due to the rapid development of virology, immunology and molecular biochemistry, the study of tumor virus has also made fast progress. Thus it is confirmed one after the other that many viruses can induce tumor and even some human viruses (such as adenovirus and herpes simplex virus) can also induce the tumor of mouse. EB virus can induce the monkey's malignant tumor. Until now, only one quarter of over six hundred animal viruses are discovered to have the characteristic of causing tumor. Of special interest is chicken's Marek disease. It is a lymphoid tumor caused by chicken's simplex virus, which can lead to the mass mortality of chickens. Now this disease can be prevented with vaccine to get significant effect. Inspired by the important progress in the research of animal tumor virus, the research about virus pathogenesis of human tumor is also continuously developing. At present, it is discovered that some human tumors, such as Burkitt lymphoid tumor, nasopharyngeal cancer, leukaemia, sarcoma, breast cancer and cervical carcinoma, are relevant to virus.

② Human tumors closely related to virus are as follows.

Burkitt lymphoid tumor: in 1964, Epsteim and other experts found a kind of new virus from suspension cell culture of lymphoid tumor. Its shape belongs to the kind of herpes virus. But its antigen is different from that of other herpes viruses. It can only reproduce in human lymphocytic system. This kind of virus is called EB virus, which can spread to all over the world through direct contact.

Nasopharyngeal cancer: the incidence rate is higher in the south of our country. Originally, EB virus is found to have relation to nasopharyngeal cancer on serology. In recent years, the important progress is that the gene and nuclear antigen of EB virus are found in epithelial cells of nasopharyngeal cancer. These results have further showed that EB virus is relevant to nasopharyngeal cancer.

Leukaemia: after finding the leukemia virus of mouse, many other animals (involving monkeys) are successively found to have the leukaemia caused by virus. Therefore, people consider that human leukaemia might be caused by C-type RNA tumor virus, and then people carry out many researches. In recent years, people discover that there is a kind of nucleic acid in human leukaemia that may generate hybridization reaction with the nucleic acid in leukemia virus of mouse as well as inverse transcriptase. C-type virosome can occasionally be seen through electron microscope.

Breast cancer: the generation of mouse's breast cancer is caused by the interaction between virus of breast cancer and the host's hereditary factors. People hold that human breast cancer may have the same pathogenesis. Mice have different germ lines of high and low incidence rate. Someone outside the country has observed the similar situation in the crowd. The inverse transcriptase is found in breast cancer patients' breast milk with virosome. These results cannot prove that virus has causal relation to human breast cancer, which needs a further research.

Cervical carcinoma: the generative organ of normal woman often has herpes simplex virus type II. According to the survey data of serological epidemiology, cervical carcinoma patients are tested a higher positive for neutralizing antibody of herpes simplex virus type II. Cell strains cultivated in cervical carcinoma have also found herpes simplex virus type II.

Herpes simplex virus type II can induce normal cell transformation and cause sarcoma in animals.

The viral pathogenesis study of human tumor has been making fast progress in recent years. Although at present it cannot be finally certain that the relation between virus and certain human tumors, this study has provided some important clues. In recent years, the viral pathogenesis study of human tumor can be mainly divided into two aspects. One is to study the relation between herpes virus and Burkitt lymphoma, nasopharyngeal cancer and cervical carcinoma; the other is to study the relation between C-type virus and leukaemia, sarcoma and Hodgkin lymphoma. If the viral pathogenesis of some human tumors could be proved, then these tumors would be prevented and controlled with vaccine as chicken's lymphoid tumor.

(3) Hormone and cancer research group: it is necessary to have a further study on the carcinogenic factors of some known cancers related to hormone. Cancer treatment should lay stress on Hormone; while cancer prevention should pay attention to the further study of hormone based on the current knowledge.

① Hormonal imbalance and tumor generation. Hormone is an important chemical substance for neuron humor to adjust the body's development and function. Various hormones maintain a dynamic equilibrium according to the law of the unity of opposites. In the case of endocrine dyscrasia caused by diseases or some reasons, hormonal imbalance leads to some hormones' sustained action on sensitive tissues. This kind of abnormal chronic irritation may cause cell hyperplasia and canceration. Hormones with carcinogenic action refer to these that can promote histiocytes growth, such as estrogen of ovary, gonadotropic hormone of pituitary, thyrotrophic hormone and galactin, etc. To give the example of breast cancer, when lacking of pituitary and ovarian hormone promoting the growth of mammary gland, mammary gland will not grow. Undeveloped mammary tissue is hard to produce tumor. Therefore, hormone is a necessary factor to induce breast cancer. Experimental studies show that hormonal imbalance can induce tumors in thyroid gland, adenohypophysis, ovary, testicle, and adrenal cortex as well as accessory organs of uterine body, uterine neck, vagina and mammary gland. Hormone takes a long time to induce tumor; and the induction often needs a certain genetic background and environmental factors to be pathogenic conditions. Furthermore, hormone can also cooperate with other carcinogenic factors to cause canceration or act as the pathogenic condition of other factors. Some hormones, such as prostatic hormone, can promote cell differentiation and strengthen immune response. Whether the hyposecretion of prostatic hormone has an effect on canceration still needs a further study.

② Hormonal pathogenesis of breast cancer: In the earliest 1896, scholars carried out surgical removals of ovary in two pre-menopausal women with breast cancer, which obviously narrow the breast tumor. Since then the relation between ovary and breast cancer has received attention. Later studies prove that removal of ovary to cause artificial menopause can reduce the incidence rate of breast cancer. Among male patients who are treated with a large dose of oestrogenic hormones, unilateral or bilateral breast cancer is reported to appear, which indicates that oestrogenic hormone may cause breast cancer. Removal of ovary before forty ages can reduce the incidence rate of breast cancer; and hereditary factors have certain effect on cancer generation. Some patients receive no response to the removal of ovary and adrenal gland. After the resection of pituitary, this breast cancer just gets palliation. The above phenomenon indicates that pituitary hormone has an effect on breast cancer. Galactin may be one of the causes of human breast cancer. But in terms of harmonic factors, breast cancer is not due to the single action of one hormone but the result of many hormones' interaction on mammary gland.

③ Hormonal pathogenesis of endometrial carcinoma: Endometrial carcinoma is more common in the women who are fat, barren or with late menopause. Long standing action of oestrogenic hormones on endometrium and lack of progesterone's periodic adjustment may be the pathogeneses of endometrial carcinoma. The growth and function of endometrium are controlled by ovarian hormone and endometrial cells contain the receptor protein of hormone. As seen from the latter half of menstruation, progesterone can reduce the level of estrogen receptor and stop the activity of endometrial cell proliferation caused by oestrogenic hormones. This shows that progestational hormone and oestrogenic hormone have the antagonistic action. Using large doses of progesterone for a long term can lead to the atrophia of endometrium, which is a basis of treating metastatic endometrial cancer with hormone therapy. About one thirds of endometrial cancers are detected to have estrogen receptors, which are related to the differential degree of cells. But progesterone receptors are not affected by cell differentiation.

④ Hormone application and cancerogenic problem: Endocrine dyscrasia can cause tumor generation of relevant organs and tissues or provide conditions for canceration. Some tumors depend on a certain dosage of hormones. Cutting off the origin of hormones and reinforcing stimulus of oppositional hormones may get curative effect. Hormone therapy has been applied in breast cancer, prostatic cancer, carcinoma of uterine body, thyroid carcinoma, leukaemia and tumor of lymphatic tissue. Some cases have got palliative effects of inhibiting cancer growth, obviously shrink primary or metastatic tumor and reduce severity.

(4) Mycotoxin and cancer research group: it is necessary to have a further study on the carcinogenic factors of some known tumors closely related to mycotoxin. Cancer treatment should lay stress on the study of relevant processing measures; while cancer prevention should pay attention to the further study of cancer prevention and treatment based on the current knowledge.

There are many metabolic products of fungus in nature, which can poison animal nervous, digestive, urinary or hematological system. These products are called Mycotoxin. Cases of human acute poisoning caused by mycotoxin have been reported a lot. In the recent ten years, some mycotoxins are gradually observed to have carcinogenic or cancer-promoting action on animals. Therefore, medical circle begin to pay more and more attention to studying the relation of fungus and its mycotoxin with human tumor.

① Experiment on cancerogenic mycotoxins: Experimental studies find that cancerogenic mycotoxins have lots of different kinds. At first feeding rates with ergot-infected grain can induce the neurofibroma of ear. Then the mouldy yellowed rice polluted by Penicillium islandicum Sopp are found in Japan; and the toxin extracted from rice can cause the hepatic cirrhosis, hepatic tumor and hepatic cancer of mice and rats. Only until 1960 when one hundred thousand turkeys were poisoned to death by groundnut flour polluted by Aspergillus flavus Liak in England and then Aflatoxin was found to have carcinogenic action on animals, cancerogenic problem of mycotoxin finally attracted wild attention. Repeated studies prove that Aspergillus flavus Liak and its derivatives have more than ten kinds, among which the best one with carcinogenic action is B_1. Mouldy grains polluted by Aflatoxin in a liver cancer-prone area of China are mixed in feed to feed rats. After six moths, the inducing rate of liver cancer is up to 80%, which also proves the carcinogenic action of mycotoxins. This kind of feed can also cause monkeys' liver cirrhosis as well as other hepatic lesions and induce liver cancer. Most of the induced liver cancers are hepatocellular cancers. Furthermore, this kind of feed can lead to the adenocarcinoma of kidney, stomach and colon; intratracheal instillation can cause squamous cell carcinoma of lung; subcutaneous injection can cause local sarcoma. There are relevant reports about causing tumors in other regions, such as lachrymal gland, mammary gland and ovary. Therefore, making a good job of mould proofing and ridding of oil and foodstuffs is important for exploring the prevention of some tumors and ensuring popular physical fitness.

In the esophageal cancer-prone area of China, Geotrichum candidum Link abstracted from edible pickled vegetable is proved to have the cancer-promoting action. Use 0.5ml fungus medium and 0.25mg / (kg · d) methyl benzyl nitrosamine to feed a series of A mice. During two to seven months, the incidence rate of proliferative lesion, papilloma and cancer in anterior stomach of A mice is obviously higher than that of other mice only fed with nitrosamine. Use the culture of Geotrichum candidum Link to feed rats for twenty months, and then papilloma in anterior stomach is induced. Some moldy food can cause precancerous lesion and early cancer in esophageal epithelium of animals. Some fungi abstracted from moldy food can increase the content of nitrite and secondary amine or produce nitrosamine in food. The above experiments expand the research field of the relation between fungus and tumor and also provide new clues for tumor pathogenesis.

So far some fungi and their toxins related to tumor generation have both carcinogenic action and cancer-promoting action. This kind of dualism deserves attention.

② The relation between cancerogenic mycotoxin and human tumor: Fungi are widespread in all over the world, which can pollute all kinds of grains and foods. Among these fungi, aspergillus, blue mold and fusarium are common to see. Toxic metabolites of fungi can exist in processed grains and foods to endanger people's health directly. Especially in the regions with higher temperature and humidity, fungi are easy to grow in grains, so the problem of Mycotoxin is rather serious.

The survey of tumor epidemiology has found that there is a relationship of some kind between the generation of some tumors and the pollution level of cancerogenic mycotoxin in food. At present, this relation has been mostly studied in the aspect of Aflatoxin. These survey reports show that the geographical distribution of positive samples of Aflatoxin and that of the incidence rate of primary liver cancer have a certain balanced relation. The regions that have more heavy pollution and larger actual intaking amount of Aflatoxin also have higher incidence rate of liver cancer. The preliminary investigation of China has found that in terms of grain contamination, the south is more serious than the north; the contaminated chance and level of corn and peanuts are higher than those of rice, wheat and beans. Different kinds of grains in different or same geographical and climatic conditions have different pollution status of Aflatoxin. While the incidence rate of liver cancer displays the appropriate relationship with the above differences. For instance, the comparable survey of liver cancer in high-incidence and low-incidence regions of China shows that the grain contaminated level of the former is more serious than that of the latter. At the same time, the comparable investigation of epidemiology and etiology between livestock liver cancer and human liver cancer in high-incidence regions also finds that liver cancer bear some relation to foods and feedstuffs polluted by Aflatoxin. These materials preliminarily explain that Aflatoxin may be related to the generation of some tumors and also point out the importance of mould proofing and detoxification of oil and foodstuffs.

Set up pilot sites of prevention work in tumor-prone regions. Through measures of mass mould proofing and ridding, carry out perspective studies and observe the interrelation between the drop of tumor incidence and the reduction of Aflatoxin contamination.

The above works are beneficial to the further discovery and clarification of the relation between fungi as well as their toxins and human tumors.

③ Measures of mould proofing and ridding: Making a good job of mould proofing and ridding of oil and foodstuffs is important for exploring the prevention of some tumors and ensuring people's physical fitness. Emphasis will be laid on mould proofing, which is a basic method for stop toxins.

The key point of mould proofing is to control the water content of foodstuffs. It is hard to reproduce fungi if the water content is 13%~14% or below. Therefore, grains need to dry out quickly as soon as they are harvested. Water content of foodstuff particle should reduce to below 13% as quickly as possible. Strengthen damp-proof measures in storage. Ted in time. Keep foodstuff particle and peanut shell in perfect, preventing fungi from invasion.

(5) Environment and cancer research group: In the present flourishing age, the standard of living of the people has been improving. All kinds of high-tech products bring not only wonderful lives but also various environmental carcinogens of chemistry, physics and biology. All kinds of carcinogens go in the human body or carcinogenic factors affect human body. People seem to be enveloped in carcinogens caused by environmental pollution.

Some people regard cancer with dread and are in a state of extreme nervousness; while others appear benumbed and unresponsive, and behave in their own way.

Cancer is not horrible. The terrible thing is that we have no early and basic knowledge of cancer prevention. Furthermore, most cancers are preventive.

During the process of seeking for the cause of cancer and occurrence conditions, human have carried out an extensive research and accumulated rich knowledge, which have found that above 80% cancers are caused by or closely related to environment.

① The relation between environment and cancer: People's living environment includes natural environment and social environment. Natural environment refers to various natural factors around people. For instance, everyone has to breathe air, drink water and eat food. These common physical environments are called the big environment.

Everybody is engaged in one kind of work and adopts a certain life style, such as occupation, life habit and hobbies make up one kind of living environment, which is called the small environment.

No matter the big environment or small environment, both of them are external environments upon which mankind depends for survival and activities.

The physiologic condition of human body is the internal environment.

Materials in external environment become closely related to internal environment through the body's ingestion, digestion, absorption, metabolism and excretion, and then have a tremendous impact on human body.

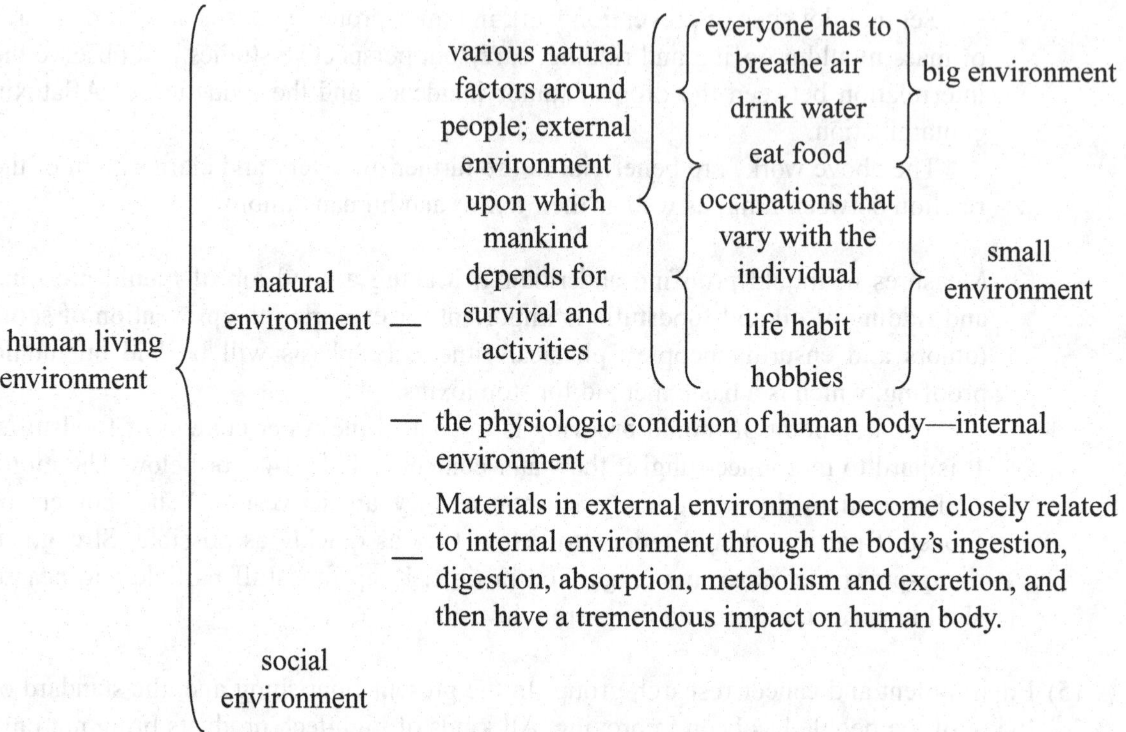

As to how to prove the relation between environmental pollution and cancer, many demonstrations have been given in history.

In 1775, English doctor Pott proved that cleaners of chimney have higher risk of suffering from scrotal skin cancer, as they always contact coal tar, which was the first historical case that combined cancer with environmental factors.

After 100 years, Germany doctor Volkman also recognized that the high rate of suffering skin cancer for workers was possibly related to the contact with coal tar.

In 1907, some scholar found that exposure to sunlight is related to skin cancer and reported firstly the epidemiologic research on sunlight and skin cancer. Researchers found that crews were always exposed to solar radiation that led to chronic skin diseases, which was often seen. Later, researchers proved that sunlight and ultraviolet rays were likely to result in skin cancer with animal model.

In 1915, the first animal model of inducing tumors by chemical agents was established. Besmearing tar repeatedly could make rabbits suffer from skin cancer, which provided experimental reasons for the theory of chemical carcinogenesis based on that cleaners of chimney were easy to suffer from carcinoma of scrotum in 1775. Later, people confirmed that and got the effective constituent by abstraction, named coal tar.

In the 1920s, bladder carcinoma was popular with the workers who produced alpha naphthylamine, ethyl naphthalene and benzidine dye. Almost all the workers who had done this suffered from bladder carcinoma later.

In 1930, the first chemical carcinogen, benzopyrene was abstracted from coal tar. The known substance of carcinogenic environment, coal tar was separated into different constituents, which were confirmed that they could result in cancer by experimental analysis with animal model.

In 1938, according to researches, it could be found that the process of chemical carcinogenesis was divided into two stages, the stage of activation and the stage of promotion. Non-specific stimulators could activate and promote the occurrence of cancer under small dose of carcinogen like besmearing tar or mastoid tumorous virus.

In 1940, researchers discovered that limitation of heat could reduce the occurrence of tumors for mice. It was proved that the intake of heat could encourage the occurrence of several kinds of tumors like breast carcinoma, liver cancer and skin cancer induced by benzoapyrene. Until today when obesity is popular worldwide, this project is attached with importance again by people.

In 1950, research on epidemiology discovered that smoking was related to lung cancer. By reviewing the lung cancer sufferers with the habit of smoking, it could be proved that smoking had close relation to lung cancer. Later, from the research on the obvious relation between smoking and the mortality of lung cancer among male doctors, it has been proved that smoking is a dangerous factor for many kinds of cancer and it can increase the mortality of cancer by 30%.

In 1958, it was been proved that food additive forbidden by reforming organization for food additive could induce the occurrence of cancer for human beings and animals.

In 1964, American surgeon Luther L Terry proposed that smoking was connected to lung cancer.

Until 1974, scientists found vinyl chloride was the major raw material of plastic industry, which was a potential strong carcinogen and could cause liver cancer.

In recent decades, according to epidemiologic research, it can be found that if workers in many occupations contact the carcinogens in manufacturing environment, the incidence rates of some parts will greatly increase. Elimination or avoiding these contacts can reduce the incidence rates gradually or even make them disappear, which plays an important role in the occurrence of tumors.

Various environmental factors outside human bodies are the major reasons resulting in the occurrence of cancer. Therefore, it is necessary to reduce the effects of these environmental, living and behavior factors to human bodies so as to get away from caner.

The following is talking about the severe cancerogenic effects of environmental pollution like air pollution, water pollution and soil pollution, etc. to human beings.

② Air pollution and cancer: Human being can not survive without air even for only a minute. Therefore, air pollution can result in the occurrence of many diseases, especially respiratory diseases including the most severe one lung cancer.

At the beginning of 20th century, lung cancer mainly happened in such occupational environments like mines, exploitation and smelting. After world war one, the morality of lung cancer began to increase. In late 1930s, with the development of modern industry air pollution, occupational carcinogens and the consumption and production of tobacco and cigarette increased greatly. Meanwhile, the morality of male who suffered from lung cancer in western industrial developed countries rose rapidly. In the UK, the death rate of lung cancer was 10/100,000 in 1930, 53/100,000 in 1950, 99.7/100,000 in 1966 and 120.3/100,000 in 1975. From 1930 to 1975, it has an increase of twelve times in 45 years.

During 1934 to 1974, lung cancer rose from the fifth to the number one place in causes of death of American male. Its mortality rate rose from 3.0/100,000 to 54.5/100,000, up 17 times as compared with before. Female lung cancer went up from the eighth to the top three. Its mortality rate rose from 2.0/100,000 to 12.4/100,000, up 5.2 times as compared with before.

In the early 1980, lung cancer in 24 countries and regions involving UK, France, Netherlands, Germany and USA and others generally occupies the number one in the cause of death of malignant tumor patients. Since the mid-20th century, the tendency of high incidence of lung cancer in western industrial developed countries has been rising.

Dangerous gases in industrial developed countries, produced from power generation, steel-making, cars, planes, fuels, energy sources and volumes of smoke, are emitted into the atmosphere and pollute air. Human respiratory tract is irritated by breathing into polluted air, which causes the continuing rise of the incidence rate and mortality rate of lung cancer.

③ Water pollution of environmental pollution and cancer: Human activity in production and life depend on water at all times. Water quality pollution is mainly caused by industrial and agricultural production as well as urban pollution discharge. In China, township enterprises are having a fast development, which worsen industrial pollution. According to the survey, many major rivers are facing a serious pollution increasingly. Fertilizers, farm chemicals and pesticides in agricultural production lead to the serious pollution of water quality.

Some rural areas of China have a habit of using pond water. The research of Qidong County in Jiangsu Province has found that the high incidence of liver cancer in this area is related to drink pond water. Fusui County in Guangxi Province also has the similar report. All of these explain that water pollution is relevant to the incidence of liver cancer. Haining County in Zhejiang Province also finds that people drinking pond water are over seven times easier to suffer from colon cancer than people drinking well water.

In recent years, due to the advance of analysis technology of water quality, more than 100 different kinds of organic substances in water are found to have actions of carcinogenesis, cancer-promoting and mutagenesis. Animal experiments have proved that drink water mixed with the following chemical compounds can cause liver cancer, such as benzene hexachloride, carbon tetrachloride, chloroform, trichloroethylene, perchlorethylene, and trichloroethane, etc. Furthermore, there are some limnetic algae toxins, such as blue-green algae has an obvious action on the promotion of liver cancer.

Mulberry fish pond area of Shunde in Guangdong Foshan is low lying and easy to generate water-logging and water accumulation, so the water quality pollution is more serious. The incidence of liver cancer of local population is higher. While neighboring residents in Siping drink deep phreatic water. The water quality is good, so the incidence of liver cancer is lower. According to the research data of WHO and International Association for Cancer Research, drinking off-standard water can induce or promote the generation of cancer. The test indicates that drink water with a large amount of nickel is easy to induce oral cancer, throat cancer and carcinoma of large intestine; water with more cadmium is easy to induce esophageal carcinoma, laryngeal carcinoma and lung cancer; water with more plumbum is easy to induce stomach cancer, intestinal cancer, oophoroma and all kinds of lymph cancer; water with more iron and zinc is easy to induce esophageal carcinoma.

④ Environmental chemical pollution and cancer—chemical carcinogenesis: Chemical carcinogen refers to chemical substances that can induce the generation of tumor.

In the mid-20th century, the problem of chemical carcinogenesis attracts widespread attention, mainly because modern tumor incidence rate and mortality rate continue to rise. The age of suffering from cancer has a younger tendency. Environmental chemical pollution is also found to have a close relation to the incidence rate of tumor. World Health Organization also indicates that 80%~90% of human cancers are relevant to environmental factors, which are mainly chemical factors.

The following chemical substances have been studied and proved to have carcinogenic action.

Chloroethylene: In 1974, people began to realize that this substance is the cause of professional cancer. Experimental study has found liver cancer, brain cancer, renal carcinoma, lung cancer and cancer of lymphatic system in experimental animals exposed to Chloroethylene. But the related personnel cannot timely realize the hazardness of these substances from experimental results. Therefore, they fail to take measures to protect workers in time. Until recently, workers start to stop using the spraying agent of Chloroethylene; and plastic factory also change manufacturing technique to prevent workers from exposure.

Here to point out that Chloroethylene is an important raw material for record, packaging material, Medical test tube, household appliances, bathroom equipment and other kinds of plastic products. Plastic products themselves have no risk, but the liver cancer risk of workers in Chloroethylene factory is 200 times higher than that of common people.

Benzene: It is a kind of harmful chemical material, which can destroy the hematopiesis of marrow. If exposed in the environment filled with benzene, people may suffer from aplastic anemia that can change into leucocythemia after a long period. The first case of "leucucythemia led by benzene" was discovered in 1928.

Researches from other countries have also proved that benzene is a sort of harmful material with occupational hazards. Italian scientists have reported before

200 years that the risk of suffering from leucocythemia for the workers in printing houses and shoemaking factories was 20 times higher than that of others.

Some activities and addictions in daily life are usually related to environmental cancerogen palycyclic aromatic closely. Palycyclic aromatic produced by smoking is the key factor of inducing lung cancer for human beings. Meanwhile, palycyclic aromatic with carcinogenicity produced in cooking foods of oil and fat including frying, grilling and smoking, etc. are threatening extremely the health for human beings, which should be attached with great importance.

In addition, benzoapyrene in asphalt and hot-mix asphalt is closely related to the high risk of cancer occurrence for roadmen and worker dealing with the water proofing of roof. Farm labors often contact several kinds of pesticides, herbicide and chemical fertilizers which contain some known carcinogens and some that can induce cancer in experimental animals and others that are proved to be mutagenic agents after short-term test. And the pesticides can enter food chain and accumulate in biological system.

⑤ The physical factors in environmental pollution and cancer—ionizing radiation: With the development of technology, frequent nuclear tests, the applications of nuclear energy and radioactive nuclides are increasing, so as the radioactive substance poured in human environment. Therefore, people pay increasingly more attention to environmental pollution by ionizing radiation.

The ionizing radiation means the rays radiated by some radioactive substance in the process of transmutation. This kind of rays can give the absorbed substance adequate energy to divide ionize molecules and atoms. Some ionizing radiations are electromagnetic radiations like X-ray and γ-ray.

The sources of artificial radiation include nuclear tests which increase the radioactive environmental pollution, the exploitation, processing and retreat of nuclear fuel, for instance, in the exploitation of mineral radon gas and radioactive dust can pollute atmosphere. As the sources of energy in the world are less and less, more and more nations have been beginning to build nuclear power stations currently. This nuclear power industry can all discharge radioactive waste gas, water and residue which will pollute environment if mishandled.

Although radioactive nuclide can be applied extensively in industry, agriculture and medicine, the radioactive waste can still pollute environment.

The major effects of ionizing radiation to human bodies are body damages including chronic radiation diseases, malignant tumors, cataract, and decrease in the capacity to bear children, etc; radiation carcinogensis with longer delitescence like leucocythemia, skin carcinoma, lung cancer and osteocarcinoma; and hereditary damages which make descendants possessed with hereditary disease.

carcinogens that enter foods from environmental pollution: With the development of technology, food processing has become increasingly industrialized. So both external environment and food processing itself can bring various external substance including chemical and biological carcinogens and pollute foods.

In the processing of raw material, adding manmade additions or using smoking, frying, baking, etc. to cook may result in the production of cancerogenic farrago in foods.

Usually finished food products are sent to customers after preservation and transportation which provide another source of carcinogens to pollute foods.

It is important to research on the sources of pollution to human foods and how to eliminate the pollution.

4. How to develop scientific research on cancer
   (1) Science: it is always the endless advancing front. The scientific researches have been always following scientific outlook on development, which is based on known medicine and facing future medicine and science, as well as rising, interdisciplinary or cross subjects. The scientific researches are to explore unknown science and knowledge based on known science. Researchers should look forward and get down to make efforts to practice scientific outlook on development in long-term and trudge forward the advanced front on the road of scientific research step by step so as to make contribution to the science of overcoming cancer.
   (2) Research: it is the exploration of truth, characters, regular rule, etc. Medical research includes theoretic research and clinical research. All clinical research of specialized clinic in Twilight Cancer Institute confirm to the following study approach: ① finding problems in clinic→ putting forward problems→ research on problems through experiments→ clinical verification to solve or explain clinical problems. ② clinic→ experiments→ clinic→ experiments again→ clinic again to solve problems. ③ all researches are based on the combination of theory and practice. The selected topics are all from clinic and find out the focus of problems and the point of break in clinic; after experimental and clinical researches, the research results can be applied in clinic to solve practical problems. All researches keep to the evidence based medicine with appreciable material of experimental researches and clinical verification using facts and data to prove.
   (3) Contents of research: the target of research is cancer, including how to recognize cancer and how to prevent and treat cancer. ① exploration of truth, characters and regular rule; ② the causes of cancer occurrence and development and the pathogenesis; ③ the biological characteristics and behaviors of cancer cells; ④ the steps and phases of metastasis; ⑤ the relation between cancer cells and host cells that decides the fortune of sufferers; ⑥ looking for new methods of preventing and treating cancer, which means the whole process including occurrence, development, metastasis and relapse as well as the prevention and treatment.

   The whole process of cancer occurrence and development is the phase with high fidelity phase before cancer early phase metaphase anaphase, namely phase of invasion and advanced phase of metastasis. Therefore, cancer metastasis is only a phase, but the whole process. It is only a phase of invasion in the occurrence and development of cancer. However, that needed to be prevented and cured is the whole process of cancer occurrence and development. Only by doing like this can overcome cancer.
   (4) Methods of research: for cancer, it is necessary to pay attention to treatment, but it is more important for precaution which can prevent cancer from the source. The solution of treatment of cancer lie in "three early", namely early discovery, early diagnosis and early treatment. That of anti-cancer relies on precaution. More than 80% of cancer cases result from environmental factors, so protecting and restoring good environment is an important part of prevent cancer. As is well known that there are cancer precaution,

control and overcome, but why the control of cancer is proposed? Because energy saving and emission reduction, antifouling and treating pollution can control the occurrence of cancer effectively. The prevention and control of cancer can use precaution of grade I, II and III. Currently, the actual grades of emission reduction and antifouling are I. At the same time, energy saving and emission reduction, antifouling and treating pollution are great pioneering works of preventing and controlling cancer which are beneficial to the nation and its people. As a result, it is necessary to enlarge the area of scientific research and face future science looking forward. Scientific research is to explore the unknown scientific knowledge and push science forward. All scientific research should be conducted according to scientific outlook on development. It is essential to renovate thoughts and change concepts under the guidance of scientific outlook on development and it is encouraged to create which will challenge traditional concepts and move forward in reforms. As cancer is the disaster for human beings, prevention and resistance of cancer are the human career.

References

[1] Zhang Tiejun, et al. Modern Study and Application of Traditional Chinese Herbs for Immunoloregulation and Liver Protection. Beijing: People's Medical Publishing House Co., Ltd, 2007: 3-10

[2] Garret M Hampton. Genomics in Cancer Drug Discovery and Development. Beijing: Science Press, 2007: 42-43

[3] Azzam F G Taktak. Outcome Prediction in Cancer. Beijing: Science Press, 2008:443-446

[4] Wan Wenwei. Clinical Application and Research of Tumor Marker. Peking University Medical Press, 2005:218-232

[5] Shen Xinfeng. Antibodies for Tumor Therapy and Their Modification Strategy. Chinese Journal of Cancer Biotherapy, 2007, 14 (2):101-103

[6] Chu Datong. Clinical Manifestation of Targeted Drugs in Individualized Therapy of Malignant Tumors. Chinese Journal of Oncology, 2010, 32:721-723

[7] Xu Binghe, Zhang Ping. Molecular Subtypes and Individualized Treatment of Breast Cancer, Chinese Journal of Oncology, 2010, 32(9):641-644

[8] Current Status of Surgical Management of Esophageal Cancer in China and the Future Strategy, Chinese Journal of Oncology, 2010, 32(6):401-403

[9] Guy de Tai. A Probe into Cancer, translated by Guo Taichu, Xi'an, Shaanxi Science and Technology Press, 1996: 154-168

[10] Hou Youxian. Prevention and Treatment of Complications in Cancer Radiotherapy. Beijing: People's Military Medical Press, 2008: 179-213

[11] Dieamar W. Siemann. Vascular-targeted Therapies in Oncology. Translated by Han Baohui, Beijing: People's Military Medical Press, 2007:67-78

[12] Feng Xiaoshan, Wang Lidong. An Introduction to Oncology. Beijing: Science Press, 2008:1-8

[13] Wu Min. Conquering Cancer. Guilin: Lijiang Press, 1996

[14] Peter Hillmen, Thomas E Witzig. Immunotherapy of Lymphoid Malignancies. Translated by Zhu Jun. Beijing: People's Military Medical Press, 2008

[15] Matsuzawa, New Methods of Anti-cancer in Japan, Translated by Ye Jianan and Ma Yonghua. Beijing: People's Military Medical Press, 2008

[16] [Switzerland] Vasella, [America] Robert Slater. Magic Cancer Bullet. Translated by Yu Gu. Beijing; CITIC Press Corporation, 2005

[17] Wang Zhenyi, Chen Zhu. Therapy of Induction, Differentiation and Apoptosis of Tumor. Shanghai: Shanghai Science and Technology Press, 1999

[18] Li Yan, Ma Hao. Molecular Targeted Cancer Therapy. Beijing: People's Medical Publishing House, 2007

[19] Chen Huanchao. Targeted Therapy of Cancer. Wuhan: Hubei Science and Technology Press:2009

[20] Wang Zhehai, Kong Li and Yu Jinming. Untoward Reaction and Countermeasures of Tumor Chemotherapy. Jinan, Shandong Science and Technology Press, 2002

[21] Li Zhen. Chemotherapy and Immunotherapy of Malignancies. Beijing: People's Medical Publishing House Co., Ltd, 1990

[22] Zhang Shengben, Zhang Lianyang. Sensitivity and Drug Resistance of Tumor Chemotherapy. Chengdu: Sichuan Science and Technology Press, 1995
[23] Cheng Shuqun, Wu Mengchao. Therapy of Tumor with Cancer Embolus in Portal Vein. Shanghai: Second Military Medical University Press, 2009
[24] Gao Jin, Zhang Jingbo. Invasion and Metastasis Basis and Clinic of Cancer. Beijing: Science Press, 2003
[25] Tang Zhaoyou. Basis and Clinic of Metastasis and Reoccurrence of Liver Cancer. Shanghai: Shanghai Scientific and Technical Education Press, 2003
[26] Wu Mengchao, Chen Han, Shen Feng. Surgical Treatment of Primary Liver Cancer: 5224-case Report attached, Chinese Journal of Surgery, 2001, 39 (6): 417-421
[27] Zhou Xinda, Tang Zhaoyou and Yu Yeqin. Review of Surgery of Liver Cancer for 40 Years. Chinese Journal of Clinical Medicine, 1996, 6: 112-114
[28] Tang Zhaoyou, Qin Lunxiu, Sun Huichuan, et al. Study on Reoccurrence and Metastasis of Liver Cancer. Chinese Journal of General Surgery. 2000, 15: 517-520
[29] Qiu Shuangjian, Wu Zhiquan, Fan Jia et al. Diagnosis and Treatment of Dissemination of Primary Liver Cancer after Operation. Chinese Journal of Clinical Medicine, 1999, 6: 118-120
[30] Sun Huichuan, Tang Zhaoyou, Ma Zengchen et al. Factors Affecting Reoccurrence Rate of Liver Cancer after Radical Removal. Chinese Journal of Hepatobiliary Surgery, 2000, 6: 58-62
[31] Wu Bingquan. Study Strategy of Cancer Metastasis. National Medical Journal of China, 1990, 70: 302-304
[32] Ling Maoying, Zhang Zhou, Gao Wansheng et al. Establishment of Metastasis Model for Experimental Lymph Path of Transplantable Ascites Carcinoma (H22) of Mice. Chinese Journal of Pathology, 1984, 13: 190-192
[33] Ma Ding. Metastasis of Tumor. Zeng Yixin. Oncology. Beijing: People's Medical Publishing House Co., Ltd, 2003
[34] Tang Zhaoyou. Clinical Hepatocellular Carcinoma. Shanghai: Shanghai Scientific and Technical Education Press, 2001: 35-44
[35] Wang Jie, Gao Tong, Xu Qing et al. Progress of Mechanism, Diagnosis and Treatment of Tumor Metastasis. Shanghai: Second Military Medical University Press, 2001: 10-16
[36] T J Vogl, M G Mack, J O Blzer. Diagnosis and Treatment of Metastatic Hepatic Carcinoma. Translated by Qian Jun. Beijing: People's Medical Publishing House Co., Ltd, 2003
[37] Robert G McKinnell. Biological Basis of Carcinoma. Translated by Gao Jing et al. Beijing: Qsinghua University Press, 2003
[38] Tang Zhaoyou. The Next Important Goal of Clinical Study on Primary Hepatic Carcinoma—Prevention and Treatment of Reoccurrence and Metastasis. Progress of Study on Carcinoma in China. Beijing: Military Medical Science Press, 1998
[39] Tang Zhensheng. Molecular Surgery and Gene Therapy. Shanghai: Shanghai Medical University Press, 1999
[40] Liu Wei, Zhang Yali. Application of RT-PCR Technique in Assay of Micrometastases in Gastro Intestinal Carcinoma. China Oncology, 2000 (2):175-177
[41] Lin Guole, Qiu Zhonghui, Xu Tong. Detection of Micrometastasis in Peripheral Blood of Patients with Colorectal Carcinoma before and during Operative Procedure. Chinese Journal of General Surgery, 2002, 17 (10): 605-607

[42] Daniel B, Longley D. Paul Harkin and Palrick G. Johnston 5-flurouracil Mechanisms of Action and Clinical Strategies. Nature Reviews Cancer, 2003, 3:330-338
[43] Oberg AN, Lindmark GE, Israelsson AC, et al. Detection of Occult Tumor Cells in Lymph Node of Colorectal Patients Using Real-time Quantitative RT-PCR for CEA and CK20Mrnas. Int J Cancer, 2004, 111 (1): 101-110
[44] Gerl R, Vaux DL. Apoptosis in the Development and Treatment of Cancer. Carcinogenesis, 2005, 26 (2):263-270
[45] Qiu Fazu. How to Realize the Innovation by Clinical Surgeons? China Journal of Surgery, 2004, 42 (12):705-706
[46] Luo Chengyu, Li Shiyong. Chemotherapeutic Failure in Micrometastasis in Peripheral Blood of Patients with Colorectal Carcinomas. Chinese Journal of Surgery, 1999, 37 (7): 421-423
[47] Luo Chengyu, Li Shiyong. Detection of Cancer Cells in Peripheral Blood of Patients with Colorectal Carcinomas and Its Clinical Implication. Chinese Journal of Experimental Surgery, 1999, 37 (4):214-215
[48] Chen Xiaoping, Qiu Fazu, Wu Zaide. Primary Hepatic Carcinoma Shall Adopt the Individualized Operation-based Comprehensive Therapy. Chinese Journal of Surgery, 2003, 41 (3): 161-162
[49] Liu Yunyi. Significance of Adjunant before and after Operation in Treatment of Primary Hepatocellular Hepatic Carcinoma through "Radical Removal". Chinese Journal of Surgery, 2003, 41 (3): 163-164
[50] Peng Jirun, Cai Shengli, Leng Xisheng et al. Mrna of MAGE Gene as Specific Markers in Detection of Tumor Cells in Peripheral Blood of Patients with Hepatocellular Carcinomas. Chinese Journal of Surgery, 2002, 40 (7): 487-490
[51] Sun Jingjing, Wu Mengchao. Molecular Mechanism of Reoccurrence and Metastasis of Hepatocellular Carcinomas. Chinese Journal of Practical Surgery, 2000, 20 (3): 176-177
[52] Liu Yinkun, Tang Zhaoyou. Progress of Related Molecular Experiment on Invasion and Metastasis of Primary Hepatocellular Carcinoma, Chinese Journal of Practical Surgery, 2000, 20 (3): 179-181
[53] Wang Qing, Feng Xiaoli, Li Zzhiying. Changes in Metastasis Characteristics of Hepatocellular Cancer Cells after Introduction of H-ras Genes. Chinese Journal of Oncology, 1997, 19 (3): 170
[54] Liao Yong, Tang Zhaoyou, Sun Fangxian et al. Effects on Growth and Metastasis of Human Hepatocellular Carcinoma in Nude Mice. National Medical Journal of China, 1996, 76 (9):650
[55] Chen Zhaocong, Liu Wenli. Gene Therapy of Carcinoma. Wuhan: Hubei Science and Technology Press, 2004
[56] Zhou Jingong. Pharmacology of Immunization with Traditional Chinese Medicine. Beijing: People's Military Medical Press, 1994: 134-157
[57] Ma Zhenya. Pharmacological Study on Immunization with Traditional Chinese Medicine. Xi'an: Shaanxi Science and Technology Press, 1986
[58] Luo Hesheng et al. Chinese Materia Medica for Immunization—Pharmacody and Clinic of Immunization with Traditional Chinese Medicine. Beijing: Joint Press of Beijing Medical University and Beijing Union Medical College, 1999: 219
[59] Li Tiemin et al. Research Progress of Immunoloregulation with Glycyrrhizin. Chinese Herbal Medicine, 1993, 24 (10):553

Appendix A

Great Progress in Study on Tumor over 100 Years

In Apr. 2007, American Association for Cancer Research (AACR) invited the famous tumor scholars all over the world to review the history of study on tumor, which is now briefly extracted as follows:

1907 It was discovered that the solar exposure was related to skin cancer and later it was proven by the animal model that sunlight and ultraviolet radiation could lead to skin cancer.

1908 The tumor was successfully transferred to another animal from one animal with cell-free concentrate. Fowl leukosis, lymphadenoma and sarcomata model was established and this discovery was later deemed as the evidence that the filterable taddecheese would lead to tumor.

1915 The first animal model of chemical-induced tumor was established. Repeated painting of tar could produce skin tumor on rabbit.

1916 It was discovered that the incidence of breast carcinoma on mice could be reduced after removal of the ovary, indicating ovarian hormone may lead to breast carcinoma.

1924 It was discovered by the study on metabolism that the tumor was manifested as anoxia metabolism.

1928 It was deemed that "gene mutation was the basic reason of producing the carcinoma".

1928 The cells of cervical carcinoma were observed through the exuviation smear of vagina. The method of detecting the suspected patient with cervical carcinoma with smear method was widely accepted by the people step by step and used as the effective detection and prevention method of the cancer until Pap smear method was applied in 1960.

1928 It was discovered that X-ray could lead to mutation. X-ray could lead to the gene mutation of common fruit fly, which was the theoretical basis of the carcinogen participation in tumorigensis.

1930 Benzopyrene, the first chemical carcinogen was separated form the coal tar and the carcinogenesis of these chemical constituents was made clear through the animal model experiment.

1932 The artificial hormone was injected to induce the breast carcinoma of mice.

1937 The leucocythemia of the mouse was transfected through transplantation of the single leukemic cell.

1938 It was discovered through study that chemical carcinogenesis process was divided into two different stages including excitation stage and promotion stage.

1939 The transplanted animal tumor could produce the blood vessel. The tumor transplanted on the ears of the rabbit could produce the vascular net, which was the early evidence of formation of the blood vessel, later the anti-angiogenesis became one target of the treatment of tumor.

1940 The heat control could reduce the incidence of tumor on the mice.

1941 The hormone dependence of prostatic carcinoma was proven. Physical castration therapy and estrogen chemical castration therapy could reduce tumor load of the metastatic prostatic carcinoma while the androgen injected could promote the metastasis.

1946 The nitrogen mustard was firstly used for tumor chemotherapy. It was observed that after contacting the nitrogen mustard, the soldiers in time of war could meet with reduction of white blood cells, enlightening the people on using the nitrogen mustard for tumor chemotherapy and the intravenously injected nitrogen mustard for treating the lymphadenoma and leukemia that could not be controlled by radiotherapy, in this way, the disease was remitted for several months. The nitrogen mustard was used for tumor treatment initially in 1949.

1948 The first chemotherapy on leukemia of children was successful. The artificial folic acid antagonist was applied to 16 children with leukemia among which 10 patients got a relieving course of 3 months.

1950 It was discovered by the study on epidemiology that smoking was related to pulmonary carcinoma.

1951 The virus spread the leucocythemia of mice. It was discovered by the study that the leucocythemia could be spread through virus from one mouse of one germ line to another mouse of another germ line and spread from one generation to the next generation vertically. Before this, it was deemed by the people that the tumor was a hereditary disease, which laid a foundation for the study on other tumor viruses and of the mice and other species in the future.

1951 Co-60 (^{60}Co) radiation equipment came out.

1951 The ultrasonic detection was firstly used for diagnosis of tumor.

1958 It was proven that the food additive prohibited by the food additive modification organ could induce the occurrence of carcinoma on human or animal.

1959 The leucocythemia induced by the food additive was related to the radioactive dose. It was proven that the radiation could induce the human carcinoma and the natural characteristics of the relation between radioactive dose and effect were also illuminated.

1963 Hodgkin lymphoma was treated with chemical method. In 1960, Hodgkin lymphoma was reported in the Sahara in Africa, which was featured in regional distribution. In those days, it was deemed that it was induced by the virus and the tumor induced by the virus was firstly successfully cured and later it was proven as Epstein virus.

1964 Luther L. Terry, an American surgeon proposed that the smoking was related to the pulmonary carcinoma.

1969 The tumor was successfully transplanted to the nude mice of different germ line.

1970 The multi-drug resistance of cell line was proposed. The multi-drug resistance of cell toxicant was the main reason of failure of chemotherapy.

1971 The growth of tumor depended on the regenerative blood vessel. Since the discovery of the tumor metastasis, it had been known that the tumor could not grow in the tissue without blood vessel. It was shown by the continuous experiments that the tumor growth factor could promote the generation of the new blood vessel and the growth of the tumor. Finally, these gene factors offered the basis for the molecular-targeted therapy of tumor.

1971 President Nixon presented an anti-cancer slogan in the address in UN.

1972 The paclitaxel, the extract from the natural vegetables could be used for chemotherapy.

1976 The virus oncogene existed in the related proto-oncogene in the normal cells. Through hybridzation technique (before DNA precedence ordering), it was discovered by the researcher that the virus oncogene existed in the chicken's cells, and so did in other families (such as mice and human kind) through study.

1977 Tamoxifen was approved for the clinical treatment of breast carcinoma.

1978 Nitrosamine in the tobacco leaf was proven as the cancerogenous substance in the cigarette. The nitrosamine derived from nicotia in the cigarette was discovered in the animal model that it was cancerogenous and soon later it was proven to be related to pulmonary carcinoma and oral carcinoma of human being.

1979 p53 gene was discovered, which was initially deemed as a kind of oncogene and finally proven as a kind of anti-oncogene by the subsequent study.

1979 Discovery of protein-tyrosine kinase (PTK) and illumination of the tyrosine phosphorylation process. One new kind of protein-tyrosine kinase (PTK) was discovered, which was related to gene products of T antigenic conversion protein and rous sarcoma virus in the polyoma virus. This discovery told us that the maladjustment of tyrosine phosphorylation process catalyzed by activated protein-tyrosine kinase could result in the malignant transformation of cells. In the following several years, the pathogenic protein-tyrosine kinase depressant was approved for clinical treatment.

1980 The degradation of peripheral collagen of the tumor impelled the metastasis of tumor. In the tumor metastasis process, it was necessary for the cancer cells to break through the epithelial layer and the true skin layer so as to invade the circulating system. It was proven by the study that tumor cells could excrete collagenase so as to degrade the peripheral collagen while the cell strains with relatively high excretion level of collagenase would be metastatic more easily.

1980 The prostate specific antigen (PSA) was discovered. Detection of PSA level in the body is the first kind of routine detection method to screen and prevent the carcinoma of prostate with tumor markers through assessing the risks of suffering the carcinoma of prostate.

1980 The importance of DNA methylation in the occurrence and development of carcinoma was revealed.

1982 The primary oncogene concept was launched. The conclusion that the oncogene in the normal cell genome could meet with variance and carcinomatosis was made through combination of the previous findings.

1982 The helicobacter pylori (Hp) was separated from the gastric ulcer of human. It was indicated by the findings over the past 10 years that the virus was cancerogenous, however, it was accepted by the people after several years that the infection of Hp would lead to the gastric ulcer while the continual Hp infection and inflammation would result in canceration.

1983 Papilloma viral infection of human was one of the pathogenic factors of cervical carcinoma. Type 16 and 18 papillomavirus of human separated from the biopsy specimen was proven to be related to the height of cervical carcinoma. This discovery would encourage the people to research, develop and use the corresponding bacterin to prevent the cervical carcinoma.

1983 American Academy of Science issued the report named "Diet, Nutrition and Carcinoma" and proposed American Association of Carcinoma to guide the healthy diet of the public so as to reduce the incidence of the carcinoma.

1990 National Institutes of Health and Department of Energy officially launched the human genome project.

1991 The specific variance of p53 gene in the hepatic carcinoma was related to the environmental carcinogen, namely aflatoxin.

1994 The carcinoma originated from the normal cells that could be transformed into cancer cells and it was shown by the survey that the stem cells in the normal tissue with clear source was most possible to develop into the cancer cells in the process of renovation.

2004 The bacterin for anti human papillomavirus (HPV) could prevent the cervical carcinoma. The type of the most common carcinogenic human papillomavirus that the bacterin can prevent mainly included HPV16 and HPV18, which could prevent 70% of the cervical carcinoma all over the world.